D1485652

URINARY STONE DISEASE

CURRENT CLINICAL UROLOGY

Eric A. Klein, MD, Series Editor

URINARY STONE DISEASE

THE PRACTICAL GUIDE
TO MEDICAL AND SURGICAL MANAGEMENT

Edited by

MARSHALL L. STOLLER, MD
MAXWELL V. MENG, MD

Department of Urology
University of California, San Francisco, School of Medicine
San Francisco, CA

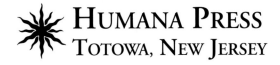 HUMANA PRESS
TOTOWA, NEW JERSEY

© 2007 Humana Press Inc.
999 Riverview Drive, Suite 208
Totowa, New Jersey 07512

humanapress.com

For additional copies, pricing for bulk purchases, and/or information about other Humana titles, contact Humana at the above address or at any of the following numbers: Tel.: 973-256-1699; Fax: 973-256-8341, E-mail: orders@humanapr.com; or visit our Website: http://humanapress.com

Due diligence has been taken by the publishers, editors, and authors of this book to assure the accuracy of the information published and to describe generally accepted practices. The contributors herein have carefully checked to ensure that the drug selections and dosages set forth in this text are accurate and in accord with the standards accepted at the time of publication. Notwithstanding, as new research, changes in government regulations, and knowledge from clinical experience relating to drug therapy and drug reactions constantly occurs, the reader is advised to check the product information provided by the manufacturer of each drug for any change in dosages or for additional warnings and contraindications. This is of utmost importance when the recommended drug herein is a new or infrequently used drug. It is the responsibility of the treating physician to determine dosages and treatment strategies for individual patients. Further it is the responsibility of the health care provider to ascertain the Food and Drug Administration status of each drug or device used in their clinical practice. The publisher, editors, and authors are not responsible for errors or omissions or for any consequences from the application of the information presented in this book and make no warranty, express or implied, with respect to the contents in this publication.

Cover design by Karen Schulz

Cover illustrations: Staghorn calculus.

This publication is printed on acid-free paper. ∞

ANSI Z39.48-1984 (American National Standards Institute) Permanence of Paper for Printed Library Materials.

Photocopy Authorization Policy:
Authorization to photocopy items for internal or personal use, or the internal or personal use of specific clients, is granted by Humana Press Inc., provided that the base fee of US $30.00 per copy is paid directly to the Copyright Clearance Center at 222 Rosewood Drive, Danvers, MA 01923. For those organizations that have been granted a photocopy license from the CCC, a separate system of payment has been arranged and is acceptable to Humana Press Inc. The fee code for users of the Transactional Reporting Service is: [978-1-58829-219-3/07 $30.00].

Printed in the United States of America.   10 9 8 7 6 5 4 3 2 1

eISBN 978-1-59259-972-1

Library of Congress Cataloging-in-Publication Data

Urinary stone disease : the practical guide to medical and surgical
management / edited by Marshall L. Stoller, Maxwell V. Meng.
        p. ; cm. -- (Current clinical urology)
  Includes bibliographical references and index.
  ISBN 1-58829-219-3 (alk. paper)
  1. Urinary organs--Calculi--Treatment.
  [DNLM: 1. Urinary Calculi--etiology. 2. Urinary
Calculi--surgery. 3. Urologic Surgical Procedures--methods. WJ 168
U738 2007] I. Stoller, Marshall L. II. Meng, Maxwell V. III. Series.
  RC916.U74 2007
  616.6'22--dc22
                              2006007610

Preface

Urinary stone disease has afflicted mankind for centuries and continues to be a significant medical ailment throughout the world. Contemporary management reflects the changes and evolution that have occurred in both medicine and, specifically, urology. Traditional open surgery has been nearly replaced by minimally invasive techniques, the result of technologic innovations, miniaturization of instruments, and interdisciplinary collaboration. Nevertheless, nephrolithiasis remains a chronic disease and our fundamental understanding of the pathogenesis, and molecular and genetic basis of stones as well as their prevention, remains rudimentary.

All large calculi were once small calculi. Where do stones originate and what facilitates their retention, allowing them to grow? Although we rely on 24-hour urinary collections, clearly our current methods of directing medical therapy have limitations. In addition, interest in disease prevention continues to grow and understanding basic questions and the underlying pathophysiology of stone disease will help optimize management strategies.

Future advances in urinary stone disease will be the result of collaboration among urologists, nephrologists, radiologists, dieticians, scientists, and partners in industry. Physicians must not be complacent with the current status quo or be overly eager to intervene because techniques are less invasive; rather, the goals should be a better understanding of the underlying disease process in order to identify those at risk, prophylax against stone development and recurrence, and improved nonsurgical therapies.

Urinary Stone Disease: The Practical Guide to Medical and Surgical Management puts together our contemporary views on the development, treatment, and prevention of urinary stone disease. We hope that the book helps improve the current care of patients but more importantly highlights areas of potential research and inspires novel approaches that will ease the burden of this disease.

Marshall L. Stoller, MD
Maxwell V. Meng, MD

Contents

Contributors

HARRISON M. ABRAHAMS, MD • *Endourology Center, Urology Associates of North Texas, Arlington, TX*

MARK ANCHETA, MD • *Resident in Anesthesia, Department of Anesthesia and Perioperative Care, University of California, San Francisco, School of Medicine, San Francisco, CA*

ELIZABETH J. ANOIA, MD • *Resident in Urology, Department of Urology, Case Western Reserve University, Cleveland, OH*

DEAN G. ASSIMOS, MD • *Professor, Department of Urology, Wake Forest University Health Sciences Center, Winston-Salem, NC*

DARREN T. BEIKO, MD • *Assistant Professor, Department of Urology, Queen's University, Kingston, Ontario Canada*

GARY C. BELLMAN, MD • *Department of Urology, Kaiser Permanente Medical Center, Los Angeles, CA*

RICHARD S. BREIMAN, MD • *Associate Clinical Professor, Department of Radiology, University of California, San Francisco, School of Medicine, San Francisco, CA*

PARAMJIT S. CHANDHOKE, MD, PHD • *Professor, Division of Urology and Renal Diseases, University of Colorado Health Sciences Center, Denver, CO*

ANDREW I. CHIN, MD • *Assistant Professor, Division of Nephrology, Department of Medicine, University of California Davis, Sacramento, CA*

HSIAO-JEN CHUNG, MD • *Division of Urology, Taipei-Veterans General Hospital, Taipei, Republic of China*

RALPH V. CLAYMAN, MD • *Professor and Chair, Department of Urology, University of California Irvine, Orange, CA*

FERGUS V. COAKLEY, MD • *Associate Professor, Department of Radiology, University of California San Francisco, School of Medicine, San Francisco, CA*

JOSEPH E. DALLERA, MD • *Division of Urology, University of Colorado Health Sciences Center, Denver, CO*

JOHN D. DENSTEDT, MD • *Professor of Urology, Division of Urology, The University of Western Ontario, London, Ontario Canada*

LOUIS EICHEL, MD • *Clinical Assistant Professor of Urology, University of Rochester; Director of Minimally Invasive Surgery, The Center for Urology, Rochester General Hospital, Rochester, NY*

ASSAAD EL-HAKIM, MD • *Department of Urology, Long Island Jewish Medical Center, New Hyde Park, NY*

GERHARD J. FUCHS, MD • *Director, Minimally Invasive Urology Institute, Cedars–Sinai Medical Center, Los Angeles, CA*

MATTHEW T. GETTMAN, MD • *Department of Urology, Mayo Clinic Rochester, Rochester, MN*

INDERBIR S. GILL, MD, MCH • *Director, Minimally Invasive Surgery Center, Glickman Urological Institute, The Cleveland Clinic Foundation, Cleveland, OH*

WILLIAM L. GITOMER, PHD • *Renal Division, Department of Medicine, University of Colorado Health Sciences Center, Denver, CO*

MANTU GUPTA, MD • *Associate Professor of Urology, Department of Urology, Columbia University College of Physicians and Surgeons; Director, Stone Center, Squier Urological Clinic, New York–Presbyterian Hospital, Columbia Presbyterian Medical Center; Director, Endourology and Minimally Invasive Urology, Saint Luke's–Roosevelt Hospital Center and New York–Presbyterian Hospital, Columbia Presbyterian Medical Center, New York, NY*

Major C. Gerry Henderson, MD • *Department of Urology, Walter Reed Army Medical Center, Washington, DC*

Ross P. Holmes, PHD • *Associate Professor, Department of Urology, Wake Forest University Health Sciences Center, Winston-Salem, NC*

Thomas W. Jarrett, MD • *Professor and Chairman, Department of Urology, The George Washington University School of Medicine, Washington, DC*

D. Brooke Johnson, MD • *Attending Urologist, Department of Urology, Dean West Clinic, Madison, WI*

William K. Johnston, III, MD • *Assistant Professor, Feinberg School of Medicine, Northwestern University; Director of Laparoscopy and Minimally Invasive Urology, Evanston Northwestern Hospital, Evanston, IL*

Christopher J. Kane, MD • *Associate Professor and Vice Chair of Urology, Department of Urology, University of California, San Francisco, San Francisco, CA*

Saeed R. Khan, PHD • *UFRF Professor, Department of Pathology, Immunology and Laboratory Medicine, Director, Center for the Study of Lithiasis, University of Florida, Gainesville, FL*

Bodo E. Knudsen, MD • *Assistant Professor, Division of Urologic Surgery, The Ohio State University Medical Center, Columbus, OH*

Dirk J. Kok, PHD • *Department of Pediatric Urology, Josephine Nefkens Institute, Erasmus University Rotterdam, Rotterdam, The Netherlands*

John S. Lam, MD • *Department of Urology, Columbia University College of Physicians and Surgeons, New York, NY*

Roger K. Low, MD • *Associate Professor, Department of Urology, University of California Davis, Sacramento, CA*

Patrick S. Lowry, MD • *Assistant Professor, Head of Endourology, Scott and White Program, Temple, TX*

Ian Mandel • *Department of Medicine, Medical College of Wisconsin, Milwaukee, WI*

Neil Mandel, PHD • *Professor, Department of Medicine, Medical College of Wisconsin, Milwaukee, WI*

Viraj A. Master, MD • *Assistant Professor, Department of Urology, Emory University, Atlanta, GA*

Freddy Mendez-Torres, MD • *Department of Urology, Tulane University School of Medicine, New Orleans, LA*

Maxwell V. Meng, MD • *Assistant Professor, Department of Urology, University of California San Francisco, San Francisco, CA*

Michael E. Moran, MD • *Clinical Associate Professor, Albany Medical College, Director of St. Peter's Kidney Stone Center, Albany, NY*

Stephen Y. Nakada, MD • *Associate Professor and Chairman, Division of Urology, The University of Wisconsin Medical School, Madison, WI*

Christopher S. Ng, MD • *Minimally Invasive Urology Institute, Cedars–Sinai Medical Center, Los Angeles, CA*

Clarita V. Odvina, MD • *Center for Mineral Metabolism and Clinical Research, University of Texas Southwestern Medical Center, Dallas, TX*

Albert M. Ong, MD • *Instructor in Urology, Fellow in Endourology, The Brady Urological Institute, Johns Hopkins Hospital, Baltimore, MD*

Charles Y. C. Pak, MD • *Center for Mineral Metabolism and Clinical Research, University of Texas Southwestern Medical Center, Dallas, TX*

Sangtae Park, MD, MPH • *Acting Assistant Professor, University of Washington, Department of Urology, Seattle, WA*

Margaret S. Pearle, MD, PHD • *Professor of Urology and Internal Medicine, Department of Urology, The University of Texas Southwestern Medical Center, Dallas, TX*

PAUL K. PIETROW, MD • *Director of Minimally Invasive Urology, Hudson Valley Urology, Poughkeepsie, NY*

GLENN M. PREMINGER, MD • *Professor, Division of Urology, Director, Comprehensive Kidney Stone Center, Duke University Medical Center, Durham, NC*

ANUP P. RAMANI, MD • *Assistant Professor, Director of Laparoscopy, Department of Urology, University of Minnesota Medical School, Minneapolis, MN*

BERENICE Y. REED, PHD • *Renal Division, Department of Medicine, University of Colorado Health Sciences Center, Denver, CO*

MARTIN I. RESNICK, MD • *Lester Persky Professor and Chairman, Department of Urology, Case Western Reserve University, Cleveland, OH*

COLONEL NOAH S. SCHENKMAN, MD • *Chief, Department of Urology, Director, Endourology and Urology Stone Center, Walter Reed Army Medical Center, Washington, DC*

BRADLEY F. SCHWARTZ, DO, FACS • *Director, Center for Urologic Laparoscopy and Endourology, Associate Professor of Urology, Southern Illinois University School of Medicine, Springfield, IL*

JOSEPH W. SEGURA, MD • *Department of Urology, Mayo Clinic, Rochester, MN (Deceased)*

OJAS SHAH, MD • *Assistant Professor, Director, Endourology and Stone Disease, Department of Urology, New York University Medical Center, New York, NY*

BIJAN SHEKARRIZ, MD • *Associate Professor, Director of Laparoscopy and Minimally Invasive Surgery, Department of Urology, Upstate Medical University, State University of New York, Syracuse, NY*

ARTHUR D. SMITH, MD • *Chairman, Professor of Urology, Department of Urology, Long Island Jewish Medical Center, New Hyde Park, NY*

G. BENNETT STACKHOUSE, MD • *Clinical Instructor, Department of Urology, University of California, San Francisco, San Francisco, CA*

MARSHALL L. STOLLER, MD • *Professor, Department of Urology, University of California, San Francisco, San Francisco, CA*

STEVAN B. STREEM, MD • *Glickman Urological Institute, The Cleveland Clinic Foundation, Cleveland, OH (Deceased)*

DANIEL SWANGARD, MD • *Director, PREPARE, Assistant Professor, Department of Anesthesia and Perioperative Care, University of California, San Francisco, School of Medicine, San Francisco, CA*

BENG JIT TAN, MD • *Department of Urology, Long Island Jewish Medical Center, New Hyde Park, NY*

YEH HONG TAN, MD • *Consultant, Department of Urology, Singapore General Hospital, Singapore*

RAJU THOMAS, MD • *Professor and Chairman, Department of Urology, Tulane University School of Medicine, New Orleans, LA*

RUBEN URENA, MD • *Department of Urology, Tulane University School of Medicine, New Orleans, LA*

RONALD M. YANG, MD • *Resident in Urology, Department of Urology, Kaiser Permanente Medical Center, Los Angeles, CA*

About the Editors

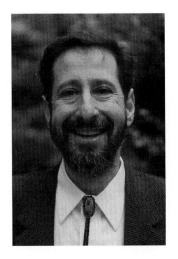

MARSHALL L. STOLLER

Dr. Stoller is currently Professor and Vice-Chairman in the Department of Urology at the University of California San Francisco. He is an expert in the management of urinary stone disease and has made numerous contributions to both the fundamental understanding of urolithiasis as well as advancing the standards of care for patients with the disease. In addition, he has been a pioneer in minimally invasive surgical techniques, neural modulation of voiding dysfunction, and holds multiple patents with medical as well as nonmedical applications.

Dr. Stoller received his undergraduate degree from the University of California at Berkeley and medical degree from the Baylor College of Medicine. His surgical and urologic training was obtained at the University of California San Francisco and with a fellowship at the University of New South Wales in Sydney, Australia.

MAXWELL V. MENG

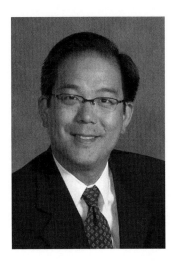

Dr. Meng is currently Assistant Professor of Urology at the University of California San Francisco. He received his training in urologic surgery, laparoscopy and endourology, and urologic oncology at UCSF. Prior to this, he studied biochemical sciences at Harvard College and received his medical degree from the Johns Hopkins School of Medicine.

His primary areas of interest are minimally invasive surgery, urologic cancers, and the combination of the two disciplines. In addition, he is investigating prostate cancer biomarkers and the utility of decision analysis for a variety urologic questions. Dr. Meng has received numerous teaching awards and is actively involved with the American Urological Association and American College of Surgeons.

I BACKGROUND

1

Stone Nomenclature and History of Instrumentation for Urinary Stone Disease

Viraj A. Master, MD, *Maxwell V. Meng*, MD, *and Marshall L. Stoller*, MD

CONTENTS

Key Words: Instrumentation; nephrolithiasis; nomenclature; stones.

"The physicians…can defend themselves when unfortunate, but if we lithotomists have a mishap, we must run for our lives"
–Pierre Franco, 16th century itinerant lithotomist

INTRODUCTION

Urinary stone disease has afflicted mankind for millennia. The oldest renal stone on record was described by Shattock in 1905 and was found in an Egyptian mummy in a tomb dating to approx 4400 bc *(1)*. This 1.5-cm calciferous calculi lay beside the first lumbar vertebra. The description of urinary stones has been a process of intense scientific investigation culminating in a burst of activity in the 19th century, when essentially all urinary stones seen commonly today were described and named. The first part of this chapter addresses some history that underlies the current names we use for urinary calculi.

The treatment of urinary stones has been the story of heady success, incorporating numerous advances in engineering, materials science, optics, physics, and, above all, the sheer inventiveness in trying to treat a pervasive disease. The second part of the chapter highlights some of the work that has gone on in the developing instrumentation applied

From: Current Clinical Urology, *Urinary Stone Disease:*
A Practical Guide to Medical and Surgical Management
Edited by: M. L. Stoller and M. V. Meng © Humana Press Inc., Totowa, NJ

to urinary stone disease, with particular emphasis on early instrumentation. Not every advance in instrumentation is reported owing to space constraints.

NOMENCLATURE OF STONES

The word "crystal" is derived from the Greek work *krystallosus*, which means "ice" and is used to refer to the solid phase of substances having a specific internal structure and enclosed by symmetrically arranged planar surfaces. The Latin word *calculus* means "pebble". The crystalline constituents of urinary calculi in the human are varied. Some of these occur geologically, whereas others are found only in the animal kingdom. A subset is found in human beings. This chapter reviews fascinating, previously published work regarding the nomenclature that underlies stone disease. The reader is especially directed to recent work by Luesmann and a comprehensive mineralogy website maintained by the Mineralogical Society of America. (http://www.mindat.org/ and http://www.minsocam.org/) *(2)*.

Although stone disease has been documented in ancient mankind *(3)* and indeed was avidly investigated by physicians and surgeons thousands of years ago, much of the scientific analysis that rigorously investigated and accurately determined the components of urinary stone disease was carried out only within the past 200 years.

Whewellite $CaC_2O_4 \cdot H_2O$

Calcium oxalate monohydrate, also known as whewellite, and occasionally synonymous with oxacalcite, is named after Professor William Whewell of Cambridge, England (Fig. 1). William Whewell (1794–1866) was one of the most important and influential figures in 19th-century Britain. Whewell, a polymath, wrote extensively on numerous subjects, including mineralogy, geology, mechanics, astronomy, political economy, theology, and architecture, in addition to his works that remain the most well known today, those in philosophy of science, history of science, and moral philosophy. In his own time his influence was acknowledged by the major scientists of the day, such as Charles Darwin and Michael Faraday, who frequently turned to Whewell for philosophical and scientific advice, and, interestingly, for terminological assistance. Whewell invented the terms "anode," "cathode," and "ion" for Faraday. On the request of the poet Coleridge in 1833 Whewell invented the English word "scientist"; before this time the only terms in use were "natural philosopher" and "man of science." Interestingly, Whewellite was first described by Henry James Brooke (1771–1857), a London wool trader and amateur mineralogist, who also discovered brookite. At Brooke's time, mineralogy nomenclature forbade individuals from attaching their names to two minerals.

Whewellite is extremely rare in nature. It is known to occur in septarium nodules from marine shale near Havre, MT, with golden calcite at Custer, SD, and as a fault filling with celestite near Moab, UT. It is found in hydrothermal veins with calcite and silver in Europe, and it often occurs in association with carbonaceous materials like coal, particularly in Saxony. It is one of the most common kidney stone minerals, however, where it typically occurs as small, smooth, botryoidal to globular, yellow-green to brown, radially fibrous crystals and is traditionally hard to fragment, as is well known to urologists.

Weddellite $CaC_2O_4 \cdot 2H_2O$

Calcium oxalate dihydrate, also known as weddellite, is named for the Weddell Sea, off Antarctica. The Weddell Sea is named after James Weddell, a great explorer, who

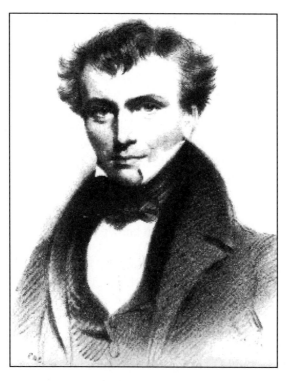

Fig. 1. Professor William Whewell, for whom whewellite is named, was professor of mineralogy and long-time master of Trinity College in Cambridge, England.

explored the most southerly portion of Antarctica in the early 19th century. There, millimeter-sized crystals were found in bottom sediments in the 1930s, and the mineral was named for the region in 1942 *(4)*. The sharp yellow crystals that urinary weddellite forms are often much larger than that however. The yellow crystals are commonly deposited on the outer surface of a smooth whewellite stone. Like whewellite, weddellite is a calcium oxalate. They differ in the amount of water that is included in their crystal structures, and this gives them very different crystal habits. Occasionally, weddellite partially dehydrates to whewellite, forming excellent pseudomorphs of grainy whewellite after weddellite's short tetragonal dipyramids.

Struvite MgNH₄PO₄ · 6H₂O

Magnesium ammonium phosphate hexahydrate, also known as struvite, is credited to Heinrich Christian Gottfried von Struve (1772–1851). Struve, also known as Baron von Struve, was a Russian diplomat and naturalist, who lived in Germany. His scientific interests included geology and mineralogy. The name struvite was coined in his honor in 1845 by Georg Ludwig Ulex, a Swedish geologist. Before that time, magnesium ammonium phosphate was sometimes referred to as guanite because the mineral was detected in bat guano. However, from the clinical realm, the scenario of the combination of phosphate stones with alkaline, ammoniacal urine and putrefaction was recognized by Marcet earlier, in 1818. Certain dogs, especially Dalmatians, can produce remarkable large, smooth, milky-white tetrahedrons of well-crystallized struvite.

Newberyite $MgHPO_4 \cdot 3H_2O$

Magnesium hydrogen phosphate trihydrate, also known as Newberyite, is named for James Cosmo Newbery (1843–1895). Newbery, who was also known as Newberry, was a 19th century Australian geologist and mineralogist, who did extensive work in the Australian outback. He was the curator of the Melbourne Museum in the late 1800s. There is an Aboriginal community named after him in Western Australia. Newberyite is rare in kidney stones. Newberyite was first identified as a crystalline component of a kidney stone in 1956 *(5)*. When it does occur, it often occurs as tiny isolated globular crystals on the surfaces of apatite–struvite stones. This probably reflects an alteration of struvite to newberyite, or perhaps a change of conditions to more acidic solutions.

Apatite $Ca_{10}(PO_4) \cdot 6H_2O$

Hydroxyapatite, or hydroxylapatite, also known as apatite, is named from the Greek word *apatao* meaning "I am misleading," in allusion to its similarity to other more valuable minerals such as the gems peridot and beryl. Apatite is a common mineral in nature. Chemically it is a complex calcium phosphate with varied, attached molecules of hydroxyl (OH), fluorine (F), and sometimes other elements. Apatite is the fundamental mineral component in bones and teeth, and when apatite has fluorine in its crystal structure, it is stronger. This is why fluorine is added to water and toothpaste. In kidney stones, the hydroxyl group is predominant, and carbonate (CO_3) substitutes for some of the phosphate, making a mineral that is relatively poorly crystallized. Apatite often forms the nucleus on which other urinary minerals are deposited. Apatite is widely found as a white powdery mineral deposit and crystallized apatite has been extensively used for fertilizer. Transparent varieties of a fine color are sometimes used for gems, although these are soft gemstones and not very valuable.

Brushite $CaHPO_4 \cdot 2H_2O$

Calcium hydrogen phosphate dihydrate, also known as brushite, was named in 1864 by G.E. Moore, in honor of George Jarvis Brush (1831–1912). Brush, something of a child prodigy, first became interested in mineralogy at the age of 15 while attending school in Connecticut. In 1855, Brush was elected full professor of metallurgy at the recently established Yale Scientific School. Brushite is a calcium phosphate compound that is very similar to the common mineral gypsum (calcium sulfate), which itself is widely used in sheetrock for home construction. Brushite is found as a common cave mineral in guano deposits and in phosphorites formed at low pH (acidic) by reaction of phosphate-rich solutions with calcite and clay. It is a soft, silky mineral, usually honey-brown and showing a fine radial fibrous structure.

Whitlockite $Ca_3(PO_4)_2$

Tricalcium phosphate, or whitlockite, was named in 1940 for Herbert Percy Whitlock (1868–1948). Whitlock was a 20th century American mineralogist and curator of the American Museum of Natural History in New York City. Whitlockite is very rarely found in the urinary system and is usually found in prostate stones. It is a calcium phosphate with small amounts of magnesium, $Ca_9(Mg,Fe)H(PO_4)_7$, and its occurrence may be stabilized by trace amounts of zinc, which perhaps accounts for its predilection for the prostate gland, which has a relatively high zinc content. The mineral is a resinous, brown material.

Lesser Known Minerals and Stones Without Eponyms

Some of the other minerals that occur extremely rarely in kidney stones include monetite (calcium phosphate), calcite (calcium carbonate), aragonite (calcium carbonate), and hannayite (magnesium phosphate). The chemical constituents of urinary calculi were first determined with uric acid stones. It was originally called the acid of calculus, or lithic acid (from the Greek, *lithos*, meaning stone), and was first isolated from the urine in 1776 by Karl Wilhelm Scheele (1742–1786). Scheele was a conundrum, who had very little formal schooling and no training at all in science, yet was a prodigious chemist, characterizing tartartic acid, murexide dye, and other substances. Even more significant than his contribution to stone disease, he characterized oxygen in 1771, two years before Priestley, but was unrecognized for his discovery, which he called "fire air" *(6)*. Ostensibly, he was an apothecary, but used all of his time in scientific experimentation and actually is believed to have died young because of his constant exposure to toxic vapors from his experiments. The uric acid stone was renamed "acide urique" by Antoine François de Fourcroy (1755–1809) and Nicholas Louis Vauquelin (1763–1829) in 1799 *(7)*.

Cystine was first isolated from a urinary calculus in 1810 by Wollaston, who also demonstrated it to be the first known amino acid *(8)*. William Hyde Wollaston (1766–1828) was, like Whewell, another true intellectual giant. Although he was formally trained as a physician, he had broad-ranging insightful interests in chemistry, mineralogy, crystallography, physics, astronomy, botany, physiology, and pathology and published notable scientific advances in all of these fields. He was recognized for his achievements by being elected President of the Royal Society. His secret method of purifying platinum enabled financial independence from medicine in 1800, so he could devote his time to scientific interests.

HISTORY OF INSTRUMENTATION

"Instrument" is defined by the Merriam-Webster dictionary as "a means whereby something is achieved, performed, or furthered." The discussion of instrumentation in the treatment of urinary stone disease generally can be seen as an orderly progression from potions and prayers to external treatments (bathing or drinking in healthful waters) *(9)*, to minimally invasive solutions (catheterization), to maximally invasive solutions (surgery), back to minimally invasive solutions (endoscopy), and finally back to oral "instruments" (medications and fruit juice) *(10)*. Another way of viewing the history of instrumentation for stone disease is a development of palliative (catheterization, cystolithotomy), to diagnostic (cystoscopy), to destructive (nephrectomy for stone disease and the sequelae of stone disease), to curative (stone removal), and finally to preventative treatments. This section highlights some aspects of the development of instrumentation as applied to urinary stone disease. Table 1 lists these major events along with some other contextual events in urology.

The ancient Egyptians removed urinary tract stones by dilating the urethra and sucking out the stones. Sir Eric Riches described the procedure as follows:

"The urethra was dilated by a wooden or cartilaginous cannula as thick as the thumb pushed in with great force alternating with blowing down the urethra; the stone was pressed down into the perineum by the fingers in the rectum until it could be reached from the urethra or sucked out by the mouth (11)."

Table 1

Important Dates in Innovation and Instrumentation in Treatment of Urolithiasis

1500 BC	The Ebers Papyrus was written. A systematic classification of remedies and medicines used in ancient Egypt. It records the use of 'bread in a rotten condition' to treat bladder diseases.
1000 BC	Vesicolithotomy first described by Susruta of India.
460 BC	Hippocrates born. He recognized the dangers of bladder stones and initiated the analysis of urine by inspection and tasting.
25 BC	The Greek physician Celsus was born. He wrote *De Medicina* and clearly described the presence and symptoms of calculi, urologic surgery, insertion of a catheter, and extraction of the stone with a lithotomy scoop.
129 AD	Galen, the Roman physician, was born in Pergamum, Asia Minor.
936 AD	Abucacis born near Cordoba. The greatest Islamic surgeon of the Middle Ages. He wrote At-Tasrif, in which surgical procedures for bladder stones were described.
1000	Avicenna recommended insertion of a louse into the urethral meatus of patients with urinary retention and this method was used for many centuries.
1535	Santo De Barletta Mariano born. An Italian surgeon who described the perineal median operation for stone in the bladder.
1556	The suprapubic cystotomy procedure was first performed by French surgeon Pierre Franco.
1688	William Cheselden born. Chief surgeon at St. Thomas' Hospital, London, who did extensive studies in lithotomy.
1742	Robert Whytt published a paper on the possibility of dissolving bladder stones with lime water and soap injections, and wrote a small book on the subject in 1752.
1795	Philip Syng Physick, the father of American surgery, was the first to perform a urethrotomy or internal longitudinal incision.
1804	Phillip Bozzini invented a cystoscope for the bladder.
1879	Max Nitze, a German urologist, developed a lens system for the cystoscope.
1810	Cystine, the first amino acid described, was isolated from urinary calculi by an English physician and chemist, Wollaston.
1815	James Archibald Jacques was born. He invented the first soft urethral catheter (Jacques catheter) while production manager of a London rubber mill.
1822	The method of bruising a urinary stone with surgical instruments (lithotrity) was first practiced.
1824	Civiale invented the definitive lithotrite.
1850	Ureteric catheterization was first performed in a woman by English surgeon Sir John Simon.
1852	Achille Etienne Malecot born. A French surgeon who designed a large-bore suprapubic urinary catheter (Malecot catheter).
1860	The Hospital for Stone in London was opened.
1871	First planned nephrectomy for renal stones by Simon in Heidelberg.
1874	Daniel Joseph McCarthy born. New York urologist who designed a panendoscope, prostatic electrotome, and several other instruments.
1877	First electrically lit cystoscope was devised by Berlin urologist Max Nitze.
1878	Rank Seymor Kidd born. London urologist who designed an operating cystoscope (Kidd cystoscope) with an electrode.
1879	Hans Christian Jacobaeus born. Sweedish internist who used a modified cystoscope to perform cautery division of pleural adhesions that led directly to the development of the thoracoscope and other similar instruments.
1880	A procedure for nephrolithotomy, in which the renal stone was removed through a lumbar incision, was performed by Sir Henry Morris of London.

Table 1 *(Continued)*
Important Dates in Innovation and Instrumentation in Treatment of Urolithiasis

1883	Henry Jacob Bigelow of Harvard modified Civiale's lithotrite to crush larger and heavier stones. He removed the fragments with a special metal catheter, to the outer end of which was attached a rubber bulb evacuator with a glass container below to receive the fragments.
1886	Operative treatment for hydronephrosis was performed by Friedrich Trendelenburg of Germany.
1887	Nitze's cystoscope was fitted with Edison's electric light by both Hartwig of Berlin and Leiter of Vienna.
1890	Urology became a separate study course from general surgery, and the first professor of urology was Guyon in Paris.
1893	The catheterization of male ureters was first done by James Brown of Johns Hopkins Hospital.
1895	Early diagnosis of stone disease became possible after the discovery of X-rays, and in 1896 Mcintyre of Glasgow visualized a kidney stone with this method.
1900	Dilatation of the ureteral orifice as treatment for ureteric calculi was first performed by Baltimore urologist H. W. Kelly.
1901	Kelling performs laparoscopy by introducing Nitze cystoscope directly through the abdominal wall.
1904	Hugh Hampton Young, a prominent American urologist, among many other inventions, devised new cystoscopes.
1906	The radiological method of visualization of the renal tract (pyelography) was introduced by Alexander von Lichtenberg of Germany.
1912	Rigid ureteroscopy (unplanned) first performed by H. H. Young.
1921	Radiological visualization of the kidneys by injecting air into the retroperitoneal space (retroperitoneal pneumatography) was devised by Rossentein and Carelli.
1929	Intravenous urography was introduced by German-born American urologist, Moses Swick.
1933	American urologist, Fredric E. B. Foley uses a double-lumened retention catheter with a balloon on the end to keep it in the bladder.
1933	A technique for recording internal body images at a predetermined plane using X-rays (tomography) was described by German physician, D. L. Bartellnk.
1933	Uroselectan, an agent in urography, was introduced by Moses Swick.
1954	Fiberoptic endoscope rod lens design is published in Nature by Harold Hopkins, a British optical physicist.
1955	Percutaneous nephrotomy is described by Goodwin.
1960	Fuller Albright noted the association between renal calculi and hyperparathyroidism. He is considered the father of endocrinology in America.
1961	Development of Nd:YAG. solid state laser.
1964	Flexible ureteroscopy described by Victor F. Marshall.
1967	Open ended silicone tubing used to bypass ureteral obstruction, described by Zimskind.
1972	Ultrasonic device to fragment kidney stones without causing bleeding (lithotripter) was invented by a Munich group including Chaussey and Eisenberger.
1976	Percutaneous pyelolithotomy described by Fernstrom.
1978	Double J ureteral stent is described by Finney.
1979	Retroperitoneoscopy for ureterolithotomy.
1980	First patient treated with SWL using Dornier HM-1 lithotripter.
1986	A tiny television camera was added to the modern laparoscope.
1988	Ureteral lithotripsy with pulsed laser by Dretler, Wickham, and Segura.
1990	Electrohydraulic lithotripsy described by Denstedt and Clayman.
1991	Laparoscopic nephrectomy by Clayman.
1992	Swiss lithoclast described.

Several remedies for bladder calculi from folk medicine are described in the Talmud (Gittin, folio 69b). One example illustrating the lack of understanding of pathophysiology was to "take a louse from a man and a woman and hang it on the penis of a man and the corresponding place in a woman; and when he urinates he should do so on dry thorns near the socket of the door" *(12)*. Surprisingly, this "remedy" remained in the medical armamentarium through the Middle Ages. The extreme suffering generated by stone disease and the importance of stone prevention is evidenced by finding recipes against kidney stones in the Croatian prayerbook *(13)*.

The use of surgical instrumentation in the treatment of urinary stone disease has a checkered history, with admonitions against surgery from the start. The great Hippocrates (460–370 BC), who was familiar with the pathology related to urinary tract stones, included a passage regarding their treatment in the original Hippocratic Oath:

> *"I will not cut persons laboring under the stone, but will leave this work to be done by men who are practitioners of this work." (Adams translation)* (14).

Of course, this statement can be interpreted two ways. Either the removal of stones was considered too lowly a craft for physicians, or conversely lithotomists must have possessed a fair degree of skill, or Hippocrates would not have recommended that only practitioners of the craft perform the delicate surgery.

Lower Urinary Tract

URETHRAL

Possibly the earliest instrument for the treatment of stone disease could be thought of as the urethral catheter. The purpose of the catheter was to bypass obstruction thus permitting drainage. The word catheter is derived from the Greek *cathienal*, "to send down," although some ascribe it incorrectly to *cathatos*, which means perpendicular *(15)*. Initially, in an effort to bypass the obstruction resulting from the calculus in the urethra or at the bladder neck, ancient Egyptians first used hollow reeds and curled-up palm leaves, but later history records Egyptians using bronze and tin for making catheters, knives, and sounds as early as 3000 BC. The ancient Hindus used tubes of gold, iron, and wood for dilating the urethra at least before 1000 BC *(16)*. The Chinese used a lacquer-coated tubular leaf of the onion plant *Allium fistulosum* to make catheters as early as 100 BC *(17)*. Metal catheters and sounds made of bronze were found in the ruins of Pompeii, which was buried in 79 AD *(18)*. Although the catheters found at Pompeii were doubly curved, all other ancient catheters and sounds had one common characteristic: they were made straight and rigid without consideration for anatomic structure of the posterior urethra. Surprisingly, the logical idea of making catheters curved was not rediscovered until literally hundreds of years later. During the 10th century, Islamic surgeons used rigid silver catheters and also catheters made of skins. Avicenna (980–1030 AD) used sea animal skins stuck together with cheese glue and also recommended lubricating the urethra with soft cheese before rigid catheterization. Many others tried different materials that were both simultaneously stiff and malleable including silver, copper, brass, ivory, pewter, and lead. Lack of the ability to create an indwelling catheter was a continuing problem with all of these designs but nevertheless provided relief to patients (Fig. 2). In the early part of the 18th century, a German anatomist, Lorenz Heister (1683–1758), had catheters made of silver in the shape of the natural curve of the prostatic urethra (Fig. 3). The true development of the modern catheter is felt to come from Heister's design and was perfected in the form of the "coude" (French, meaning

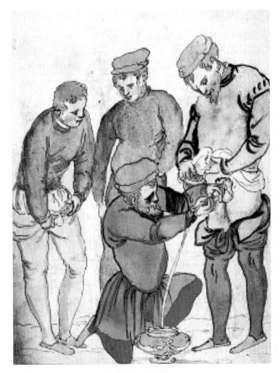

Fig. 2. Sixteenth century itinerant barber-surgeons catheterized grateful patients to relieve obstruction caused by bladder stones, as illustrated in a Italian medical picture book by Henricus Kullmaurer and Albert Meher.

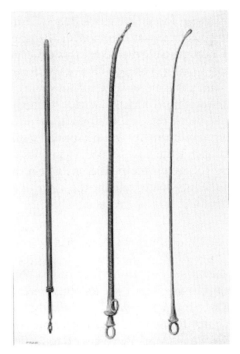

Fig. 3. Silver catheters showing evolution in design with the two on the right being bent to simulate the natural curve of the prostatic urethra.

elbow [noun], or bent [adjective]) catheter by the eminent French surgeon Louis Mercier (1811–1882), although the literature still contains spurious assertions that a certain Emile Coude was responsible *(19)*.

The first flexible catheters were made of wax-impregnated cloth and molded on a silver sound created by Frabricius, professor of surgery in Padua, in 1665. These catheters were not very durable and softened rapidly, thus losing the ability to maintain a patent lumen. Modern flexible catheters, basic prototypes of the ones used today, were first made with the introduction of elastic gum, derived from the latex sap of the *Hevea* tree species in 1735 *(20)*. These were far more comfortable than the rigid catheters, but still suffered from problems of extreme stickiness in hot weather and brittle stiffening in cold weather. The ability to transform this elastic gum into a durable and versatile substance that did not have temperature dependence was discovered by Charles Goodyear in 1839, who termed this process vulcanization. After methods were developed for stabilizing the natural latex and preventing it from coagulating, rubber products could be made over a mold dipped into a vat of latex. This rubber catheter was relatively durable, flexible, and therefore easily introduced and comfortably retained. Its introduction marked the true beginning of the modern urinary catheter. This catheter still required external appliances to hold it in place, such as taping it to the penile shaft or suturing to the labia in women. In 1822, Ducamp used submucosal layers of ox intestines, which were tied on to the catheters as inflatable balloons to hold a catheter in place. In 1853 Reybard devised a catheter that incorporated a separate balloon channel. A growing surge of transurethral surgery led to the need to secure hemostasis and finally resulted in F. E. B. Foley, an American urologist, devising the modern balloon catheter in the 1930, which was distributed by Bard in 1933 *(21)*. Modern 20th-century developments in catheters have centered mostly on the use of different materials, like silicone, to reduce urethral toxicity from latex.

A Parisian instrument maker, Joseph Frederick Benoit Charriere (1803–1876), devised a sizing system for urologic instruments commonly called the French scale in the United States, which is based on progressive diameter sizes differing from each other by one-third of a millimeter, i.e., 1 mm = 3 French (Fr) or 0.039 inches *(22)*.

It was known for millennia that merely pulling out stones lodged in the penile urethra could result in irreversible urethral injury. In fact, Celsus himself, devotes a large section of his book, *De Medicina*, to the removal of urethral calculi. He describes first using a scoop, but failing that, urethrolithotomy was performed with a sharp knife. The urethra and skin edges were left open to heal by secondary intention. An ingenious prevention of fistula formation was to stretch the penile shaft skin distally and push the glans proximally so that after the incision to remove the stone, the relaxed skin would result in nonoverlapping urethral and skin openings *(23)*.

BLADDER

Perineal Lithotomy

The operation for bladder stone is one of the oldest recorded surgical techniques apart from trepanning and circumcision *(20)*. Patients were understandably reluctant to undergo surgery, given the absence of anesthesia and the very high procedure-related mortality, as described in the following paragraphs. Only severe, prolonged, insufferable pain related to the stone made patients submit to the acute pain of the knife. The literature is replete with descriptions of special instruments, knives, lancets, and gorgets with unique blades for opening the bladder through the prostatic urethra. Medial litho-

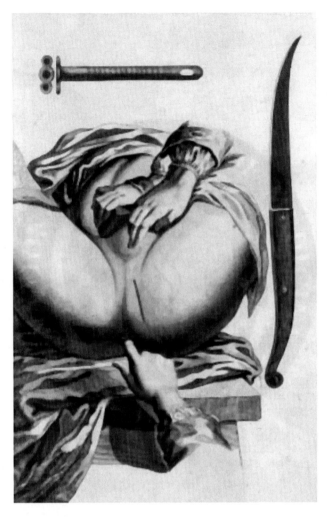

Fig. 4. Lithotomy using instruments of the "lesser" apparatus. Note the lateral incision for lithotomy. Note the sharp bistoury on the right and the cannula at top, which were designed by M. Fourbert in the 18th century.

tomy (cutting on the gripe) is the oldest variety of the perineal operation, but even Celsus, in approx 50 AD, recognizing the great danger of rectal injury, deflected the inferior end of the perineal incision toward the left ischial tuberosity before incising the bladder. In perineal lithotomy of the "small apparatus" a staff or sound was passed through the urethra into the bladder (Fig. 4). This sounding was the method employed to confirm the presence and location of vesical stone. With the patient in a semisitting posture, the tip of the sound was maneuvered to bring the stone down to the lowest point in the bladder. When the perineal incision was made the surgeon felt for the groove on the convex side of the staff as a guide for the incision into the membranous urethra and prostate. When an assistant held the urethral staff, the surgeon could cut directly onto the stone. Perineal lithotomy using the "grand apparatus" of Mariano Santo came next in 1535 (Fig. 5). Instruments, forceps, and scoops, rather than the finger, were inserted

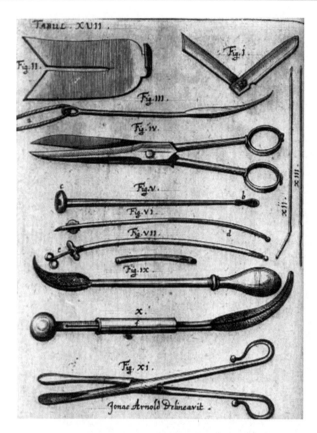

Fig. 5. Elements of the "major" apparatus used for lithotomy in the 17th century. Note the multiplicity of knives, spatulas, and hooks used for cystolithotomy in the later period compared with that in Figure 4, which just used a knife and a cannula.

through the perineal incision to engage and extricate the stone. In the main, it can be said that the additional apparatus not only complicated the procedure but added to the operative risk *(24)*. The sole objective of lithotomy was to relieve the patient of strangury by extracting the stone as quickly as possible through a perineal incision. Operations were frequently performed in the home. The patient was purged and often bled before as well as after operation. Bleeding immediately beforehand had the advantage of producing shock and considerable diminution in sensitivity to pain. As many as five or more cases were often scheduled for one session. Pouteau, the great 18th-century French surgeon, described the scenes as an "auto-da-fe affair" (act-of-faith affair). The courage and agony of the patient on the lithotomy table, known as the scaffold or Bed of Misery (Fig. 6), and the boldness and skill of the surgeon were the magnetic attractions that drew onlookers, both rich and poor (Fig. 7). After the terror and pain of the operation, the patient usually had a sense of relief as urine escaped through the lithotomy wound without initiating attacks of vesical colic. Perineal lithotomy provided the surgeon a fine opportunity to indulge in showmanship. Sir Astley Cooper often did the operation in less than a minute and the average maximum time in a surgical editorial in 1828 was about 6 min *(24)*.

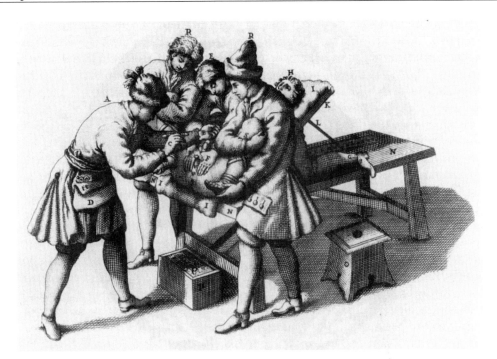

Fig. 6. Lithotomist at work, ca. 1700. Two assistants are holding the legs in lithotomy position, while a third pushes on the suprapubic region to keep the stone fixed in place at the bladder neck.

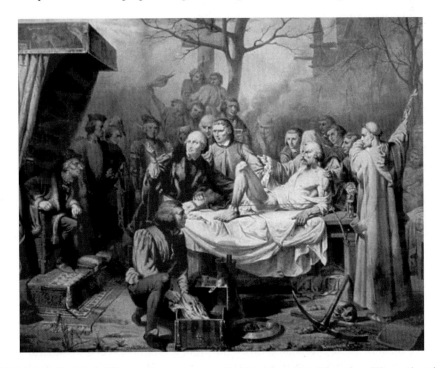

Fig. 7. Lithograph titled, "The earliest operation for the stone," by Rivoulon. The patient is lying on a platform and the physician is performing an operation before a large crowd, which includes King Louis XI of France, seen seated on the left, intently watching the showmanship. This fanciful lithograph has little relation to the pain the patient suffered during the stone removal.

From the mid-16th century well into the 18th, a brand of self-made stone cutters, "specialists" who acquired art through apprenticeship, were the chief lithotomists. Without formal training, they usually practiced poor operative technique and some were charlatans *(25)*. Mortality was high, approx 18 to 53%. Extravasation of infected urine into the paravesical tissues was often the reason for death, rather than hemorrhage. Those who cut too widely were known to lacerate the internal pudendal artery, often resulting in exsanguination. Interestingly, there were a few outliers, most spectacularly, Pouteau, a notable French surgeon of the 18th century, whose mortality rate was only 2.5%. This was achieved a century before the development of antisepsis by his strict adherence to the importance of keeping hands clean and the use of disposable paper dressings. Strangely, published accounts of mortality even during the antiseptic era were almost as high as the nonantiseptic era, in the range of 10% *(24)*. One hypothesis is that the open wound management after vesical incision essentially allowed for irrigation of the wound by urine. It is interesting that the morbidity and mortality associated with this operation was so high that some of the first informed-consent documents were associated with lithotomy *(26)*. The first suprapubic lithotomy for removal of a bladder stone was carried out in 1561 by Franco, who performed removal of an egg-sized stone in a 2-yr-old boy, but did not achieve acceptance as a safe modality at the time, likely because of the frequent risk of peritoneal injury and septic death *(27)*.

Celsus, Franco, and Cheselden stand out in their periods as the greatest contributors to the development of lithotomy. The first truly sterile operation for stone was Joseph Lister's median lithotomy for vesical calculus on June 4, 1881. He swabbed the wound with zinc chloride and left it open, but provided a drainage tube to facilitate the escape of urine. The patient recovered quickly.

Urinary incontinence, occasionally reported after perineal lithotomy in the male, was so frequent following urethrovesical lithotomy in the female that the procedure came to be abandoned. Urethral dilatation was substituted because of the distensibility and shortness of the female urethra.

Lithotrity/Lithoprisy

The dangers and difficulties of lithotomy were an important spur that drove the development of alternative minimally invasive methods of bladder stone extraction. Ammonius, in 247 BC, is credited with fragmentation of bladder stones by impaling them with an ice pick-like device passed through a catheter *(11)*. After engaging the stone, a hammer was used on the pick to fragment the stone. This idea was apparently unpopular and there is no mention of stone fragmentation for several centuries. Some lithotomists, such as Elderton in 1819, unsuccessfully tried to fix stones in place by loops of wire passed through a straight catheter. When the stone was engaged a drill bow was used to break up the stone *(11)*. Interestingly, some famous self-performed operations for urinary stones did involve lithotrity-type maneuvers, such as that of Colonel Martin of Lucknow, a layman who in 1782 ingeniously devised instrumentation to file his stone to small pieces, which he was then able to void *(28)*. The first truly effective drilling instrument was made by Civale of France and used in 1824. This instrument, known as a trilabe or lithontripteur, consisted of two straight metal tubes, one inside the other; the inner had three curved arms that projected when the outer sheath was retracted and by which the stone was seized. It was held in position by advancing the outer sheath. An iron rod with a sharp point was passed through the inner tube to bore a hole into the stone This was uncomfortable for the patient and treatment sessions were limited to 5 min with

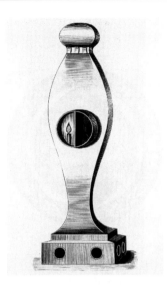

Fig. 8. The "lichtleiter" or light conductor of Bozzini. One can see the candle used for illumination immediately next to the eyepiece for viewing.

several sessions required to break the stone into small enough fragments that the patient could void *(29)*. With this minimally invasive approach, mortality was reduced to a mere 3%. Ambroïse Paré put teeth in the blades of his crushing forceps and a thumbscrew in the handle so as to increase the power of the instrument to crush large stones, but this also increased mortality. The introduction of ether anesthesia in 1842 allowed surgeons to perform longer and more precise operations. Bigelow in 1878 added to the development of this procedure by the use of suction irrigation and renamed the lithotrity procedure litholapaxy. The use of anesthesia coupled with suction enabled complete removal of the stone in a single session, which could last 2 h. However, without the ability to visualize the stone, this technique was not popularized until cystoscopy was developed, whereupon the lithotrite was combined with a cystoscope into a single instrument.

Cystoscopy

The desire to look into the cavities of the body to diagnose and treat disease occupied many medical specialists throughout the 18th century, especially as the alternative was extensive surgery, not yet possible without the development of anesthesia. The first instruments designed for urologic evaluation were designed for the female, because of the shorter length and greater diameter of the urethra. Initially various specula were developed to inspect the female urethra, mostly by dilating it, but they were painful when widely opened and provided only a limited viewing ability *(30)*. The biggest hindrance to viewing ability was insufficient illumination. To solve this problem, in 1805 Phillip Bozzini, from Germany, developed the "lichtleiter," or light conductor *(31)*. This instrument, made of silver and covered in sharkskin, contained a tallow candle balanced on a spring to keep the position of the flame constant (Fig. 8). The observer applied his eye to the body of the instrument and was able to see past the mirror down a series of fittings, or specula: a narrow tube for the urethra, a bigger one for the rectum, a four-valved one

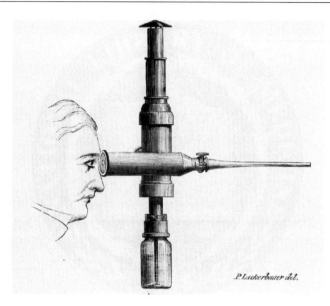

Fig. 9. "L'endoscope" of Desormeaux devised in 1865.

for the vagina, and a fitting with a mirror on the end for laryngoscopy. Bozzini, an obstetrician, wanted to use endoscopy for operating on the uterus and to remove foreign bodies and stones from the bladder *(32)*. The lichtleiter was successfully tested in Vienna, but it was also clear that candlelight did not have enough illumination to view the bladder. Moreover, because of local medical politics, further development was blocked. The lichtleiter certainly accomplished one goal—it spurred the development of endoscopy by other physicians. Although many other physicians worked on developing endoscopic instrumentation, the next leap forward was by Desormeaux, who in 1853 introduced his "l'endoscope" (Fig. 9). This instrument had the advantage of a stronger light source (initially a paraffin or kerosene lamp), the use of a mirror as a light reflector, and the ability to introduce working instruments. He was able to make sketches of the bladder and bladder calculi using this device. Additionally, he diagnosed and treated urethritis, carried out direct vision internal urethrotomy, and even removed a papilloma from the urethra. One major problem with this device was the constant fear of burning the surgeon's face or the patient's legs. Francis Cruise of Dublin, a friend of Desormeaux, encased the instrument in a mahogany box, which allowed for safety from heat but made it even more unwieldy. The second problem was that illumination still could not reliably provide for inspection of the entire bladder. Nevertheless, this research spurred others to develop analogous instruments such that in 1861, Joseph Grunfeld, a dermatologist, was able to remove a bladder papilloma.

Investigators focused their attention on changing the light source from an external source to an internal source, which would prove pivotal to the advancement of endoscopy. In 1867, Julius Bruck, a dentist from Dresden used an electrically heated platinum loop, inserted into the rectum, to transilluminate the bladder, although Gustave Trouve of Paris is also credited with this work. Cooling of the loop was a problem, resulting in rectal burns.

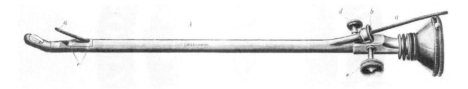

Fig. 10. Maximilian Nitze's cystoscope, showing the probe channel, urethral probe, and bulb illumination.

Finally, in 1877 the potential of Bruck's theoretical advance was realized, and, in combination with other advances, essentially established the form of a clinically useful cystoscope as it is used today. The 28-yr-old urologist responsible for this synthesis was Maximilian Nitze of Berlin. Nearly 90 yr had passed since Bozzini first described his lichtleiter. Nitze, working with a mechanic and an optician, devised an instrument with a platinum wire light source at the tip that also had a glass optic system similar to that of a microscope, allowing for a larger, magnified view of the bladder. This instrument still produced a good deal of heat and required water cooling. However, once Edison invented the incandescent electric bulb in 1880, Nitze, as well as Joseph Leiter, produced the first practical cystoscope in the late 1880s, which was an affordable instrument (Fig. 10). Additional major design changes took place in the early 1900s and included the use of water instead of air to distend the bladder and the use of hemispherical lenses to increase the viewing area *(33)*. The development of fiberoptic instrumentation and the use of the Hopkins "rod-lens" in the 1950s enabled the clarity of endoscopic images that we see today. Reviewing this remarkable story, one notes the consistent theme running through this development, the integration of advancements in physics and optics by surgeons themselves to make better instruments.

In terms of specific use of instrumentation for stone disease, Kelly published the use of endoscopy to remove a ureteral calculus, albeit small, in 1895. Kolischer later used a primitive endoscope and ureteral catheter to inject sterile oil below a stone in order to facilitate stone passage *(32)*.

The history of flexible urological instrumentation is a recent one. Basil Hirschowitz, a South African gastroenterologist, again in collaboration with the physicist Hopkins, produced a flexible fiberoptic endoscope, which enabled him to perform endoscopy in 1957 on a dental student's wife who was suffering from a duodenal ulcer *(34)*. Interestingly and fortuitously for urologists, American Cystoscope Makers Inc. (ACMI) was the only company interested in commercializing this instrument. The first reported use of flexible instrumentation in the urinary tract was actually ureteroscopy and is detailed later *(35)*.

LITHOTRIPTICS

With the severe complications of sepsis, hemorrhage, rectal injury, and death from surgery, many patients turned to various substances said to be capable of dissolving stones in vivo. These drugs, taken orally or injected into the bladder with special devices (Fig. 11), were called lithotriptics, literally "stone-breakers *(36)*." One of the most famous, or rather infamous, was sold by Mrs. Joanna Stephens. This resourceful lady has been reviled as perpetrating a fraud on England in 1739 by her claims of being able to

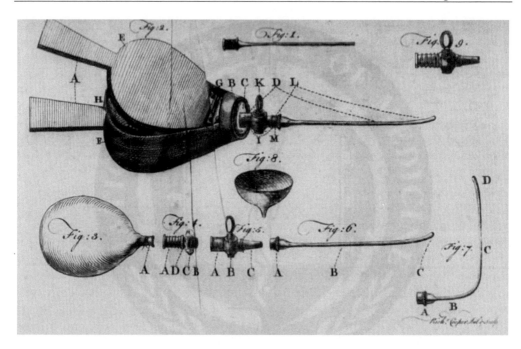

Fig. 11. Bellows designed for the administration of lithotriptic bladder irrigation solution.

dissolve vesical calculi by medication (Mrs. Stephen's Cure for the Stone) *(37)*. This concoction of hers, containing crushed eggshells, snails, and soap, had many famous advocates and an equal number of detractors. Such was the magnitude of the problem in 18th century England that a grateful Parliament awarded her 5000 pounds, a princely sum in that era. In summary, medications of this class mainly contained lime as the active ingredient and worked far better in vitro than in vivo, as a result this kind of "remedy" fell into disuse.

Upper Urinary Tract

IMAGING

Imaging instruments have been critical in making diagnosis of urinary calculi. The first seminal event was the introduction of the X-ray. Roentgen introduced imaging technology on November 8, 1895, calling the source of energy "X-rays" because of their unknown origins, although they were then identified as high-energy electromagnetic radiation, which gave physicians a noninvasive method of looking for suspected urinary calculi. The first radiograph showing a renal calculus was obtained by a Scottish physician (otolaryngologist), John Macintyre in 1896. Specific anatomic detail as well as functional dynamic activity of the urinary tract was made possible by the synthesis of an iodinated compound, uroselectan, by Moses Swick and others in 1928 *(38,39)*. The ultimate imaging "instrument" impacting urological surgery was the advent of CT scanning in the 1970s *(40)*. Interestingly, in this landmark article, although calculi are clearly identified, the authors state, "The clinical merit of this observation [finding calculi] is presently unknown."

Diagnostic Applications

Endoscopic evaluation of the upper urinary tract was an act of serendipity *(41)*. It was first performed using a 9.5-Fr pediatric cystoscope in 1912 and reported in 1929 by Hugh Hampton Young and Robert W. McKay *(42)*. His description of this procedure, performed in a 2-mo-old child with massively dilated ureters secondary to posterior urethral valves, is succinct and illuminating, "In one case in which it was possible to introduce the cystoscope into a dilated ureter, we were able, by using the extra-long straight cystoscope, which is employed in Young's cystoscopic lithotrite, to introduce the cystoscope to the pelvis of the kidney, and when withdrawn the greatly dilated ureter with its convolutions and tortuosities and valvelike septa were seen." However, it was not until 1977 that the development and use of routine rigid ureteroscopy was reported by E. S. Lyon and by T. M. Goodman. Lyon performed distal ureteroscopy in four women, including ureteroscopic resection, after dilation of the ureteral orifice up to 16 Fr with Jewett sounds, simultaneously passing the sound alongside a pediatric cystoscope through the female urethra. Once the orifice was dilated, an 11-Fr cystoscope or 14-Fr resectoscope was used. An average of 4 cm of distal ureter could be visualized in this fashion. Goodman, who performed ureteroscopy in two men and one woman, did not dilate the orifice, but on one occasion did create a ureteral meatotomy to achieve access to ureteral tumor to cauterize it. He was actually able to fulgurate a ureteral tumor in this fashion, thereby using ureteroscopy as a therapeutic tool for the first time *(43,44)*. With the development of the rod lens system by Harold Hopkins in 1960, smaller diameter ureteroscopes could be constructed that have improved optical clarity and allow for the introduction of working channels. The rod lens system was also marked by having increased durability, a problem that plagued early ureteroscopes. The first rigid urologic endoscope used in clinical practice was made by Wolf and its use was reported in 1979. This instrument had a working length of 23 centimeters, as it was based on the design of a pediatric cystoscope, and sheath sizes from 13 to 16 Fr. The size of this instrument allowed for the directed ureteroscopic extraction of calculi for the first time *(45)*. The rapid introduction of longer (39 cm) and narrower (9 Fr) rigid ureteroscopes soon followed, which allowed for instruments to reach into the renal pelvis *(46)*.

It is interesting that the introduction of flexible ureteroscopy and its publication actually predated rigid ureteroscopy. V.F. Marshall first performed flexible ureteropyeloscopy in 1960 by introducing a 9-Fr ureteroscope through a ureterostomy into the renal pelvis to visualize stones. Subsequently, his associates used this instrument placed through a 26-Fr cystoscope to visualize a left ureteral stone 9 cm from the ureteral orifice *(35)*. This instrument was not capable of directed deflection and was only used diagnostically (Fig. 12). With increasing improvements in fiberoptic technology, a small-caliber 2-mm-tipped actively deflectable 70-cm ureteroscope was used by Takagi and colleagues to perform transurethral ureteroscopy, including visualization of the renal pelvis and calyces. This instrument did not have an irrigation channel so visualization was often impaired as surgeons relied on mannitol-induced forced diuresis *(47,48)*.

Therapeutic Instrumentation

Intracorporeal Instrumentation

Electrohydraulic lithotripsy (EHL) was the first use of a shock wave in a liquid medium for the fragmentation of urinary stones. It was invented in 1955 by L. A. Yutkin, a Russian engineer. Unfortunately for patients, he was a victim of Stalinist persecution

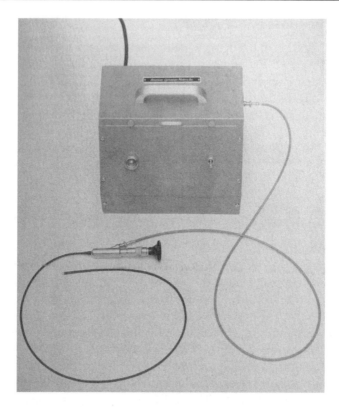

Fig. 12. Flexible ureteroscope designed by V. F. Marshall. Note the lack of an irrigating channel.

and was banished for 10 yr, thus delaying the clinical introduction of this technology. EHL essentially functions as an underwater spark plug producing both a powerful shock wave and a cavitation bubble when the device is about 1 mm away from a stone. Later, the physicist Jutkin in Leningrad showed that underwater electrical discharges between electrode tips could destroy plates of china *(49)*. His colleague, Goldberg, a urologist from Riga, used electrohydraulic shock waves, delivered via a cystoscope, to destroy a bladder stone in a patient. It was quickly used to treat ureteral calculi as well. In 1978, Raney used a 9-Fr EHL probe to blindly fragment distal ureteral stones successfully *(50)*.

Other intracorporeal stone fragmentation instruments were being developed at approximately the same time. Ultrasound was first used experimentally for fragmenting urinary stones by William P. Mulvaney in 1953 *(51)*. This device consisted of a metal probe attached to a piezoelectric plate. When electric current was delivered to the plate, the tip vibrated and resulted in stone fragmentation and also heat production, which caused thermal damage. The final advance in this instrument was a combination of irrigation, coupled with suction, so that heat buildup would not occur.

The ruby laser was developed in 1960 and was able to fragment urinary calculi, but produced unacceptable thermal tissue damage *(52)*. Many other lasers were used, including the clinical use of the flashlamp-pumped tunable dye laser. The laser most used for urinary stone disease is currently the Holmium:YAG laser because of its versatility and cost-effectiveness *(53)*.

Extracorporeal Instrumentation

The first attempts to disintegrate human calculi by acoustic energy (extracorporeal shock wave lithotripsy [SWL]) used a setup without direct contact between the transducer and the stone surface, and the first reported fragmentation of biliary calculi in an in vitro model appeared in 1950 from Harold Lamport and Herbert Newman. Urinary calculi could not be fragmented with this particular noncontact setup. Finally, an in vitro contact-free approach combined with pulsed acoustical energy was derived using an electrode-ellipsoid system by Lamport and Newman in the 1950s *(49)*. Later, the German aerospace firm Dornier developed an interest in understanding the effects of shock waves, which was prompted by observations of aircraft metal fatigue as well as shock wave-related injuries sustained by tank crews struck by shells. Experimentally, focused shock waves were created by an underwater spark discharge. Dornier scientists discovered that when metallic spheres were bombarded with shock waves, small pit marks would appear beneath water droplets on the sphere's surface. Sometime later, a Dornier engineer experienced a sensation similar to an electrical shock when he touched a target body at exactly the same moment that it was hit by a high-velocity projectile, although unlike an electrical shock, his skin was not injured at the point of contact *(54)*. As the story goes, the wife of one of these engineers suggested studying the effect of shock waves on kidney stones *(55)*. In the 1970s a research program in Munich, led by F. Eisenberger and C. Chaussey, showed that shock waves could be created and passed through biologic media without causing harm. Dogs were implanted with urinary stones and then successfully treated. The first human was treated in 1980 using the Dornier HM-1 (Human Machine-1). The first reports describing this technology by Chaussey and colleagues for successful clinical use appeared in 1980 *(56,57)*. The first commercial lithotriper was the HM-3, which was produced in 1984. Further refinements in this instrument have been directed at producing machines that produce weaker shock waves so that less anesthesia is necessary, as well as making machines portable. More detailed accounts of the interesting development of SWL are found elsewhere *(55,58)*.

Percutaneous

Willard E. Goodwin first reported the use of percutaneous trocar nephrostomy in 1955 using static X-ray images and 12-gauge needles with polyethylene tubing for drainage *(59)*. With this enormous advance, a Swedish team including a urologist B. Johannson and a radiologist, I. Fernstrom, performed the first percutaneous nephrolithotomy in 1973, and reported it in 1976 *(60)*. This was a heroic undertaking, lasting approx 2 wks, quite unlike the percutaneous single-stage procedures of today. After the initial needle placement into a "strategically chosen calyx," increasingly larger semirigid polypropylene tubes were placed as dilators. These tubes were warmed over steaming water generated by a teapot to make them malleable and were upsized every other day. In this way, it took 10–14 d of successive dilations to create a 20-Fr channel. After this, a Dormia basket was inserted and the stone removed under fluoroscopic guidance. Subsequent modifications in instrumentation followed because of the variable shape of stones, requiring, on occasion, the local silversmith to make forceps of the requisite shape. The potential power of this technology was advanced quickly in the early 1980s by P. Alken and Michael Marberger in Germany, by J. E. A. Wickham and Ronald A. Miller in England and by Joseph W. Segura and Ralph V. Clayman in the United States *(61)*. The end result of a great deal of effort was to create the ability to widen tracts in a single session and to remove stones under direct vision, including the use of flexible nephroscopy. Essentially by a process of steady miniaturization, instrumentation and techniques used in the lower urinary tract, such as litholopaxy using ultrasonic disintegration and EHL, were then used successfully in the upper tracts *(62)*.

Laparoscopic

Laparoscopy was first performed in 1901 to observe the effect of pneumoperitoneum on the abdominal organs. Georg Kelling (1866–1945), a surgeon from of Dresden, introduced a Nitze cystoscope into a dog's abdominal cavity and found with pressures of 100 mmHg organs were smaller and colorless. He attempted to use it on two patients, one of whom was having an intraabdominal hemorrhage, which he thought he could arrest with "lufttamponade" (pneumoperitoneum). The patients refused and it was a further 9 yr before the first clinical use in a human by Hans Christian Jacobaeus *(63)*.

During the 1960s gynecologists began to carry out small surgical interventions on a regular basis, which mainly consisted of endoscopic sterilization first performed by R. Palmer of Paris. Kurt Semm, a gynecologist, performed the first laparoscopic appendectomy in 1980. The pace of introduction and implementation of this instrumentation was rapid. In September 1985, Erich Muhe, a general surgeon from Germany, used Semm's instruments to remove the first gallbladder in the world laparoscopically *(64)*. The first major solid organ to be removed was performed by Ralph Clayman and colleagues, who performed a right laparoscopic radical nephrectomy *(65)*.

The use of laparoscopic instrumentation for ureterolithotomy was first reported by John Wickham in 1979 *(66)*. Incidentally, it was Wickham who first coined the term, "minimally invasive surgery" *(64)*. Laparoscopic instrumentation for ureterolithotomy was used as an alternative to open surgery in the setting of a salvage procedure after failed shock wave lithotripsy or endoscopic procedures.

It is fascinating to examine the "cross-pollination" of different surgical specialties in advancing instrumentation. For example, the cystoscope was used for thoracoscopy. Surgeons then used the thoracoscope therapeutically to release pleural adhesions, which provided impetus to perform transurethral procedures. Laparoscopic instrumentation designed for relatively simple gynecologic operations like tubal ligation was modified and advanced for extirpative general surgical procedures like cholecystectomy and finally to major organ removal like nephrectomy and ultimately to laparoscopic reconstructive surgery like pyeloplasty. Similarly, the first cardiac catherization experiment was performed by Werner Forssmann using a ureteral catheter to place into his own left arm vein *(15)*.

REFERENCES

1. Modlin M. A history of urinary stone. S Afr Med J 1980; 58: 652–655.
2. Leusmann DB. Whewellite, weddellite and company: where do all the strange names originate? BJU Int 2000; 86: 411–413.
3. Morris AG, Rodgers AL. A probable case of prehistoric kidney stone disease from the northern Cape Province, South Africa. Am J Phys Anthropol 1989; 79: 521.
4. Bannister FA, Hey MH: Report on some crystalline components of the Weddell Sea. Discovery Rep 1936; 13: 60.
5. Lonsdale K, Sutor DJ. Newberyite in ancient and modern urinary calculi: identification and space group. Science 1966; 154: 1353.
6. Website: http://85.1911encyclopedia.org/S/SC/SCHEELE_KARL_WILHELM.htm. Accessed: July, 2006.
7. Rosenfeld L. The chemical work of Alexander and Jane Marcet. Clin Chem 2001; 47: 784.

8. Wollaston WH. On cystic oxide: a new species of urinary calculus. Trans R Soc Lond 1810; 100: 223.

9. Nenov D, Nenov V, Lazarov G, Tchepilev A. Treatment of renal stones in Bulgaria in ancient times ("Hissarya" baths). Am J Nephrol 1999; 19: 163,164.

10. Seltzer MA, Low RK, McDonald M, Shami GS, Stoller ML. Dietary manipulation with lemonade to treat hypocitraturic calcium nephrolithiasis. J Urol 1996; 156: 907–909.

11. Riches E. The history of lithotomy and lithotrity. Ann R Coll Surg Engl 1968; 43: 185–199.

12. Rosner F. Earlier therapies for urinary stones. JAMA 1986; 256: 1294.

13. Tiselius HG. A few comments on the recipes against kidney stones in the Croatian prayerbook. Scand J Urol Nephrol 1998; 32: 250.

14. Bloom DA. Hippocrates and urology: the first surgical subspecialty. Urology 1997; 50: 157–159.

15. Cule J. Catheters: forerunners of Foley. Nurs Mirror 1980; 150: Suppl i–vi.

16. Thomas GJ. Urological instruments. In: History of Urology, vol. 2., (E. G. Ballenger, ed.), Williams and Wilkins, Baltimore, MD, 1933.

17. Bloom DA, McGuire EJ, Lapides J. A brief history of urethral catheterization. J Urol 1994; 151: 317.

18. Nacey J, Delahunt B. The evolution and development of the urinary catheter. Aust N Z J Surg 1993; 63: 815–819.

19. Cockett AT, Cockett WS. Case against the catheter: Emile Coude. Urology 1978; 12: 619–620.

20. Murphy LJ. The History of Urology. Charles C. Thomas, Springfield, OH, 1972.

21. Zorgniotti AW. Frederic E. B. Foley. Early development of balloon catheter. Urology 1973; 1: 75.

22. Tucker RA. History of sizing of genitourinary instruments. Urology 1982; 20: 346–349.

23. Gentile DP. "Urethrolithotomy": an ingenious approach of the ancients. J Urol 1984; 132: 359, 360.

24. Wangensteen OH, Wangensteen SD, Wiita J. Lithotomy and lithotomists: progress in wound management from Franco to Lister. Surgery 1969; 66: 929–952.

25. Backhouse N. Trial and error in the development of urology. Nurs Mirr 1974; 139: 63.

26. Bacic J. A urological operation in 1365. Br J Urol 1998; 82: 86–89.

27. Ellis H. A history of bladder stone. J R Soc Med 1979; 72: 248–251.

28. Murphy LJ. Self-performed operations for stone in the bladder. Br J Urol 1969; 41: 515–529.

29. Shah J, Whitfield HN. Urolithiasis through the ages. BJU Int 2002; 89: 801–810.

30. Herman JR. Urethral specula. Urology 1977; 9: 345H.

31. Bush RB, Leonhardt H, Bush IV, Landes RR. Dr. Bozzini's Lichtleiter. A translation of his original article (1806). Urology 1974; 3: 119–123.

32. Reuter MA, Reuter HJ. The development of the cystoscope. J Urol 1998; 159: 638–640.

33. Shah J. Endoscopy through the ages. BJU Int 2002; 89: 645.

34. Hisrschowitz BI. A personal history of the fiberscope. Gastroenterology 1979; 76: 864.

35. Marshall VF. Fiber optics in urology. J Urol 1964; 91: 110–114.

36. Viseltear AJ. Attempts to dissolve bladder stones by direct injection. Bull Hist Med 1969; 43: 477–481.

37. Viseltear AJ. Joanna Stephens and the eighteenth century lithontriptics; a misplaced chapter in the history of therapeutics. Bull Hist Med 1968; 42: 199–220.

38. Swick M. Radiographic media in urology. The discovery of excretion urography: historical and developmental aspects of the organically bound urographic media and their role in the varied diagnostic angiographic areas. Surg Clin North Am 1978; 58: 977–994.

39. Loughlin KR, Hawtrey CE. Moses Swick, the father of intravenous urography. Urology 2003; 62: 385–389.

40. Sagel SS, Stanley RJ, Levitt RG, Geisse G.: Computed tomography of the kidney. Radiology 1977; 124: 359.

41. Young HH: Hugh Young A Surgeon's Autobiography. Harcourt Brace, New York, NY, 1940.

42. Young HH, McKay RW. Congenital valvular obstruction of the prostatic urethra. Surg Gynecol Obstet 1929; 48: 509.

43. Goodman TM. Ureteroscopy with pediatric cystoscope in adults. Urology 1977; 9: 394.

44. Lyon ES, Kyker JS, Schoenberg HW. Transurethral ureteroscopy in women: a ready addition to the urological armamentarium. 1978. J Urol 2002; 167: 859,860; discussion 861.

45. Lyon ES, Banno JJ, Schoenberg HW. Transurethral ureteroscopy in men using juvenile cystoscopy equipment. J Urol 1979; 122: 152, 153.
46. Conlin MJ, Marberger M, Bagley DH. Ureteroscopy. Development and instrumentation. Urol Clin North Am 1997; 24: 25–42.
47. Takagi T, Go T, Takayasu H, Aso Y, Hioki R. A small caliber fiberscope for visualization of the urinary tract, biliary tract and spinal canal. Surgery 1968; 64: 1033.
48. Takagi T, Go T, Takayasu H, Aso Y. Fiberoptic pyeloureteroscope. Surgery 1971; 70: 661.
49. Delius M, Brendel W. Historical roots of lithotripsy. J Lithotr Stone Dis 1990; 2: 161–163.
50. Raney AM. Electrohydraulic ureterolithotripsy. Urology 1978; 12: 284.
51. Mulvaney W. Attempted disintegration of calculi by ultrasound. J Urol 1953; 70: 704.
52. Mulvaney WP, Beck CW. The laser beam in urology. J Urol 1968; 99: 112.
53. Grocela JA, Dretler SP. Intracorporeal lithotripsy. Instrumentation and development. Urol Clin North Am 1997; 24: 13–23.
54. Newman J. Advances in lithotripsy and stone disease treatment. Radiol Technol 1996; 67: 479.
55. Lingeman JE. Extracorporeal shock wave lithotripsy: development, instrumentation and current status. Urol Clin North Am 1997; 24: 185.
56. Chaussy C, Brendel W, Schmiedt E.: Extracorporeal induced destruction of kidney stones by shock waves. Lancet 1980; II: 1265.
57. Chaussy C, Schmiedt E, Jocham D, Brendel W, Forssmann B, Walther V. First clinical experience with extracorporeally induced destruction of kidney stones by shock waves. 1981. J Urol 2002; 167: 844–847; discussion 848.
58. Dretler SP. Extra-corporeal shockwave lithotripsy. In: Stone Disease: Diagnosis and Management. (S. N. Rous, ed.), Grune and Stratton, Orlando, FL, 1987, p. 289.
59. Goodwin WE, Casey WC, Woolf W. Percutaneous trocar (needle) nephrostomy in hydronephrosis. JAMA 1955; 157: 891.
60. Kinn AC, Fernstrom I, Johansson B, Ohlsen H.: Percutaneous nephrolithotomy—the birth of a new technique. Scand J Urol Nephrol Suppl 1991; 138: 11–14.
61. Castaneda-Zuniga WR, Clayman R, Smith A, Rusnak B, Herrera M, Amplatz K. Nephrostolithotomy: percutaneous techniques for urinary calculus removal. 1982. J Urol 2002; 167: 849–853; discussion 854.
62. Korth KH, Hohenfellner R, Altwein JE: Ultrasound litholapaxy of a staghorn calculus. J Urol 1977, 117: 242.
63. Litynski GS, Paolucci V. Origin of laparoscopy: coincidence or surgical interdisciplinary thought? World J Surg 1998; 22: 899–902.
64. Litynski GS. Endoscopic surgery: the history, the pioneers. World J Surg 1999; 23: 745–753.
65. Clayman R, Kavoussi LR, Soper NJ, et al. Laparoscopic nephrectomy. N Engl J Med 1991; 324: 1371.
66. Wickham JE. The surgical treatment of renal lithiasis. In: Urinary Calculus Disease. (J. E. Wickham, ed.), Chruchill Livingstone, New York, NY, 1979, pp. 145–198.

2 Epidemiology and Incidence of Stone Disease

Joseph E. Dallera, MD
and Paramjit S. Chandhoke, MD, PhD

CONTENTS

TYPES OF STONES
INCIDENCE, PREVALENCE, AND LIFETIME PREVALENCE
AGE, SEX, AND RACE
RISK FACTORS FOR STONE DISEASE
PEDIATRIC STONE DISEASE
PREGANCY
STONE DISEASE IN PATIENTS WITH SPINAL CORD INJURY
RECURRENCE FOLLOWING SWL
REFERENCES

Key Words: Epidemiology; nephrolithiasis; incidence.

TYPES OF STONES

Urinary stones are polycrystalline aggregates consisting of varying amounts of crystal and organic matrix components. Although urolithiasis is inclusive of renal, ureteral, and bladder stones, the following discussion will pertain only to symptomatic renal and ureteral stones, as they are the most common. The most common urinary stone types are calcium oxalate, calcium phosphate, uric acid, struvite (magnesium ammonium phosphate), and cystine. In an analysis of 14,557 renal and ureteral stones, 52% were purely calcium oxalate, 13% purely calcium phosphate, 15% a mixture of calcium oxalate and phosphate, 4% struvite, 8% uric acid, and 8% other compounds *(1)*. As the majority of stones are of the calcium variety, it is likely that most epidemiological studies of nephrolithiasis pertain to this compositional form. Of the less common stone varieties, struvite stones are commonly associated with urinary tract infections, most notably secondary to urease splitting organisms such as *Proteus* and *Klebsiella*. Uric acid stones, associated with hyperuricosuric patients, are found in patients with gout, dehydration, and exces-

From: Current Clinical Urology, *Urinary Stone Disease:*
A Practical Guide to Medical and Surgical Management
Edited by: M. L. Stoller and M. V. Meng © Humana Press Inc., Totowa, NJ

sive purine intake. Finally, cystine stones are a rare form associated with inborn errors of metabolism resulting in abnormal absorption of dibasic amino acids in the small bowel and proximal renal tubule.

A more recent variety of urolithiasis is found secondary to treatment with indavir, a protease inhibitor used as a primary treatment for the human immunodeficiency virus *(2)*. Indavir was approved by the Federal Drug Administration in 1996 and is formulated as a sulfate salt. It has been reported that as much as 20% of the drug is excreted unchanged in the urine *(3)*. Compositional analysis of indavir stones often reveal pure Indavir, but may also include other constituents such as calcium oxalate. The significance of this compositional variance, in contrast to all other stone types, is that pure indavir stones may not be visible on noncontrast computed tomography scans *(4)*. In a recent study of 105 patients undergoing treatment with indavir for 1 yr, a stone incidence of 12% with a median duration of time from treatment to acute stone episode of 22 wk was reported *(4)*.

INCIDENCE, PREVALENCE, AND LIFETIME PREVALENCE

It is important to define the terms incidence, prevalence, and lifetime prevalence of stone disease to ensure proper comparisons between epidemiological studies. The *incidence* of stone disease is defined as the number of new stone patients in a given population over a defined period of time (usually a year). *Prevalence* is defined as the number of stones present in a screened population at a particular point in time. Finally, *lifetime prevalence* is defined as the presence of a stone at any point in a patient's history. Therefore, surveys that ask if a person has "ever had a kidney stone" imply a lifetime prevalence of urolithiasis.

In a 25-yr study of the incidence of stone disease from 1950 to 1974 among the population in Rochester, MN, the overall rate for males was 109.5 per 100,000 and the rate for females was 36.0 per 100,000 *(5)*. In a more recent prospective study by Curhan et al., the incidence of stone disease was found to be 300 per 100,000 in males and 100 per 100,000 in females *(6,7)*. This suggests a possible increase in the incidence of stone disease over the last three decades. In an Italian study conducted between 1993 and 1994, the incidence was calculated at 168 per 100,000 inhabitants *(8)*. Finally, a Japanese study determined the incidence of stone disease in 1995 to be 100.1 per 100,000 for males and 55.4 per 100,000 for females *(9)*. In comparison to a similar study conducted in 1965 (81.3 per 100,000 for males and 29.5 per 100,000 for females), Yoshida et al. concluded that there was a steady increase in the annual incidence of stone disease in Japan over a 30-yr period *(9)*.

Estimates of lifetime prevalence have been determined by several studies in the United States. In a study by Soucie et al., the lifetime prevalence of stone disease was found to be 10% for men and 4% for women *(10)*. Similarly, a study by Curhan et al. found a lifetime prevalence of 8.7% in men *(6)*. However, in considering lifetime prevalence of stone disease, it is necessary to discuss variations based on gender, race, geography, and diet. These factors will be discussed subsequently.

AGE, SEX, AND RACE DEPENDENCE

Symptomatic calcium stone disease is most common from the third to sixth decades of life. However, variations are evident depending on gender and stone type. In a 25-yr study of the population of Rochester, MN, the incidence of stone disease in men increased significantly after the age of 35, most notably between the ages of 50 and 70.

In women the rate remained relatively constant over the entire 25-yr period *(5)*. Therefore, the overall male to female ratio of the incidence of stone disease increased from 1.8:1 to 3.8:1 over the entire study period. With respect to age, men and women have a similar incidence of stone disease during early life (second and third decades) and late life (seventh decade and older) *(11)*. However, between the third and seventh decades of life, men have an incidence of symptomatic stones two to five times that of women. It should be noted that these figures pertain to symptomatic kidney and ureteral stones as the prevalence and age frequency of asymptomatic stones is unknown. It is possible that the incidence of asymptomatic stone disease is similar between men and women *(12)*.

Epidemiological studies of the lifetime prevalence of stone disease have been conducted primarily within the Caucasian population. Several studies among the African American, Hispanic, and Asian populations, however, suggest the male predominance of stone disease may not be maintained outside of the Caucasian population. In a study of 444 patients with stone disease in 1994, women made up 68% and 62% of the African American and Hispanic stone populations, respectively *(13)*. Another racial comparison study revealed that African American men have a 0.4, Hispanic men a 0.66, and Asian men a 0.56 lifetime prevalence of stone disease relative to Caucasian men *(10)*. In comparison to Caucasian women, African American women were found to have a 0.61, Hispanic women a 0.85, and Asian women a 0.54 relative lifetime prevalence of stone disease *(10)*.

RISK FACTORS FOR STONE DISEASE

Climate and Geography

Many epidemiological studies have recorded a geographic variability in the prevalence of stone disease. It has been postulated that this variability may be owing to variations in climate and sun exposure, although others have questioned the role of diet and water quality as well. The most convincing evidence to date, however, reveals temperature and sun exposure to play important roles in the geographic variability of stone disease. It is believed that individuals living in hot climates have an increased lifetime prevalence of stone disease secondary to dehydration. Further, individuals living in areas with increased sun exposure are likely to have absorptive hypercalciuria secondary to elevated vitamin D synthesis. In a 1994 study by Soucie et al., the lifetime prevalence of stone disease increased in the United States from north to south and west to east *(10)*. Further, it was determined in a later study that correction for ambient temperature, sunlight, and consumption of several beverages eliminated the geographic variation in lifetime prevalence of stone disease *(14)*. In contrast, a recent study of 1179 postmenopausal women with stone disease found no association between temperature and stone disease *(15)*. Therefore, other factors likely play an important role in the geographic variability of stone disease and must be considered.

Similar to geographical location, a person's occupation may influence their risk for nephrolithiasis. As warm climates seem to predispose to stone formation, so do occupations involved with warm working environments. However, the situation of occupation is independent of the effects of sun exposure and vitamin D synthesis. Epidemiological studies have shown an increased risk of stone disease in cooks and machinists. A 1993 study of machinists working in a hot environment revealed a prevalence of 8.5% compared with age- and sex-matched controls working in a normal temperature, which had a prevalence of 2.4% *(16)*. Not surprisingly, uric acid stones were the most common stone type found in the machinists. However, it is unknown if the mechanism for increased urinary excretion of uric acid is secondary to hypercatabolism resulting from heat stress or a state of chronic dehydration.

Diet

Diet has long been suspected to affect the incidence of stone disease. Specific dietary factors, which have been shown to have a role in stone disease, include animal protein, supplemental calcium, sodium, oxalate, and fruit juices. Excessive animal protein intake has been shown to lead to an increase in urinary excretion of calcium and uric acid, and a decrease in urinary citrate. Additionally, a recent study suggests that a diet rich in animal protein leads to an increase in urinary oxalate excretion in recurrent idiopathic calcium stone formers (17). In contrast to this view that excessive animal protein intake leads to an increased incidence of stone disease, a 1996 prospective study showed a low protein diet group to have a risk of stone formation 5.6 times higher than the control group (18).

Studies investigating the role of calcium intake and stone formation differentiate dietary calcium intake from supplemental calcium, used most commonly by women (19). In contrast to traditional belief, recent studies have shown an inverse relationship between dietary calcium intake and the incidence of stone disease (20). However, there also seems to be a direct relationship between the use of supplemental calcium in women and the incidence of urolithiasis (21). These studies hypothesize that dietary calcium binds to dietary oxalate and reduces the intestinal absorption of oxalate, thus reducing the risk for calcium oxalate stone formation. Based on this hypothesis, women are advised to take supplemental calcium only with meals. Although these epidemiological studies provide convincing evidence regarding dietary calcium and the incidence of urolithiasis, they are largely based in individuals with no previous history of kidney stones.

Other epidemiological studies implicate sodium and certain fruit juices with an increase in the incidence of nephrolithiasis. Increased sodium intake has been linked to increased urinary calcium excretion, and thus to increased calcium stone formation. Increases in sodium intake of 100 mmol may produce an increase in urinary calcium of 1 mmol (22).

In a recent randomized clinical trial conducted in recurrent stone formers, Borghi et al. compared the recurrence of stone disease in patients either on a low calcium diet (400 mg/d) or a diet low in protein and sodium but with a normal calcium intake (23). Although no differences were noted in stone recurrence at 3 yr between these two groups, patients on a low calcium diet had twice the stone recurrence rate at 5 yr compared with patients on a normal calcium, low protein, and low sodium diet (23).

Family History

A positive family history of urolithiasis is associated with an increased risk of urinary stone disease. Epidemiological studies have shown a familial component to the incidence of stone disease that is independent of dietary and environmental factors. It has been reported that the relative risk of stone formation in men with a positive family history was 2.57 compared with those with a negative family history (24). Further, patients with a positive family history also have a higher risk for stone recurrence. Studies that have attempted to identify the genetic component of familial nephrolithiasis suggest that the responsible genes affect calcium, oxalate, and citrate transport within the intestine and kidney (25). Recent work has also suggested the possibility of allelic variations in the vitamin D receptor, which may be responsible for familial cases of stone disease *(26)*. However, further investigation is necessary to positively identify the specific genetic components responsible for the observed familial inheritance of nephrolithiasis.

Hypertension

Many epidemiological studies have reported an increase in the incidence of urolithiasis in patients with hypertension. Similarly, the rate of hypertension among known stone formers is higher than the general population. In a study of 132 patients with stable hypertension and 135 normotensive patients, all free of stone disease, 14.3% of the hypertensives and 2.9% of the normotensives developed stone disease within 7 yr *(27)*. Hypertensives were 5.5 times more likely to develop urolithiasis compared with the normotensive study population. Although the majority of hypertensive stone formers were also overweight (body mass index >26), the levels of urinary oxalate remained significantly elevated in the hypertensive group after controlling for body mass index. The pathophysiological mechanisms responsible for this link between hypertension and urolithiasis are unknown.

PEDIATRIC STONE DISEASE

Urolithiasis in the pediatric population is relatively rare in the United States, although it remains a significant health issue in certain parts of the world. The incidence in the USA has been reported as 1 per 1000 to 1 per 7600 hospital admissions, varying with the geographic "stone belt" as observed in adults *(28)*. In the UK and Europe, the etiology of pediatric urolithiasis has been shown to be urinary tract infection in 30–90% of cases, whereas metabolic disturbances are the most common cause in the United States. Infectious stones represent 24% of pediatric urolithiasis in the USA *(28)*.

In contrast to adult stone disease, the pediatric population shows only a slight male preponderance of stone disease, with some studies showing an equal incidence between boys and girls. In several epidemiological studies analyzing race and pediatric stone disease, it was noted that approx 10% of children with stone disease are African American and approx 80% are Caucasian *(28)*.

Similar to the adult population, the most common metabolic etiology of pediatric stone disease is hypercalciuria. Further, a positive family history of stone disease has been reported in 52% of children with idiopathic hypercalciuria. Other studies have found abnormalities in urinary citrate and oxalate concentrations in children with urolithiasis. In a study of 78 children between 1 and 15 yr of age with calcium stones, hypocitraturia was 4.3 times more common than in healthy controls *(29)*.

Increased urinary calcium excretion is also seen in children with primary hyperparathyroidism, sarcoidosis, distal renal tubular acidosis, immobilization, and vitamin D excess, thus predisposing to calcium stone disease. Other associated risk factors for urolithiasis in children include prematurity and the use of furosemide in the neonatal period.

PREGNANCY

Physiological changes during pregnancy include an increase in glomerular filtration rate, which leads to increased urinary concentrations of calcium, sodium, and uric acid. Despite this effect of pregnancy, epidemiological studies have shown the incidence of urinary stone disease during pregnancy to be the same as that in the nonpregnant popu-lation. Urolithiasis has been shown to affect from 1 in 1240 to 1 in 3300 pregnancies (30,31). Further, in a study of women with a known history of urolithiasis, whom sub-sequently became pregnant, there was no change in the rate of symptomatic stone disease (31). Although multiparous women are affected more commonly than primiparae, the incidence becomes similar when adjusted for age.

Approximately 80% of pregnant women with stone disease present during the second and third trimesters. In a study of 57 pregnant women with stone disease, 20% presented in the first trimester, 40% presented in the second trimester, and 40% presented in the third trimester (31). The mean gestational age at presentation was 23 wk. Similar to the nonpregnant population, the most common presenting chief complaint in the gravid patient is flank pain. Abdominal pain, nausea, vomiting, and hematuria are less common presenting symptoms. Rarely, pregnant women with stone disease may present in preterm labor. In the study of 57 pregnant women with urolithiasis, 84% presented with flank pain, 23% presented with low abdominal pain, and 23% presented with gross hematuria (31).

STONE DISEASE IN PATIENTS WITH SPINAL CORD INJURY

Urolithiasis is a common complication in patients with a spinal cord injury (SCI), and is thought to be secondary to a neurogenic bladder, immobilization, and subsequent urinary tract infections. Evidence for this includes the finding that greater than 90% of stones in patients with SCI are struvite stones. However, the percentage of struvite stones increases with time from injury, suggesting that urinary tract infections play an increas-ingly important role in stone formation in later years. The incidence of first time stone disease in spinal cord patients has been reported as 7% within 10 yr of injury. In a cohort study of 8314 patients with SCI, the incidence of stone disease was 31 per 1000 person-years in the first 3 mo, 8 per 1000 person-years after the first year, and less than 4 per 1000 person-years after the eighth year (32). This decreasing trend in the risk for stone disease following spinal cord injury has also been reported in other epidemiological studies. Therefore, it appears that the greatest risk for urolithiasis following spinal cord injury is within the first year after injury.

Other factors that affect the incidence of stone disease include race, gender, age, geography, and the extent of the cord lesion. In the cohort study of 8314 SCI patients, the 5-yr incidence was 6% for Caucasians, 2% for Hispanics, and 3% for African Ameri-cans (33). Further, patients older than 55 yr at time of injury had a twofold increased risk for stone formation within the first year when compared with patients 25–34 yr old. An increased risk has also been associated with decreasing latitude and increasing annual temperature (33).

RECURRENCE FOLLOWING SHOCKWAVE LITHOTRIPSY

It is unknown if microscopic residual stone debris following shockwave lithotripsy (SWL) predisposes to recurrence of stone disease. The incidence of stone recurrence in patients who are radiographically stone free following SWL is reported as 6–22% during the first year of follow-up and 28–35% after 2 yr of follow-up (34–36). In contrast, the reported incidence of stone recurrence following percutaneous nephrolithotomy is 4.2% after 1 yr and 22.6% after 2 yr of follow-up. The incidence of stone recurrence following SWL is dependent on whether or not medical management is instituted following treatment. It has been reported that the recurrence rate is 0.09 stones/patient/year in patients undergoing medical treatment and 0.67 stones/patient/year in those not undergoing medical treatment *(37)*. Several epidemiological studies have attempted to identify risk factors for recurrence following SWL. Although male gender and history of multiple stones have been implicated as risk factors for recurrence following SWL, further study is necessary to identify other important risk factors.

REFERENCES

1. Gault MH, Chafe L. Relationship of frequency, age, sex, stone weight and composition in 15,624 Stones: comparisons of results for 1980–1983 and 1995–1998. J Urol 2000; 164: 302–307.
2. Reiter WJ, Schon-Pernerstorfer H, Dorfinger K, Hofbauer J, Marberger M. Frequency of urolithiasis in individuals seropositive for human immunodeficiency virus treated with indinavir is higher than previously assumed. J Urol 1999; 161: 1082–1084.
3. Indavir Sulfate (Crixivan) package insert. Merck and Co., West Point, Pennsylvania, PA 1996.
4. Wu DS, Stoller ML. Indinavir urolithiasis. Current Opinion Urol 2000; 10: 557–561.
5. Johnson CM, Wilson DM, O'Fallon WM, Malek RS, Kurland LT. Renal stone epidemiology: a 25-year study in Rochester, Minnesota. Kid Int 1979; 16: 624–631.
6. Curhan GC, Rimm EB, Willet WC, Stampfer MJ. Regional variation in nephrolithiasis incidence and prevalence among United States men. J Urol 1994; 151: 838–841.
7. Curhan GC, Curhan SG. Diet and urinary stone disease. Current Op Urol 1997; 7: 222.
8. Serio A, Fraioli A. Epidemiology of nephrolithiasis. Nephron 1999; 81S: 26–30.
9. Yoshida O, Terai A, Ohkawa T, Okada Y. National trend of the incidence of urolithiasis in Japan from 1965–1995. Kid Int 1999; 56: 1899–1904.
10. Soucie JM, Thun MJ, Coates RJ, McClellan W, Austin H. Demographic and geographic variability of kidney stones in the United States. Kid Int 1994; 46: 893–899.
11. Gault MH, Chafe L. Relationship of frequency, age, sex, stone weight and composition in 15,624 stones: comparisons of results for 1980–1983 and 1995–1998. J Urol 2000; 164: 302–307.
12. Curhan GC, Willett WC, Peizer FE, Stampfer MJ. Twenty-four hour urine chemistries and the risk of kidney stones among women and men. Kid Int 2001; 59: 2290–2298.
13. Michaels EK, Nakagawa Y, Miura N, Pursell S, Ito H. Racial variation in gender frequency of calcium urolithiasis. J Urol 1994; 152: 2228–2231.
14. Soucie JM, Coates RJ, McClellan W, Austin H, Thun M. Relation between geographic variability in kidney stones prevalence and risk factors for stones. Am J Epi 1996;143(5): 487–495.
15. Hall WD, Pettinger M, Oberman A, et al. Risk factors for kidney stones in older women in the Southern United States. Am J Med Sci 2001; 322(1): 12–18.
16. Borghi L, Meschi T, Amato F, Novarini A, Romanelli A, Cigala F. Hot occupation and nephrolithiasis. J of Urol 1993; 50: 1757–1760.
17. Nguyen QV, Kalin A, Drouve U, Casez JP, Jaeger P. Sensitivity to meat protein intake and hyperoxaluria in idiopathic calcium stone formers. Kid Int 2001; 59(6): 2273–81.
18. Hiatt RA, Ettinger B, Caan B, Quessenberry CP, Duncan D, Citron J. Randomized control trial of a low animal protein, high fiber diet in the prevention of recurrent calcium oxalate kidney stones. Am J Epidemiol 1996; 144: 25.
19. Sowers MR, Jannausch M, Wood C, Pope SK, Lachance LL, Peterson B. Prevalence of renal stones in a population-based study with dietary calcium, oxalate, and medication exposures. Am J Epi 1998; 147(10): 914–920.
20. Curhan GC, Willet WC, Rimm EB, Stampher MJ. A prospective study of dietary calcium and other nutrients and the risk of symptomatic kidney stones. N Eng J Med 1993; 328: 833.
21. Curhan GC, Curhan SG. Diet and urinary stone disease. Current Op Urol 1997; 7: 222.
22. Cappuccio FP, Kalaitzidis R, Duneclift S, Eastwood JB. Unraveling the links between calcium excretion, salt intake, hypertension, kidney stones, and bone metabolism. J Neprhol 2000; 13: 3, 169–177.
23. Borghi L, Schiani T, Meschi T, et al. Comparison of two diets for the prevention of recurrent stones in idiopathic hypercalciuria. N Eng J Med 2002; 346: 77–84.

24. Curhan GC, Willett WC, Rimm EB, Stampfer MJ. Family history and risk of kidney stones. J Am Soc Nephrol 1997; 8: 10, 1568–1573.

25. Goodman HO, Brommage R, Assimos DG, Holmes RP. Genes in idiopathic calcium oxalate stone disease. World J Urol 1997; 15: 3, 186–194.

26. Jackman SV, Kibel AS, Ovuworie CA, Moore RG, Kavoussi LR, Jarrett TW. Familial calcium stone disease: Taq1 polymorphism and the vitamin D receptor. J Endourology 1999; 13: 4, 313–316.

27. Borghi L, Meschi T, Guerra A, et al. A. Essential hypertension and stone disease. Kid Int 1999; 55: 2397–2406.

28. Santos-Vistoriano M, Brouchard BH, Cunningham III, RJ. Renal stone disease in children. Clin Ped 1998; 37: 583–600.

29. Tekin A, Tekgul S, Atsu N, Sahin A, Ozen H, Bakkaloglu M. A study of the etiology of idiopathic calcium urolithiasis in children: hypocitruria is the most important risk factor. J Urol 2000; 164: 162–165.

30. Swanson SK, Heilman RL, Eversman WG. Urinary tract stones in pregnancy. Surg Clin N Amer 1995; 75(1): 123–142.

31. Butler EL, Cox SM, Eberts EG, Cunningham FG. Symptomatic nephrolithiasis complicating pregnancy. Ob Gyn 2000; 96(5): 753–756.

32. Chen YY, Roseman JM, DeVivo MJ, Huang CT. Geographic variation and environmental risk factors for the incidence of initial kidney stones in patients with spinal cord injury. J Urol. 2000; 164: 21–26.

33. Chen Y, DeVivo MJ, Roseman JM. Current trend and risk factors for kidney stones in persons with spinal cord injury: a longitudinal study. Spinal Cord 2000; 38: 346–353.

34. Sun BY-C, Lee YH, Jiaan, BP, Chen KK, Chang LS, Chen KT. Recurrence rate and risk factors for urinary calculi after extracorporeal shock wavy lithotripsy. J Urol 1996; 156: 903.

35. Kamihira O, Ono Y, Katoh N, Yamada S, Mizutani K, Ohshima S. Long-term stone recurrence rate after extracorporeal shock wave lithotripsy. J Urol 1996; 156: 1267–1271.

36. Carr LK, Honey RJD, Jewett MAS, Ibanez D, Ryan M, Bombardier C. New stone formation: a comparison of extracorporeal shock wave lithotripsy and percutaneous nephrolithotomy. J Urol 1996; 155: 1565–1567.

37. Fine JK, Pak CYC, Preminger GM. Effect of medical management and residual fragments on recurrent stone formation following shockwave lithotripsy. J Urol 1995; 153: 27–33.

3 The Genetics of Stone Disease

Berenice Y. Reed, PhD and William L. Gitomer, PhD

CONTENTS

Key Words: Nephrolithiasis; genetics; molecular biology; gene.

INTRODUCTION

The lifetime risk of stone formation is estimated at 5–10%; hence, stone disease represents one of the most frequent causes of hospitalization in the United States *(1)*. Various intrinsic and extrinsic factors are associated with risk for stone formation. Among intrinsic factors are race, sex, and genetics *(2,3)*. Over the past decade significant advances have occurred in our understanding of the underlying genetic lesions that are associated with many forms of stone disease. However, it is interesting to note that most advances in the identification of genetic defects have been made in the rarer forms of stone disease. Progress toward understanding the genetic contribution in the more common forms of calcium oxalate stone disease has been impeded by the fact that many forms of this disease are complex, associated with phenotypic variability, and further compounded by multifactorial inheritance. A recent review of the literature indicates that 27 individual chromosomal loci have been associated with various forms of urolithiasis *(4)*. All modes of inheritance are represented among the various genetic stone diseases.

Varied approaches have been applied for studying stone diseases. A distinct phenotype associated with a specific enzyme defect permits direct search for and analysis of the associated gene. A deficiency of the hepatic peroxisomal enzyme, alanine glyoxalate

From: Current Clinical Urology, *Urinary Stone Disease:*
A Practical Guide to Medical and Surgical Management
Edited by: M. L. Stoller and M. V. Meng © Humana Press Inc., Totowa, NJ

Table 1
Frequency and Classification of Various Renal
Stones Associated With Genetic Disorders

Stone classification	%
Calcium (oxalate or phosphate)	91
Uric Acid	7
Cystine	1
Other	<1

aminotransferase (AGT) leads to identification of mutations in the corresponding gene (*AGXT*) in primary hyperoxaluria type 1 *(5)*. In instances where no candidate gene is indicated, a positional cloning approach has also been successful. In three families with familial absorptive hypercalciuria (AH) the defect was mapped to chromosome 1q23-24 by linkage analysis *(6)*. Sequence analysis of genes within the linkage interval lead to identification of several AH-associated base substitutions in a gene encoding an adenylate cyclase homologous to the rat testis bicarbonate-sensitive adenylate cyclase *(7)*. Identification of a specific defect in other diseases has involved a combination of both candidate gene and positional cloning methods. This strategy permitted identification of mutations in the dibasic amino acid transporter SLC3A1 in cystinuria *(8,9)*. The following discussion of gene defects associated with stone diseases will be grouped according to the composition of stones. By this classification calcium-containing stones are the most common, accounting for 90% of all analyzed stones (Table 1).

CALCIUM CONTAINING STONES

Hypercalciuria

Hypercalciuria is the most common finding in patients with stone disease *(10)*. Classification of hypercalciuria according to the primary organ affected leads to the description of three major types: *absorptive*, related to intestinal hyperabsorption of calcium; *resorptive*, owing to increased bone resorption associated with primary hyperparathyroidism; and *renal*, associated with renal leak of calcium *(11)*. The complexity of the underlying physiological defects, which may affect kidney, intestine, and bone, has complicated the search for gene defects linked with this disorder. However, in spite of this complexity, a number of gene defects have been discovered that result in hypercalciuria.

Absorptive Hypercalciuria

This condition, previously referred to as idiopathic hypercalciuria, results from intestinal hyperabsorption of calcium. This increases the renal calcium load resulting in hypercalciuria and formation of stones predominantly composed of calcium oxalate or mixed calcium oxalate and calcium phosphate *(10)*. The disorder is heterogeneous *(12,13)* and stone formation multifactorial, leading to difficulty in identification of a specific genetic lesion in this disorder. An autosomal dominant pattern of inheritance has been demonstrated in the familial form of this disorder *(14,15)* following analysis of large kindreds. Adoption of a candidate gene approach has been of limited success.

Several studies have focused on the vitamin D receptor (VDR) gene as a candidate for the gene defect in this disorder although with different conclusions. In a rat model for AH, increased VDR numbers have been demonstrated in bone, intestine, and kidney *(16,17)*. However, conflicting results have emerged from human investigations. Although an increased number of vitamin D receptors have been demonstrated on peripheral blood lymphocytes of some patients with AH *(18)*, no abnormality of the VDR gene nor link between VDR alleles frequency and the AH phenotype was demonstrated for these patients *(19,20)*. Linkage analysis of the chromosome 12 map region associated with the VDR and 1, α-hydroxylase genes in three families demonstrated no linkage between these genes and the AH phenotype *(21)*. However, other studies have shown an association between the *Fok I* polymorphism of the VDR and calcium oxalate stone disease *(22)*, whereas the *TaqI* allele of the VDR was recently shown to be a risk factor for severe stone disease and recurrent stone formation by Nishijima *(23)*. Other investigations have also demonstrated an association between the aggressiveness of calcium stone disease in hypercalciuric subjects and polymorphisms of the VDR *(24,25)*.

In a study of 47 French-Canadian pedigrees with idiopathic hypercalciuria, Scott et al. identified a susceptibility locus near the VDR gene *(26)*. Other studies from the same group have evaluated and eliminated the calcium-sensing receptor gene and the *CYP1a* (1,α-hydroxylase) genes as candidates in calcium stone forming patients *(27,28)*. Study of patients with severe chromosomal abnormalities can frequently indicate an association between symptoms and genes located within the aberrant chromosomal region. Imamura et al. studied two nonrelated Japanese girls with an unbalanced translocation and deletion of 4q33-qter *(29)*. Both girls had an exaggerated calciuric response to an oral calcium load and sporadic hypercalciuria, one with stone formation. Based on the presentation, these researchers concluded that the AH locus mapped within the 4q33-qter region.

We have previously mapped one susceptibility gene for AH to chromosome 1q24 *(6)*. A linkage study performed on three families with a severe form of AH revealed one locus associated with the AH phenotype of hypercalciuria and intestinal calcium hyperabsorption located at chromosome 1q 23-24. Subsequent analyses of genes from this region led to the identification of base substitutions in a new gene related to AH. The new gene was named the *AH* related adenylate cyclase gene *(AHRAC)(7)*. This gene was shown to be homologous with a rat gene encoding a bicarbonate sensitive adenylate cyclase described by Buck et al. *(30)*. The human gene, made up of 33 exons, encodes a protein of 1610 amino acids containing two adenylate cyclase catalytic domains *(7)*. The gene is ubiquitously expressed within tissues, including the three tissues associated with AH, namely, bone, intestine, and kidney. The frequency of occurrence of the base substitutions in the *AHRAC* gene was studied in 80 nonrelated AH patients and 132 healthy normal volunteers and it was demonstrated that six base substitutions occurred with significantly increased frequency in the AH population. The estimated risk for AH associated with any single base change was between 2- and 3.5-fold. Many patients had multiple base changes with corresponding increase in estimated risk of stone formation to 11.5-fold when five base changes were present within the gene (Table 2). There was also a strong correlation between sequence variation in the *AHRAC* gene and vertebral bone density among AH patients. Bone loss is a frequent complication of AH occurring in approx 30% of patients *(31)*.

Polymorphisms in several other genes have been associated with calcium oxalate stone formation. Interleukin-1 involvement has been implicated in bone mineral loss associated with idiopathic hypercalciuria *(32,33)*. Chen et al. reported an association

Table 2
Multiple Base Substitutions in Absorptive
Hypercalciuria Related Adenylate Cyclase (AHRAC)
Increases Estimated Risk for Absorptive Hypercalciuria

Number of base substitutions	Estimated risk[*]
3–4	4.0–4.5
5	11.5

[*]Estimated risk based on odds ratio.

between stone disease and polymorphism in the interleukin-1β receptor antagonist gene *(34)*. However, no significant differences were noted between the hypercalciuric and normocalciuric subsets of their stone forming patients. A second study from the same group examined a polymorphism located in the 3´-untranslated region of the urokinase gene in a group of stone formers and found an association between this polymorphism and a threefold increase in risk for calcium oxalate stone formation *(35)*. Another investigation suggested a polymorphism in the calcitonin receptor gene as a genetic marker for urinary stone disease based on an odds ratio of 5.6 *(36)*. Although the results relating to the genetics of hypercalciuric nephrolithiasis may appear incongruous, they may be explained based on the known heterogeneity of the disease *(12,13)*. The literature is further confounded by the use of the term "idiopathic hypercalciuria," which may encompass hypercalciuria of intestinal, renal, or bone origin.

X-Linked Nephrolithiasis (Dent's Disease)

X-linked nephrocalcinosis, also known as Dent's disease, is a renal tubular disorder characterized by low-molecular-weight proteinuria, hypercalciuria, nephrocalcinosis, nephrolithiasis, and eventual renal failure. Stones formed by patients are composed of calcium oxalate or calcium phosphate. Clinically the presentation of disease is variable, which lead to the description of three separate syndromes of X-linked nephrolithiasis, Dent's disease, hypophosphatemic rickets type III, and idiopathic low-molecular-weight proteinuria *(37–39)*. Inactivating mutations in the renal chloride channel gene *CLCN5* were identified in these syndromes *(40,41)*. The human gene was initially mapped by linkage analysis to chromosome Xp11.22 *(42–45)*. A microdeletion at Xp11.22 occurring in a patient with Dent's disease facilitated the cloning and identification of a gene encoding a new member of the voltage-gated chloride channels (CLC-5), which was deleted in patients with the microdeletion *(43)*. The human *CLCN5* gene comprising 12 exons spanning 30 Kb of DNA was mapped to chromosome Xp11.22 and shown to encode a 746 amino acid protein *(46,47)*. CLC-5 is expressed in proximal tubule and the intercalated cells of the cortical collecting duct *(48–51)* where it is colocalized with the brush border proton pump *(52)*. In the cell, CLC-5 has been localized to the subapical endosomes, where colocalization with the vacuolar H^+-ATPase has led to the suggestion of a role in counter-ion acidification of the endosomes *(52,53)*. An animal model for Dent's disease was created by Piwon et al. by targeted disruption of the *CLCN-5* gene *(54,55)*. These mice had impaired apical membrane vesicular endocytosis in the proximal tubule. Defective recycling of low-molecular-weight proteins is one consequence of impaired vesicular trafficking and explains the low-molecular-weight proteinuria in affected patients. However, hypercalciuria and stone formation have been suggested to arise from secondary effects of defective endocytic transport. Piwon postulated that decreased endocytosis of parathyroid hormone (PTH) results in increased stimulation of PTH receptors, with consequent stimulation of hydroxylation of 25-hydroxy vitamin D_3 to its active form *(54)*. An alternative postulate was suggested by Yu involving impaired internalization of the calcium channel (EcaC) *(56)*.

Renal Tubular Acidosis

Nephrocalcinosis/nephrolithiasis is most commonly associated with distal renal tubular acidosis (dRTA) type 1 where these symptoms occur in approximately two-thirds of patients *(57)*. In dRTA hydrogen-ion secretion is impaired in the distal nephron, leading to a metabolic acidosis and often hypokalemia. Stones formed are composed of calcium phosphate and result from a number of urinary abnormalities, including increased urinary calcium and phosphate excretion, high urinary pH, and decreased excretion of citrate *(58)*. In familial dRTA, affected children usually present with failure to thrive and growth retardation. Both autosomal dominant and recessive inheritance patterns occur with more severe phenotype and earlier onset associated with the recessive form of the disorder. The recessive form of dRTA is frequently accompanied by sensorineural hearing loss.

Bruce et al. first described mutations in the red cell Cl^-/HCO^3 anion exchanger (Band 3, AE1) gene in a study of four families with autosomal dominant dRTA *(59)*. The gene *(AE1)* is located on chromosome 17q21-22. The encoded protein is the major intrinsic membrane protein in the red cell. The protein is also expressed at high levels in the intercalated cell of the collecting duct in the kidney *(57)*. The renal transcript comprises 20 exons with transcription initiation in exon 3. The kidney protein lacks 65 amino acids present at the amino terminus of the red cell protein *(60)*. Several mutations in *AE1* have been described in the dominant form of dRTA *(59,61,62)*. Interestingly, these mutations appear to have little effect on anion transport in the red cell. Heterologous expression of mutated *AE1* in *Xenopus* oocytes caused approx 50% reduction in Cl^-/Cl^- or Cl^-/HCO^3- exchange as compared with wild type *(61,62)*. Although mutations occurring throughout *AE1* effect expression of the erythroid mRNA and result in hereditary spherocytosis, there appears to be little effect of these mutations on transport in the kidney. *AE1* mutations associated with dRTA appear to be limited to the regions of the gene coding for transmembrane domains and have little or no effect on red cell transport *(58)*. There appears to be a lack of correlation between genotype and phenotype both complete and incomplete (without metabolic acidosis) RTA being present within the same family *(63)*. *AE1* mutations have also been described in recessive dRTA within Asian populations *(64,65)*. Recessive and compound heterozygous mutations of *AE1* are not associated with anemia exhibiting either loss of function or diminished function associated with the kidney form of *AE1* alone *(58)*.

A gene linked to the recessive form of dRTA was mapped to chromosome 2p13 following genome-wide screening *(66)*. Subsequently, the B1 subunit of the VH⁺-ATPase was remapped to this linkage interval. The ATP6B1 gene *(ATP6B1)* contains 14 exons, which encode a 513 amino acid peptide. Karet identified 15 mutations distributed throughout the gene in 19 of 62 evaluated kindreds *(66)*. Linkage mapping in additional families with recessive dRTA but without hearing loss led to the identification of a further locus on chromosome 7q33-34 associated with recessive dRTA *(67)*. Eight mutations in a new gene *ATP6NB1*, which encodes a further subunit of the VH$^+$-ATPase were identified in affected kindreds *(68)*. Further mutations in both the *ATP6B1* and *ATP6NB1* genes have recently been reported *(69)*. In addition to elucidation of the specific gene defect associated with various forms of dRTA, molecular studies have also provided new insight into the mechanism of acid secretion in the kidney underlining the important synergism between molecular and cellular biology.

Hypophosphatemia

Renal phosphate leak resulting in hypophosphatemia leads to elevation of 1,25(OH)$_2$ vitamin D with consequences of increased intestinal calcium absorption, parathyroid suppression, and hypercalciuria. The type 2a sodium-phosphate cotransporter (NPT2a) is localized in the apical membrane of the renal proximal tubular cells where it represents the rate-limiting step in phosphate resorption in the kidney and is consequently a candidate gene for the defect in hypophosphatemia *(70)*. Screening of the *NPT2a* gene in 20 patients with urolithiasis and bone loss revealed two mutations in the *NPT2a* gene *(71)*. Expression of the mutant protein in *Xenopus* oocytes revealed diminished sodium dependent phosphate uptake in oocytes expressing the mutant protein *(71)*. Mutations in the *NPT2a* gene have been ruled out in two other forms of familial hypophosphatemia— X-linked hypophosphatemic rickets, which is associated with mutation of an endopeptidase on the X chromosome *PHEX* gene *(72)*, and autosomal dominant hereditary rickets, which is associated with mutation of the fibroblast growth factor 23 gene *(73)*.

Other Stone Diseases Related to Hypercalciuric Nephrolithiasis

Mutation of the calcium-sensing receptor (CASR) has been associated with several familial syndromes related to hypercalciuria with stone formation. The CASR is a plasma membrane G protein-coupled receptor that is expressed in the parathyroid-producing chief cells of the parathyroid gland and the kidney tubule-lining cells. PTH secretion and renal cation handling are modified through changes in Ca^{2+} concentration detected by the CASR *(74)*. The gene encoding the CASR (*CASR*) has been mapped to chromosome 3q13.3-q21 by Janicic et al. and is made up of six exons *(75)*. Multiple mutations have been described in the *CASR* and were recently reviewed by Hendy *(76)*. Activating mutations in the *CASR* have been described in familial hypocalcemia with hypercalciuria *(76,77)*. Pearce et al. concluded that depending on the site of the mutation in the CASR gene it is possible to modify the response of the CASR, effectively changing the set point for Ca^{2+} sensing and secretion of parathyroid hormone *(77)*. An inactivating mutation in the cytoplasmic tail of the CASR was recently described in a Swedish family with hypercalciuric hypercalcemia *(78)*.

PRIMARY HYPEROXALURIA TYPE 1

Primary hyperoxaluria type1 (PH1) is a rare autosomal recessive disorder. In North America it accounts for 0.7% of end-stage renal disease in children, whereas the prevalence in Mediterranean countries is much higher; in Tunisia it accounts for 13.5% of children with end stage renal disease *(79)*. The disease is caused by a deficiency of the peroxisomal enzyme AGT *(80)*. AGT catalyzes the conversion of glyoxlate to glycine. Functional deficiency of the enzyme allows glyoxylate to be oxidized to oxalate in the peroxisome by glycolate oxidase or by lactate dehydrogenase in the cytoplasm. Glyoxylate is also reduced to glycolate by glyoxylate reductase in the cytoplasm

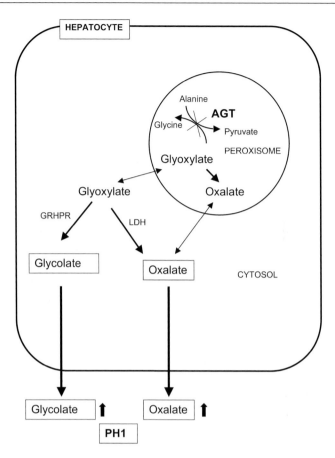

Fig. 1. Metabolic defect associated with PH1. AGT, alanine glyoxylate aminotransferase. GRHPR, glyoxylate reductase/D-glycerate dehydrogenase/hydroxypyruvate reductase. LDH, lactate dehydrogenase. Elevated metabolites are indicated in large type.

(Fig. 1). The primary clinical manifestations of the disorder are related to increased excretion of oxalate and glycolate. Oxalate is excreted by the kidney and the increased concentration of oxalate results in formation of insoluble calcium oxalate (CaOx) deposits in the kidney (nephrocalcinosis) or urinary tract resulting in urolithiasis or nephrolithiasis, leading to eventual renal failure. Following renal failure, systemic oxalosis occurs with CaOx deposition throughout the body. The gene encoding AGT (*AGXT*) was mapped to chromosome 2q 36-37 and comprises 11 exons, which encode a 1600-bp cDNA *(81)*. To date more than 30 separate mutations have been identified in *AGXT* associated with PH1 *(82)*. There is considerable heterogeneity of phenotype associated with PH1, the most common presentation occurring in infancy with progression to renal failure in childhood or early adulthood. The spectrum of disease ranges from extreme cases of renal failure during infancy to renal failure in late adulthood *(83)*. Similar heterogeneic diversity exists at the enzyme level in PH1. Some patients have no enzymatic or immunoreactive AGT, whereas others retain 30–50% of the normal catalytic activity. In these patients AGT activity falls within the range of activity associated with heterozygotes *(84)*. The variability of AGT activity in PH1 has made clinical diagnosis based on enzyme assay difficult. Numerous mutations and polymorphisms have been identified in *AGXT*. The most common mutations are associated with amino acid substitutions G170R and I244T and account for 30% and 9%, respectively, of the disease alleles encountered *(84,85)*. Many polymorphisms have also been described, the most common being the amino acid substitutions P11L and I340M, which segregate with a frequency of 20% in normal European and North American populations *(84,86)*. A unique mistargeting defect is associated with the occurrence of the *P11L* polymorphism and the *G170R* mutation. The *P11L* polymorphism creates a weak mitochondrial targeting sequence the strength of which increases in the presence of the *G170R* mutation *(86)*. In patients expressing 30–50% of normal enzyme activity, disease is associated with mistargeting of the enzyme to the mitochondrion instead of the peroxisome in hepatocytes. Lumb et al. have examined the synergism between the *P11L* polymorphism and four of the most common disease-associated mutations using an in vitro expression system *(82)*. They demonstrated a threefold reduction in specific activity of the enzyme associated with the *P11L* polymorphism. Expression of AGT containing the *G41R, F152I, G170R*, or *I244T* mutations resulted in a soluble and catalytically active enzyme. However, in the presence of the *P11L* polymorphism all mutations resulted in protein destabilization and aggregation into inclusion bodies in the *Escherichia coli* expression system *(82)*. They also demonstrated that the *G82E* mutation abolished enzyme activity by interfering with cofactor binding. Despite the fact that the kidney is the primary organ affected by PH1, liver transplantation is required for cure of the disease as AGT is a hepatic enzyme. In PH1 associated with a mistargeting defect, liver transplantation allows replacement of the enzyme within the correct organ and appropriate peroxisomal expression results within the transplant. Limited therapeutic benefit has been associated with renal transplant alone owing to persistence of the liver defect, which allows formation of further CaOx precipitates in the transplanted kidney *(5)*. In a worldwide study of the outcome of PH1, Cochat demonstrated 33% morbidity associated with patients undergoing transplantation as compared with 71% of patients without transplantation *(87)*.

Primary Hyperoxaluria Type 2

Primary hyperoxaluria type 2 (PH2) is a rare monogenic disorder, which is inherited as an autosomal dominant trait. The disease is caused by a deficiency of the enzyme glyoxylate reductase (GRHPR) (also called D-glycerate dehydrogenase or hydroxypyruvate reductase) *(88),* which catalyzes the conversion of glyoxylate to glycolate (Fig. 2). When the enzyme is deficient, more glyoxylate is oxidized to oxalate. Glyoxylate reductase also catalyzes the reduction of hydroxypyruvate to D-glycerate; in PH2 hydroxypyruvate is reduced to L-glycerate. Clinically PH2 is characterized by increased oxalate and L-glycerate excretion. The presence of L-glycerate and absence of glycolic acid in the urine serves to distinguish PH2 from PH1. Increased oxalate excretion results in nephrolithiasis and nephrocalcinosis and can progress to renal failure although PH2 generally has a less severe phenotype than PH1 *(89)*. The cDNA encoding the GRHPR has been identified as an 1198-bp clone made up of nine exons, which encodes a 328 amino acid protein *(90)*. The corresponding gene was mapped to chromosome 9cen within the reference interval D9S1874-D9S273 *(91)*. Cramer et al. used a combination of single-stranded conformational polymorphism and sequence analyses to identify a single-nucleotide deletion in exon 2 of the GRHPR gene in four patients with PH2 *(92)*. The deletion results in a frameshift mutation and protein truncation. Five additional mutations were

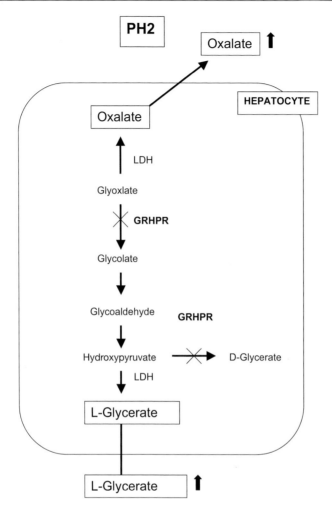

Fig. 2. Metabolic defect associated with PH2. GRHPR, glyoxylate reductase/d-glycerate dehydrogenase/hydroxypyruvate reductase. LDH, lactate dehydrogenase . Elevated metabolites are indicated in large type.

identified in 11 patients with PH2 by Webster et al., confirming the association between the GRHPR gene and PH2 (92).

CYSTINE-CONTAINING STONES

Cystinuria, one of the inborn errors of metabolism first discussed by Garrod (93), is an autosomal recessive or incompletely recessive familial transport disorder, which is characterized by an exaggerated renal excretion of cystine and the dibasic amino acids arginine, lysine, and ornithine (reference 94 and references cited within). Because of the low solubility of cystine in urine, the increased excretion results in the formation of cystine stones (95). Clinically, a patient who excretes >250 mg cystine/g creatinine/d is classified as being cystinuric (96).

Table 3
Phenotypic Differentiation of Cystinuric Subtypes

Cystinuric subtype	Active transport of dibasic amino acids in intestinal biopsies from homozygotes			Change in plasma after cystine load in homozygotes	Urinary dibasic amino acids in heterozygotes
	cys_2	lys	arg		
I	−	−	−	no change	normal
II	±	−	nd[*]	no change	elevated
III	+	+	+	increase	elevated

Adapted from 97.
[*]nd = not determined.

Phenotypic Subtyping of Cystinurics

Since the initial studies of Rosenberg, et al. (97,98), cystinuria has been classified into subgroups based on physiological observations of affected individuals and obligate carriers of the disease (Table 3). Type I cystinuria is inherited in an autosomal recessive manner, with homozygous patients excreting increased amounts of cystine and other dibasic amino acids and heterozygous carriers having normal urinary amino acid profiles (96). Cystinuria types II and III are inherited in an incompletely recessive manner(97,98) with heterozygotes having elevated, although usually not pathological, urinary excretion of dibasic amino acids. The observed aminoaciduria is generally more pronounced in type II heterozygotes than type III heterozygotes, although there is overlap between the two subgroups (97,98). Intestinal handling of dibasic amino acids further differentiates the three subtypes of cystinuria. Intestinal biopsies from type III, but not type I, cystinurics exhibit active transport of cystine, lysine, and arginine, whereas biopsies from type II cystinurics exhibit only a slight active transport of cystine and no transport of lysine (97). In addition, an oral cystine load in patients with type III cystinuria will cause a temporal increase in plasma cystine concentration, but not in patients with type I or II presentations (97,98).

Renal Cystine Transporters

The increase in urinary dibasic amino acids observed in cystinuria is a consequence of a defect in the renal reuptake mechanism(s) for these amino acids because the plasma concentrations remain normal or slightly below normal (99). Two renal transport systems for cystine have been described. One of the transporters, located in the proximal straight tubule (100), has a high affinity for cystine with a relatively low maximum rate of transport, whereas the other transporter, located in the proximal convoluted tubule (101), has a low affinity for cystine and a high maximum rate of transport. The high affinity system has an apparent K_m for cystine of 12 μM and a maximum transport velocity of 19 μmol cystine/L intracellular water/min, (102) and has been shown to catalyze hetero-exchange of dibasic amino acids with neutral amino acids(103). The low affinity transporter has a K_m for cystine of 550 μM and a 13-fold greater maximum velocity than the high affinity system ($V = 256\,\mu$mol cystine/L intracellular water/min) (102). The two transporters also differ in their specificity for dibasic amino acids and their dependence on Na^+. The high affinity system will also transport arginine, lysine, and ornithine, and does not require Na$^+$ *(102,104)*, whereas the low affinity transporter is specific for cystine *(102)* and is Na$^+$-dependent *(104)* with an apparent K$_m$ for Na$^+$ of 36 m*M (102)*. Because only the high affinity transporter also transports arginine, lysine, and ornithine, it has been proposed that this is the transporter system most likely involved in cystinuria *(105)*.

Genes Coding for Renal Cystine Transporters

Of the two cystine transporters described biochemically, only the high-affinity/low-capacity transporter has been cloned *(106–108)*. The transporter is a heterodimer *(109,110)* consisting of a heavy subunit and a light subunit. There are a number of recent reviews that extensively describe these proteins and their involvement with cystinuria *(111–114)*.

The heavy subunit (rBAT) is coded for by the SLC3A1 gene *(106,107)* located on chromosome 2p *(8)*. The structure of the gene within the genomic DNA consists of 10 exons *(115,116)*. More than 40 mutations *(see* references *112, 113* and references therein) within this gene that have been identified and in all instances in which the patients have been subtyped the SLC3A1 mutations have been shown to occur only in type I cystinurics *(117–119)*.

The light subunit b$^{(0,+)}$AT is coded for by the SLC7A9 gene *(108)*, which is located on chromosome 19q *(120–122)*. The gene consists of 13 exons (108) and 35 mutations have been reported in this gene. However, unlike the *SLC3A1* gene, mutations within this gene have been found in all subtypes of cystinuria *(108)*.

Taken together identified mutations within these two genes can account for approx 80% of cystinuric patients studied. Whether the other approx 20% of patients have disease causing mutations within unscreened portions of the SLC3A1 and SLC7A9 genes (i.e., the introns and promoter regions) or the disease is caused by mutations in an as yet unidentified gene *(123)* remains to be determined.

STONE FORMATION CAUSED BY ABERRATIONS IN NUCLEOTIDE METABOLISM

The last group of stone disease to be discussed is all related because the stones formed are all composed of products of purine nucleotide metabolism (Fig. 3). Stone formation has been shown to be caused by either direct defects in the enzymes of nucleotide metabolism, as in the formation of xanthine, 2,8-dihydroxyadenine, and uric acid stones, or indirect effects of the urinary environment, such as uric acid stones in which a severe decrease in urinary pH below 5.5 leads to stone formation.

Uric Acid Stones

PARTIAL HYPOXANTHINE GUANINE PHOSPHORIBOSYLTRANSFERASE DEFICIENCY

Lesch–Nyhan syndrome (LNS, 124, OMIM 300322) and Kelley–Seegmiller syndrome (KSS, 125, OMIM 300323) are X-linked recessive diseases that result from mutations in hypoxanthine guanine phosphoribosyltransferase (HPRT). The two syndromes differ in the amount of residual HPRT activity with LNS having <1.5% wild-type HPRT activity and KSS having at least 8% wild-type HPRT activity *(126)*. Even though, the clinical presentation of LNS (abnormal metabolic and neurologic symptoms) is much more severe than KSS, uric acid stones are uncommon in LNS, whereas they are

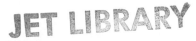

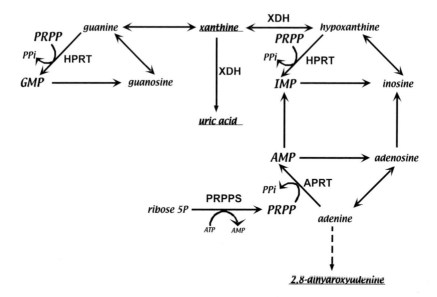

Fig. 3. Interrelationship of the purine salvage pathways of guanine, adenine, and hypoxanthine. Compounds underlined form renal stones when appropriate genetic defects are present (*see* text for details). PRPP, 5-phosphoribosyl-1-pyrophosphate; HPRT, hypoxanthine guanine phosphoribosyltransferase; XDH, xanthine dehydrogenase; APRT, adenine phosphoribosyltransferase; PRPPS, phosphoribosylpyrophosphate synthetase.

often one of the sole presenting symptoms of KSS *(126)*. Additionally, the occurrence of partial HPRT deficiency in patients presenting with uric acid stones and/or gout is quite rare with Yu et al. *(127)* reporting only seven cases (five from the same family) of partial HPRT deficiency out of 425 cases examined.

The gene coding for HPRT is located at the chromosomal locus Xq26-q27 *(128)* and contains nine exons spanning a region of 44 kb *(129)*. HPRT, part of the purine nucleotide salvage pathway, catalyzes the condensation of PRPP with either guanine or hypoxanthine to form GMP and IMP, respectfully (Fig. 3). Diminished activity of the enzyme leads to increased flux through the xanthine dehydrogenase catalyzed reaction and thus increased uric acid formation. A large number of mutations have been reported in the HPRT gene *(126)*; however, in most instances as stated previously, only those mutations causing a less severe decrease in enzyme activity are associated with uric acid stone formation *(126)*.

Phosphoribosylpyrophosphate Synthetase 1 Superactivity

Greatly increased activity of phosphoribosylpyrophosphate synthetase (PRPPS) has been shown to be associated with increased uric acid production, gout, and uric acid stone formation *(130)*. PRPPS catalyzes the formation of PRPP from the condensation of ATP and ribose 5-P (Fig. 3). The increase in enzyme activity has been shown to be caused by either an insensitively to allosteric regulation by ADP and GDP *(131)*, which is present in the wild type enzyme, or an overexpression of the enzyme protein *(132)*. Two isoforms of PRPPS have been identified—PRPPS 1 and PPRPS 2. The two enzymes are located on opposite arms of the X chromosome with the PRPPS 1 locus at Xq22-q24 and the

PRPPS 2 locus at Xp22.3-p22.2 *(133)*. To date only mutations in PRPPS 1 have been associated with increased enzyme activity and uric acid stone formation *(134)*. A consequence of the superactivity of PRPPS 1 is an increase in the *de novo* and salvage pathways of purine, pyrimidine, and pyridine nucleotides, which in turn leads to increased uric acid production *(134)*.

IDIOPATHIC INHERITED URIC ACID STONE FORMATION

In the early 1960s there were two reports of familial uric acid nephrolithiasis that were inherited in an autosomal dominate manner *(135,136)*. These individuals did not have gout or hyperuricemia but did exhibit an excessively low urinary pH (<5.5) and an early onset of stone disease *(135,136)*. Whether this is a defect directly involving either uric acid synthesis or transport, or a defect in the regulation of urinary acidification is not known. Of interest is the recent report of a linkage analysis study in a small, isolated founder population of a Sardinian village with an increased prevalence of uric acid stone formation relative to Western populations. The authors identified two chromosome loci with evidence of linkage for susceptibility genes for uric acid stones. The strongest linkage was found at 10q21-q22, where a lod score of 3.07 was obtained for chromosomal marker D10S1652. In addition suggestive, but not definitive, evidence was obtained for linkage at chromosomal locus 20q13.1-q13.3 using multipoint non-parametric analysis *(137)*. However, screening of the two regions for likely candidate genes for uric acid lithiasis using data from the Human Genome Project yielded no likely candidate genes.

Adenine Phosphoribosyltransferase Deficiency

Adenine phosphoribosyltransferase (APRT) deficiency results in the increased formation and urinary excretion of 2,8-dihydroxyadenine *(138)* as a consequence of a defect in the salvage pathway for the conversion of adenine to AMP (Fig. 3). The low solubility of 2,8-dihydroxyadenine leads to stone formation. APRT deficiency is inherited in an autosomal recessive manner *(138)* and the chromosomal loci for the gene coding for APRT is 16q22.2-q23.2 *(139)*. The gene for APRT consists of five exons spanning 2.5 kb of genomic DNA *(140)*. A number of mutations in the gene have been identified *(141)* and based on the residual amount of enzyme activity APRT deficiency has been divided into two subtypes. Type-1 patients, who are predominantly Caucasian, have no residual enzyme activity *(142)* whereas type-2 patients, who are predominantly Japanese, have up to 25% residual enzyme activity *(143)*. Both the clinical and enzymatic presentations of APRT deficiency are heterogeneous and a number of individuals with mutations are asymptomatic *(144)*.

Xanthinuria

Xanthinuria results from a deficiency in the activity of xanthine dehydrogenase (XDH; *see* Reference *145*) that leads to over excretion of xanthine and, as a consequence of its low solubility, xanthine stone formation. Xanthinuria has been divided into two subtypes based on enzyme deficiencies. Type-1 xanthinuria is the result of the sole deficiency of XDH, which catalyzes the conversion of hypoxanthine to xanthine and xanthine to uric acid (*see* Reference *145*; Fig. 3). In type-2 xanthinuria, XDH deficiency is coupled to aldehyde oxidase deficiency *(146)*. It has been proposed that the defect in type-2 xanthinuria is not caused by mutations in either the XDH or AO genes but is caused by disruption of the mechanism by which an essential sulfur atom is inserted into the active sites of both enzymes *(146)*. Type-1 patients can metabolize allopurinol, whereas type-2 patients cannot (147). It should be noted that xanthinuria, like hyperoxaluria, is primarily a hepatic disease because XDH is found predominately in the liver and as such, as with hyperoxaluria, specific attention should be given to the hepatic defect when treating the presenting renal disease.

The gene coding for XDH has been localized to the chromosomal locus 2p23-p22 *(148)* and has been to shown to consist of 36 exons spanning 60 kb of genomic DNA *(149)*. Only three unique mutations in the gene have been reported *(150)*.

CONCLUSION

Genetic studies have greatly facilitated our understanding of the underlying disease process in numerous stone-forming disorders. However, sometimes identification of a specific gene defect does not unlock the door to the understanding of the pathophysiology of a disease process. Once a gene has been identified often the most complex problem is the elucidation of the biochemical role of the related protein. Given the availability of suitable families for genetic study and careful clinical phenotype evaluation genome-wide screening can be undertaken fairly rapidly. Characterization of a mutant protein may often require intricate and time-consuming biochemical and physiological studies. In conclusion one significant benefit arising from identification of disease associated genes is the option of genetic testing as an aid to clinical diagnosis.

REFERENCES

1. Clark JY, Thompson IM, Optenberg SA. Economic impact of urolithiasis in the United States. J Urol. 1995; 154: 2020.
2. Curhan GC, Willett WC, Rimm EB, Stampfe MJ. Family history and risk of kidney stones. J Am Soc Nephrol. 1997; 8: 1568
3. Manthey DE, Teichman J. Nephrolithiasis. Emergency Med Clin North Am. 2001;19: 633–654.
4. Mc Kusick catalog, OMIM data base http//www.3.ncbi.nlm.nih.gov:80/Omim/
5. Danpure CJ. Genetic disorders and urolithiasis. Urol Clin N. Am 2000; 27: 287–299.
6. Reed BY, Heller HJ, Gitomer WL Pak CYC. Mapping a gene defect in absorptive hypercalciuria to chromosome 1q 23.4 to 1q 24. J Clin Endocrinol Metab 1999; 84: 3907.
7. Reed BY, Gitomer WL, Heller HJ, et al. Identification of a gene with base substitutions associated with the absorptive hypercalciuria phenotype and low spinal bone density. J Clin Endocrinol Metab 2002; 87: 1476.
8. Pras E, Arber N, Aksentijevich I, et al. Localization of a gene causing cystinuria to chromosome 2p. Nat Genet 1994; 6: 415.
9. Calonge MJ, Gasparini P, Chillaron J, et al. Cystinuria caused by mutations in rBAT, a gene involved in the transport of cystine. Nat Genet 1994; 6: 420.
10. Pak CYC, Britton F, Peterson R, et al. Ambulatory evaluation of nephrolithiasis: classification, clinical presentation and diagnostic criteria. Am J Med 1980; 69: 19.
11. Pak CYC, Ohata M, Lawrence ED, Snyder W. The hypercalciurias: causes, parathyroid functions and diagnostic criteria. J Clin Invest 1974; 54: 387.
12. Breslau NA, Preminger GM, Adams BV, Otey J, Pak CYC. Use of ketokonazole to probe the pathogenic importance of 1,25-dihydroxyvitamin D in absorptive hypercalciuria. J ClinEndocrinol Metab 1992; 75: 1446.
13. Broadus AE, Insogna KL, Lang R, Ellison AF, Dreyer BE. Evidence for disordered control of 1,25-dihydroxyvitamin D production in absorptive hypercalciuria. N Engl J Med 1984; 311: 73.
14. Coe F, Parks JH, Moore ES. Familial idiopathic hypercalciuria. New Engl J Med 1979; 300: 337.

15. Pak CYC, McGuire J, Peterson R, Britton F, Harrod MJ. Familial absorptive hypercalciuria in a large kindred. J Urol 1981; 126: 717.

16. Kreiger NS, Stathopoulos VM, Bushinsky DA. Increased sensitivity to $1,25(OH)_2D_3$ in bone from genetic hypercalciuric rats. Am J Physiol 1996; 271(1 Pt 1): C130.

17. Li X-Q, Tembe V, Horowitz GM, Bushinsky DA, Favus MJ. Increased intestinal vitamin D receptor in genetic hypercalciuric rats: a cause of intestinal calcium hyperabsorption. J Clin Invest 1993; 91: 661.

18. Zerwekh JE, Yu X-P, Breslau NA, Manologas S, Pak CYC. Vitamin D receptor quantitation in human mononuclear cells in health and disease. Mol Cell Endocrinol 1993; 96: 1.

19. Zerwekh JE, Hughes MR, Reed BY et al. Evidence for normal vitamin D receptor mRNA and genotype in absorptive hypercalciuria. J Clin Endocrinol Metab 1996; 80: 2960.

20. Zerwekh JE, Reed BY, Heller HJ, Gonzalez GB, Haussler MR, Pak CYC. Normal vitamin D receptor concentration and responsiveness to 1,25-dihydroxyvitamin D_3 in skin fibroblasts from patients with absorptive hypercalciuria. J Min Electrolyte Metab 1998; 24: 307.

21. Reed B, Heller HJ, Lemke M, et al. Linkage analysis in absorptive hypercalciuria: Lack of linkage to the vitamin D receptor or $1,25(OH)_2$ 1-α-hydroxylase loci. In: Proceedings 8th International Symposium on Urolithiathis. (Pak CYC, Resnick MI, Preminger GM, eds.), Millet, 1996, pp. 540–542.

22. Chen W-C, Chen H-Y, Lu H-F, Hsu C-D,Tsai F-J. Association of the vitamind D receptor gene start codon *Fok* I polymorphism with calcium oxalate stone disease. BJU International 2001; 87: 168.

23. Nishijima S, Sugaya K, Naito A, Morozumi M, Hatano T, Ogawa Y. Association of vitamin D receptor gene polymorphism with urolithiasis. J Urol 2002; 167: 2188.

24. Ruggiero M, Pacini S, Amato M, Chiarugi V. Association between vitaminD receptor gene polymorphism and nephrolitiasis. Min Electrolyte Metab 1999; 25: 185.

25. Jackman SV, Kibel AS, Ovuworie CA, Moore RG, Kavoussi LR, Jarrett TW. Familial calcium stone disease: Taq1 polymorphism and the vitamin D receptor. J Endourol 1999; 13: 313.

26. Scott P, Ouimet D, Valiquette L, et al. Suggestive evidence for a susceptibility gene near the vitamin D receptor locus in idiopathic calcium stone formation. J Am Soc Nephrol 1999; 10: 1007.

27. Petrucci M, Scott P, Ouimet D, et al. Evaluation of the calcium-sensing receptor gene in idiopathic hypercalciuria and calcium nephrolithiasis. Kid Int 2000; 58: 38.

28. Scott P, Ouimet D, Proulx Y, Trouve ML, Guay G, Gagnon B. The 1 alpha-hydroxylase locus is not linked to calcium stone formation or calciuric phenotypes in French-Canadian families. J Am Soc Nephrol 1998; 9: 425.

29. Imamura K, Tonoki H, Wakui K, et al. 4q33-qter deletion in absorptive hypercalciuria: Report of two unrelated girls. Am J Med Genetics 1998; 7: 52.

30. Buck J, Sinclair ML, Schapal L, Cann MJ, Levin LR. Cytosolic adenylate cyclase defines a unique signaling molecule in mammals. Proc Natl Acad Sci 1999; 96: 79.

31. Pietchmann F, Breslau NA, Pak CYC. Reduced vertebral bone density in hypercalciuric nephrolithiasis. J Bone Min Res 1992; 7: 1383.

32. Paciifici R, Rothstein M, Rifas L, et al. Increased monocyte interleukin-1 activity and decreased vertebral bone density in patients with fasting idiopathic hypercalciuria. J Clin Endocrinol Metab 1990; 71: 138.

33. Weisinger JR, Alonzo E, Bellorin-Font E, et al. Possible role of cytokines on the bone mineral loss in idiopathic hypercalciuria. Kid Int 1996; 49: 244.

34. Chen W-C, Wu H-C, Chen H-Y, Wu M-C, Hsu C-D, Tsai F-J. Interleukin-1b gene and receptor antagonist gene polymorphisms in patients with calcium oxalate stones. Urol Res 2001; 29: 321.

35. Tsai F-J, Lin C-C, Lu H-F, Chen H-Y, Chen W-C. Urokinase gene 3´-UTR T/C polymorphism is associated with urolithiasis. Urology 2002; 59: 458.

36. Chen W-C, Wu H-C, Lu H-F, Chen H-Y, Tsai F-J. Calcitonin receptor gene polymorphism: A possible genetic marker for patients with calcium oxalate stones. Eur Urol 2001; 39: 716.

37. Frymoyer P A, Scheinman SJ, Dunham PB, Jones DB, Hueber P, Schroeder ET. X-linked recessive nephrolithiasis with renal failure. New Engl J Med 1991; 325: 681.

38. Wrong O, Norden AGW, Feest TJ. Dent's disease: a familial proximal renal tubular syndrome with low-molecular weight proteinuria, hypercalciuria, nephrocalcinosis, metabolic bone disease, progressive renal failure, and a marked male predominance. Q J Med 1994; 87: 473.

39. Igarashi T, Hayakawa H, Shiraga H, et al. Hypercalciuria nephrocalcinosis in patients with idio-pathic low molecular weight proteinuria in Japan: is this identical to Dent's disease in the United Kingdom? Nephron 1995; 69: 242.

40. Lloyd SE, Gunther W, Pearce SH, et al Characterization of renal chloride channel, CLCN5, muta-tions in hypercalciuric nephrolithiasis (kidney stones) disorders. Hum Mol Genet 1997; 6: 1233.

41. Lloyd SE, Pearce SHS, Fisher SE, et al. A common molecular basis for three inherited kidney stone diseases. Nature 1996; 379: 445.

42. Scheinman SJ, Pook MA, Wooding C, Pang JT, Frymoyer PA, Thakker RV Mapping the gene causing X-linked recessive nephrolithiasis to Xp11.22 by linkage studies. J Clin Invest 1993; 91: 2351.

43. Pook MA, Wrong O, Wooding C, Norden AG, Feest TG, Thakker RV. Dent's disease a renal Fanconi syndrome with nephrocalcinosis and kidney stones is associated with a microdeletion involving DXS255 and maps to Xp11.22 Hum. Mol Genet 1993; 2: 2129.

44. Scheinman SJ, Pook MA, Wooding C, Pang JT, Frymoyer PA, Thakker RV. Mapping the gene causing X-linked recessive nephrolithiasis to Xp11.22 by linkage studies. J Clin Invest 1993; 91: 2351.

45. Blair HJ, Ho M, Monaco AP, Fisher S, Craig IW, Boyd I. High-resolution comparative mapping of the proximal region of the mouse X chromosome Genomics 1995; 28: 305.

46. Fisher SE, Black GCM, Lloyd SE, et al. Cloning and characterization of a chloride channel gene which is expressed in kidney and is a candidate for Dent's disease (X-linked hereditary nephroli-thiasis). Hum Mol Genet 1994; 3: 2053.

47. Fisher SE, Van Bakel I, Lloyd SE, Pearce SHS, Thakker RV, Craig IW. Cloning and character-ization of CLCN5, the human kidney chloride channel gene implicated in Dent disease (X-linked hereditary nephrolithiasis) Genomics 1995; 29: 598.

48. Luyckx VA, Goda FO, Mount DB, et al. Intrarenal and subcellular localization of rat CLC5. Am J Physiol 1998; 275(5 Pt 2): F761.

49. Gunther W, Luchow A, Cluzeaud F, Vandewalle A, Jentsch TJ. CLC-5 the chloride channel mutated in Dent's disease, colocalizes with the proton pump in endocytically active kidney cells. Proc Natl Acad Sci 1998; 95: 8075.

50. Devuyst O, Christie PT, Courtoy PJ, Beauwens R, Thakker RV. Intra-renal and subcellular dis-tribution of the chloride channel CLC-5, reveals a pathophysiological basis for Dent's disease. Hum Mol Genet 1999; 8: 247.

51. Sakamoto H, Sado Y, Naito I. et al Cellular and subcellular immunolocalization of CLC-5 channel in mouse kidney: colocalization with H+-ATPase. Am J Physiol 1999; 277(6 Pt 2): F957.

52. Gunther W, Luchow A, Cluzeaud F, Vandewalle A, Jentsch TJ. ClC-5, the chloride channel mutated in Dent's disease, colocalizes with the proton pump in endocytically active kidney cells. Proc Natl Acad Sci USA 1998; 95: 8075.

53. Nykjaer A, Dragun D, Walther D, et al. An endocytic pathway essential for renal uptake and activation of the steroid 25-(OH) D3. Cell 1999; 96: 507.

54. Piwon N, Gunther W, Schwake M, Bosr MR, Jentsch TJ. ClC-5 Cl⁻ -channel disruption impairs endocytosis in a mouse model for Dent's disease. Nature 2000; 408: 12,174.

55. Wang SS, Devuys O, Courtoy PJ, et al. Mice lacking renal chloride channel, CLC-5, are a model for Dent's disease, a nephrolithiasis disorder associated with defective receptor-mediated endocy-tosis. Hum Mol Genet 2000; 9: 2937.

56. Yu ASL. Role of CLC-5 in the pathogenesis of hypercalciuria: recent insights from transgenic mouse models. Curr Opin Nephrol Hyperten 2001; 10: 415.

57. Brenner RJ, Spring DB, Sebastian A, et al. Incidence of radiographically evident stone disease, nephrocalcinosis, and nephrolithiasis in various types of renal tubular acidosis. N Engl J Med 1982; 307: 217.

58. Alper SL. Genetic diseases of acid base transporters. Ann Rev Physiol 2002; 64: 899.

59. Bruce LJ, Cope DL, Jones GK, et al. Familial distal renal tubular acidosis is associated with mutations in the red cell anion exchanger (Band 3, AE1) gene. J Clin Invest 1997; 100: 1693.

60. Kollert-Jons A, Wagner S, Hubner S, Appelhans H, Drenckhahn D. Anion exchanger 1 in human kidney and oncocytoma differs from erthyroid AE1 in its NH₂ terminus. Am J Physiol Renal Physiol 1993; 265: F813.

61. Jarolim P, Shayakul C, Prabakaran D, et al. Autosomal dominant distal renal tubular acidosis is associated in three families with heterozygosity for the R589H mutation in AE1 (band 3) Cl$^-$/HCO3$^-$ -exchanger. J Biol Chem 1998; 273: 6380.

62. Karet FE, Gainza FJ, Gyory AZ, et al. Mutations in the chloride-bicarbonate exchanger gene AE1 cause autosomal dominant but not autosomal recessive distal renal tubular acidosis. Proc Natl Acad Sci USA 1998; 95: 6337.

63. Weber S, Soergel M, Jeck N, Konrad M. Atypical distal renal tubular acidosis confirmed by mutation analysis. Pediatr Nephrol 2000; 15: 201.

64. Tanphaichitr VS, Sumboonnanonda A, Ideguchi H, et al. Novel AE1 mutations in recessive distal renal tubular acidosis: loss-of-function is rescued by glycophorin A. J Clin Invest 1998; 102: 2173.

65. Bruce LJ, Wrong O, Toye AM et al. Band 3 mutations, renal tubular acidosis and South-East Asian ovalocytosis in Malaysia and Papua New Guinea: loss of up to 95% band 3 transport in red cells. Biochem J 2000; 350: 41.

66. Karet FE, Finberg KE, Nelson RD, et al. Mutations in the gene encoding B1 subunit of H+-ATPase cause renal tubular acidosis with sensoineural deafness. Nature Genetics 1999; 21: 84.

67. Karet FE, Finberg KE, Nayir A, et al. Localization of a gene for autosomal recessive distal renal tubular acidosis with normal hearing (rdRTA2) to 7q33-34. Am J Hum Genet 1999; 65: 1656.

68. Smith AN, Skaug J, Choate KA, et al. Mutations in ATP6N1B encoding a new kidney vacuolar proton pump 116-kD subunit, cause recessive distal renal tubular acidosis with preserved hearing. Nat Genet 2000; 26: 71.

69. Stover EH, Bavalia C, Eady N, Borthwick KJ, Smith AN, Karet FE. Novel ATP6B1 and ATP6N1B mutations in autosomal recessive distal renal tubular acidosis. J Am Soc Nephrol 2001; 12: 560A (Abstr).

70. Murer H, Hernando N, Forster I, Biber J. Proximal tubular phosphate resorption molecular mechanisms. Physiol Rev 2000; 80: 1373.

71. Prie D, Huar V, Bakouh N, et al. Nephrolithiasis and osteoporosis associated with hypophosphatemia caused by mutations in the type 2a sodium-phosphate cotransporter. N Engl J Med 2002; 347: 983.

72. The HYP Consortium. A gene (PEX) with homologies to endopeptidases is mutated in patients with X-linked hypophosphatemic rickets. Nat Genet 1995; 11: 130.

73. The ADHR Consortium. Autosomal dominant hypophosphatemic rickets is associated with mutations in FGF23. Nat Genet 2000; 26: 345.

74. Brown EM, Gamba G, Riccardi D, et al. Cloning and characterization of an extracellular Ca^{2+}sensing receptor from bovine parathyroid. Nature 1993; 366: 575.

75. Janicic N, Soliman E, Pausova Z, et al. Mapping of the calcium-sensing gene (CASR) to human chromosome 3q13.3-21 by fluorescence in situ hybridization and localization to rat chromosome 11 and mouse chromosome 16. Mammalian Genome 1995; 6: 798.

76. Hendy GN, D'Souza-Li L, Yang B, Canaff L, Cole DEC. Mutations in the calcium-sensing receptor (CASR) in familial hypocalciuric hypercalcemia, neonatal severe hyperparathyroidism, and autosomal dominant hypocalcemia. Hum Mut 2000; 16: 281.

77. Pearce SHS, Williamson C, Kifor O, et al. A familial syndrome of hypocalcemia with hypercalciuria due to mutations in the calcium-sensing receptor. N Engl J Med 1996; 335: 1115.

78. Carling T, Szabo E, Bai M, et al. Familial hypercalcemia and hypercalciuria caused by a novel mutation in the cytoplasmic tail of the calcium receptor. J Clin Endocr Med 2000; 85: 2042.

79. Kamoun A, Lakhoua R. End stage renal disease of the Tunisian child: Epidemiology, etiologies and outcomes. Pediatr Nephrol 1996; 10: 479.

80. Danpure CJ, Jennings R. Peroxisomal alanine:glyoxylate aminotransferase deficiency in primary hyperoxaluria type 1. FEBS Lett 1986; 201: 20.

81. Purdue PE, Lumb MJ, Fox M, et al. Characterization and chromosomal mapping of a genomic clone encoding the human alanine:glyoxylate aminotransferase. Genomics 1991; 10: 34.

82. Lumb MJ, Danpure CJ. Functional synergism between the most common polymorphism in the human alanine: glyoxylate aminotransferase and four of the most common disease-causing mutations. J Biol Chem 2000; 275: 36,415.

83. Danpure CJ, Jennings PR, Fryer P, Purdue PE, Allsop J. Primary hyperoxaluria type1: Genotypic and phenotypic heterogeneity. J Inher Metab Dis 1994; 17: 487.

84. Danpure CJ, Rumsby G. Strategies for the prenatal diagnosis of primary hyperoxaluria type 1. Prenat Diagn 1996; 16: 587.

85. Tarn AC, von-Schnakenburg C, Rumsby G. Primary hyperoxaluria type 1: Diagnostic relevance of mutations and polymorphisms in the alanine:glyoxylate aminotransferase gene (AGXT). J Inher Metab Dis 1997; 5: 689.

86. Purdue PE, Takada Y, Danpure CJ. Identification of mutations associated with peroxisome-to-mitochondrion mistargeting of alanine/glyoxalate aminotransferase in primary hyperoxaluria type 1. J Cell Biol 1990; 111: 2341.

87. Cochat P, Nogueira PCK, Mahmoud MA, Jamieson NV, Scheinman JI, Rolland M-O. Primary hyperoxaluria in infants: medical ethical and economic issues. J Pediat 1999; 135: 746.

88. Williams HE, Smith LH, Jr. L-glyceric aciduria: a new genetic variant of primary hyperoxaluria. N Engl J Med 1968; 278: 233.

89. Chelbeck P, Milliner D, Smith LH, Jr. Long term prognosis in primary hyperoxaluria type ll (L-glyceric aciduria). Am J Kidney Dis 1994; 23: 255.

90. Cramer SD, Lin K, Holmes RP. Towards identification of the gene responsible for primary hyperoxaluria type ll: A cDNA encoding human d-glycerate dehydrogenase. J Urol 1998; 159 (suppl): 173.

91. Cramer SD, Ferree PM, Lin K, Milliner DS, Holmes RP. The gene encoding hydroxypyruvate reductase (GRHPR) is mutated in patients with primary hyperoxaluria type ll. Hum Molec Genet 1999; 8: 2063.

92. Webster KE, Ferree PM, Holmes RP, Cramer SD. Identification of missense, nonsense, and deletion mutations in the GRHPR gene in patients with primary hyperoxaluria type ll (PH2). Hum Genet 2000; 107: 176.

93. Garrod AE. The Croonian Lectures on Inborn Errors of Metabolism. Lecture III. Lancet 1908; 2: 142.

94. Segal S, Their SO. Cystinuria. In: The Metabolic and Molecular Basis of Inherited Disease. 7th Ed. (Scriver CR, Beaudet AL, Sly WS, Valle D, eds.), McGraw-Hill; New York, NY, 1995; p. 3581.

95. Wollaston WH. On cystic oxide: A new species of urinary calculus. Phil Trans Roy Soc, London, 1810; 100: 223.

96. Harris H, Mittwoch U, Robson EB, Warren FL. Pattern of amino acid excretion in cystinuria. Ann Hum Genet 1955; 19: 196.

97. Rosenberg LE, Downing SE, Durant JL, Segal S. Cystinuria: biochemical evidence for three genetically distinct diseases. J Clin Invest 1966; 45: 365.

98. Rosenberg LE, Durant JL, Albrecht I. Genetic Heterogeneity in cystinuria: Evidence for allelism. Trans Assoc Am Phys 1966; 79: 284.

99. Dent CE, Senior B, Walshe JM. The pathogenesis of cystinuria. II. Polarographic studies of the metabolism of sulphur-containing amino-acids. J Clin Invest 1954; 33: 1216.

100. Furriols M, Chillarón J, Mora C, et al. rBAT, related to L-cystine transport, is localized to the microvilli of proximal straight tubules, and its expression is regulated in kidney by development. J Biol Chem 1993; 268: 27060.

101. Völkl H, Silbernagl S. Mutual inhibition of L-cystine/l-cysteine and other neutral amino acids during tubular reabsorption. A microperfusion study in rat kidney. Pflügers Arch 1982; 395: 190.

102. Foreman JW, Hwang S-M, Segal S. Transport interactions of cystine and dibasic amino acids in isolated rat renal tubules. Metabolism 1980; 29: 53.

103. Chillarón J, Estévez R, Mora C, et al. Obligatory amino acid exchange via systems b$^{o,+}$-like and y^{+}L-like. A tertiary active transport mechanism for renal reabsorption of cystine and dibasic amino acids. J Biol Chem 1996; 271: 17761.

104. McNamara PD, Pepe LM, Segal S. Cystine uptake by rat renal brush-border vesicles. Biochem J 1981; 194: 443.

105. Dent CE, Rose GA. Amino acid metabolism in cystinuria. Q J Med 1951; 20: 205.

106. Lee W-S, Wells RG, Sabbag RV, Mohandas TK, Hediger MA. Cloning and chromosomal localization of a human kidney cDNA involved in cystine, dibasic, and neutral amino acid transport. J Clin Invest 1993; 91: 1959.

107. Bertran J, Werner A, Chillarón J, et al. Expression cloning of a human renal cDNA that induces high affinity transport of L-cystine shared with dibasic amino acids in Xenopus oocytes. J Biol Chem 1993; 268: 14842.

108. Font MA, Feliubadalo L, Estivill X, et al. Functional analysis of mutations in SLC7A9, and genotype-phenotype correlation in non-type I cystinuria. Hum Mol Genet 2001; 10: 305.

109. Wang Y, Tate SS. Oligomeric structure of a renal cystine transporter: implications in cystinuria. FEBS Lett 1995; 368: 389.

110. Pfeiffer R, Loffing J, Rossier G, et al. Luminal heterodimeric amino acid transporter defective in cystinuria. Mol Biol Cell 1999; 10: 4135–4147.

111. Palacin M, Fernandez E, Chillaron J, Zorzano A. The amino acid transport system b(o,+) and cystinuria. Mol Membrane Biol 2001; 18: 21.

112. Pras E. Cystinuria at the turn of the millennium: clinical aspects and new molecular developments. Mol Urol 2000; 4: 409.

113. Ito H, Egoshi K, Mizoguchi K, Akakura K. Advances in genetic aspects of cystinuria. Mol Urol 2000; 4: 403.

114. Goodyer P, Boutros M, Rozen R. The molecular basis of cystinuria: an update. Exp Nephrol 2000; 8: 123.

115. Pras E, Sood R, Raben N, Aksentijevich I, Chen X, Kastner DL. Genomic organization of SLC3A1, a transporter gene mutated in cystinuria. Genomics 1996; 36: 163.

116. Purroy J, Bisceglia L, Calonge MJ, et al. Genomic structure and organization of the human rBAT gene (SLC3A1). Genomics 1996; 37: 249.

117. Gasparini P, Calonge MJ, Bisceglia L, et al. Molecular genetics of cystinuria: identification of four new mutations and seven polymorphisms, and evidence for genetic heterogeneity. Am J Hum Genet 1995; 57: 781.

118. Gitomer WL, Reed BY, Ruml LA, Sakhaee K, Pak CYC. Mutations in the genomic deoxyribonucleic acid for SLC3A1 in patients with cystinuria. J Clin Endocrin Metab 1998; 83: 3688.

119. Saadi I, Chen XZ, Hediger M, et al. Rozen, R. Molecular genetics of cystinuria: mutation analysis of SLC3A1 and evidence for another gene in type I (silent) phenotype. Kidney Int 1998; 54: 48.

120. Bisceglia L, Calonge MJ, Totaro A, et al . Localization, by linkage analysis, of the cystinuria type III gene to chromosome 19q13.1. Am J Hum Genet 1997; 60: 611–616.

121. Wartenfeld R, Golomb E, Katz G, et al. Molecular analysis of cystinuria in Libyan Jews: exclusion of the SLC3A1 gene and mapping of a new locus on 19q. Am J Hum Genet 1997; 60: 617–624.

122. Stoller ML, Bruce JE, Bruce CA, Foroud T, Kirkwood SC, Stambrook PJ. :Linkage of type II and type III cystinuria to 19q13.1: codominant inheritance of two cystinuric alleles at 19q13.1 produces an extreme stone-forming phenotype. Am J Med Genet 1999; 86: 134.

123. Leclerc D, Wu Q, Ellis JR, Goodyer P, Rozen R. Is the SLC7A10 gene on chromosome 19 a candidate locus for cystinuria? Mol Genet Metab 2001; 73: 333.

124. Nyhan WL, Olivier WJ, Lesch M. A familial disorder of uric acid metabolism and central nervous system function. J Pediatr 1965; 67: 257.

125. Kelley WN, Rosenbloom FM, Henderson JF, Seegmiller JE. A specific enzyme defect in gout associated with overproduction of uric acid. Proc Natl Acad Sci 1967; 57: 1735.

126. Online Mendelian Inheritance in Man, OMIM™. Johns Hopkins University, Baltimore, MD. MIM Number: {MIM 300322}: {4/11/2001}: World Wide Web URL: http://www.ncbi.nlm.nih.gov/omim/

127. Yu T-F, Balis ME, Krenitsky TA, et al. Rarity of X-linked partial hypoxanthine-guanine phosphoribosyltransferase deficiency in a large gouty population. Ann Intern Med 1972; 76: 255.

128. Pai GS, Sprenkle JA, Do TT, Mareni CE, Migeon BR. Localization of loci for hypoxanthine phosphoribosyltransferase and glucose-6-phosphate dehydrogenase and biochemical evidence of nonrandom X chromosome expression from studies of a human X-autosome translocation. Proc Natl Acad Sci USA 1980; 77: 2810.

129. Patel PI, Framson PE, Caskey CT, Chinault AC. Fine structure of the human hypoxanthine phosphoribosyltransferase gene. Mol Cell Biol 1986; 6: 393.

130. Sperling O, Eliam G, Persky-Brosh S, De Vries A. Accelerated erythrocyte 5-phosphribosyl-1-pyrophosphate synthesis: a familial abnormality associated with excessive uric acid production and gout. Biochem Med 1972; 6: 310.

131. Sperling O, Persky-Brosh S, Boer P, De Vries A. Human erythrocyte phosphoribosylpyrophosphate synthetase mutationally altered in regulatory properties. Biochem Med 1973; 7: 389.

132. Becker MA, Taylor W, Smith PR, Ahmed M. Overexpression of the normal phosphoribosyl-pyrophosphate synthetase 1 isoform underlies catalytic superactivity of human phosphoribosyl-pyrophosphate synthetase. J Biol Chem 1996; 271: 19894.

133. Becker MA, Heidler SA, Bell GI, et al. Cloning of cDNAs for human phosphoribosylpyrophosphate synthetases 1 and 2 and X chromosome localization of PRPS1 and PRPS2 genes. Genomics 1990; 8: 555.

134. Online Mendelian Inheritance in Man, OMIM™. Johns Hopkins University, Baltimore, MD. MIM Number: {MIM 311850}: {3/1/1999}: World Wide Web URL: http://www.ncbi.nlm.nih.gov/omim/

135. de Vries A, Frank M, Atsmon A. Inherited uric acid lithiasis. Am J Med 1962; 33: 880.

136. Gutman AB, Yu TF. Urinary ammonium excretion in primary gout. J Clin Invest 1965; 44: 1474.

137. Ombra MN, Forabosco P, Casula S, et al. Identification of a new candidate locus for uric acid nephrolithiasis. Am J Hum Genet 2001; 68: 1119.

138. Kelley WN, Levy RI, Rosenbloom FM, Henderson JF, Seegmiller JE. Adenine phosphoribosyl-transferase deficiency: a previously undescribed genetic defect in man. J Clin Invest 1968; 47: 2281–2289.

139. Fratini A, Simmers RN, Callen DF, et al. A new location for the human adenine phosphoribosyl-transferase gene (APRT) distal to the haptoglobin (HP) and fra(16)(q23) (FRA16D) loci. Cytogenet Cell Genet 1986; 43: 10.

140. Broderick TP, Schaff DA, Bertino AM, Dush MK, Tischfield JA, Stambrook PJ. Comparative anatomy of the human APRT gene and enzyme: nucleotide sequence divergence and conservation of a nonrandom CpG dinucleotide arrangement. Proc Natl Acad Sci USA 1987; 84: 3349.

141. Online Mendelian Inheritance in Man, OMIM™. Johns Hopkins University, Baltimore, MD. MIM Number: {MIM 102600}: {11/30/2000}: World Wide Web URL: http://www.ncbi.nlm.nih.gov/omim/

142. Debray H, Cartier P, Temstet A, Cendron J. Child's urinary lithiasis revealing a complete deficit in adenine phosphoribosyl transferase. Pediatr Res 1976; 10: 76.

143. Fox IH, Meade JC, Kelley WN. Adenine phosphoribosyltransferase deficiency in man: report of a second family. Am J Med 1973; 55: 614.

144. Simmonds HA, Sahota AS, Van Acker KJ. Adenosine phosphoribosyltransferase deficiency and 2,8-dihydroxyadenine lithiasis. In: The Metabolic and Molecular Basis of Inherited Disease. 7th Ed. (Scriver CR, Beaudet AL, Sly WS, Valle D, eds.), McGraw-Hill, New York, NY, 1995; p. 1707.

145. Dent CE, Philpot GR. Xanthinuria: an inborn error of metabolism. Lancet I: 1954; 182.

146. Online Mendelian Inheritance in Man, OMIM™. Johns Hopkins University, Baltimore, MD. MIM Number: {MIM 603592}: {2/26/1999}: World Wide Web URL: http://www.ncbi.nlm.nih.gov/omim/

147. Simmonds HA, Reiter S, Nishino T. Hereditary xanthinuria. In: The Metabolic and Molecular Bases of Inherited Disease. Vol. 2, (Scriver CR, Beaudet AL, Sly WS, Valle D, eds.), McGraw-Hill, New York, NY, 1995; p. 1781.

148. Xu P, Zhu XL, Huecksteadt TP, Brothman AR, Hoidal JR. Assignment of human xanthine dehy-drogenase gene to chromosome 2p22. Genomics 1994; 23: 289.

149. Xu P, Huecksteadt TP, Hoidal JR. Molecular cloning and characterization of the human xanthine dehydrogenase gene (XDH). Genomics 1996; 34: 173.

150. Online Mendelian Inheritance in Man, OMIM™. Johns Hopkins University, Baltimore, MD. MIM Number: {MIM 278300}: {5/18/2001}: World Wide Web URL: http://www.ncbi.nlm.nih.gov/omim/

4 Theories of Stone Formation

Hsiao-Jen Chung, MD, *Harrison M. Abrahams,* MD,
Maxwell V. Meng, MD, *and Marshall L. Stoller,* MD

CONTENTS

Key Words: Nephrolithiasis; etiology; saturation; crystal.

INTRODUCTION

Water is a pivotal element in digestion, circulation, elimination, and regulation of body temperature. A critical function of the urinary system is the maintenance of normal composition and volume of body fluid; this is accomplished by glomerular filtration, tubular reabsorption, and tubular secretion of soluble and filterable plasma components. By such means, urine contains water, electrolytes, minerals, hydrogen ions, end products of protein metabolism, and other compounds not useful to the metabolism, energy requirements, or structure of the body. Under normal circumstances, urine will not contain solid particles (stones).

Why do humans suffer from urinary stone disease? Although urinary stones have been noted in human remains as old as 7000 years *(1)*, the underlying etiology of stone formation remains a mystery. The development of urinary calculi is most likely a multifactorial process and cannot be fully addressed by current theories. Fundamental knowl-

From: Current Clinical Urology, *Urinary Stone Disease:*
A Practical Guide to Medical and Surgical Management
Edited by: M. L. Stoller and M. V. Meng © Humana Press Inc., Totowa, NJ

edge of these theories is too complicated to entirely fit in this short chapter. Discussions in the subsequent sections provide readers simplified general ideas developed from current studies of urinary stone formation. This chapter will discuss the possible pathogenesis of urinary stone formation, including the topics of basic physical chemistry, nucleation, crystal aggregation and growth, epitaxy, matrix, and crystal retention.

BASIC PHYSICAL CHEMISTRY

When a small amount of sodium chloride is added to a glass of pure water at a given pH and temperature, all of the sodium chloride will dissolve. With the addition of more and more sodium chloride, a point will be reached at which the sodium chloride will no longer dissolve. This type of solution is called a saturated solution. In a saturated solution, equilibrium exists between the dissociated ions and the solid compound. Some of the solute is continuously crystallizing out of solution, and at the same time, a similar amount of the solid dissolves into the solution. The equilibrium expression for this reaction is (2):

$$K_{eq} = [Na^+][Cl^-]/[NaCl] \qquad (1)$$

As long as solid sodium chloride remains, its effect on the equilibrium does not change. The solubility product constant (K_{sp}) is useful in predicting whether a precipitate will form under specified conditions (2). The solubility product is a simplified equation that only factors in the ionic concentrations.

$$K_{sp} = K_{eq}[NaCl] = [Na^+][Cl^-] \qquad (2)$$

In a real world situation, every ion in solution will interact with every other so the solubility is altered accordingly. Strictly speaking, it is the ionic activities, and not the ionic concentration, that govern the solubility principles described previously. Solubility product (solubility ion product) is therefore defined as the ion product at saturation at a specific temperature. The ion product is a mathematical expression for overall ionic activities (3).

If the numerous components of the urine and urinary stones are factored into the equation, the concept becomes more complicated. Urine contains many electrically active ions and small and macromolecular organic components. Some urinary constituents, referred to as inhibitors of crystal formation, enable the urine to retain more ions in solution than at the level of saturation (1). For example, nephrocalcin can inhibit the precipitation of calcium oxalate crystals in urine (4). This state is termed supersaturation, operationally defined as the solute concentration in solution above that which would ordinarily result in precipitation if the solution were held at equilibrium (3). In the study of urolithiasis, the term formation product (formation ion product) is used to depict the saturation ion product point at which the spontaneous crystal nucleation will occur. When listing a formation product, environmental factors such as temperature, pH, time of onset of nucleation, method of detection of nucleation, and surface of reaction container must be specified, along with any unusual circumstances, such as cavitations from stirring, strong magnetic or electric fields, and method of supersaturation generation (3). Formation product is dependent on many factors making it difficult to reproduce experimentally. Hence, it is graphically represented as a band-shaped region (Fig. 1).

Figure 1 illustrates the states of saturation as a general example of urinary stone components. If the concentration product is less than the solubility product, the solution is termed undersaturated, and crystal nucleation will not occur. The metastable region

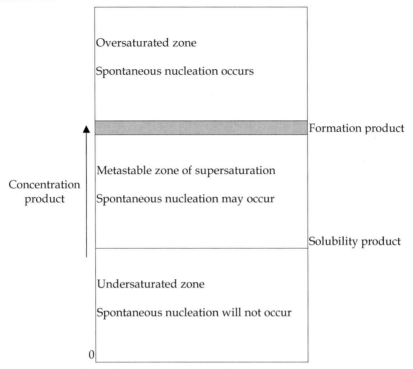

Fig. 1. States of saturation. (*See* text for details.)

is the area between the solubility product and the formation product. Spontaneous nucleation may occur in this region. A solution with a concentration product that is greater than the formation product is quite unstable, and crystal nucleation will occur spontaneously.

One method to help prevent urinary stone formation is to avoid supersaturation. It is important therefore to understand the states of urinary supersaturation in urinary-stone patients. Calculation of urinary supersaturation is based on thermodynamics. From a thermodynamic standpoint, urinary stone crystal formation is a spontaneous process and occurs in the direction that decreases free energy. If there is available free energy, the crystallization will occur. This driving force, expressed as free energy (ΔG), can be written:

$$\Delta G = RT \ln (A_i/A_o) \tag{3}$$

in which R is the universal gas constant, T is the temperature (in degrees Kelvin), and A_i and A_o are the activities of the un-ionized salt species in solution at any given condition and equilibrium, respectively *(5,6)*. The ratio A_i/A_o is termed relative supersaturation, namely, the actual concentration product divided by the solubility product. Activity (A) is related to concentration (C) through an activity coefficient (f) by:

$$A = fC \tag{4}$$

In the above equations, only one salt is considered. Manual calculation of the relative supersaturation of a salt in urine, which always contains multiple constituents, would be tedious and impractical. To solve this problem, Finlayson developed a Fortran IV computer program, EQUIL, for calculating ion equilibrium for solutions as complex as urine *(5)*. A BASIC language version of EQUIL, called EQUIL2, was also published *(7)*.

Results of the calculation by these programs are suggested to be reasonably accurate *(5,7)*. These computer programs are useful for calculating not only urinary ion equilibrium but ion equilibrium in a variety of other solutions commonly used in biological laboratories. However, kinetic considerations, such as how fast the crystallization process occurs, are not factored into these programs nor consideration of aggregation, retention, nucleation, and the role of matrix *(7)*. Despite these shortfalls, the EQUIL and EQUIL2 are powerful tools in the study of urinary stone formation. Many commercial laboratories evaluating 24-h urinary constituents use these equations to calculate and predict supersaturations.

NUCLEATION

Although the precise pathogenesis of urinary stone formation is unknown, most believe it is related to crystal formation, especially in the early stages. Many crystalline substances have been identified in urinary stones. The principal components are calcium oxalate monohydrate ($CaOx \cdot H_2O$, whewellite), calcium oxalate dihydrate ($CaOx \cdot 2H_2O$, weddellite), basic calcium hydrogen phosphate ($Ca_5(PO_4)_3OH$, apatite), calcium hydrogen phosphate ($CaHPO_4 \cdot 2H_2O$, brushite), magnesium ammonium phosphate ($Mg(NH_4)(PO_4) \cdot 6H_2O$, struvite), uric acid, and cystine *(8)*. Urine is often saturated with respect to the most common stone components. Even though all urinary stones are made of crystals, not every stone former has crystalluria in their voided specimen *(9)*. Conversely, crystalluria is very common in nonstone formers *(10–15)*. There are overlaps of the severity of crystalluria between stone formers and nonstone formers. Robertson and Peacock, however, showed that stone formers tend to excrete larger crystal clumps than nonstone formers *(11)*. In addition, stone formers generally had calcium oxalate dihydrate crystalluria, whereas nonstone formers generally had calcium oxalate monohydrate crystalluria. The clinical significance of these findings is unknown.

Calcium oxalate is a major component of renal calculi. It is intriguing that calcium oxalate crystalluria is typically in the dihydrate form whereas, in renal stones, it is most commonly present in the monohydrate form. Calcium oxalate may exist in the monohydrate (COM), dihydrate (COD), or trihydrate (COT) configurations. Calcium oxalate monohydrate is the most stable and the COT is the most unstable thermodynamically. There is supporting evidence that the COT is the first nucleated crystal phase of calcium oxalate. Subsequently, COT is converted to COD and then to COM *(16–18)*. COT is so unstable that it is rarely detected in urine and urinary stones. COD can be transformed to COM in a relatively short period of time (3.5 d) *(19)*. Their solubility differs with COT being the most soluble, COD intermediate, and COM being the least soluble. Despite the fact that COM is the most stable crystal phase, COD can exist in urine for a prolonged time; why this is so is unknown. Several factors in urine, however, favor the presence of the COD. For example, the rate of transformation from COD to COM is reduced by magnesium *(20,21)*. Polyphosphate markedly inhibits the crystallization of COM but has a much smaller effect on the formation of COD and COT *(18)*. Some macromolecules in urine favor formation of COD crystals *(22)*.

Crystals in the urine result from nucleation, the initial step whereby the urinary constituent transforms from a liquid to a solid phase in a supersaturated solution. When the concentration product of the ions of the stone components is greater than the formation product, ions begin to cluster close together to form the earliest nonsoluble crystal structure. This cluster structure is a loose association and is initially not compact *(23)*.

Gradually the structure becomes more and more organized and finally resembles an orderly crystal lattice structure *(24)*. The term, nucleation, is used to depict this process.

There are two types of nucleation: homogeneous and heterogeneous. When the process occurs spontaneously in a pure solution, homogeneous nucleation results. Because impurities are always present in human urine, homogeneous nucleation is unlikely to occur in vivo. The surfaces provided by the impurities can serve as a nidus in the nucleation process, leading to heterogeneous nucleation. Heterogeneous nucleation will generally occur at a lower supersaturation level than that required for the induction of homogeneous nucleation. The role of heterogeneous nucleation in stone formation is not well understood. Nevertheless, several studies have reported that most stones are a mixture of several different crystals with one or two prominent constituents *(25–28)*. These are indirect clues to support the inclusion of heterogeneous nucleation in the process of stone formation.

A large proportion of urinary stones contain a mixture of calcium oxalate and calcium phosphate. Crystallization of calcium oxalate is thought to start through the process of heterogeneous nucleation, which is facilitated by a good fit for the calcium oxalate lattice. Calcium phosphate may act as a nidus in this example *(29–31)*. It has been demonstrated that seed crystals of hydroxyapatite have the ability to induce the growth of COM crystals from a metastable supersaturated solution of calcium oxalate *(32)*. Conversely , seed crystals of COM cannot induce the growth of hydroxyapatite crystals *(32)*. Hydroxyapatite is thermodynamically the most stable form of calcium phosphate in alkaline urine. It is probably transformed from dicalcium phosphate dihydrate *(33)*, which is the most stable form in acidic urine *(34)*. Dicalcium phosphate dihydrate also has been found to induce the heterogeneous nucleation of calcium oxalate crystals *(35)*. These findings support the theory that renal stones composed of calcium salts start by a heterogeneous nucleation in metastable supersaturated urine.

Formed crystals either can be excreted in the urine as crystalluria or grow and/or aggregate to become clinically significant stones. If one takes into consideration the speed of crystal nucleation and aggregation, and the transit time of urine through the kidney (glomeruli to papillae, takes approx 2–3 min), one recognizes that crystal nucleation alone cannot explain urinary stone formation. Indeed, Finlayson and Reid calculated the required time for free crystals to nucleate and grow, and concluded that before free calcium oxalate particles could grow large enough to be trapped within the renal tubules, they would be excreted in the urine rather than develop into calculi *(36)*. Different types of crystals tend to nucleate in different parts of the nephron. Crystal nucleation of calcium carbonate, calcium phosphate, and calcium oxalate are more likely to occur in the loop of Henle, the late distal tubule, and the collecting ducts, respectively *(37,38)*. Although crystal nucleation is thought to be one of the prerequisites for urolithiasis, it alone cannot explain stone disease, in which the stones are much larger than the crystal nuclei. There must, therefore, be other mechanisms for crystals to grow and be retained in the kidney to form stones before they are excreted in the urine.

CRYSTAL AGGREGATION AND GROWTH

Crystal nuclei will bind to each other to form larger particles. This process is called aggregation or agglomeration. When one large particle is broken into many small particles in solution, energy must be consumed to overcome the forces holding the small particles together. Conversely, the aggregation of small particles into large aggregates is favored from a thermodynamic perspective *(23)*. According to Randolph and Drach, aggregation is different from agglomeration *(3)*. Aggregation, by their definition, is the grouping of two or more particles held together by strong intermolecular forces, which cannot be dispersed by shear forces. The definition of agglomeration, on the other hand, is the grouping of two or more particles held together by weak cohesive forces, which can be broken up by dispersion with shear forces or water solvents. Most authors use the term aggregation, when referring to the binding of urinary crystals.

Despite the fact that aggregation is thermodynamically favored in nature, it does not always occur. Aggregation or disaggregation depends on the final combined effect of opposing forces. Van der Waals forces, viscous binding, and solid bridges help to hold particles together, whereas electrostatic repulsion (zeta potential) tends to disaggregate crystal particles. Van der Waals forces are attractive forces between molecules *(2)*. There are three principal types of intermolecular (van der Waals) forces: dipole–dipole attractions; hydrogen bond forces; and London forces *(2)*. The van der Waals force is inversely proportional to the distance between two particles to the sixth power when they are at a short distance from each other, or inversely proportional to the squared distance between them at a further distance *(39)*. The viscous binding is derived from the "sticky" properties imparted by hydrophilic molecules on the particle surface. This occurs when adsorbed substances on the particles adhere to each other. The zeta potential reflects the repulsive force between two particles; it is the electric potential at the interface between a colloid particle and its surrounding solution *(39)*. Human urine is a colloid system consisting of urinary stone components and macromolecular organic particles. The macromolecular organic particles are responsible for stabilizing this colloid system *(39)*. For example, COM in water has a zeta potential of approx +20 mV *(40)*. In urine, however, the zeta potential of COM shifts to approx -5 mV. It is believed that the adsorption of negatively charged urinary components such as citrate, pyrophosphate, and acidic polymers results in the reduction of the zeta potential of COM. Further reduction in COM zeta potential (approx -20 mV) can be induced by the adsorption of Tamm-Horsfall protein derived from normal subjects *(39)*. Reductions of the zeta potential lead to energy barriers that minimize COM crystal aggregation. Shear forces can either enhance or inhibit aggregation. For example, shear forces increase the probability of particle collision, which favors aggregation but also at the same time disrupts aggregated particles *(41)*. Aggregation is influenced by the saturation of the solution, although it can occur in supersaturated as well as undersaturated solutions *(24,42)*.

Crystal aggregation likely plays an important role in urinary stone formation. Several pieces of evidence support this theory. Crystalline clumps are frequently seen in the center of calculi, particularly in whewellite/weddellite, uric acid, and brushite stones *(25)*. Highly aggregated structures are noted in microscopic examinations and ultrastructural analyses of renal stones. Iwata et al. developed a partial dissolution method and used a scanning electron microscope to examine the internal architecture of COM urinary calculi *(43)*. They found all calculi have three distinct zones. A core zone is composed of randomly aggregated platelike crystals with frequent rosette formations. An intermediate area is composed of radially arranged piles of sheetlike crystals. The peripheral layer shows concentric laminations and each layer of lamination is composed of minute crystals. Khan and Hackett also studied architectural details and intercrystalline associations of urinary calculi and demonstrated that all stones have a central nucleus region and a peripheral zone *(44)*. The former contains an aggregate of discernible individual crystals. The peripheral region, on the other hand, consists of concentric layers of either discrete crystals or solid striated material.

Robertson et al. found that recurrent calcium stone formers tend to excrete larger calcium oxalate crystals (10–20 μm in diameter) than those (3–4 μm in diameter) in nonstone formers *(12)*. Moreover, the crystals of stone formers often fused into polycrystalline aggregates 20–300 μm in diameter. In a study, measuring the effects of urines from healthy subjects and from calcium oxalate stone formers, Kok et al. demonstrated that the urines from stone formers had a similar effect on the solubility, but a significantly lower ability to inhibit the crystal growth and the crystal aggregation *(45)*. They concluded that defective inhibition of the kinetic process of crystal aggregation constitutes a major physiochemical mechanism of calcium oxalate renal stone formation, which appears to be modulated by urinary citrate concentrations. Subsequent studies have suggested that Tamm-Horsfall protein from stone formers bear functional abnormalities resulting in decreased ability to inhibit calcium oxalate crystal aggregation *(39,46,47)*. Furthermore, a single crystal can never reach a size large enough to be retained within the kidney by crystal growth alone *(48)* but the speed of aggregation is rapid enough to allow development of significantly sized particles within seconds *(42)*. These observations reveal the potential role of crystal aggregation in urinary stone formation.

EPITAXY

Multicomponent urinary stones are frequently observed. These stones, when sectioned, have distinct concentric rings. Different layers contain different components but each layer has a homogeneous crystalline composition *(25)*. Although the mechanism of growth in these multicomponent stones is not fully understood, epitaxy has been suggested to play a significant role.

During the process of multicomponent stone formation, the molecules on the surface of one layer must bind to the molecules of a different component in a specific order such that the growth of the new component can be incorporated and promoted. For this to happen, the regular and predictable crystal lattices of the two different components must be chemically compatible and supportive of each other at the contact zone. Epitaxy describes the process of oriented growth of one crystalline lattice over another crystalline lattice whose dimensions are similar *(49)*. In general, epitaxy can be considered a special type of heterogeneous nucleation. The major forces holding these structures together can be explained by analyzing the crystal structures of the common components of renal calculi. In cation-containing structures, such as whewellite, weddellite, brushite, apatite, and monosodium urate monohydrate, the major force is cation–anion attraction. In the noncation-containing structures, such as uric acid, uric acid dihydrate, and L-cystine, the major force is a hydrogen bonding network *(49)*.

A clinical example to support the theory of epitaxy is the association of hyperuricosuria with calcium oxalate stone formation. It has been well documented that patients with hyperuricosuria may form calcium-salt stones even if they are normocalciuric and otherwise have no other risk factors for stone formation *(50,51)*. It is postulated that monosodium urate or uric acid first crystallizes because of hyperuricosuric supersaturation. These crystals either act as seed crystals for inducing epitaxy of calcium oxalate or adsorb normally occurring macromolecular inhibitors of calcium oxalate crystallization in urine that may not have been sufficiently supersaturated for the spontaneous nucleation of calcium oxalate crystals *(52,53)*. Based on a crystallographic dimensional comparison for a substrate crystal of uric acid and an epitaxial layer of calcium oxalate monohydrate, the crystalline lattice of both components match *(49)*. This theoretical comparison of the dimensions of the prominent crystal growth faces was first published by Lonsdale in 1968 *(54)*. Mandel et al. extended the calculation of the percentage misfit. The criteria used by them included the lengths of the two lattice vectors in the selected two-dimensional slice through the three-dimensional structure, the angles between these two lattice vectors defining the possible contact face, and a parameter indicating the general complexity of the associated atomic pattern on the potential contact plane *(49)*. In addition, they analyzed the atomic structures of the two contacting crystal lattices. The atomic overlay at the interface is excellent in the calcium oxalate monohydrate–uric acid system. The two-dimensional misfit in this system is predicted to be less than 5% *(49)*. Clinically, treatment of hyperuricosuria with allopurinol or purine restriction has been found to reduce the recurrence rate of hyperuricosuric calcium-based stones *(50,51,55,56)*.

MATRIX

Analysis of urinary stones reveals that they are not simply composed of crystals but rather contain a noncrystalline protein-like component, termed matrix. The percentage of matrix, by weight, in urinary stones varies. In general, most solid urinary stones have a matrix content of about 3% by weight *(57)*. Matrix stones, however, may contain up to 65% of matrix *(58,59)*. Although the matrix can be found throughout a urinary stone, it is not evenly distributed. Warpehoski and colleagues reported that matrix from the core of calcium oxalate stones weighed an average of 2.7% but total matrix weight was 5.7% when the outer zone of the stones was analyzed *(60)*.

Chemical analysis of stone matrix reveals approx 65% is hexosamine and 10% is bound water *(61)*. Many other compounds have been isolated from matrix, such as matrix substance A *(62)*, a protein containing large amounts of γ-carboxyglutamic acid *(63)*, nephrocalcin *(64)*, Tamm-Horsfall glycoprotein *(65)*, renal lithostatine *(66)*, albumin *(61)*, glycosaminoglycans *(67–69)*, and free carbohydrates *(70)*.

Nephrolithiasis is one of the manifestations of pathological calcification, which by definition includes all calcium salt deposits in soft tissues as well as concretions of calcium salts in the secretory and excretory passages of the body. In humans, calcium salts are deposited normally in the formation of bone. In the process of bone formation, osteoblasts produce the extracellular organic matrix, which initially lacks mineral deposits *(71)*. Deposits of inorganic mineral salts then begin to appear throughout the matrix. These deposits increase in size and number and begin to coalesce, thereby progressively displacing water until the matrix becomes completely mineralized. Whether the stone matrix has a role in the promotion of urinary stone formation, like the bone matrix described previously, or whether it is incorporated by nonspecific adsorption is unknown *(72)*. Many studies have been conducted to identify the role of matrix in urinary stone formation *(67,68,73–75)*. Although several encouraging findings have been reported, there is still no satisfactory theory to explain the importance of urinary stone matrix in the development of urinary stones.

INHIBITORS AND PROMOTERS

This review of the pathogenesis of urinary stone formation would be incomplete without mentioning inhibitors and promoters. Urine contains substances that influence crystallization processes, and therefore regulate stone formation. Substances that reduce the crystallization are called inhibitors whereas those that increase crystallization are termed promoters. Inhibitors and promoters of urinary stones will be discussed in subsequent chapters.

CRYSTAL RETENTION

Previous sections in this chapter have explained theories about crystal precipitation, growth, and aggregation. None of these elements would result in urinary stone formation if the nucleated crystals were flushed out by urinary flow. Crystal retention is therefore a key factor. Crystal retention will result if the crystals grow large enough to be trapped in renal tubules or if they adhere to urothelium before excretion. The earliest evidence of crystal retention was the finding of macroscopic plaques of subepithelial deposits of calcium crystals in renal papillae by Randall in 1940 *(76)*. He proposed that these calcific deposits originate in damaged renal tubule epithelial basement membranes and later erode into the urinary collecting system. These plaques, now known as Randall's plaques, are thought to serve as a nidus for urinary stone formation *(77,78)*. The incidence of calcified papillary plaques was 19.6% of cadaveric renal units *(76)*. Stoller et al., by using high resolution radiography, demonstrated papillary calcifications in 57% of radiographically imaged cadaveric kidneys *(77)*. They also showed a correlation between a history of hypertension and papillary calcifications. To further investigate the association between papillary calcifications and urinary stone formation, the presence, pattern, and distribution of Randall's plaques were mapped endoscopically in patients *(78)*. This study revealed the incidence of plaques varied with the primary composition of extracted stones. In addition, the incidence of papillary plaques was significantly more common in patients with calcium oxalate (88%) and calcium phosphate stones (100%) than in patients without a history of urinary stone disease (43%) *(78)*. These findings suggest that the presence of papillary plaques is associated with calcium nephrolithiasis and may contribute to the pathogenesis of calcium urinary stones.

Many groups have investigated the concept of crystal retention leading to our current understanding. Normal urothelium has been shown to bear a protective mechanism against nucleation and adhesion of calcium oxalate crystals *(79)*. Chemically injured urothelium will lose this property resulting in the adherence of calcium oxalate crystals *(79–81)*. Gill and associates have demonstrated that heparin, a sulfated heteropolysaccharide of glucuronic acid and glucosamine, could restore the anticrystal adherence property of injured urothelium *(81)*. Other sulfated polysaccharides, sulfated glycosaminoglycans, and monosaccharides were, however, not effective in the restoration of protection against calcium oxalate crystal adhesion. The glycosaminoglycan layer of normal urothelium plays an important role against bacterial adherence and is also responsible for preventing crystal adherence *(82,83)*. The exact mechanism of action is unknown but it has been postulated that the sulfur groups on glycosaminoglycan molecules will bind large quantities of water molecules forming a "water barrier" on the cell surface thereby inhibiting calcium oxalate crystal and bacterial adherence *(84)*. Pantazopoulos et al. have demonstrated that treating chemically injured urothelium with sodium pentosanpolysulfate, a semisynthetic glycosaminoglycan with an electric charge similar to that of natural glycosaminoglycan, and carbenoxolone sodium, an ester of β-glycyrrentinic acid and succinic acid having the ability of increasing production of glycosaminoglycan, could restore the protective property of urothelium to prevent crystal adhesion *(85)*. It has been postulated that the crystal adherence reaction is mediated through cell surface substances, termed crystal-binding molecules *(86)*. Several compounds, including phosphatidylserine *(87,88)*, sialic acid *(89)*, collagen type IV *(90)*, osteopontin *(91)*, and hyaluronan *(86)*, have been shown to be candidates of crystal-binding molecules. Despite decades of research focusing on crystal–cell interaction, the definite crystal-binding molecules and the mechanisms of urothelial injury in recurrent stone formers are awaiting to be elucidated.

The crystal–renal cell interaction is supported by clinical observations and laboratory studies *(92)*. For example, endocytosis of calcium oxalate crystals was observed in a patient with type 1 primary hyperoxaluria *(93)*. In studies using monkey renal epithelial cells as a model of the distal tubular epithelium, COM crystals were endocytosed by the cells and cellular proliferation was induced *(94,95)*. The interaction is influenced by the type of crystal *(22)*, the presence of a crystal coat *(96)*, the type of cell surface *(97)*, and the surface electric charge *(89,98)*. Once adhered, the particles are subsequently internalized into the epithelial cells through endocytosis; altered gene expression, cytoskeletal alterations, and cellular proliferation can then occur *(92)*.

CONCLUSIONS

Urinary stone formation likely starts after crystallization, which is induced by urinary supersaturation. Supersaturation alone cannot explain the process of stone formation. Urine is a complex solution with frequent changes in pH. The presence of multiple inorganic and organic constituents and interactions between promoters and inhibitors, all modulate the already complicated pathogenesis of stone formation. Crystalline material is nucleated somewhere inside the nephron. Crystals of calcium phosphate are predominantly formed in the proximal and distal renal tubules, whereas, calcium oxalate is the primary crystallization product in the collecting ducts *(38,99)*. The formed calcium phosphate crystals flow toward collecting ducts and likely serve as nidi and induce heterogeneous nucleation of calcium oxalate. These particles grow via crystal aggregation into the size range of, or even greater than, the inner diameter of the collecting ducts and thus might be retained *(100)*. The aggregated particles may also adhere to the renal epithelium through the mechanism of crystal–renal cell interaction or may be retained by anatomic abnormalities, such as ectatic tubules or ureteropelvic junction obstruction. Either way, these particles will have chance to grow into clinically significant stones, which may be unable to pass through the urinary tract in a spontaneous fashion. There is insufficient evidence to understand the entire process of urinary stone formation, however, the processes described above help explain how a crystal will form, grow, aggregate with other crystals, and ultimately be retained in the kidney.

REFERENCES

1. Menon M, Resnick MI: Urinary lithiasis: etiology, diagnosis, and medical management. In: Campbell's Urology, 8th Ed., vol. 4, (Walsh PC, Retik AB, Vaughan ED, Jr, et al., eds.). Saunders, Philadelphia, PA, 2002; pp. 3229–3305.
2. Dickerson RE, Gray HB, Darensbourg MY, et al. Chemical Principles, 4th Ed. Benjamin/Cummings, Menlo Park, CA, 1984; pp. 158–212.
3. Randolph AD, Drach GW. A proposal of standardized nomenclature in the study of crystallization in biological systems, e.g. urolithiasis. Presented at the Proceedings of the Fourth International Symposium on Urolithiasis Research, Williamsburg, VA, 1980.

4. Worcester EM. Inhibitors of stone formation. Semin Nephrol 1996; 16: 474.

5. Finlayson B. Calcium stones: Some physical and clinical aspects. In: Calcium Metabolism in Renal Failure and Nephrolithiasis, (David D, ed.). John Wiley, New York, NY, 1977; pp. 337–382.

6. Finlayson B. Physicochemical aspects of urolithiasis. Kidney Int 1978; 13: 344.

7. Werness PG, Brown CM, Smith LH, et al. EQUIL2: a BASIC computer program for the calculation of urinary saturation. J Urol 1985; 134: 1242.

8. Tiselius HG. Solution chemistry of supersaturation. In: Kidney Stones: Medical and Surgical Management. (Coe FL, Favus MJ, Pak CYC, et al., eds.) Lippincott-Raven, Philadelphia, 1996; pp. 33–64.

9. Cifuentes Delatte L. Crystalluria. In: Stones: Clinical Management of Urolithiasis. (Roth RA, Finlayson B, eds.) Williams & Wilkins, Baltimore, MD, 1983; pp. 23–52.

10. Werness P G, Bergert JH, Smith LH. Crystalluria. J Crystal Growth 1981; 53: 166.

11. Robertson WG, Peacock M. Calcium oxalate crystalluria and inhibitors of crystallization in recurrent renal stone-formers. Clin Sci 1972; 43: 499.

12. Robertson WG, Peacock M, Nordin BE. Calcium crystalluria in recurrent renal-stone formers. Lancet 1969; 2: 21.

13. Elliot JS, Rabinowitz IN, Silvert M. Calcium oxalate crystalluria. J Urol 1976; 116: 773.

14. Elliot JS, Rabinowitz IN. Calcium oxalate crystalluria: crystal size in urine. J Urol 1980; 123: 324.

15. Fleisch H. Inhibitors and promoters of stone formation. Kidney Int 1978; 13: 361.

16. Gardner GL. Kinetics of the dehydration of calcium oxalate trihydrate crystals in aqueous solution. J Colloid Interface Sci 1976; 54: 298.

17. Tomazic BB. Nancollas GH. A study of the phase transformation of calcium oxalate trihydrate-monohydrate. Invest Urol 1979; 16: 329.

18. Tomazic BB, Nancollas GH. Crystal growth of calcium oxalate hydrate: a comparative kinetic study. J Colloid Interface Sci 1980; 75: 149.

19. Nakai H, Yanagawa M, Kameda K, et al. Transformation of calcium oxalate dihydrate crystals in solution: why is not calcium oxalate dihydrate detected in urinary calculi? Presented at the Proceedings of the Eighth International Symposium on Urolithiasis, Dallas, TX, 1996.

20. Hesse A, Berg W, Schneider HJ, et al.: A contribution to the formation mechanism of calcium oxalate urinary calculi. II. In vitro experiments concerning the theory of the formation of Whewellite and Weddellite urinary calculi. Urol Res 1976; 4: 157.

21. Berg W, Hesse A, Schneider HJ. A contribution to the formation mechanism of calcium oxalate urinary calculi. III. On the role of magnesium in the formation of oxalate calculi. Urol Res 1976; 4: 161.

22. Wesson JA, Worcester EM, Kleinman JG, et al. Inhibitor proteins in urine favor formation of calcium oxalate dihydrate crystals, which have a smaller affinity for renal tubule cells than monohydrate. Presented at the Proceedings of the Eighth International Symposium on Urolithiasis, Dallas, TX, 1996.

23. Garten VA, Head RB. Homogeneous nucleation and phenomenon of crystalloluminescence. Phil Mag 1966; 14: 1243.

24. Kok DJ. The role of crystallization processes in calcium oxalate urolithiasis: University of Leiden 1991.

25. Mandel NS, Mandel GS. Physicochemistry of urinary stone formation. In: Renal Stone Disease. (Pak CYC, ed.) Martinus Nijhoff, Boston, MA, 1987; pp. 1–24.

26. Prien EL. Studies in urolithiasis: II. relationships between pathogenesis, structure, and composition and calculi. J Urol 1949; 61: 821.

27. Sutor DJ, Wooley SE. Composition of urinary calculi by x-ray diffraction: collected data from various localities. IX-XI. Br J Urol 1971; 43: 268.

28. Brien G, Schubert G, Bick C. 10,000 analyses of urinary calculi using X-ray diffraction and polarizing microscopy. Eur Urol 1982; 8: 251.

29. Pak CY. Physicochemical basis for formation of renal stones of calcium phosphate origin: calculation of the degree of saturation of urine with respect to brushite. J Clin Invest 1969; 48: 1914.

30. Lanzalaco AC, Singh RP, Smesko SA, et al. The influence of urinary macromolecules on calcium oxalate monohydrate crystal growth. J Urol 1988; 139: 190.

31. Baumann JM. Can the formation of calcium oxalate stones be explained by crystallization processes in urine? Urol Res 1985; 13: 267.
32. Meyer JL, Bergert JH, Smith LH. Epitaxial relationships in urolithiasis: the calcium oxalate monohydrate-hydroxyapatite system. Clin Sci Mol Med 1975; 49: 369.
33. Nancollas GH, Mohan MS. The growth of hydroxyapatite crystals. Arch Oral Biol 1970; 15: 731.
34. Berg C, Tiselius HG. The effects of citrate on hydroxyapatite induced calcium oxalate crystallization and on the formation of calcium phosphate crystals. Urol Res 1989; 17: 167.
35. Meyer, J. L., Bergert, J. H., Smith, L. H.: Epitaxial relationships in urolithiasis: the brushite-whewellite system. Clin Sci Mol Med 1977; 52: 143.
36. Finlayson B, Reid F. The expectation of free and fixed particles in urinary stone disease. Invest Urol 1978; 15: 442.
37. Coe F, Parks JH. Defenses of an unstable compromise: crystallization inhibitors and the kidney's role in mineral regulation. Kid Int 1990; 38: 625.
38. Luptak J, Bek-Jensen H, Fornander A-M, et al. Crystallization of calcium oxalate and calcium phosphate at supersaturation levels corresponding to those in different parts of the nephron. Scanning Microsc 1994; 8: 47.
39. Boeve ER, Cao LC, De Bruijn WC, et al. Zeta potential distribution on calcium oxalate crystal and Tamm-Horsfall protein surface analyzed with Doppler electrophoretic light scattering. J Urol 1994; 152: 531.
40. Curreri P, Onoda GY, Finlayson B. An electrophoretic study of calcium oxalate monohydrate. J Colloid Interface Sci 1979; 69: 170.
41. Hess B, Kok DJ. Nucleation, growth, and aggregation of stone-forming crystals. In: Kidney Stones: Medical and Surgical Management. (Coe FL, Favus MJ, Pak CYC, et al., eds.). Lippincott-Raven, Philadelphia, PA, 1996; pp. 3–32.
42. Blomen LJMJ. Growth and agglomeration of calcium oxalate crystals, [dissertation] University of Leiden, 1982.
43. Iwata H, Nishio S, Wakatsuki A, et al. Architecture of calcium oxalate monohydrate urinary calculi. J Urol 1985; 133: 334.
44. Khan SR, Hackett RL. Role of organic matrix in urinary stone formation: an ultrastructural study of crystal matrix interface of calcium oxalate monohydrate stones. J Urol 1993; 150: 239.
45. Kok DJ, Papapoulos SE, Bijvoet OL. Crystal agglomeration is a major element in calcium oxalate urinary stone formation. Kid Int 1990; 37: 51.
46. Wiggins RC. Uromucoid (Tamm-Horsfall glycoprotein) forms different polymeric arrangements on a filter surface under different physicochemical conditions. Clin Chim Acta 1987; 162: 329.
47. Hess B, Nakagawa Y, Parks JH, et al. Molecular abnormality of Tamm-Horsfall glycoprotein in calcium oxalate nephrolithiasis. Am J Physiol 1991; 260: F569.
48. Burns JR, Finlayson B, Gauthier J. Calcium oxalate retention in subjects with crystalluria. Urol Int 1984; 39: 36.
49. Mandel NS, Mandel GS. Epitaxis in renal stones. In: Renal Tract Stone: Metabolic Basis and Clinical Practice. (Wickham JEA, Colin Buck A, eds.). Churchill Livingstone, Edinburgh, UK, 1990; pp. 87–101.
50. Coe FL, Raisen L. Allopurinol treatment of uric-acid disorders in calcium-stone formers. Lancet 1973; 1: 129.
51. Coe FL, Kavalach AG. Hypercalciuria and hyperuricosuria in patients with calcium nephrolithiasis. N Engl J Med 1974; 291: 1344.
52. Pak CY, Waters O, Arnold L, et al. Mechanism for calcium urolithiasis among patients with hyperuricosuria: supersaturation of urine with respect to monosodium urate. J Clin Invest 1977; 59: 426.
53. Coe FL, Strauss AL, Tembe V, et al. Uric acid saturation in calcium nephrolithiasis. Kid Int 1980; 17: 662.
54. Lonsdale K. Epitaxy as a growth factor in urinary calculi and gallstones. Nature 1968; 217: 56.
55. Coe FL. Treated and untreated recurrent calcium nephrolithiasis in patients with idiopathic hypercalciuria, hyperuricosuria, or no metabolic disorder. Ann Intern Med 1977; 87: 404.
56. Smith MJ. Placebo versus allopurinol for renal calculi. J Urol 1977; 117: 690.

57. Boyce W, King J, Jr. Crystal-matrix interrelations in calculi. J Urol 1959; 81: 351.
58. Allen TD, Spence HM. Matrix stones. J Urol 1966; 95: 284.
59. Mall JC, Collins PA, Lyon ES. Matrix calculi. Br J Radiol 1975; 48: 807.
60. Warpehoski MA, Buscemi PJ, Osborn DC, et al. Distribution of organic matrix in calcium oxalate renal calculi. Calcif Tissue Int 1981; 33: 211.
61. Boyce WH. Organic matrix of human urinary concretions. Am J Med 1968; 45: 673.
62. Boyce WH, King JS, Jr, Fielden ML. Total nondialyzable solids (TNDS) in human urine. VIII. Immunological detection of a component peculiar to renal calculous matrix and to urine of calculous patients. J Clin Invest 1962; 41: 1180.
63. Lian JB, Prien EL, Jr, Glimcher MJ, et al. The presence of protein-bound gamma-carboxyglutamic acid in calcium-containing renal calculi. J Clin Invest 1977; 59: 1151.
64. Nakagawa Y, Ahmed M, Hall SL, et al. Isolation from human calcium oxalate renal stones of nephrocalcin, a glycoprotein inhibitor of calcium oxalate crystal growth. Evidence that nephrocalcin from patients with calcium oxalate nephrolithiasis is deficient in gamma-carboxyglutamic acid. J Clin Invest 1987; 79: 1782.
65. Grant AM, Baker LR, Neuberger A. Urinary Tamm-Horsfall glycoprotein in certain kidney diseases and its content in renal and bladder calculi. Clin Sci 1973; 44: 377.
66. Verdier JM, Dussol B, Casanova P, et al. [Renal lithostathine: a new protein inhibitor of lithogenesis]. Nephrologie 1993; 14: 261.
67. Roberts SD, Resnick MI. Glycosaminoglycans content of stone matrix. J Urol 1986; 135: 1078.
68. Nishio S, Abe Y, Wakatsuki A, et al. Matrix glycosaminoglycan in urinary stones. J Urol 1985; 134: 503.
69. Yamaguchi S, Yoshioka T, Utsunomiya M, et al. Heparin sulfate in the stone matrix and its inhibitory effect on calcium oxalate crystallization. Urol Res 1993; 21: 187.
70. King JS, Boyce WH. Amino acid and carbohydrate composition of the mucoprotein matrix in various calculi. Proc Soc Exp Biol Med 1957; 95: 183.
71. Frost HM. The Physiology of Cartilaginous, Fibrous, and Bony Tissue. Charles C. Thomas, Springfield, OH, 1972.
72. Roberts SR, Resnick MI. Urinary stone matrix. In: Renal tract stone: metabolic basis and clinical practice. Wickham JEA, Colin Buck A. Churchill Livingstone, Edinburgh, OH, 1990; 59–70.
73. Kimura Y, Kisaki N, Ise K. The role of the matrix substance in formation of urinary stones. Urol Int 1976; 31: 355.
74. Leal JJ, Finlayson B. Adsorption of naturally occurring polymers onto calcium oxalate crystal surfaces. Invest Urol 1977; 14: 278.
75. Khan SR, Finlayson B, Hackett RL. Stone matrix as proteins adsorbed on crystal surfaces: a microscopic study. Scan Electron Microsc 1983; 379–385.
76. Randall A. Etiology of primary renal calculus. Int Abst Surg 1940; 71: 209.
77. Stoller ML, Low RK, Shami GS, et al. High resolution radiography of cadaveric kidneys: unraveling the mystery of Randall's plaque formation. J Urol 1996; 156: 1263.
78. Low RK, Stoller ML. Endoscopic mapping of renal papillae for Randall's plaques in patients with urinary stone disease. J Urol 1997; 158: 2062.
79. Gill WB, Ruggiero KJ, Fromes MC. Elevation of the metastable limits and absence of container surface nucleation for calcium oxalate crystallization in a urothelial-lined system as compared to glass containers. Invest Urol 1980; 18: 158.
80. Gill WB, Ruggiero K, Straus FH, 2nd. Crystallization studies in a urothelial-lined living test tube (the catheterized female rat bladder). I. Calcium oxalate crystal adhesion to the chemically injured rat bladder. Invest Urol 1979; 17: 257.
81. Gill WB, Jones KW, Ruggiero KJ. Protective effects of heparin and other sulfated glycosaminoglycans on crystal adhesion to injured urothelium. J Urol 1982; 127: 152.
82. Parsons CL, Greenspan C, Mulholland SG. The primary antibacterial defense mechanism of the bladder. Invest Urol 1975; 13: 72.
83. Parsons CL, Greenspan C, Moore SW, et al. Role of surface mucin in primary antibacterial defense of bladder. Urology 1977; 9: 48.
84. Parsons CL, Mulholland SG, Anwar H. Antibacterial activity of bladder surface mucin duplicated by exogenous glycosaminoglycan (heparin). Infect Immun 1979; 24: 552.

85. Pantazopoulos D, Karagiannakos P, Sofras F, et al. Effect of drugs on crystal adhesion to injured urothelium. Urology 1990; 36: 255.

86. Asselman M, Verkoelen CF. Crystal-cell interaction in the pathogenesis of kidney stone disease. Curr Opin Urol 2002; 12: 271.

87. Bigelow MW, Wiessner JH, Kleinman JG, et al. Surface exposure of phosphatidylserine increases calcium oxalate crystal attachment to IMCD cells. Am J Physiol 1997; 272: F55.

88. Wiessner JH, Hasegawa AT, Hung LY, et al. Mechanisms of calcium oxalate crystal attachment to injured renal collecting duct cells. Kid Int 2001; 59: 637.

89. Lieske JC, Leonard R, Swift H, et al. Adhesion of calcium oxalate monohydrate crystals to anionic sites on the surface of renal epithelial cells. Am J Physiol 1996; 270: F192.

90. Kohri K, Kodama M, Ishikawa Y, et al. Immunofluorescent study on the interaction between collagen and calcium oxalate crystals in the renal tubules. Eur Urol 1991; 19: 249.

91. Yamate T, Kohri K, Umekawa T, et al. Interaction between osteopontin on madin darby canine kidney cell membrane and calcium oxalate crystal. Urol Int 1999; 62: 81.

92. Lieske JC, Toback FG. Interaction of urinary crystals with renal epithelial cells in the pathogenesis of nephrolithiasis. Semin Nephrol 1996; 16: 458.

93. Lieske JC, Spargo BH, Toback FG. Endocytosis of calcium oxalate crystals and proliferation of renal tubular epithelial cells in a patient with type 1 primary hyperoxaluria. J Urol 1992; 148: 1517.

94. Lieske JC, Toback FG. Regulation of renal epithelial cell endocytosis of calcium oxalate mono-hydrate crystals. Am J Physiol 1993; 264: F800.

95. Lieske JC, Walsh-Reitz MM, Toback FG. Calcium oxalate monohydrate crystals are endocytosed by renal epithelial cells and induce proliferation. Am J Physiol 1992; 262: F622.

96. Tamura M, Kohjimoto Y, Ebisuno S, et al. The effects of human urine on the adhesion of calcium oxalate crystals to MDCK cells. Presented at the Proceedings of the Eighth International Symposium on Urolithiasis, Dallas, TX, 1996.

97. Bigelow MW, Kleinman JG, Wiessner JH, et al. Calcium oxalate crystal attachment to IMCD membranes: dependence on membrane composition and structure. Presented at the Proceedings of the Eighth International Symposium on Urolithiasis, Dallas, TX, 1996.

98. Lieske JC, Leonard R, Toback FG. Adhesion of calcium oxalate monohydrate crystals to renal epithelial cells is inhibited by specific anions. Am J Physiol 1995; 268: F604.

99. Kok DJ. Intratubular crystallization events. World J Urol 1997; 15: 219.

100. Kok DJ, Khan SR. Calcium oxalate nephrolithiasis, a free or fixed particle disease. Kidney Int 1994; 46: 847.

5 Structure and Compositional Analysis of Kidney Stones

Ian Mandel and Neil Mandel, PhD

Key Words: Nephrolithiasis; crystal; stone composition.

INTRODUCTION

It is well established that human urine is supersaturated with respect to ions and molecules, which can crystallize as clinical crystalluria with a potential for stone development. Regardless of the specific site of crystallization within the nephron, crystals can either pass from the kidney into the bladder and be excreted or attach to cells in the late collecting duct and grow into mature kidney stones. The crystalline composition of a stone reflects the urine chemistry and abnormalities in tubular physiology during the process of stone development. Accurate knowledge of the composition of the stone is critical to elucidating the underlying etiology of the patient's clinical disorder(s) that precipitated the stone disease.

Crystalline material is the primary constituent of most human urinary tract stones. All stones contain macromolecules and other cellular components from the urine, termed matrix, and the amount of matrix normally approaches 2–5%, although some stones can be composed entirely of matrix. Most human stones contain more than one crystalline component and are termed multicomponent stones. The presence of multicomponent

From: Current Clinical Urology, *Urinary Stone Disease:*
A Practical Guide to Medical and Surgical Management
Edited by: M. L. Stoller and M. V. Meng © Humana Press Inc., Totowa, NJ

Table 1

The Chemical Name, Composition, Mineral Name, and Abbreviation
of the Most Common Components of Human Urinary Tract Calculi

Chemical name	Mineral name	Chemical formula	Abbreviation
Oxalates			
• Calcium oxalate monohydrate	Whewellite	$CaC_2O_4 \cdot H_2O$	WH
• Calcium oxalate dihydrate	Weddellite	$CaC_2O_4 \cdot (2+x)H_2O$	WE
Phosphates			
• Basic calcium phosphate	Apatite	$Ca_5(PO_4)_3(OH)$	AP
• Calcium hydrogen phosphate	Brushite	$CaHPO_4 \cdot 2H_2O$	BR
• Magnesium ammonium phosphate hexahydrate	Struvite	$MgNH_4PO_4 \cdot 6H_2O$	ST
Purines			
• Uric acid		$C_5H_4N_4O_3$	UA
• Monosodium urate monohydrate		$NaC_5H_3N_4O_3 \cdot H_2O$	MSU
Other			
• L-Cystine		$(-SCH_2CHNH_2COOH)_2$	CY

Table 2
Relative Frequency of Occurrence of Admixed Stones [a]

Country No. Stones	USA (13) 1,000	Glasgow (15) 149	Berlin (11) 10,000	USA (5) 3,833
WH	13.7	4	24.9	23.4
WE	0.4	1	0.6	4.7
WH/WE	18.6	21	33.2	29.4
WH/WE/AP	22.4	45[b]	13.5	5.2
WH/AP	7.2	45[b]	2.9	2.7
WE/AP	4.7	45[b]	0.3	1.3
AP	3.4	5	1.1	6.6
ST/AP	15.5	14	7.0	6.4
ST	0.4	—	0.3	4.3
WH/ST/AP	—	3	1.4	0.0
UA	4.7	—	2.4	5.2
UA/UD	—	1	3.9	1.6
WH/UA	—	—	2.9	1.5
WH/UA/UD	—	—	1.8	0.2
BR	—	2	0.4	1.2
CY	2.2	1	0.2	0.4

[a] No. stones represents number of samples included in study.

[b] Frequency of occurrence of both whewellite and weddelite mixed with apatite reported as a single group.

stones suggests multiple physiologic conditions that must be unraveled in the process of defining the optimal medical management and the avoidance of stone recurrence.

The major crystalline components of human urinary tract stones are listed in Table 1. Prevalence of crystalline admixtures from multiple studies of multicomponent stones is presented in Table 2. Currently, there are two analysis methods that are routinely used for stone analysis, namely X-ray powder diffraction crystallography (XRD) and Fourier transform infrared spectroscopy (FTIR). These two analysis methods differentiate stone crystalline composition based on either the uniqueness of crystalline structures or subtle energy differences associated with the motion of atoms in chemical bonds found in the various stone components. It is worthwhile to first address the chemistry of stone components and aspects of various crystalline structures seen in stones before discussing the unique aspects and capabilities of the two primary methods of stone analysis.

CHEMISTRY AND STRUCTURES FOUND IN STONES

The primary component of human stones, calcium oxalate, crystallizes in two different chemical and crystallographic forms: a monohydrate and a dihydrate structural complex. Calcium oxalate is a calcium salt of a dicarboxylic acid, oxalic acid. The differences in the degree of water of crystallization included in the crystalline lattice results in two different crystalline structures, leading to different growth morphologies, different atomic structures on the crystal surfaces of the two hydrated structures, and different effective biologic activities.

The second major class of components of stones includes phosphate salts. Four different calcium phosphate salts and two magnesium phosphate salts are found in stones. The calcium phosphate salts vary in calcium-to-phosphate ratio, hydroxyl-vs-hydrogen ion content, and the degree of water of crystallization included in the crystalline lattice structure. The magnesium phosphate salts differ by inclusion of either ammonium or hydrogen ions and the degree of water of crystallization in the crystalline lattice structure. Similarities in chemistry, but differences in crystalline structures, often create challenges in composition analysis using infrared spectroscopic analysis that are focused at differentiating chemistry.

All of the calcium and magnesium salts have different crystalline structures and are easily differentiated by XRD methods of analysis, but sensitivity of detection can complicate and challenge a complete analysis. Similarly, the purine structural moieties include subtle chemical and structural variations of the uric acid-like six/five-member aromatic ring structure. Addition of carbonyl groups to the purine ring moiety separates related structures such as hypoxanthine, xanthine, and uric acid. The salts of the purine organic acids and variations in the degree of water of crystallization induce additional chemical and structural variation in the identification criteria for definitive compositional analysis. The preceding description regarding the method of analysis for the oxalates and phosphates in stones is also applicable to the purines and their salts. Similar chemistry leads to very subtle differences in infrared spectra, but they lead to significant differences in XRD data. The miscellaneous components are sufficiently unique that analyses by either the XRD or the FTIR method is straightforward, assuming accurate standards are available.

Need for instrumentation sensitivity and more importantly accurate standards for comparison are critical for successful stone analysis using either XRD or FTIR analysis methods. The two methods of analysis used separately have unique capabilities depending on the type of stone being analyzed. It is clear that the two analysis methods used collectively yield the highest degree of certainty in compositional analysis of urinary tract stones.

CRYSTALLURIA AND STONE MORPHOLOGY

Determination of crystalluria and probable crystalline composition must be accomplished using freshly voided urine and a polarizing microscope. The different crystalline components found in crystalluria reveal different growth morphologies when viewed with a polarizing microscope *(1,2)*. Many of the crystals demonstrate birefringence so observation of growth morphology is often more definitive. Calcium oxalate monohydrate can be observed as ovals or dumbbells and calcium oxalate dihydrate as bipyramids. Apatite crystals usually appear as an amorphous precipitate, and frequently grow as clumps of very small crystallites. Struvite crystals grow in a characteristic coffin lid shape. Uric acid crystals appear as flat parallelepiped plates, and cystine crystals appear as hexagonal plates. The most common growth morphologies of mature stones composed of components listed in Table 1 are described in the following sections.

Calcium Oxalate Monohydrate

These stones are frequently hard, dark brown, and often have a dull gray exterior. When sectioned, the stones often appear to grow in radial fashion from a nidus with wedges rounding off at their extremities creating a generally smooth exterior.

Calcium Oxalate Dihydrate

Pure dihydrate stones are usually small and spherical consisting of a tan or yellow cluster of platelets. The platelets are sharp and are arranged in various orientations.

Admixed monohydrate/dihydrate stones frequently have many of the characteristics of a dihydrate stone because dihydrate most frequently appears on the exterior of the admixed stone. These stones are normally larger than pure dihydrate stones, are often spherical, and have a cluster of yellow platelets surrounding a hard dark brown interior. The platelets are sharp and in various orientations. Occasionally, the interior is light brown in color and has a granular consistency.

Apatite

Pure apatite stones are usually small, white in color with a very fine granular surface, and they have a soft white chalklike interior. Occasionally, these stones are also light brown with a smooth shiny surface.

The most frequently occurring stone admixture of apatite or calcium oxalate monohydrate and calcium oxalate dihydrate is generally smooth, spherical, and has light brown platelets on the surface. The interior is normally layered with both white and light brown sections. Frequently, papillary casts are observed on one side of the stone with apatite located in the cast because it is often the first crystalline substance deposited. The dihydrate plates are normally observed on the opposing side from the papillary casts.

Struvite

Pure struvite stones are usually off-white to light brown in color with a rough textured surface. When sectioned, the interior of the stone contains white concentric rings, and occasionally the interior contains white porous granulated material. Struvite stones frequently grow in a staghorn shape.

Admixed struvite/apatite stones are usually light brown in color with a coarse, granular surface. The interior is normally intermixed with white and light brown layers.

Brushite

Pure brushite stones are normally clusters of beige, nodular material surrounding a crystalline interior with a cauliflower-like growth pattern. Occasionally, the surface has a yellow or white tinge.

Uric Acid

Uric acid stones are spherical with a smooth yellow-orange surface. When sectioned, the interior of the stone appears as orange concentric rings with little to no macroscopic substructure.

Uric Acid Dihydrate

The surface of uric acid dihydrate stones is often dark orange and the stone is composed of small spherical regions. When sectioned, the stones have a well-defined nidus with thick concentric rings composed of small needles that radiate from the center of the stone.

L-*Cystine*

Pure L-cystine stones are homogeneously composed of very small yellow spheroids.

Matrix

Matrix stones are noncrystalline and take on a variety of shapes and colors. The stones are composed of a variety of organic molecules including urinary macromolecules and membrane fragments *(3)*.

Other

Other substances that have been reported in stones include the drugs sulfamethoxazole, crixivan, guaifenesin, triamterene and 5-fluorocytosine, xanthine, 2,8-dihydroxyadenine, gypsum, and silicates following antacid therapy. Growth morphology for these components is often variable.

STONE ANALYSIS

XRD *(1–5)* and FTIR *(6–8)* are the most frequently used methods of stone analysis. Both XRD and FTIR methods require a very comprehensive and accurate library of standard diffraction or spectroscopic patterns for comparative analysis. The focus of these methods is the identification of the crystalline mineral composition of the stone with little emphasis on the macromolecular or other noncrystalline entities that may be present. XRD should be viewed as a semiquantitative method of analysis. XRD analysis should be presented in rank order of relative amounts of the stone components in multicomponent stones. FTIR spectral libraries allow for the reporting of relative percentage compositional analyses in multicomponent stones using computer algorithms that mathematically admix spectra of pure components at specified percent admixtures. Computer addition of spectra from components with significantly different infrared absorption characteristics can artificially and inappropriately skew spectral standard comparison methodology.

Virtually all crystal structures are unique is some structural aspect and their diffraction patterns can be differentiated from other structures and diffraction patterns. Highly sensitive and accurate XRD instruments are often necessary to differentiate some of the structures seen in stones as their chemistry and crystal structures can be similar.

The XRD data for the most common components of human kidney stones are presented in Table 3. The diffraction data are presented in crystallographic language as interplanar d-spacings in Ångstroms (d[Å]) associated with the distances between atoms in the structure and as diffraction intensities either relative to a weak vs strong scale or on a maximum of 100 scale *(4,9,10)*.

In practice, the experimental XRD patterns are compared with those for the standard patterns presented in Table 3. All diffraction lines of a given standard pattern, especially the strongest lines, must be matched with diffraction lines in the sample pattern. If some lines of a given intensity are thought to match a standard, then all lines with equal or greater intensity must also match the standard lines. Remaining unmatched lines are used to determine any other crystalline components in the sample. With the advent of high resolution XRD cameras utilizing focusing monochromators and high flux X-ray generators, the ability to detect minor stone components has greatly increased as the diffraction patterns appear sharper and diffraction lines are easily differentiated from

Table 3
XRD Interplanar Spacings and Relative Intensities of the Components of Human Urinary Calculi

COM		COD		AP		BR		ST		UA		MSU		CY	
d (Å)	I	d (Å)	I	d (Å)	I	d (Å)	I	d (Å)	I	d (Å)	I	d (Å)	I	d (Å)	I
5.93	100	8.70	12	8.15	29	7.59	100	5.90	38	6.56	38	10.60	8	4.70	
5.79	25	6.31	100	5.26	6	4.24	100	5.60	45	5.63	20	9.30	30	4.68	100
4.64	7	6.15		4.08	8	3.80	8	5.38	22	4.91	48	7.50	25	4.63	
4.52	6	4.40	45	3.89	10	3.04	75	4.60	6	4.76	6	5.28	10	4.45	5
3.78		3.89	14	3.44	45	2.93	70	4.25	100	3.86		4.88	22	4.20	7
	13	3.09	18	3.17	10	2.85	15	4.14	34	+	55	4.63	4	3.32	8
3.65	100	3.07		2.81	100	2.60	30	3.29	24	3.70	5	3.45	15	3.18	19
3.00	10	2.81	20	2.78	62	2.56	6	3.02	10	3.28	14	3.38	20	3.13	30
2.97	46	2.77		2.72	58			2.96		3.18	70	3.26	5	3.06	16
2.91	12	2.75	85	2.63	31			+	16	3.09	100	3.12	100+	2.71	
2.89	10	2.41	14	2.53	5			2.95		2.87		3.01	1	2.70	32
2.84	14	2.39	14	2.40	7			2.92	46	+	25	2.87	12	2.68	
2.48	30	2.33	10	2.26	20			2.80	26	2.86		2.84	8	2.60	17
2.41	5			2.15	9			2.72	8	2.80		2.78	5		
2.34	90			2.06	7			2.69	37	+	10	2.63	40		
				2.00	5			2.66	37	2.79		2.59	5		
				1.94	30					2.57	18				
				1.89	15										
				1.87	5										
				1.81	20										

neighboring diffraction lines separated by as little as 0.01–0.03 Å interplanar spacings. The increased sensitivity has allowed for the identification of smaller amounts of poorly crystalline materials such as apatite. However, the most severe limitation of XRD is sensitivity when a very limited amount of sample is available. Also, if the stone material is a drug, or drug metabolite whose XRD pattern or single crystal structure has not been published, XRD methods fail to definitively characterize the sample. In those cases, the XRD method can only tell you what the stone is not composed of.

In FTIR spectral analysis, spectral data is related to the vibrational motions of atoms in bonds (e.g., bond stretching, bond contracting, or bond wagging, etc.). Classically, the powdered sample is admixed with powdered potassium bromide, compressed into a nearly transparent wafer, and the IR beam is passed through the wafer. Recently, advances in other sample preparation methods have allowed powdered samples to simply be ground to ensure optimal sampling of a multicomponent stone and then the IR beam is directed at the sample surface (attenuated total reflectance). The reflected IR beam containing spectral data specific to the sample is then recorded. Standard IR patterns for common stone components are presented in Figures 1–8. The IR pattern contains absorption bands representing specific energies (presented as wavelengths in units of cm-1, or more commonly known as wavenumbers) corresponding to molecular motions in molecules. It is therefore possible to differentiate molecular motions in similar organic groups. The IR pattern of a mixed component stone is frequently very complex, but the advent of computer controlled IR spectrometers, especially modern FTIR spectrometers has allowed for computer assisted pattern stripping and comparative standards library matching. Frequently, the assignment of weak absorbance bands in the spectra to specific structures is very difficult and often requires careful background and noise level adjustments in the computer data smoothing functions. The specific choice of mathematical calculations used in the standards library search/match routines can provide markedly different results, so operator training and experience is critical.

The real benefit of FTIR is the high sensitivity of the new computer controlled spectrometers that can take many repetitive spectra of the same sample and mathematically enhance the sample signal to experimental noise ratio. It is often possible to obtain a definitive FTIR spectra with less material than is needed for XRD. FTIR is the method of choice for the characterization of noncrystalline samples or drug related samples because the IR absorbance is related to independent chemical bonds and IR data related to a majority of the molecule is still definitive. Metabolism of a drug resulting in an altered chemical structure in a stone compared with the ingested molecule has far less impact in FTIR analysis compared with XRD. The drawback to FTIR is that the differentiation of spectral signals from more than one component with similar molecular bonds can be difficult. All too often the operator of modern FTIR instruments may rely too heavily on the computer-assisted analysis of the spectra as the computer algorithms scan and interpolate data from computer based spectral libraries. In the case of weak spectra or multicomponent stones, the computer often indicates a positive identification, but in fact the component identification is false.

The analysis of stone composition with microscopic inspection (including polarizing microscopy) is very inaccurate and unfortunately too frequently used for the routine analysis of stones *(3,11,12)*. The assumption is that all components of stones always appear the same regardless of unique urine chemistry and different admixtures with other

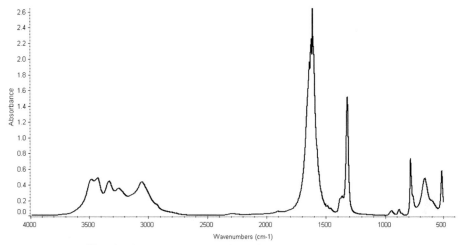

Fig. 1. The FTIR spectra of calcium oxalate monohydrate.

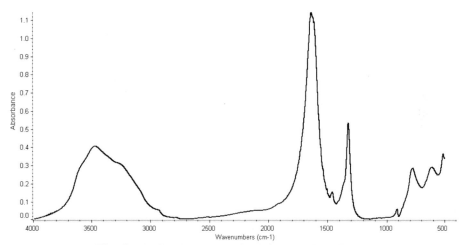

Fig. 2. The FTIR spectra of calcium oxalate dihydrate.

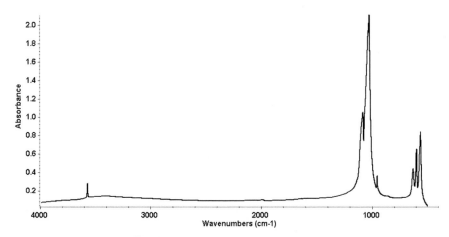

Fig. 3. The FTIR spectra of hydroxyapatite.

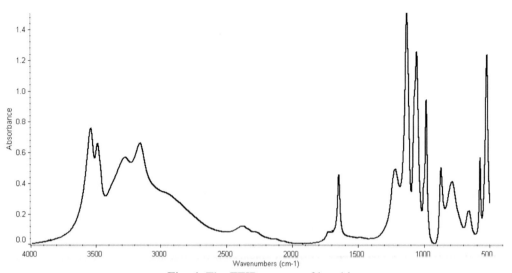

Fig. 4. The FTIR spectra of brushite.

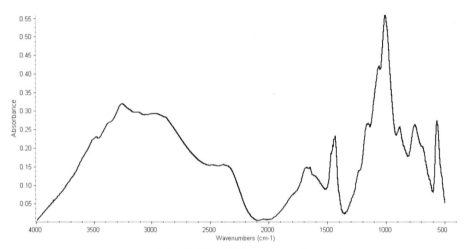

Fig. 5. The FTIR spectra of struvite.

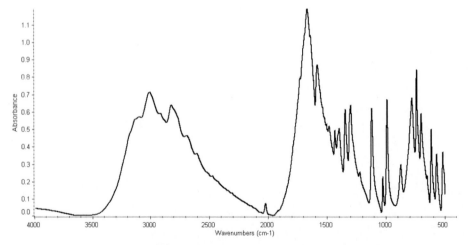

Fig. 6. The FTIR spectra of uric acid.

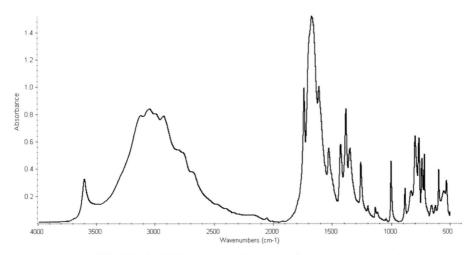

Fig. 7. The FTIR spectra of monosodium urate monohydrate.

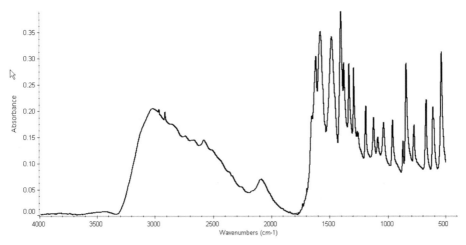

Fig. 8. The FTIR spectra of cystine.

stone components. This is not a sound assumption. After fracturing the calculi to reveal the internal structure, samples are taken from various portions of the stone and are visually inspected and identified using a polarizing microscope. This technique is not capable of identifying small amounts of crystalline materials in admixed samples. A significant contribution to the potentially low level of accuracy using this method is that the accuracy is entirely dependent on the level of sophistication and experiences of the technicians conducting the analyses *(12)*.

CONCLUSIONS AND RECOMMENDATIONS

Numerous treatises have been written on the crystalline composition of renal calculi and the frequency of occurrence of the varied crystalline components in stones observed in industrialized countries *(3,5,13–17)*. The majority of urinary stones are admixtures of two or more components. The admixture of calcium oxalate or apatite accounts for 45% *(15)* to 9.2% *(5,17)* and the incidence of pure whewellite stones varies from 24.9% *(11)* to 4% *(25)*. Although the actual percentages vary among the different studies, the most frequent stone compositions are whewellite/weddellite, pure whewellite, apatite/whewellite/weddellite, and apatite/struvite. Calcium oxalate was present in $73 \pm 7\%$ of all stones analyzed in these studies.

Because most stones are multicomponent, the method employed in the analysis of stone material should be capable of resolving all components of the stone, especially all the crystalline components. The literature on stone analysis methods clearly supports the use of XRD or FTIR as the prime choices. The use of both methods to obtain supportive and the most accurate compositional data is ideal. For XRD and FTIR, the accuracy of the analysis is very strongly dependent on the quality of standard spectra. Most laboratories conducting stone analyses prepare their own standards libraries. Unfortunately, many analysis laboratories use patient stone material to create their standard spectra. As their stones are analyzed by the same method as they are using to analyze other stone samples, their unknowns become their standard. As virtually no stone is composed of only one pure crystalline component, such spectral libraries are very inaccurate and the potential for skewed and inaccurate stone analysis is highly probable. Preparation of synthetic stone components for the generation of standards and verification of composition by alternative methods is the only correct way to prepare a standards library for either XRD or FTIR, especially for FTIR. Commercial libraries should only be used for supplemental data in those rare instances when experimental data cannot be correlated with defined stone component standards, especially for identification of nonbiologic or false stones.

One issue not yet resolved in the literature is the level of accuracy one should accept in analysis reports. Specifically, rank order of compositional analysis in multicomponent stones analyzed by XRD is probably the best one can expect. In FTIR analyses, although it is possible to generate computer aided admixed spectral standards at any percent admixture, many years of experience and cross-correlating analysis results with accurately weighed admixtures of pure standards suggests that percent compositional analysis should be quoted at 10% or more for accuracy.

The issue of stone composition analysis accuracy is certainly clouded by the fragmented samples now seen by most analysis labs with the common utilization of lithotripsy. Virtually no laboratories can be assured that they have received the entire voided sample or if the sample they have received for analysis accurately represents overall stone composition. Accuracy of analysis by other methods such as microscopic evaluation that is quoted as approaching or exceeding the XRD or FTIR levels should be questioned for scientific basis.

In conclusion, high resolution XRD and FTIR spectroscopic methods of analysis are currently the only two methods that should be considered for the accurate and complete characterization of crystals in urine and for the compositional analysis of kidney stones. Frequently, the use of both XRD and FTIR is beneficial and occasionally necessary for an accurate analysis of multicomponent stones. The accuracy of these methods of analysis is very much dependent on the quality and completeness of a standards library as well as on the experience of the instrument operator, especially in the use of computer-based match routines supporting both XRD and FTIR instruments.

ACKNOWLEDGMENTS

This work was supported in part by the Department of Veterans Affairs as Merit Review grants (NM), a VA Research Career Scientist Award (NM), local and national funding for the National VA Crystal Identification Center, and by National Institutes of Health grants DK30579 (NM), DK62739 (NM), and DK64616 (NM).

REFERENCES

1. Mandel N. Urinary tract calculi. Lab Med 1986; 17: 449–458.
2. Mandel NS, Mandel GS. Physicochemistry of urinary stone formation. In: Renal Stone Disease, (Pak CYC, ed.). Martinus Nijhoff, Boston, MA, 1987; pp. 1–24.
3. Herring LC. Observations on the analysis of ten thousand urinary calculi. J Urol 1962; 88: 545–562.
4. Sutor DJ, Scheidt S. Identification standards for human urinary calculus components, using crystallographic methods. Br J Urol 1968; 40: 22–28.
5. Mandel NS, Mandel GS. Urinary tract stone disease in the United States veteran population. II. Geographic analsysis of variations in composition. J Urol 1989; 142: 1516–1521.
6. Hesse A, Molt K. Technik der infrarotspektroskopischen harnsteinanalyse. J Clin Chem Clin Biochem 1982; 20: 861–873.
7. Berthelot M, Cornu G, Daudon M, Helbert M, Laurence C. Computer-aided infrared analysis of urinary calculi. Clin Chem 1987; 33: 2070–2073.
8. Lehmann CA, McClure GL, Smolens I. Identification of renal calculi by computerized infrared spectroscopy. Clinica Chimica Acta 1988; 173: 107–116.
9. Mandel NS, Mandel GS. Structures of crystals that provoke inflammation. In: Advances in Inflammation Research, (Weissmann G, ed.). Raven Press, New York, NY, 1982; pp. 73–94.
10. JCPDS Powder Diffraction Files. International Centre for Diffraction Data. Swarthmore, PA, 1985.
11. Brien G, Schubert G, Bick C. 10,000 analyses of urinary calculi using x-ray diffraction and polarizing microscopy. Eur Urol 1982; 8: 251–256.
12. Prien EL. Crystallographic analysis of urinary calculi: a 23-year survey study. J Urol 1963; 80: 917–924.
13. Prien EL. Studies in urolithiasis: II. Relationships between pathogenesis, structure, and composition and calculi. J Urol 1949; 61: 821–836.
14. Lonsdale K, Sutor DJ, Wooley S. Composition of urinary calculi by x-ray diffraction. Collected data from various localities. I. Norwich (England) and district, 1773–1961. Br J Urol 1968; 40: 33–36.
15. Sutor DJ, Wooley SE. Composition of urinary calculi by x-ray diffraction: Collected data from various localities. IX. Glasgow, Scotland. Br J Urol 1971; 43: 268–272.
16. Bastian HP, Gebhardt M. Die harnsteinanalyse. Therapiewoche 1976; 26: 5935–5938.
17. Mandel NS, Mandel GS. Urinary tract stone disease in the United States veteran population. II. Geographic frequency of occurrence. J Urol 1989; 142: 1513–1515.

II | METABOLISM

6 Calcium Physiology

G. Bennett Stackhouse, MD and Marshall L. Stoller, MD

CONTENTS

Key Words: Nephrolithiasis; calcium metabolism; absorption; renal handling.

INTRODUCTION

An understanding of extracellular calcium handling in the body is helpful for those who treat stone disease. Calcium is a component in the majority of urinary stones. Researchers and clinicians seek to broaden their knowledge of calcium handling and of derangements in calcium metabolism in an effort to uncover the etiology of a patient's stone disease and to prevent further recurrence.

Calcium is a divalent cation found in many food sources and is essential for life. Calcium is important as a building block in bony skeletal crystals, and plays an important role in multiple physiologic cascades. Extracellular calcium is important to neuromuscular excitability, and extreme variations in extracellular calcium concentrations can lead to tetany (if calcium levels fall) or flaccidity and arrhythmias (if calcium is too high). Muscular contractions via actin and myosin require intracellular calcium. Calcium also plays a role in the clotting cascade, especially in converting fibrinogen and prothrombin to fibrin and thrombin. Many other systems require calcium for normal function. Our

From: Current Clinical Urology, *Urinary Stone Disease:*
A Practical Guide to Medical and Surgical Management
Edited by: M. L. Stoller and M. V. Meng © Humana Press Inc., Totowa, NJ

Abbreviations

Ca^{++}-ATPase	Calcium adenosine triphosphatase
CaBP	Calcium binding protein, calbindin
CaM	Calmodulin
CaR	Calcium receptor
CTR	Calcitonin receptor
DRI	Dietary reference intake
OPG	Osteoprotegrin
PMCA	Plasma membrane calcium adenosine triphosphatase
PTH	Parathyroid hormone
PTHrP	Parathyroid hormone-related protein
RANK	Receptor activator of NF-κB
RANKL	Receptor activator of NF-κB ligand
TRPC	Transient receptor potential channels
VDR	Vitamin D receptor
VDR_{nuc}	Vitamin D nuclear receptor
VDR_{mem}	Vitamin D membrane receptor

understanding of calcium metabolism has grown from clinical studies of pathophysiologic states such as rickets and hyperparathyroidism, from elegant animal physiology models, and more recently from modern microbiologic techniques. It is important to note that much of this work has been done with nonhuman tissue sources, but appears to be applicable to humans. This chapter is a brief summary of current concepts and theory regarding calcium handling. Further research will be needed to clarify areas that remain controversial or unclear at present.

Calcium Metabolism Overview

Calcium is absorbed through the intestine wall and stored as apatite crystals in bone matrix and in intracellular organelles. Calcium is continually liberated from and stored in bony apatite crystals through osteoblast and osteoclast activity. Homeostasis of calcium levels in both the intracellular and extracellular compartments is maintained within a very narrow range. Intracellular calcium is generally maintained at 50–100 nM, and extracellular concentration is 1.1–1.3 mM (8.6–10.5 mg/dL.) Outside this physiologic range of extracellular calcium concentrations, deleterious effects occur within multiple systems, most notably the neuromuscular and cardiac systems. Calcium is filtered by the renal glomerulus and largely reabsorbed in the renal tubule and collecting duct. Calcium is not secreted by the kidney. Variations in renal reabsorption rates from the urinary lumen allow for net excretion of calcium from the body. Feedback mechanisms to the parathyroid gland and to the renal proximal tubule allow control of parathyroid hormone secretion and vitamin D activation to modify bone turnover, calcium absorption, and net calcium excretion to maintain homeostasis.

Calcium transport across epithelial surfaces in both the intestine and kidney is a function of several analogous processes, with similar proteins involved. Both intestinal calcium absorption and renal calcium reabsorption use active cellular and passive paracellular systems to move calcium from the lumen (intestinal lumen or renal tubular lumen) to the extracellular space. In both enterocytes and renal cells, active cellular calcium (re)absorption can be divided into three distinct regions: (1) calcium transport into the cell at the apical (luminal) membrane, (2) transcellular calcium transport to the basolateral membrane, and (3) calcium extrusion from the cell into the extracellular compartment. Current research is still defining the similarities and differences of calcium transport across the epithelia of the kidney and intestine (1), as will be shown subsequently in this chapter.

Calcium Pathophysiology Overview

Derangements of calcium and calcium handling can lead to multiple disease processes. Changes in extracellular calcium levels have profound effects. Elevated extracellular calcium can lead to flaccidity, atony, and death. Depressed extracellular calcium leads to tetany. Defects in calcium handling can lead to dystrophic calcifications, hypo- or hypercalcemia. Abnormalities of hormonal control of calcium lead to chronic disease processes. Vitamin D deficiency can lead to rickets and osteomalacia. Hyperparathyroidism results in osteopenia, nephrolithiasis, and pathologic fractures. Calcium is also a prime constituent in the majority of urinary stones in the Western world. Elevated levels of urine calcium are found in a significant number of patients suffering from stone disease. Understanding calcium metabolism may be important for prevention and treatment of urolithiasis.

CALCIUM ABSORPTION FROM THE INTESTINAL TRACT

Overview of Gastrointestinal Calcium Absorption

The Western daily diet contains about 1000 mg of calcium. The dietary reference intake for calcium is 1000 mg/d for adults, 1300 mg/d for adolescents, and 1200 mg/d for elderly persons (2). About 70% of this daily intake is complexed to sulfates, oxalates, phosphates, and other moieties in a non-ionic form in the intestinal lumen and cannot be absorbed. This non-ionized calcium is excreted in the stool. Calcium that remains ionized or bound to small organic molecules is available for absorption across the intestinal mucosa through both active and passive processes. This absorption is mediated via cellular and paracellular pathways, as reviewed by Bronner and summarized here (3). The paracellular pathways involve passive diffusion of calcium down a concentration gradient from the bowel lumen into the paracellular spaces. This mechanism is the predominating means of calcium absorption from the gastrointestinal tract when total oral calcium intake is high. When total calcium intake is lower, more active absorption may be required to maintain homeostasis, and the proportional amount of calcium absorbed through active cellular pathways will increase. Calcitriol serves to regulate active absorption (see "Transcellular Absorption of Calcium" following) and increases active absorption in times of low total calcium intake.

Active processes predominate in the duodenum and jejunum, whereas passive absorption takes place mostly in the ileum but occurs to a lesser extent throughout the intestinal tract. The proportion of calcium absorbed through passive processes in a given bowel segment is inversely related to the rate of intestinal propulsion and directly related to the sojourn time of chyme in that bowel segment. The pH of chyme within differing bowel segments may also affect how much calcium remains ionized and available for absorption.

Calcium absorption is under hormonal control, with the primary hormone being 1,25 dihydroxy vitamin D (calcitriol). In times of high calcium intake, passive absorption is favored by the high concentration gradient, and the relatively high serum calcium availability downregulates calcitriol production. This decreases active absorptive processes.

Paracellular Absorption of Calcium

Paracellular pathways involve calcium movement through tight junctions into narrow spaces between cells. This is the predominant mechanism of intestinal calcium absorption, especially when calcium is plentiful in the diet. Calcium ions and small molecules complexed to calcium are diffusible between cells *(4)*. Tight junctions are found where epithelial cell borders come into close contact at the apex of the cells, and serve to restrict paracellular movement and to define apical and lateral surfaces of the cells. They are made of integral membrane proteins and junctional adhesion molecules. Recent research suggests that particular ion channels are inserted into tight junctions to facilitate selective passage of certain ions *(5)*.

Regulation of paracellular movement is not well elucidated. Passive paracellular movement is influenced by the electrochemical gradient from the lumen to the intercellular space. Factors that indirectly affect passive movement include structural changes to the tight junctions. Tight junctions are modulated by hormones, growth factors, cytokines, toxins, and possibly phosphorylation *(3)*.

Transcellular Absorption of Calcium

Calcium is absorbed in the intestine via cellular and paracellular pathways. Paracellular absorption occurs throughout the small and large intestine, but mainly in the ileum. Cellular absorption occurs mostly in the duodenum and jejunum *(6)*. Cellular pathways involve three distinct steps for moving calcium ions from the intestinal lumen across the enterocyte to the extracellular space: (1) calcium transport from the intestinal lumen into the cell, (2) movement across the intracellular space, and (3) extrusion of calcium out of the basolateral membrane of the cell into the intercellular space (Fig. 1). This overall process is under the hormonal control of calcitriol, via its interaction with the vitamin D receptor (VDR).

Transport From the Intestinal Lumen Into the Cell

Because the intracellular calcium concentration is usually lower than the intestinal lumen calcium concentration, this first step of calcium movement into the cell is most often down a chemical gradient. This movement must be regulated, as the intracellular calcium concentrations are very low (50–100 nM) and unregulated movement of calcium from the lumen would rapidly raise the intracellular levels to supraphysiologic levels. The membrane transport mechanism was originally labeled CaT1. CaT1 appears to be regulated by calcitriol. Experiments in VDR knockout mice show that calcitriol dependent absorption accounts for approx 90% of total movement across the cell apical lumen *(7)*. Further work has identified CaT1 as a transient receptor potential channel, TRPV6 *(8)*. Other names for TRVP6 in the literature include ECaC2 and CaT-like. A closely related protein to TRPV6 is TRPV5, which appears to be more important in the renal epithelium and will be discussed below. TRPV6 is part of a family of transient receptor potential channels (TRPC). TRPV6 appears to be inactivated by high levels of intracellular calcium, and at high intracellular calcium concentrations it is bound by

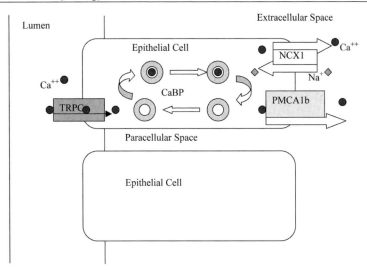

Fig. 1. Calcium transport across epithelial cells. Two TRPCs (transient receptor potential channels) are important for calcium homeostasis. TRPV5 is the dominant form in the renal tubule, whereas TRPV6 is dominant in intestinal segments. CaBP, Calcium binding protein (calbindin) refers to a family of calcium binding transport proteins. Calbindin-D9k is predominant in enterocytes. Calbindin-D28k appears to be more important in renal tubular cells. PMCA1b, a calcium adensosine triphosphatase. NCX1, sodium calcium exchange protein.

calmodulin (CaM). The activity of TRPV6 appears to be modulated by S100A10-Annexin2 complex. S100A10 complexes with Annexin2 as a heterotetramer, and is present in multiple cellular processes. It appears to have a regulatory function for TRPV5 and TRPV6 (9). Binding and regulation of these TRPCs may help control calcium entry into the cell.

Kinetic studies by Bronner et al. show that movement of calcium across the apical cell membrane may be via a dual mechanism—a carrier mediated mechanism that involves use of active transport molecules to move calcium across the cell membrane, and a channel mediated mechanism that relies on opening and closing porous channels to allow calcium to diffuse into the cell along electrochemical gradients (3). Subsequent work implies that the dynamics attributed to CaT1 correspond well to the carrier mediated portion of the dual mechanism postulate of calcium absorption. The channel mediated portion is regulated by intracellular calcium concentration. The channel mediated mechanism has not been verified, and further work is needed to determine the significance of this "dual mechanism" in humans.

CALCIUM MOVEMENT ACROSS THE CELL TO THE BASOLATERAL MEMBRANE

After entry into the cell, calcium is transported across the cell to the basolateral membrane. This must be tightly regulated to allow extrusion from the basolateral membrane at the same rate as influx from the apical membrane, to avoid changes in intracellular calcium level. Evidence indicates that >90% of calcium crossing the cytosol is bound to members of the calcium binding protein family (CaBP), calbindins, during intracellular movement. Binding to calbindins serves to buffer intracellular calcium levels, as the bound calcium is not ionic, free, metabolically active intracellular calcium.

The maximum capacity for transcellular calcium transport is directly related to the calbindin content of the cell. This transport in the intestinal luminal cell involves calcium binding to calbindin-D 9K. The expression of calbindin-D 9k has been well studied, and expression in the duodenum is higher than in other intestinal segments. Expression of calbindin-D 9k is regulated by calcitriol, and decreases in older animals *(10)*. It is not clear whether calbindin-D 9k binding alone is capable of transporting/buffering calcium across the cytosol. It appears that calcium may also be transported across the cytosol in calcium enriched vesicles, formed near the apical membrane via disruption of actin filaments. Calcium ions then are bound to CaM, and the actin filaments are repaired. The calcium enriched vesicles fuse with lysosomes and may then be transported across the cells via a microtubular network.

CALCIUM EXTRUSION INTO THE EXTRACELLULAR SPACE

On reaching the basolateral membrane, the calcium must be extruded from the cell into the extracellular space. This must occur against an electrochemical gradient. Two cellular mechanisms have been proposed for this activity. One is a plasma membrane calcium adenosine triphosphatase pump ($Ca^{++}ATPase$, specifically PMCA1b), and the other is a sodium–calcium exchange pump (NCX). In the intestine the majority of calcium is extruded by the PMCA1b. This pump is activated by calcium, CaM, and calbindin-D. A smaller proportion is extruded by the NCX, a Na^+Ca^{++} exchange pump. Three NCX genes have been identified in mammals thus far—*NCX1, NCX2*, and *NCX3*. NCX1 appears to be the active pump in intestinal and renal tissues. In renal tissue it represents the predominate means of extrusion from the basolateral membrane.

NCX1 is regulated by membrane potential, phosphokinase C activation, hydrogen ions, nucleotides, and parathyroid hormone (PTH). Direct actions of PTH on the intestine are debated. It is not clear whether PTH augments the NCX1 protein activity or whether it increases NCX1 mRNA expression. NCX1 mRNA expression is also regulated by calcitriol *(11)*.

Potassium dependent sodium–calcium exchange pumps (NCKX) have also been identified and are expressed in renal and intestinal tissue, but it is not currently known what role they play in calcium extrusion at the basolateral membrane *(12,13)*.

Regulation of Intestinal Calcium Absorption

Calcitriol regulates expression of the calcium binding proteins (calbindins) and therefore regulates the rate of calcium transport across the cell. Calcitriol also serves to activate the Ca^{++}-ATPase pump, regulating the extrusion of calcium from the enterocyte into the extracellular space *(14)*. Classic teaching is that PTH participates only by stimulating calcitriol production, thereby leading to increased intestinal absorption of calcium and phosphate from the intestine. This has been challenged by some authors who propose that PTH may have direct effects on calcium uptake and transport in the intestine *(15)*. See section "Calcium Regulating Hormones" for further discussion of hormonal controls of intestinal calcium absorption.

BONY STORAGE OF CALCIUM

Overview of Calcium Metabolism in Bone

In addition to providing a structural frame for the body, bones serve as a reservoir for calcium. The total body calcium store is about 1.2 kg. Ninety nine percent of this calcium is stored as apatite in bone, and 1% is in cells or in plasma. Bony calcium stores are not static. The actions of parathyroid hormone on the bony reservoir are crucial for the daily regulation of serum calcium levels. Bones are continually remodeled through osteoblast and osteoclast activity. During the course of a typical day, 300 mg of calcium is resorbed from bone and 300 mg is added to bone. This resorption and new bone formation not only serves to regulate homeostasis in extracellular calcium levels; it is also critical in bony remodeling.

Osteoblast Activity

Osteoblast activity lays down new apatite crystals, binding and storing calcium and phosphate. Calcium is an agonist for osteoblastic activity. Elevated extracellular calcium levels may promote bone formation, however reports of the calciumsensing receptor (CaR) in osteoblasts give conflicting evidence for the importance of CaR in regulation of osteoblastic activity (16,17). Osteoblastic activity may be regulated by calcyclin, a calcium-binding intracellular protein (18).

Osteoclast Activity

Osteoclasts are large multinucleated cells formed by fusion of osteoclast precursor cells. The precursor cells differentiate from hematopoietic stem cells. Osteoclast activity involves resorption of bone and is well summarized by Väänänen (19). Both calcitriol and PTH are needed to increase osteoclast activity and mobilize calcium from bone by breakdown of apatite crystals. Interestingly, calcitriol and PTH also increase absorption of calcium from the intestine and raise serum calcium levels, thus they also cause more calcium to become available for new bone formation. Calcitonin inhibits osteoclast activity and serves to lower serum calcium levels by causing a net increased apatite formation. CaR is also present in osteoclasts and in osteoclast precursors. Stimulation of CaR by high levels of calcium inhibits osteoclast activity and increases the rate of apoptosis (20). Stimulation of CaR in precursor cells appears to inhibit formation of osteoclasts. Conversely, stimulation of VDR by calcitriol in osteoclast precursors promotes osteoclast differentiation and increases osteoclast numbers (21). Other hormones are known to affect osteoclast differentiation, including estrogen and macrophage colony stimulating factor.

Hormonal Regulation of Bony Calcium Stores

Hormonal regulation of bony calcium stores provides for rapid correction of extracellular calcium fluctuations and maintenance of homeostasis. This regulation serves to increase or decrease the relative activities of osteoblasts and osteoclasts to store calcium as apatite or to liberate more calcium into the extracellular space. The interaction between osteoblasts and osteoclasts is complex and regulated. Osteoblasts express receptor activator of NF-κB ligand (RANKL) and they also express and extrude osteoprotegrin (OPG). OPG functions as a "decoy" ligand for RANKL. OPG can bind and effectively block RANKL, preventing it from binding to receptor activator of NF-κB (RANK). Osteoclast precursors express RANK as a surface protein. RANKL–RANK interaction leads osteoclast precursors to differentiate into osteoclasts. This RANKL–RANK interaction is blocked by excess OPG. Calcitriol stimulates RANKL expression and represses OPG production. PTH and prostaglandins also stimulate RANKL expression (22) (Fig. 2).

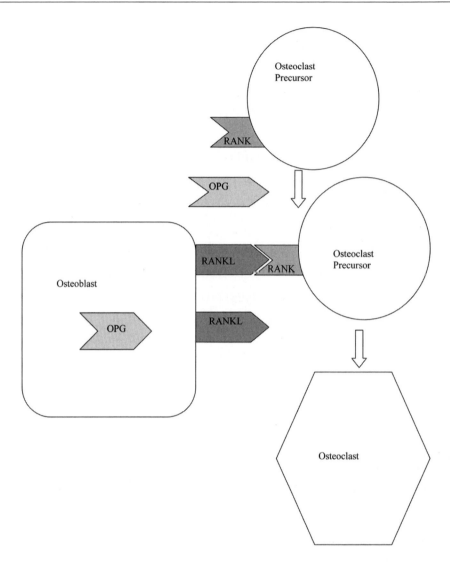

Fig. 2. Osteoblast/osteoclast interaction. Osteoblasts express RANKL, but also actively secrete OPG, which serves as a competitive inhibitor or "decoy" to bind RANKL. Expression of OPG is under hormonal control, and serves to regulate the availability of RANKL. Osteoclast precursors express RANK. When RANKL is available to bind to RANK, osteoclast differentiation and maturation is promoted. OPG, osteoprotegrin; RANK, receptor activator of NF-κB; RANKL, receptor activator of NF-κB ligand *(21)*.

CELLULAR CALCIUM

Calcium is used as a cellular activator throughout the body. The concentration of free ionized calcium within the cell is regulated by protein binding, chelation, transport into cellular organelles, and transport out of the cells. Primary organelles with large calcium stores include the mitochondria, the Golgi apparatus, the sarcoplasmic reticulum, and the endoplasmic reticulum. A full review of intracellular calcium handling is beyond the scope of this chapter, but useful reviews are published *(23,24)*.

Extracellular Calcium

Extracellular calcium is available for use by multiple systems in the body, and is tightly regulated within a narrow window of concentration. Serum levels reflect the extracellular plasma level of calcium and are generally 8.6–10.5 mg/dL. Calcium in plasma is 45% ionized, 40% bound to protein, and 15% complexed to anions. Ionized and complexed calcium are diffusible across membranes and are filtered at the renal glomerulus. Albumin accounts for 90% of the protein-binding of calcium. This protein binding is pH dependent, with acidosis leading to decreased binding sites and increased serum ionized calcium, and alkalosis yielding increased protein binding sites and decreased ionized calcium.

Ionized calcium is detected by the CaR and is the regulated form of calcium. It is the active form in neuromuscular function and in other organs.

CALCIUM EXCRETION FROM THE KIDNEYS

Overview of Calcium Excretion

Calcium is not actively secreted by the nephron; thus calcium excretion is the difference between the amount of calcium filtered and the amount reabsorbed. Filtration is a more passive process, so excretion is controlled by regulation of reabsorption. Reabsorption occurs from the proximal tubule to the collecting duct. The bulk of this is a passive paracellular process, but in the distal tubule and collecting duct active processes requiring cellular energy expenditure predominate. In these distal segments, hormonal control of the active processes determines net calcium excretion.

Glomerular Filtration of Calcium

The ionized calcium and the calcium complexed to small anions are filterable at the renal glomerulus. The majority (98–99%) of this filtered calcium is then reabsorbed in the nephron. The remainder that is not reabsorbed represents the excreted fraction. The filtered load is the product of the glomerular filtration rate and the serum calcium concentration.

Renal Reabsorption of Calcium

Most (85%) of calcium reabsorptive activity takes place in the proximal tubule and in the thick ascending limb of the loop of Henle (25), through paracellular pathways. In this portion of the nephron, sodium is actively reabsorbed, and is followed passively by chloride and water. Calcium also appears to be passively reabsorbed through paracellular pathways in this portion of the collecting tubule. A small amount of calcium is actively reabsorbed in this region as well. Active transport moves calcium against its concentration gradient and requires expenditure of energy. In the proximal tubule, active transport is provided by $Ca^{++}ATPase$ and a $Na^+–Ca^{++}$ exchanger, which is a carrier protein that relies on the intracellularly directed sodium gradient. In the thin loop of Henle there is little calcium transport. The thick ascending limb of the loop of Henle uses both passive and active reabsorption. In this region, movement of anions out of the tubular fluid leaves an electrical gradient that promotes passive movement of positively charged calcium ions through paracellular channels.

Fifteen percent of the filtered load is reabsorbed in the distal portion of the nephron and collecting duct. In this portion of the nephron, calcium is reabsorbed against an electrochemical gradient. The tight junctions in this distal region are impermeable to calcium, so paracellular transport is not possible. The active reabsorption appears to occur in three parts. The first is at the apical or luminal surface of the cell, and involves calcium movement through membrane bound protein channels. The second step involves movement of calcium through the cytosol to the basolateral membrane of the cell. The final step involves extrusion of the calcium out into the extracellular fluid compartment.

The membrane bound protein channels were at first only putative. These were originally described as CaT1 channels, but two of these have now been identified and cloned, named TRPV5 *(26)* and TRPV6 *(8)*. It appears that in renal tissue, TRPV5 is the more metabolically active and important form. These TRPVs allow entry of calcium from the tubular fluid into the cell. They are subject to negative feedback inhibition by calcium *(27)*. The calcium transported into the cell via TRPV5 and TRPV6 is then bound by calbindin D proteins. The specific calbindin protein thought to be involved is CaBP28K. These proteins serve to transport the calcium from the apical to the basolateral surface of the cell. Because the calcium is bound to them, they also serve as a buffer to prevent the intracellular calcium levels from rising. The CaBP28K moves the calcium to the basolateral membrane, where they are extruded via a Na^+–Ca^{++} exchanger (NCX1) and by PMCA. In renal tissue, NCX1 appears to be the predominant mechanism of calcium extrusion through the basolateral membrane, unlike in intestinal tissue where PMCA dominates.

CALCIUM REGULATING HORMONES
Introduction

Calcium regulating hormones (calciotropic hormones) include vitamin D, PTH, and calcitonin *(28)*. PTH serves as the serum calcium raising hormone. Calcitonin serves as a serum calcium lowering hormone. Each of these calcium regulating hormones will be discussed in detail under its own heading following. Table 1 summarizes the effects of calcium regulating hormones.

Vitamin D

Vitamin D, not a true vitamin, is actually a steroid derived hormone critical for calcium regulation, immune system function, and may play a role in tumor prevention. Vitamin D was discovered during investigations into the etiology of rickets and osteomalacia. It is essential for optimal calcium and phosphate metabolism, and insufficient vitamin D is epidemiologically associated with rickets, hypertension, diabetes mellitus, autoimmune disease, and cancer. Comprehensive reviews of vitamin D metabolism are available *(21,29)*. The active forms of vitamin D are 1,25 dihydroxy vitamin D_3(calcitriol) and 24R,25$(OH)_2$-vitamin D_3 (24R,25$(OH)_2D_3$). Calcitriol is the dominant metabolically active form of vitamin D in terms of calcium homeostasis. 24R,25$(OH)_2D_3$ is important in bone fracture healing, but has not been implicated in day-to-day calcium homeostasis *(30)*. Calcitriol is formed from vitamin D in the diet or from the action of ultraviolet light converting 7-dehydrocholesterol to vitamin D_3 in the skin. Hydroxylation to 25, hydroxy vitamin D_3 then occurs in the liver. This step is mediated by parts of the cytochrome P-450 system; in particular CYP2R1 is the most likely 25-hydroxylase *(31)*. In the kidney proximal tubule, this 25 hydroxy vitamin D3 is further hydroxylated by 1-α-hydroxylase to 1,25 dihydroxyvitamin D_3 (calcitriol) *(21)*. 1-α-Hydroxylase is found in other tissues *(32)*

Table 1

Effects of Calcium Regulating Hormones

Hormone	Serum calcium	Intestinal absorption	Renal calcium excretion	Bone metabolism
Calcitriol	• Elevates	• Increases calcium absorption by enterocytes	• Works with PTH to increase reabsorption, decreasing excretion	• Promotes osteoclast activity, releasing calcium and phosphate into the serum
Parathyroid	• Elevates	• Most researchers believe no direct effect, but serves to increase calcitriol levels, leading indirectly to increased intestinal absorption	• Works with calcitriol to increase reabsorption, decreasing excretion	• Promotes osteoclast activity, releasing calcium and phosphate into the serum
Calcitonin	• Lowers			• Inhibits osteoclast activity, leading to a net increase in bony apatite formation

and may perform this function outside the kidney in certain physiologic and pathologic states such as pregnancy and renal failure. 1-α-Hydroxylase activity is regulated by PTH and by serum calcium levels. Tight regulation of calcitriol production
is necessary because of calcitriol's potent role in calcium homeostasis. For this reason, measurement of 25 hydroxy vitamin D_3 is a more useful indicator of dietary
vitamin D status, as the hepatic 25-hydroxylation is not tightly regulated (33).

After release in the plasma, calcitriol is bound to vitamin D binding protein and is
delivered to target organ cells. Calcitriol effects are mediated through two separate
VDRs. The nuclear receptor, VDR_{nuc} is responsible for regulating gene transcription
when stimulated by calcitriol. VDR_{nuc} is a 50-kDa receptor bound to the nuclear membrane, and has been cloned and studied. There is also a putative membrane receptor,
$VDR_{mem1,25}$, that is a rapid-reacting receptor that opens calcium and chloride ion channels and activates MAP-kinase. This receptor has not yet been cloned, but research
indicates that it is 60 kDa and it is expressed in enterocytes (34), chondrocyte matrix
vesicles (35), and elsewhere. Calcitriol causes increased gastrointestinal absorption of
calcium and phosphate, resorption of bone by osteoclasts, and also induces formation of
calcibindin D in cells throughout the body. Calbindin D refers to a group of proteins that
promote binding and transmembrane transport of calcium in the intestinal cells and in
the proximal tubule of the kidney. Calcitriol appears to work in concert with PTH in bone
and in the renal tubule to achieve its effects. The net effect of calcitriol on calcium
metabolism is to increase ionized calcium availability in the extracellular space.

Parathyroid Hormone

PTH is a peptide hormone secreted by chief cells of the parathyroid gland. It is
composed of 84 amino acids. The actions of PTH are complex and have been summarized in the literature (36). A closely related hormone, parathyroid hormone-related
peptide (PTHrP), is important in lactation, early development (37), and placental transport of calcium (38), but does not appear to play an important regulatory role in calcium
homeostasis. Release of PTH is stimulated in response to low circulating calcium levels,
and also in response to elevated extracellular phosphate levels. This release of PTH from
chief cells is mediated by CaR discussed later in this chapter.

PTH acts on the target cells through the PTH/PTHrP receptor. This receptor has been
characterized (39), and is the predominant PTH receptor used for extracellular calcium
homeostasis. Other PTH receptors have been described but they appear to have functions apart from extracellular calcium regulation (40,41). The 34 amino acids at the
N-terminus of PTH and PTHrP appear to form the stimulatory region for the PTH/
PTHrP receptor. The secondary and tertiary structure of this N-terminus region has been
investigated and conflicting evidence is present regarding the active conformation. In
any event, receptor ligand binding appears to result in the synthesis of cyclic adenosine
monophosphate and activation of protein kinase A. There is also evidence in rat cell
models that activation of the PTH/PTHrP receptor results in activation of phospholipase
C and elevates intracellular levels of inositol triphosphate and free calcium (42), and
evidence of signaling through the mitogen-activated protein kinase pathway (43). Taken
together, the presence of multiple signal cascades resulting from stimulation of the
PTH/PTHrP receptor and the existence of at least two agonists (PTH and PTHrP) for the
receptor may point to multiple functions mediated by the PTH/PTHrP receptor in different organs.

In the kidney, PTH stimulates 1-α-hydroxylase in proximal tubules to convert vitamin D_2 to calcitriol. PTH indirectly increases intestinal absorption of calcium and phosphate through activation of calcitriol, but also experimentally through direct action on PTH receptors in intestinal villi. This direct action of PTH on the intestine is controversial at present and not accepted by all researchers (44). PTH is a direct agonist of osteoclast activity, raising extracellular calcium levels by osteoclastic breakdown of apatite crystals in bone. In the kidney, PTH increases calcium reabsorption at the distal convoluted tubule. In the proximal tubule PTH acts to decrease expression of sodium-phosphate co-transporters (NPT-2a and NPT-2c). This decreased expression serves to inhibit phosphate reabsorption.

Thus, the net effect of PTH release is to elevate serum calcium and phosphate levels through bone resorption, and to decrease renal calcium excretion but increase renal phosphate excretion.

Calcitonin

Recent research regarding calcitonin has been well summarized (45). Calcitonin is a 32-amino acid peptide hormone made by the parafollicular (C cells) of the thyroid gland. There is significant divergence of calcitonin amino acid sequence across different species, resulting in differing potencies of calcitonins and care must be made when applying nonhuman research to human clinical conditions. Elevated serum calcium levels cause parafollicular cells of the thyroid gland to release calcitonin. Calcitonin is active in multiple tissues and organs, and has biologically diverse roles. Calcitonin is also synthesized in several other nonthyroid organ tissues, but these other sites do not link calcitonin synthesis with serum calcium levels, and they do not appear to participate in calcium homeostasis.

Calcitonin interacts with the calcitonin receptor (CTR). The CTR gene has been identified in humans, and has at least 14 exons (46). The messenger RNA transcript is subject to multiple alternative splicings, leading to several different isoforms of the receptor in humans. The most common isoforms appear to have similar binding affinities to human calcitonin, but differ in their intracellular signaling.

Activation of CTR leads to coupling with different G proteins, largely dependent on cellular function. This coupling can activate adenylate cyclase and leads to elevated cyclic adenosine monophosphate levels, and can also activate phospholipase C, leading to elevated intracellular inositol triphosphate, free calcium, and activated protein kinase C (43). Just as was seen in the discussion of PTH/PTHrP receptors in the preceding section, this multiplicity of cellular signaling pathways probably reflects the various roles of calcitonin in stimulating different cell types.

In regards to extracellular calcium homeostasis, calcitonin inhibits osteoclast activity (47), inhibits osteoclast precursor cell differentiation, and increases renal calcium excretion. By inhibiting osteoclast activity, calcitonin causes serum calcium levels to fall. This osteoclast inhibition appears to be a slower process in adult humans than in growing animals, and calcitonin may be less involved in minute-to-minute calcium homeostasis in adults than other calcium regulating hormones. Administration of large doses of calcitonin to normal human adults has little effect on serum calcium levels. On the other hand, administration of calcitonin to human adults with pathologic states involving increased bone resorption such as Paget disease has been shown to significantly lower serum calcium levels (48). Interestingly, calcitonin causes lysosomal degradation of

CTRs in osteoclasts, making them more "resistant" to the effects of calcitonin. Clinically this is seen as therapeutic loss of responsiveness to exogenously administered calcitonin (49).

CALCIUM RECEPTORS AND CHANNELS

Calcium sensing receptor (CaR) is a G-coupled protein receptor (GCPR) found throughout the body (50). An excellent review of this receptor is available (51). This receptor serves to sense the level of extracellular calcium concentration. It is active in the chief cells of the parathyroid, where it helps regulate release of PTH. It is also expressed in bone, renal, and intestinal tissues. It is a 1078-amino acid protein with an extracellular domain with the N-terminus, and transmembrane domain, and an intracellular domain with the carboxyl-terminus (52,53). Calcium is the major agonist for this receptor throughout the body, and it is sensitive to very slight changes in concentration. Magnesium is also an agonist at high concentration, although in most parts of the body this would be a supraphysiologic effect. In the renal tubule approaching the thick ascending limb of the loop of Henle, the magnesium concentration may be great enough to allow it to act as an agonist (54). Spermine and spermidine are also weak agonists of this receptor. This may be important in the central nervous system where spermine concentrations are high enough to be agonistic (55).

Because calcium is an agonist, extracellular calcium ions can serve as calcium regulating hormones. The parathyroid glands express CaR on the cell surface membrane. The CaR in the chief cells of the parathyroid gland serve to induce the inverse relationship between serum calcium levels and serum PTH levels. This allows rapid correction of variation in extracellular calcium levels by immediate secretion of PTH. In this regard, the CaR acts analogously to a thermostat, regulating calcium within a very narrow range.

The CaR belongs to the GCPR family C, group II. Mutations in CaR lead to metabolic derangements of calcium metabolism. Heterozygous mutations involving loss of function in CaR result in familial hypocalciuric hypercalcemia. Homozygous mutations involving loss of CaR function cause neonatal severe primary hyperparathyroidism. Mutations of CaR may also lead to gain of function, resulting in autosomal dominant hypoparathyroidism.

CONCLUSION

Calcium metabolism is critical to homeostasis, and understanding calcium metabolism will be crucial to understanding the pathophysiology of nephrolithiasis. Current research is expanding our knowledge of these key pathways at an increasing rate. As we understand more about calcium metabolism, more therapeutic targets will be identified. Medical management of stone formers is focused on interventions to urinary constituents and urine physical properties. As clinicians seek to change urinary calcium excretion, urinary pH, urinary sodium excretion, urine volume production, and use other medical therapeutic interventions, the complex regulatory pathways of calcium metabolism must be understood.

REFERENCES

1. Hoenderop JGJ, Nilius B, Bindels RJM. Calcium absorption across epithelia. Physiol Rev 2005; 85: 373–422.

2. Institute of Medicine. Dietary reference intakes for energy, carbohydrate, fiber, fat, fatty acids, cholesterol, protein, and amino acids. National Academy Press, Washington, DC, 2002.
3. Bronner F. Mechanisms of intestinal calcium absorption. J Cell Biochem 2003; 88: 387–393.
4. Goodenough DA. Plugging the leaks. Proc Natl Acad Sci USA 1999; 96: 319–321.
5. Tang VW, Goodenough DA. Paracellular ion channel at the tight junction. Biophys J 2003; 84: 1660–1673.
6. Pansu D, Bellaton C, Bronner F. The effect of calcium intake on the saturable and non-saturable components of duodenal calcium transport. Am J Physiol 1981; 240: G32–G37.
7. Van Cromphaut SJ, Dewerchim NM, Hoenderop JGJ, et al. Duodenal calcium absorption in vitamin D receptor knock out mice: Functional and molecular aspects. Proc Natl Acad Sci USA 2001; 98: 13,324–13,329.
8. Peng JB, Chen XZ, Berger UV, et al. Molecular cloning and characterization of a channel-like transporter mediating intestinal calcium absorption. J Biol Chem 1999; 274: 22,739–22,746.
9. Van de Graaf SF, Hoenderop JG, Gkika D, et al. Functional expression of the epithelial Ca2+ channels (TRPV5 and TRPV6) requires association of the S100A10-annexin 2 complex. EMBO J 2003; 22: 1478–1487.
10. Armbrecht HJ, Boltz MA, Bruns ME. Effect of age and dietary calcium on intestinal calbindin D-9k expression in the rat. Arch Biochem Biophys 2003; 420: 194–200.
11. Hoenderop JG, Dardenne O, Van Abel M, et al. Modulation of renal Ca2+ transport protein genes by dietary Ca2+ and 1,25-dihydroxyvitamin D3 in 25-hydroxyvitamin D3-1alpha-hydroxylase knockout mice. FASEB J 2002; 16: 1398–1406.
12. Cai X, Lytton J. Molecular cloning of a sixth member of the K+-dependent Na+/Ca2+ exchanger gene family, NCKX6. J Biol Chem 2004; 279: 5867–5876.
13. Li XF, Kraev AS, Lytton J. Molecular cloning of a fourth member of the potassium-dependent sodium-calcium exchanger gene family, NCKX4. J Biol Chem 2002; 277: 48,410–48,417.
14. Bronner F. Current concepts of calcium absorption: an overview. J Nutr 1992; 122:641–643.
15. Nemere I, Larsson D. Does PTH Have a Direct Effect on Intestine? J Cellular Biochemistry 2002; 86:29–34.
16. Chattopadhyay N, Yano S, Tfelt-Hansen J, et al. Mitogenic action of calcium-sensing receptor onrat calvarial osteoblasts. Endocrinology 2004; 145: 3451–3462.
17. Pi M, Garner SC, Flannery P, Spurney RF, Quarles LD. Sensing of extracellular cations in CasRdeficient osteoblasts. Evidence for a novel cation-sensing mechanism. J Biol Chem 2000; 275: 3256–3263.
18. Tu Q, Pi M, Quarles LD. Calcyclin mediates serum response element (SRE) activation by an osteoblastic extracellular cation-sensing mechanism. J Bone Miner Res 2003; 18:1825–1833.
19. Vaananen K. Mechanism of osteoclast mediated bone resorption—rationale for the design of new therapeutics. Adv Drug Deliv Rev 2005; 57(7): 959–971.
20. Lorget F, Kamel S, Mentaverri R, et al. High extracellular calcium concentrations directly stimulate osteoclast apoptosis. Biochem Biophys Res Commun 2000; 268: 899–903.
21. Dussa A S, Brown A J, and Slatopolsky E. Vitamin D. AJP–Renal 2005; 289: 8–28.
22. Nakagawa N, Kinosaki M, Yamaguchi K, et al. RANK is the essential signaling receptor for osteoclast differentiation factor in osteoclastogenesis. Biochem Biophys Res Commun 1998; 253: 395–400.
23. Saris N-E L, Carafoli E. A historical review of cellular calcium handling, with emphasis on mitochondria. Biochemistry (Moscow) 2005; 70(2): 187–194.
24. Tiruppathi C, Minshall RD, Paria BC, Vogel SM, Malik AB. Role of Ca2+ signaling in the regulation of endothelial permeability. Vascul Pharmacol 2002; 39(4–5): 173–185.
25. Suki WN: Calcium transport in the nephron. Am J Physiol (Lond) 1979; 237: F1–F6.
26. Hoenderop JG, van der Kemp AW, Hartog A, et al. Molecular identification of the apical Ca2+ channel in 1, 25-dihydroxyvitamin D3-responsive epithelia. J Biol Chem 1999; 274: 8375–8378.
27. Nilius B, Prenen J, Vennekens R, et al. Modulation of the epithelial calcium channel, ECaC, by intracellular Ca2. Cell Calcium 2001; 29: 417–428.
28. Tfelt-Hansen J, Schwarz P, Brown EM, Chattopadhyay N. The calcium-sensing receptor in human disease. Front Biosci 2003; 8: s377–s390.

29. DeLuca HF. Overview of general physiologic features and functions of vitamin D. Am J Clin Nutr. 2004; 80(6 Suppl): 1689S–1696S.

30. Norman AW, Okamura WH, Bishop JE, Henry HL. Update on biological actions of 1a,25(OH)2-vitamin D3 (rapid effects) and 24R,25(OH)2-vitamin D3. Mol Cell Endocrinol 2002; 197: 1–13.

31. Cheng JB, Levine MA, Bell NH, Mangelsdorf DJ, Russell DW. Genetic evidence that the human CYP2R1 enzyme is a key vitamin D 25-hydroxylase. Proc Natl Acad Sci USA 101: 2004; 7711–7715.

32. Hewison M, Zehnder D, Chakraverty R, Adams JS. Vitamin D and barrier function: a novel role for extra-renal 1a-hydroxylase. Mol Cell Endocrinol 2004; 215: 31–38.

33. Holick MF. The cutaneous photosynthesis of previtamin D3: a unique photoendocrine system. J Invest Dermatol 1981; 77: 51–58.

34. Lieberherr M., Grosse B, Duchambon P, Dru¬® eke T. A functional cell surface type receptor is required for the early action of 1,25-dihydroxyvitamin D3 on the phosphoinositide metabolism in rat enterocytes. J Biol Chem; 1989; 264: 20,403–20,406.

35. Pedrozo HA, Schwartz Z, Rimes S, et al. Physiological importance of the 1,25(OH)2D3 membrane receptor and evidence for a membrane receptor specific for 24,25(OH)2D3. J Bone Miner Res 1999; 14: 856–867.

36. Gensurea RC, Gardella TJ, Jüppner H. Parathyroid hormone and parathyroid hormone-related peptide, and their receptors. Biochem Biophys Res Comm 2005; 328: 666–678.

37. Kronenberg HM. Developmental regulation of the growth plate, Nature 2003; 423 (6937): 332–336.

38. Rodda CP, Kubota M, Heath JA, et al. Evidence for a novel parathyroid hormone-related protein in fetal lamb parathyroid glands and sheep placenta: comparisons with a similar protein implicated in humoral hypercalcaemia of malignancy. J Endocrinol 1988; 117(2): 261–271.

39. Juppner H. Molecular cloning and characterization of a parathyroid hormone/parathyroid hormone-related peptide receptor: a member of an ancient family of G protein-coupled receptors. Curr Opin Nephrol Hypertens 1994; 3(4): 371–378.

40. Usdin TB, Bonner TI, Hoare SR, The parathyroid hormone 2 (PTH2) receptor. Receptors Channels 2002; 8 (3–4): 211–218.

41. Inomata N, Akiyama M, Kubota N, Juppner H. Characterization of a novel parathyroid hormone (PTH) receptor with specificity for the carboxyl terminal region of PTH-(1–84), Endocrinology 1995; 136(11): 4732–4740.

42. Abou-Samra AB, Juppner H, Force T, et al. Expression cloning of a common receptor for parathyroid hormone and parathyroid hormonerelated peptide from rat osteoblast-like cells: a single receptor stimulates intracellular accumulation of both cAMP and inositol trisphosphates and increases intracellular free calcium, Proc. Natl. Acad. Sci. USA 1992; 89(7): 2732–2736.

43. Offermanns S, Iida-Klein A, Segre GV, Simon MI. G alpha q family members couple parathyroid hormone (PTH)/PTH-related peptide and calcitonin receptors to phospholipase C in COS-7 cells. Mol Endocrinol 1996; 10(5): 566–574.

44. Nemere I, Larsson D. Does PTH have a direct effect on intestine? J Cell Biochem 2002; 86: 29–34.

45. Findlay DM, Sexton PM. Calcitonin. Growth Factors. 2004; 22(4): 217–224.

46. Zolnierowicz S, Cron P, Solinas-Toldo S, Fries R, Lin HY, Hemmings BA. Isolation, characterization, and chromosomal localization of the porcine calcitonin receptor gene. Identification of two variants of the receptor generated by alternative splicing. J Biol Chem 1994; 269: 19,530–19,538.

47. Chambers TJ, Magnus CJ. Calcitonin alters behaviour of isolated osteoclasts. J Pathol 1982; 136: 27–39.

48. Martin TJ, Moseley JM, Sexton PM. Calcitonin, In: Endocrinology, 4th Ed., (DeGroot LJ, Jameson JL, eds.). W.B. Saunders, Philadelphia, PA, 2001; pp. 999–1008.

49. Sexton PM, Findlay DM, Martin TJ. Calcitonin. Curr Med Chem 1999; 6: 1067–1093.

50. Brown EM, Gamba G, Riccardi D, et al. Cloning and characterization of an extracellular Ca2+-sensing receptor from bovine parathyroid. Nature 1993; 366: 575–80.

51. Tfelt-Hansen J, Brown EM. The calcium-sensing receptor in normal physiology and pathophysiology: a review. Crit Rev Clin Lab Sci 2005; 42(1): 35–70.

52. Aida K, Koishi S, Tawata M, Onaya T. Molecular cloning of a putative Ca+ -sensing receptor cDNA from human kidney. Biochem Biophys Res Commun 1995; 214: 524–529.
53. Garrett JE, Capuano IV, Hammerland LG, et al. Molecular cloning and functional expression of human parathyroid calcium receptor cDNAs. J Biol Chem 1995; 270: 12,919–12,925.
54. Hebert SC, Brown EM, Harris HW. Role of the Ca2+-sensing receptor in divalent mineral ion homeostasis. J Exp Biol 1997; 200 (Pt 2): 295–302.
55. Brown EM, MacLeod RJ. Extracellular calcium sensing and extracellular calcium signaling. Physiol Rev 2001; 81: 239–297.

7 Management of Patients With Hyperoxaluria

Ojas Shah, MD, Ross P. Holmes, PhD, and Dean G. Assimos, MD

CONTENTS

Key Words: Nephrolithiasis; oxalate; absorption.

INTRODUCTION

Oxalate excretion is a prerequisite for the formation of calcium oxalate stones and the development of hyperoxaluric states. In this chapter, we review the aspects of oxalate physiology germane to these conditions, the clinical manifestations of these entities, as well as therapy.

OXALATE PHYSIOLOGY

Oxalate is a simple dicarboxylic acid and is a major component of the most common type of renal calculus. The oxalate concentration in urine affects its supersaturation with calcium oxalate and an increase will promote crystal formation, a key event in calculogenesis. The oxalate in urine is derived from two sources: the diet and endogenous synthesis. Oxalate is a common component of plants and an unavoidable constituent of

From: Current Clinical Urology, *Urinary Stone Disease:*
A Practical Guide to Medical and Surgical Management
Edited by: M. L. Stoller and M. V. Meng © Humana Press Inc., Totowa, NJ

human diets. It is a metabolic end product in humans that is linked to a variety of vital pathways, including gluconeogenesis, glycolysis, ureagenesis, pentose–phosphate pathway, glyoxylate pathway, serine pathway, and xylulose pathway *(1)*.

Oxalate is freely filtered through the glomerulus and secretory fluxes may also occur *(2–5)*. Oxalate transport in proximal tubular cells may be complex because it seem to plays a role as a recycling substrate that functionally links the transcellular absorption of chloride to that of other anions such as bicarbonate and sulfate *(6,7)*. At the basolateral membrane, oxalate enters the cell in exchange for sulfate or bicarbonate *(6–8)*. At the luminal brush border membrane, oxalate can be transported out of the cell in exchange for chloride and may be transported back into the cell in exchange for sulfate *(6, 7)*. There is also evidence that oxalate exchange may occur in the distal tubule *(9)*. Various anion exchange proteins mediate these processes *(10,11)*.

Oxalate is absorbed all along the gastrointestinal tract, including the stomach *(12)*. Absorptive and secretory pathways for oxalic acid regulated by substances that direct the net oxalate ion flux have been identified in the proximal and distal segments of rat colon *(13–16)*. Cations such as calcium and magnesium complex with oxalate in the alimentary tract and limit its absorption. The free anionic form of oxalate is thought to be the one that is absorbed. Recent oxalate loading studies in healthy volunteers have demonstrated that oxalate absorption varies tremendously, with 2–18% of a dietary oxalate load in normal individuals being absorbed *(17)*. In addition, the time sequences of absorption studies suggest that a significant amount of oxalate is absorbed in the small intestine in humans. Oxalate is also degraded in the colon by oxalate-degrading bacteria such as *Oxalobacter formigenes* and other organisms *(18)*. The actual role that this bacterium plays in altering intestinal oxalate content and oxalate absorption has not been well characterized.

A role for the intestinal absorption of dietary oxalate in stone formation was suggested by the studies of Curhan and associates *(19,20)*. A low-calcium intake was shown to be a significant risk factor for stone development. The explanation for this finding is that calcium complexes with oxalate in the alimentary tract thus limiting oxalate absorption. Metabolic studies in humans support this theory. We demonstrated a 34% increase in urinary oxalate excretion in normal adult subjects when dietary calcium is reduced from 1002 mg to 391 mg/d while other dietary constituents are unchanged, which is consistent with this theory *(21)*. In addition, Liebman and Chai found that supplemental calcium decreased the absorption of an oxalate load in humans by more than 50% *(22)*.

Studies have shown that supraphysiologic concentrations of oxalate can damage cultured renal tubular cells through free-radical-induced oxidative stress *(23–27)*. Exposure of a line of human renal epithelial cells, HK-2, to oxalate resulted in a programmed sequence of events that led to an increase in membrane permeability, alterations in cell morphology and viability, and the re-initiation of DNA synthesis *(23)*. It has been hypothesized that this concentration-dependent damage promotes a release of lipid-rich cellular membranes that act as a nidus for crystal nucleation and retention, which likely leads to lithogenesis *(28–31)*. Although there is currently no evidence that such events occur in human stone formers, stones do contain lipids in their matrix *(32)*.

The roles of oxalate and calcium in the lithogenic process have nearly always been attributed to their impact on the supersaturation of urine with calcium oxalate. Some studies have demonstrated that supersaturation of calcium oxalate in stone formers does not differ significantly from that in nonstone formers *(33,34)*. However, Borghi et al. have shown that oxalate-loading in calcium oxalate stone formers was associated with

Table 1
Oxalate Content of Various Foods

	Oxalate, mg/100 g	Oxalate per serving, mg (serving size, g)	
Spinach	645.0	645.0	(100)
Fibre One cereal	142.0	43.0	(30)
Bran flakes	141.0	42.0	(30)
Green beans (steamed)	33.0	33.0	(100)
Potato (raw)	27.1	27.1	(100)
Snack bar (Butterfinger)	53.5	24.0	(45)
Peanut butter	95.8	19.2	(20)
Tea (brewed)	7.5	18.8	(250)
Celery	61.2	18.4	(30)
Chocolate (American)	42.5	13.0	(30)
Ravioli	6.5	13.0	(200)
White bread	14.3	8.0	(56)
Carrots (raw)	5.7	5.7	(100)
Potato chips	9.4	3.0	(30)
White rice (steamed)	2.1	2.1	(100)
Broccoli (steamed)	1.8	1.8	(100)
Strawberry jelly	5.3	1.1	(20)
Corn flakes	1.9	0.6	(30)
Mustard	12.1	0.6	(5)
Apple (raw)	0.5	0.5	(100)
Peaches (canned)	0.3	0.3	(100)
Grape jelly	1.5	0.3	(20)

an increased potential for crystal nucleation as compared to controls (35). Supersaturation and nucleation of calcium oxalate are insufficient to explain the formation of stones alone, but an increased tendency to nucleation may precipitate subsequent events that are responsible for the formation of stones (36). Additionally, the upper limit of metastability in urine samples and the ability of urine components to inhibit crystal growth may be more sensitive indices in providing discrimination between the urine of stone formers and normal individuals (34).

SOURCES OF URINARY OXALATE

It was previously thought that the contributions of urinary oxalate were 40–50% hepatic synthesis, 40–50% breakdown of ascorbic acid (vitamin C), and the remaining 10–20% dietary (37). However, we and others have shown that dietary oxalate is a major contributor to urinary oxalate excretion in most humans and may account for 50% or more of the daily urinary oxalate excreted. We have demonstrated that when normal adults are placed on an oxalate-free formula diet, oxalate excretion decreases about 50% from the levels on self-selected diets, indicating that dietary oxalate is a major contributor of urinary oxalate in most individuals (21,22). Dietary oxalate originates almost exclusively from plant-derived foods (Table 1).

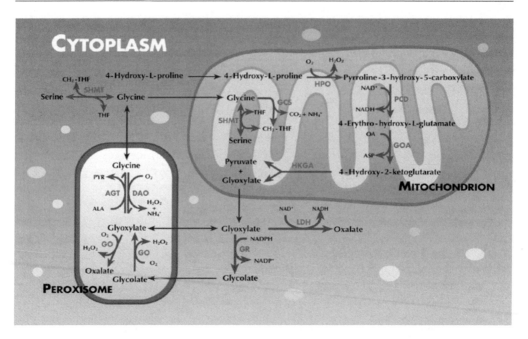

Fig. 1. Pathways associated with oxalate synthesis in hepatocytes. Transport processes are shown as the thin, dark arrows and enzymatic reactions as the thicker, lighter arrows. AGT, alanine:glyoxylate aminotransferase; DAO, D-amino acid oxidase; GCS, glycine cleavage system; GO, glycolate oxidase; GOA, glutamate oxaloacetate aminotransferase; GR, glycolate reductase; HKGA, 4-hydroxy-2-ketoglutarate lyase; HPO, hydroxyproline oxidase; LDH, lactate dehydrogenase; PCD, pyrroline-3-hydroxy-5-carboxylate dehydrogenase; SHMT, serine hydroxymethyltransferase.

Endogenous oxalate synthesis occurs in the liver. A variety of precursor molecules, including serine, glycine, hydroxyproline, ethylene glycol, and several carbohydrates, can lead to production of oxalate via pathways that converge on glycolate and glyoxylate *(38)*. The key steps are depicted in Fig. 1. This includes the oxidation of glycolate to glyoxylate catalyzed by glycolate oxidase and oxidation of glyoxylate to oxalate primarily by lactate dehydrogenase. Alanine glyoxylate aminotransferase (AGT), a very important enzyme located in the hepatic peroxisomal compartment in normal humans, diverts glyoxylate from oxalate synthesis by a transamination process, with alanine converted to pyruvate as glyoxylate is converted to glycine *(1)*.

There is still an ongoing debate on whether ascorbic acid metabolism contributes significantly to the urinary oxalate pool. Ascorbic acid is converted into oxalate by a process in the liver involving diketogluconic acid as an intermediate, with two carbons of ascorbic acid being converted into oxalate *(39)*. This conversion of diketogluconate to oxalate is nonenzymatic, although the extent to which it occurs is controversial. Little is known about the factors controlling this metabolism. The intake of high doses of ascorbic acid has been demonstrated to increase urinary oxalate excretion in normal adult individuals and stone-formers *(41)*.

Table 2
Diseases Associated With Enteric Hyperoxaluria

Diseases involving bowel mucosa
- Crohn's disease
- Ulcerative colitis
- Celiac sprue

Surgical interruption
- Jejunoileal bypass
- Ileal resection

Other causes of malabsorption and steatorrhea
- Pancreatic insufficiency or resection
- Biliary obstruction or diversion
- Primary biliary cirrhosis
- External biliary drainage
- Bacterial overgrowth
- Blind loop syndrome

HYPEROXALURIA: DEFINITION

The definition of hyperoxaluria has varied in reports in the literature. We analyzed urinary oxalate excretion in 100 normal adults and 100 adult stone-formers on self-selected diets. We found a fairly distinct difference at 30 mg of oxalate/g of excreted creatinine (42). We therefore define hyperoxaluria as anything greater than this level. The use of creatinine in this ratio limits inaccuracy caused by collection error and corrects for differences in body size. Other investigators have used different criteria for defining hyperoxaluria; e.g., greater than 43 mg/d in men and 32 mg/d in women (43). There are also varied reports of the prevalence of this metabolic disorder in stone formers, with estimates ranging from approx 8–30% (42,44).

There are three types of hyperoxaluria: enteric, primary, and idiopathic. We will discuss the etiology, manifestation, and treatment options for each.

ENTERIC HYPEROXALURIA

Enteric hyperoxaluria is caused by a variety of functional and anatomic small bowel problems (Table 2) (37,45–50). It is encountered in approx 5% of patients evaluated in specialized metabolic stone clinics and should be suspected in any patient with hyperoxaluria and small bowel abnormality (1). These patients typically also have low urine volume and diminished calcium, magnesium, and citrate excretion.

Various theories about the mechanism of enteric hyperoxaluria have been postulated. Oxalate normally complexes with calcium to form an insoluble salt or crystal that is excreted in feces. The saponification of calcium and magnesium with excess intraluminal fatty acids, secondary to their malabsorption, leaves more free oxalate to be absorbed by the intestine. Gregory et al. demonstrated increased oxalate absorption in a group of patients who underwent small bowel bypass surgery for treatment of morbid obesity (46). These patients absorbed an average of 38% of an oxalate load, compared with 6% in normal controls. In addition, there is an increased delivery of bile acids and salts to the colon, which has been demonstrated to increase oxalate uptake in this bowel segment

Table 3
Treating Hyperoxaluria With Medical Therapies

Enteric
- Fluid therapy:
  50 mL/kg body weight every 24 h in adults; higher relative intake in children
- Low-fat, low-oxalate diet
- Calcium citrate supplementation
- Magnesium oxide or magnesium gluconate can be substituted or added
- Cholestyramine therapy
- Potassium citrate to correct associated hypocitraturia
- Correct underlying bowel pathology when possible

Primary
- Type 1:
  — Fluid therapy (as described above for enteric hyperoxaluria)
  — Pyridoxine therapy
  — Orthophosphate therapy (not in patients with renal insufficiency)
  — Magnesium oxide therapy (select cases)
  — Potassium citrate therapy (select cases)
  — Sodium citrate therapy (select cases)
  — In patients with progressive renal damage leading to failure, combined renal
    and liver transplantation
- Type 2:
  — Medical therapy similar to type I
  — Role of transplantation not well defined

Idiopathic
- Fluid therapy (as described above for enteric hyperoxaluria)
- Low-oxalate diet
- Adequate calcium consumption
- Pyridoxine therapy for patients who do not respond to diet restrictions

in animal models *(51)*. The mechanism of this phenomenon has not been identified. Patients subjected to contemporary bariatric surgery may also develop this problem.

Treatment

If correction or treatment of the underlying bowel pathology is possible, this should be the initial approach for treatment of patients with enteric hyperoxaluria (Table 3). These individuals should be encouraged to increase their fluid intake because they are frequently dehydrated. They should also limit consumption of fat and high oxalate containing foods.

The administration of calcium salts with meals is recommended for most patients. The supplemental calcium promotes enteric complexation with oxalate thus limiting oxalate absorption. Calcium citrate (Citracal, 250 mg), at an initial dose of one to two tablets three times a day with meals, is the preferred agent as it will also help correct hypocitraturia *(45,46,52,53)*. The dose may need to be escalated based on follow-up 24-h urine assessments.

Magnesium oxide or magnesium gluconate may be substituted or added to this regimen. This should be considered in patients who have high normal or increased urinary calcium excretion and in those with concomitant hypomagnesemia *(54–56)*.

Cholestyramine therapy can be used when there is bile acid malabsorption to bind fatty acids, bile acids, and oxalate *(57,58)*. Other citrate salts, preferably potassium citrate, can also be given to correct associated hypocitraturia *(59,60)*. The liquid form of potassium citrate is preferred as these patients typically have rapid gastrointestinal transit.

Specific therapies of steatorrhea in certain conditions can be used: gluten-free diet in celiac sprue, pancreatic enzyme replacement in pancreatic insufficiency, and antibiotics in bacterial overgrowth.

PRIMARY HYPEROXALURIA

The primary hyperoxalurias result from endogenous overproduction of oxalate. There are two main types of primary hyperoxaluria, type I (PH1) and II (PH2). Both are rare autosomal recessive disorders caused by defects in hepatic enzyme systems important in the metabolism of glyoxylate. The marked oxalate production in both disorders may result in calcium oxalate stone formation, nephrocalcinosis, systemic oxalosis, and, in some, end-stage renal disease.

Primary Hyperoxaluria 1

PH1 is caused by a defect in glyoxylate metabolism attributable to low or absent activity of the liver-specific peroxisomal enzyme AGT *(61)*. Except for the AGT defect, peroxisomes in PH1 are normal in almost every respect *(62)*. The functional deficiency of AGT in PH1 results in a failure to detoxify glyoxylate within the peroxisomes (Fig. 1). Instead of being transaminated to glycine, glyoxylate is oxidized to oxalate and reduced to glycolate *(10,61,62)*. As a result, urinary excretion of glycolate and oxalate is significantly increased.

The gene encoding for AGT is located on chromosome 2q37.3 *(10,63,64)*. Several mutations and polymorphisms have been identified thus far and there is considerable molecular heterogeneity among patients. Half of the patients exhibit no detectable AGT activity, whereas the other half exhibits residual (2–48%) AGT activity *(10,62)*. However, even patients with residual activity can become ill and do not differ clinically from patients without AGT activity. Danpure et al. demonstrated that this occurs because AGT is mistargeted from the peroxisomes to the mitochondria *(10,62,64)*. Such patients exhibit residual enzymatic activity, with only 10% or less of the AGT localized in peroxisomes. This mistargeting defect is observed in approx 30% of all patients with PH1 *(10,65)*. A number of mechanisms have been suggested to explain the lack of catalytic activity in those with immunochemically detectable AGT. These include: (1) presence of a common P11L polymorphism, which decreases the specific activity of AGT; (2) the presence of the P11FL polymorphism in conjunction with the PH1 specific mutation, which leads to AGT protein destabilization and aggregation into inclusion bodies; (3) naturally occurring amino acid substitutions that lead to peroxisome-to-mitochondrion AGT mistargeting; and (4) interference with cofactor binding *(66)*. These may be caused by synergism between certain disease-associated mutations and the common nondisease causing AGT polymorphism, P11L.

PH1 typically manifests in patients early in life and should be suspected when oxalate excretion is greater than 1–2 mmol/1.73 m^2/24 h (normal reference range 0.11–0.46 mmol/24 h/1.73 m^2) and elevated glycolate excretion (normal range 21–168 µmol per mmol of creatinine) (1,10,65,67). Glycolate levels are elevated in approximately two-thirds of patients with PH1. Therefore findings of normal values do not exclude this diagnosis (10,65). Liver biopsy can be performed to establish a definitive diagnosis. The AGT activity and immunoreactivity in hepatic tissue are measured (10,65). A search for disease associated AGT mutations can also be undertaken. The latter approach can be used for prenatal diagnosis using chorionic villous sampling (68). The diagnosis can now be established in some patients with polymerase chain testing of blood to screen for certain AGT gene mutations associated with PH1.

Recurrent urolithiasis and nephrocalcinosis are the main manifestations, and the combination of the two conditions is characteristic for PH1 and may lead to progressive loss of renal function. Half of the patients with PH1 exhibit their first symptoms by age 5 (71,72). Approximately 40% of PH1 patients will eventually develop end-stage renal disease (ESRD) (1). The calculi of PH1 patients almost exclusively consist of calcium oxalate monohydrate (whewellite) (69,70).

Systemic oxalosis occurs when the critical saturation point for plasma oxalate (levels >30 µmol/L) is reached, typically early in renal insufficiency (73). Deposition occurs in every organ and tissue except the liver and can lead to significant morbidity. The skeleton is the most crippling site of calcium oxalate deposition. The lesions are characteristic both in X-rays (radiodense metaphyseal bands, a "bone-within-bone" appearance, and diffuse demineralization with a coarse trabecular pattern) and in histologic assessments (intraosseous tophi of calcium oxalate and granulomas replacing bone marrow) (74). Clinical manifestations of oxalate osteopathy are pain, spontaneous fractures, and erythropoietin-resistant anemia (74,75). Additional sites of oxalate deposits are the retina, media of the arteries (with subsequent ischemia and gangrene), peripheral nervous system (neuropathy), the heart, thyroid gland, and skin (livedo reticularis) (76).

TREATMENT

The goals of therapy are to decrease oxalate production and increase the urinary solubility of calcium oxalate. Without treatment, the outlook for patients with PH1 is extremely poor. Latta and Brodehl reviewed 330 patients with PH1 and found that 50% of 330 patients had ESRD by the age of 15 yr and 80% by the third decade (77). Dialysis does not remove sufficient oxalate to match its production in these patients (78–80). If initiated when renal function is satisfactory, treatment of PH1 may improve the long-term outcome of these patients (67).

Fluid therapy is a key factor in the management of patients with PH1. It has been recommended that adults with PH1 consume greater than 50 mL/kg body weight every 24 h; a higher relative intake is recommended for pediatric patients (67). It is extremely important for close follow-up monitoring and to maintain preventative measures to avoid episodes of dehydration.

Pyridoxine is an essential cofactor in the AGT enzyme pathway and approx 30% of PH1 patients respond to pyridoxine therapy (81). Pharmacologic doses of pyridoxine (dose ranges from 2.5 to 20 mg/kg/d) are able to significantly reduce (by at least 30%) oxalate excretion in one-third of patients (67,83–87). To follow pyridoxine responsiveness, reliable baseline urinary oxalate values are needed. A trial of pyridoxine therapy for at least 3 mo is warranted, although the effects usually occur in 1–2 wk in most cases

(76). Very high doses of pyridoxine should be avoided as this may cause peripheral neuropathy *(76)*. The mechanism of pyridoxine's action has not been defined. Pyridoxine responsiveness is associated with the G17OR and F1521 mutations, the latter causing mistargeting of AGT.

Orthophosphate therapy has been used in combination with pyridoxine to reduce stone formation and attenuate calcium oxalate deposition in patients with PH1 *(67)*. Its mechanism of action is thought to be caused by a resultant increase in pyrophosphate concentration, a known inhibitor of calcium oxalate crystallization, and perhaps to decreased calcium excretion *(1)*. A clinical trial of this combination in 25 patients lead to a significant decrease in stone events and prevented renal deterioration in most patients at a mean follow-up of 10.3 yr *(67)*. Orthophosphate should not be used in patients with renal insufficiency.

Magnesium oxide, sodium citrate, and potassium citrate therapy have also been used in PH1, but the true efficacy of these agents has not been determined. Citrate not only binds calcium but also is an inhibitor of calcium oxalate crystal nucleation and growth *(88)*. Although there is clinical and experimental evidence of the beneficial effects of this therapy, it has been difficult to conclusively prove *(89,90)*. Magnesium is another potential inhibitor of calcium oxalate crystallization because it binds to oxalate.

Patients with PH1 who develop renal failure are best managed by combined liver and renal transplantation. Renal transplantation alone does not correct the basic hepatic enzyme abnormality and therefore recurrent disease is a potential problem. Broyer et al. reviewed the European experience where primarily cadaveric renal transplantation was performed. The 3-yr graft and patient survivals were 20% and 74%, respectively *(91)*. Saborio and Scheinman reported on the experience in the United States where living-related renal transplantation was primarily undertaken. The 6-yr actuarial graft and patient survivals were 51% and 84%, respectively. However the 10-yr graft survival rate was only 35% *(92)*.

Because the metabolic defect is in the liver, total hepatectomy is required before liver and renal transplantation. The first successful, combined liver and kidney transplant for a patient with PH1 was performed in 1984 *(93)*. The actuarial 5-yr graft and patient survival rates for this approach in some series have been approx 70% and 80%, respectively. However, recent studies demonstrated that patient survival is better after renal transplantation. Poor prognostic factors for graft and patient survival include presence of systemic oxalosis, young age (<5 yr), and history of >2 yr of dialysis. In addition, the renal function of survivors remains stable over time, between 40 and 60 mL/min/1.73 m^2 after 5–10 yr *(87, 94–96)*.

Some investigators have performed pre-emptive hepatic transplantation in those afflicted with PH1. However this approach is controversial. If liver transplantation was a simple procedure with minimal risks and there were no shortage of organs, preemptive transplantation would probably be an acceptable treatment option in patients with PH1. However, there are ethical issues including the risk of graft loss and complications related to the transplant in a patient who might have done well for several years longer without such an aggressive intervention. There is also concern about the potential long-term effects of immunosuppressive drugs including renal toxicity and malignancy. Isolated liver transplantation can only be successful if renal function is adequate (glomerular filtration rate greater than the 40–50 mL/min) *(76)*. If the glomerular filtration rate is <40 mL/min/1.73 m^2, there is a significant risk of eventual renal failure *(97)*. Results of preemptive liver transplantation have thus far been reasonable *(97)*.

Other approaches have been considered for patients with PH1. We evaluated the short-term efficacy of (L)-2-oxothiaolidine-4-carboxylate (OTZ) therapy. OTZ is a cysteine precursor that is converted to cysteine within the cell and forms a stable adduct with the aldehyde group of glyoxylate, which could potentially decrease oxalate synthesis. Administration of OTZ has been demonstrated to reduce oxalate excretion in rats and normal human subjects *(98,99)*. However, it did not result in a reduction in two patients with PH1 perhaps caused by the extremely large glyoxylate pool. The utilization of agents that inhibit glycolate oxidase, a key enzyme in oxalate synthesis, has been proposed as another therapeutic approach.

The identification and characterization of the AGT gene has stimulated interest in gene therapy for those afflicted with PH1 *(63)*. Intraportal infusion of recombinant viruses or macromolecular DNA as gene vectors has been suggested *(1)*. The other approach involves the surgical removal or ablation of hepatic tissue, isolation of hepatocytes or stem cells, *ex vivo* transfection of these cells, and infusion of the transfected hepatocytes into the portal vein *(100–102)*. A major hurdle to overcome is the large size of the hepatic target which makes vector delivery quite difficult. The ability to maintain the corrective gene will also need to be established. Surgical or pharmacologic strategies to reduce the targeted hepatic mass will be necessary to facilitate adequate gene delivery; another impediment.

Primary Hyperoxaluria (PH2)

PH2 results from a deficiency in glyoxylate reductase (GR) activity which leads to an increased oxalate synthesis and urinary excretion *(103–106)*. The responsible gene, GRHPR, is mapped to the centromeric region of chromosome 9 *(107)*. Although the liver has the highest GR activity, the enzyme is ubiquitously expressed in all tissues, perhaps indicating that all tissues synthesize glyoxylate. As with PH1, a range of different mutations has been identified, although one mutation predominates in Caucasians *(108)*. Clinical manifestations are not as severe as in PH1, although ESRD can result *(109)*. The metabolic features of PH2 are increased urinary excretion of L-glycerate and oxalate. The conservative stone prevention treatments used with PH1 patients can also be applied to PH2 patients. However the efficacy of pyridoxine therapy and liver transplantation has not been established. Owing to the ubiquitous expression of GR activity, liver transplantation may not be as effective.

Another group of patients with hyperoxaluria in the primary hyperoxaluria range has been identified which do not have the metabolic characteristics of PH1 and PH2 *(110)*. The mechanisms of this novel form of hyperoxaluria have not yet been defined.

Idiopathic Hyperoxaluria

Idiopathic hyperoxaluria is the most common type of hyperoxaluria. Patients frequently have other coexistent metabolic abnormalities that should also be addressed.

Dietary modifications should be initially considered for treatment (Table 3). Given that a significant amount of urinary oxalate is derived from dietary sources, patients should refrain from consuming high oxalate containing foods (Table 1). Approximately one-third of patients with idiopathic hyperoxaluria are protein sensitive, with increased animal protein consumption leading to increased urinary oxalate excretion *(111,112)*. Therefore, animal protein restriction should be considered for this reason as well as the promotion of other beneficial changes such as a reduction in calcium and uric acid excretion and an increase in citrate excretion. Normal dietary calcium consumption is important as reduced calcium intake is associated with an increase in oxalate excretion *(21)*. Supplementation of meals with calcium should also be considered, particularly in those patients who do not like to, or cannot, consume dairy products.

Pyridoxine therapy is an option for those patients with poor response to dietary restrictions. The results with this therapy have been conflicting, however a trial of this agent should be considered because there are no other known treatment options and the side effects are minimal *(113–118)*.

POTENTIAL FUTURE THERAPY

Probiotic Therapy

Campieri and colleagues reported that the urinary oxalate excretion decreased when hyperoxaluric stone-formers were administered lactic acid bacteria *(119)*. Although the results need to be corroborated, this suggests that probiotic therapy may play a future role in the management of this patient population. The utilization of *O. formigenes* for this purpose has been undertaken. There are several reasons why this approach has been proposed. This anaerobic bacterium is not pathogenic. A higher percentage of nonstone formers have *O. formigenes* fecal colonization as compared to stone formers *(120)*. An inverse correlation between colonization and urinary oxalate excretion has been reported *(120)*. Some investigators have suggested that there is also an inverse correlation between stone activity and fecal colonization with this organism *(121)*. The administration of this bacterium to rats promoted a decrease in urinary oxalate excretion *(121,122)*. A pilot study suggested that the oral administration of this bacterium promoted a similar response in humans *(123)*. Although antegrade or retrograde (enema) colonization of subjects lacking this bacterium in the colon may prove to be beneficial, the daily oral administration of this organism with meals may allow for oxalate degradation in the small bowel, an area where the majority of oxalate absorption is thought to occur. Preliminary results have demonstrated that giving this bacterium to patients with PH1 may promote a reduction in oxalate excretion. This is hypothesized to be due to stimulating oxalase secretion within the gut. An expanded ongoing study will hopefully define the utility of this approach.

Enzymatic Therapy

Another approach for limiting oxalate absorption is the development of methods to degrade this organic acid in the intestinal tract. Administering capsules containing oxalate-degrading enzymes such as oxalate decarboxylase could possibly accomplish this.

The control of oxalate and its effects at the renal level may be used to treat certain calcium oxalate stone formers in the future. Brandle and colleagues have reported on the development of an inhibitor of renal oxalate secretion (EO8) which is thought to have an action on the oxalate/sulfate exchanger in the basolateral membrane of the proximal tubule *(124)*. EO8 significantly reduced oxalate clearance in rats without inducing an increase in plasma oxalate. This indicates that EO8 might influence oxalate transport in the gastrointestinal tract and liver where similar transporters exist.

Phytotherapy/Complementary Medicine

Phytotherapy may prove to be beneficial for patients with hyperoxaluria. Investigators have found that banana stem extract significantly reduces oxalate excretion in rats by unknown mechanisms *(126)*. Some investigators have hypothesized that its high level of oxalate oxidase could potentially degrade oxalate in the alimentary tract and therefore decrease enteric oxalate absorption *(127)*. We anticipate that other complementary agents will surface in the future, but the actual benefit will need to be established in well-controlled studies.

CONCLUSIONS

The therapy of hyperoxaluric patients should be directed by the underlying causes. Future innovations should facilitate the management of individuals afflicted with hyperoxaluric states.

REFERENCES

1. Assimos DG, Goodman HO, Holmes RP. Hyperoxaluria: Advances in medical therapy. Contemp Urol. 1997; 47–60.
2. Senekjian HO, Weinman EJ. Oxalate transport by proximal tubule of the rabbit kidney. Am J Physiol. 1982; 243(3): F271–275.
3. Greger R, Lang F, Oberleithner H, Deetjen P. Handling of oxalate by the rat kidney. Pflugers Arch. 1978; 374(3): 243–248.
4. Weinman EJ, Frankfurt SJ, Ince A, Sansom S. Renal tubular transport of organic acids. Studies with oxalate and para- aminohippurate in the rat. J Clin Invest. 1978; 61(3): 801–806.
5. Williams HE, Johnson GA, Smith LH, Jr. The renal clearance of oxalate in normal subjects and patients with primary hyperoxaluria. Clin Sci. 1971; 41(3): 213–218.
6. Karniski LP, Lotscher M, Fucentese M, Hilfiker H, Biber J, Murer H. Immunolocalization of sat-1 sulfate/oxalate/bicarbonate anion exchanger in the rat kidney. Am J Physiol. 1998; 275(1 Pt 2): F79–87.
7. Karniski LP, Aronson PS. Anion exchange pathways for Cl- transport in rabbit renal microvillus membranes. Am J Physiol. 1987; 253(3 Pt 2): F513–521.
8. Brandle E, Bernt U, Hautmann RE. In situ characterization of oxalate transport across the basolateral membrane of the proximal tubule. Pflugers Arch. 1998; 435(6): 840–849.
9. Lohi H, Kujala M, Makela S, et al. Functional characterization of three novel tissue-specific anion exchangers SLC26A7, -A8, and -A9. J Biol Chem. 2002; 277(16): 14,246–14,254.
10. Danpure CJ. Primary hyperoxaluria. In: The Metabolic and Molecular Bases of Inherited Diseases, (Scriver CR, Beaudet AL, Sly WS, et al., eds.). McGraw-Hill, New York, NY, 2001; pp. 3323–3367.
11. Scheid CR, Koul H, Hill A, Lieske JC, Toback G, Menon M. Oxalate ion and calcium oxalate crystal interactions with renal epithelial cells. In: Kidney Stones: Medical and Surgical Management, (Coe FL, Favus MJ, Pak CYC, Parks JH, Preminger GM, eds.). Lippincott-Raven, Philadelphia, PA, 1996; pp. 120–143.
12. Hautmann RE. The stomach: a new and powerful oxalate absorption site in man. J Urol. 1993; 149(6): 1401–1404.
13. Freel RW, Hatch M, Earnest DL, Goldner AM. Oxalate transport across the isolated rat colon. A re-examination. Biochim Biophys Acta. 1980; 600(3): 838–843.
14. Hatch M, Freel RW, Goldner AM, Earnest DL. Oxalate and chloride absorption by the rabbit colon: sensitivity to metabolic and anion transport inhibitors. Gut. 1984; 25(3): 232–237.
15. Hatch M, Freel RW, Vaziri ND. Characteristics of the transport of oxalate and other ions across rabbit proximal colon. Pflugers Arch. 1993; 423(3–4): 206–212.
16. Hatch M, Freel RW, Vaziri ND. Mechanisms of oxalate absorption and secretion across the rabbit distal colon. Pflugers Arch. 1994; 426(1–2): 101–109.

17. Hesse A, Schneeberger W, Engfeld S, Von Unruh GE, Sauerbruch T. Intestinal hyperabsorption of oxalate in calcium oxalate stone formers: application of a new test with [13C2]oxalate. J Am Soc Nephrol. 1999; 10 Suppl 14: S329–333.

18. Allison MJ, Dawson KA, Mayberry WR, Foss JG. Oxalobacter formigenes gen. nov., sp. nov.: oxalate-degrading anaerobes that inhabit the gastrointestinal tract. Arch Microbiol. 1985; 141(1): 1–7.

19. Curhan GC, Willett WC, Speizer FE, Spiegelman D, Stampfer MJ. Comparison of dietary calcium with supplemental calcium and other nutrients as factors affecting the risk for kidney stones in women. Ann Intern Med. 1997; 126(7): 497–504.

20. Curhan GC, Willett WC, Rimm EB, Stampfer MJ. A prospective study of dietary calcium and other nutrients and the risk of symptomatic kidney stones. N Engl J Med. 1993; 328(12): 833–838.

21. Holmes RP, Goodman HO, Assimos DG. Contribution of dietary oxalate to urinary oxalate excretion. Kidney Int. 2001; 59(1): 270–276.

22. Liebman M, Chai W. Effect of dietary calcium on urinary oxalate excretion after oxalate loads. Am J Clin Nutr. 1997; 65(5): 1453–1459.

23. Bhandari A, Koul S, Sekhon A, et al. Effects of oxalate on HK-2 cells, a line of proximal tubular epithelial cells from normal human kidney. J Urol. 2002; 168(1): 253–259.

24. Thamilselvan S, Khan SR. Oxalate and calcium oxalate crystals are injurious to renal epithelial cells: results of in vivo and in vitro studies. J Nephrol. 1998; 11 Suppl 1: 66–69.

25. Thamilselvan S, Byer KJ, Hackett RL, Khan SR. Free radical scavengers, catalase and superoxide dismutase provide protection from oxalate-associated injury to LLC-PK1 and MDCK cells. J Urol. 2000; 164(1): 224–229.

26. Scheid C, Koul H, Hill WA, et al. Oxalate toxicity in LLC-PK1 cells: role of free radicals. Kidney Int. 1996; 49(2): 413–419.

27. Scheid C, Koul H, Hill WA, et al. Oxalate toxicity in LLC-PK1 cells, a line of renal epithelial cells. J Urol. 1996; 155(3): 1112–1116.

28. Koul HK, Koul S, Fu S, Santosham V, Seikhon A, Menon M. Oxalate: from crystal formation to crystal retention. J Am Soc Nephrol. 1999; 10 Suppl 14: S417–421.

29. Khan SR, Glenton PA. Increased urinary excretion of lipids by patients with kidney stones. Br J Urol. 1996; 77(4): 506–511.

30. Khan SR, Maslamani SA, Atmani F, et al. Membranes and their constituents as promoters of calcium oxalate crystal formation in human urine. Calcif Tissue Int. 2000; 66(2): 90–96.

31. Bigelow MW, Wiessner JH, Kleinman JG, Mandel NS. Calcium oxalate-crystal membrane interactions: dependence on membrane lipid composition. J Urol. 1996; 155(3): 1094–1098.

32. Khan SR, Shevock PN, Hackett RL. Presence of lipids in urinary stones: results of preliminary studies. Calcif Tissue Int. 1988; 42(2): 91–96.

33. Asplin JR, Parks JH, Coe FL. Dependence of upper limit of metastability on supersaturation in nephrolithiasis. Kidney Int. 1997; 52(6): 1602–1608.

34. Asplin JR, Parks JH, Chen MS, et al. Reduced crystallization inhibition by urine from men with nephrolithiasis. Kidney Int. 1999; 56(4): 1505–1516.

35. Borghi L, Meschi T, Guerra A, Bergamaschi E, Mutti A, Novarini A. Effects of urinary macromolecules on the nucleation of calcium oxalate in idiopathic stone formers and healthy controls. Clin Chim Acta. 1995; 239(1): 1–11.

36. Borghi L, Guerra A, Meschi T, et al. Relationship between supersaturation and calcium oxalate crystallization in normals and idiopathic calcium oxalate stone formers. Kidney Int. 1999; 55(3): 1041–1050.

37. Williams HE, Wandzilak TR. Oxalate synthesis, transport and the hyperoxaluric syndromes. J Urol. 1989; 141(3 Pt 2): 742–749.

38. Nath R, Thind SK, Murthy MS, Talwar HS, Farooqui S. Molecular aspects of idiopathic urolithiasis. Mol Aspects Med. 1984; 7(1–2): 1–176.

39. Baker EM, Saari JC, Tolbert BM. Ascorbic acid metabolism in man. Am J Clin Nutr. 1966; 19(6): 371–378.

40. Wandzilak TR, D'Andre SD, Davis PA, Williams HE. Effect of high dose vitamin C on urinary oxalate levels. J Urol. 1994; 151(4): 834–837.

41. Traxer O, Huet B, Pak CYC, Pearle MS. Stone forming risk of ascorbic acid. J Endourol. 2000; 14 (Suppl 1): A9.

42. Goodman HO, Holmes RP, Assimos DG. Genetic factors in calcium oxalate stone disease. J Urol. 1995; 153(2): 301–307.

43. Nemeh MN, Weinman EJ, Kayne LH, Lee DBN. Absorption and excretion of urate, oxalate, and amino acids. In: Kidney Stones: Medical and Surgical Management, (Coe FL, Favus MJ, Pak CYC, Parks JH, Preminger GM, eds.). Lippincott-Raven, Philadelphia, PA, 1996; pp. 303–319.

44. Levy FL, Adams-Huet B, Pak CY. Ambulatory evaluation of nephrolithiasis: an update of a 1980 protocol. Am J Med. 1995; 98(1): 50–59.

45. Clayman RV, Buchwald H, Varco RL, DeWolf WC, Williams RD. Urolithiasis in patients with a jejunoileal bypass. Surg Gynecol Obstet. 1978; 147(2): 225–230.

46. Gregory JG, Park KY, Schoenberg HW. Oxalate stone disease after intestinal resection. J Urol. 1977; 117(5): 631–634.

47. Earnest DL. Enteric hyperoxaluria. Adv Intern Med. 1979; 24: 407–427.

48. Earnest DL, Johnson G, Williams HE, Admirand WH. Hyperoxaluria in patients with ileal resection: an abnormality in dietary oxalate absorption. Gastroenterology. 1974; 66(6): 1114–1122.

49. Kaye MC, Streem SB, Hall PM. Enteric hyperoxaluria associated with external biliary drainage. J Urol. 1994; 151(2): 396, 397.

50. Ogilvie D, McCollum JP, Packer S, et al. Urinary outputs of oxalate, calcium, and magnesium in children with intestinal disorders. Potential cause of renal calculi. Arch Dis Child. 1976; 51(10): 790–795.

51. Dobbins JW, Binder HJ. Effect of bile salts and fatty acids on the colonic absorption of oxalate. Gastroenterology. 1976; 70(6): 1096–1100.

52. Harvey JA, Zobitz MM, Pak CY. Calcium citrate: reduced propensity for the crystallization of calcium oxalate in urine resulting from induced hypercalciuria of calcium supplementation. J Clin Endocrinol Metab. 1985; 61(6): 1223–1225.

53. Rudman D, Dedonis JL, Fountain MT, et al. Hypocitraturia in patients with gastrointestinal malabsorption. N Engl J Med. 1980; 303(12): 657–661.

54. Hessov I, Hasselblad C, Fasth S, Hulten L. Magnesium deficiency after ileal resections for Crohn's disease. Scand J Gastroenterol. 1983; 18(5): 643–649.

55. Gerlach K, Morowitz DA, Kirsner JB. Symptomatic hypomagnesemia complicating regional enteritis. Gastroenterology. 1970; 59(4): 567–574.

56. Galland L. Magnesium and inflammatory bowel disease. Magnesium. 1988; 7(2): 78–83.

57. Caspary WF, Tonissen J, Lankisch PG. 'Enteral' hyperoxaluria. Effect of cholestyramine, calcium, neomycin, and bile acids on intestinal oxalate absorption in man. Acta Hepatogastroenterol (Stuttg). 1977; 24(3): 193–200.

58. Smith LH, Fromm H, Hofmann AF. Acquired hyperoxaluria, nephrolithiasis, and intestinal disease. Description of a syndrome. N Engl J Med. 1972; 286(26): 1371–1375.

59. Pak CY, Fuller C, Sakhaee K, Preminger GM, Britton F. Long-term treatment of calcium nephrolithiasis with potassium citrate. J Urol. 1985; 134(1): 11–19.

60. Barcelo P, Wuhl O, Servitge E, Rousaud A, Pak CY. Randomized double-blind study of potassium citrate in idiopathic hypocitraturic calcium nephrolithiasis. J Urol. 1993; 150(6): 1761–1764.

61. Danpure CJ, Jennings PR, Watts RW. Enzymological diagnosis of primary hyperoxaluria type 1 by measurement of hepatic alanine: glyoxylate aminotransferase activity. Lancet. 1987; 1(8528): 289–291.

62. Danpure CJ, Jennings PR, Fryer P, Purdue PE, Allsop J. Primary hyperoxaluria type 1: genotypic and phenotypic heterogeneity. J Inherit Metab Dis. 1994; 17(4): 487–499.

63. Purdue PE, Lumb MJ, Fox M, et al. Characterization and chromosomal mapping of a genomic clone encoding human alanine:glyoxylate aminotransferase. Genomics. 1991; 10(1): 34–42.

64. Takada Y, Kaneko N, Esumi H, Purdue PE, Danpure CJ. Human peroxisomal L-alanine: glyoxylate aminotransferase. Evolutionary loss of a mitochondrial targeting signal by point mutation of the initiation codon. Biochem J. 1990; 268(2): 517–520.

65. Cochat P. Primary hyperoxaluria type 1. Kidney Int 1999; 55(6): 2533–2547.

66. Lumb MJ, Danpure CJ. Functional synergism between the most common polymorphism in human alanine:glyoxylate aminotransferase and four of the most common disease- causing mutations. J Biol Chem. 2000; 275(46): 36,415–36,422.

67. Milliner DS, Eickholt JT, Bergstralh EJ, Wilson DM, Smith LH. Results of long-term treatment with orthophosphate and pyridoxine in patients with primary hyperoxaluria. N Engl J Med. 1994; 331(23): 1553–1558.

68. Rumsby G. Experience in prenatal diagnosis of primary hyperoxaluria type 1. J Nephrol. 1998; 11 Suppl 1: 13–14.

69. Neuhaus TJ, Belzer T, Blau N, Hoppe B, Sidhu H, Leumann E. Urinary oxalate excretion in urolithiasis and nephrocalcinosis. Arch Dis Child. 2000; 82(4): 322–326.

70. Daudon M, Estepa L, Lacour B, Jungers P. Unusual morphology of calcium oxalate calculi in primary hyperoxaluria. J Nephrol. 1998; 11 Suppl 1: 51–55.

71. Kopp N, Leumann E. Changing pattern of primary hyperoxaluria in Switzerland. Nephrol Dial Transplant. 1995; 10(12): 2224–2227.

72. Cochat P, Deloraine A, Rotily M, Olive F, Liponski I, Deries N. Epidemiology of primary hyperoxaluria type 1. Societe de Nephrologie and the Societe de Nephrologie Pediatrique. Nephrol Dial Transplant. 1995; 10(Suppl 8): 3–7.

73. Hoppe B, Kemper MJ, Bokenkamp A, Langman CB. Plasma calcium-oxalate saturation in children with renal insufficiency and in children with primary hyperoxaluria. Kidney Int. 1998; 54(3): 921–925.

74. Schnitzler CM, Kok JA, Jacobs DW, et al. Skeletal manifestations of primary oxalosis. Pediatr Nephrol. 1991; 5(2): 193–199.

75. Toussaint C, De Pauw L, Vienne A, et al. Radiological and histological improvement of oxalate osteopathy after combined liver-kidney transplantation in primary hyperoxaluria type 1. Am J Kidney Dis. 1993; 21(1): 54–63.

76. Leumann E, Hoppe B. The primary hyperoxalurias. J Am Soc Nephrol. 2001; 12(9): 1986–1993.

77. Latta K, Brodehl J. Primary hyperoxaluria type I. Eur J Pediatr. 1990; 149(8): 518–522.

78. Marangella M, Petrarulo M, Vitale C, et al. Serum calcium oxalate saturation in patients on maintenance haemodialysis for primary hyperoxaluria or oxalosis-unrelated renal diseases. Clin Sci (Lond). 1991; 81(4): 483–490.

79. Hoppe B, Graf D, Offner G, et al. Oxalate elimination via hemodialysis or peritoneal dialysis in children with chronic renal failure. Pediatr Nephrol. 1996; 10(4): 488–492.

80. Watts RW, Veall N, Purkiss P. Oxalate dynamics and removal rates during haemodialysis and peritoneal dialysis in patients with primary hyperoxaluria and severe renal failure. Clin Sci (Lond). 1984; 66(5): 591–597.

81. Gibbs DA, Watts RW. The action of pyridoxine in primary hyperoxaluria. Clin Sci. 1970; 38(2): 277–286.

82. Marangella M. Transplantation strategies in type 1 primary hyperoxaluria: the issue of pyridoxine responsiveness. Nephrol Dial Transplant. 1999; 14(2): 301–303.

83. Leumann E, Matasovic A, Niederwieser A. Pyridoxine in primary hyperoxaluria type I. Lancet. 1986; 2(8508): 699.

84. Smith LH, Jr., Williams HE. Treatment of primary hyperoxaluria. Mod Treat. 1967; 4(3): 522–530.

85. Watts RW, Veall N, Purkiss P, Mansell MA, Haywood EF. The effect of pyridoxine on oxalate dynamics in three cases of primary hyperoxaluria (with glycollic aciduria). Clin Sci (Lond). 1985; 69(1): 87–90.

86. Alinei P, Guignard JP, Jaeger P. Pyridoxine treatment of type 1 hyperoxaluria. N Engl J Med 1984; 311(12): 798, 799.

87. Leumann E, Hoppe B. What is new in primary hyperoxaluria? Nephrol Dial. Transplant 1999; 14(11): 2556–2558.

88. Coe FL, Parks JH. New insights into the pathophysiology and treatment of nephrolithiasis: new research venues. J Bone Miner Res. 1997; 12(4): 522–533.

89. Leumann E, Hoppe B, Neuhaus T. Management of primary hyperoxaluria: efficacy of oral citrate administration. Pediatr Nephrol. 1993; 7(2): 207–211.

90. Leumann E, Hoppe B, Neuhaus T, Blau N. Efficacy of oral citrate administration in primary hyperoxaluria. Nephrol Dial Transplant. 1995; 10(Suppl 8): 14–16.

91. Broyer M, Brunner FP, Brynger H, et al. Kidney transplantation in primary oxalosis: data from the EDTA Registry. Nephrol Dial Transplant. 1990; 5(5): 332–336.

92. Saborio P, Scheinman JI. Transplantation for primary hyperoxaluria in the United States. Kidney Int. 1999; 56(3): 1094–1100.

93. Watts RW, Calne RY, Rolles K, et al. Successful treatment of primary hyperoxaluria type I by combined hepatic and renal transplantation. Lancet. 1987; 2(8557): 474, 475.

94. Cochat P, Gaulier JM, Koch Nogueira PC, et al. Combined liver-kidney transplantation in primary hyperoxaluria type 1. Eur J Pediatr. 1999; 158 Suppl 2: S75–80.

95. Jamieson NV. The European Primary Hyperoxaluria Type 1 Transplant Registry report on the results of combined liver/kidney transplantation for primary hyperoxaluria 1984–1994. European PH1 Transplantation Study Group. Nephrol Dial Transplant. 1995; 10(Suppl 8): 33–37.

96. Jamieson NV. The results of combined liver/kidney transplantation for primary hyperoxaluria (PH1) 1984-1997. The European PH1 transplant registry report. European PH1 Transplantation Study Group. J Nephrol. 1998; 11 Suppl 1: 36–41.

97. Nolkemper D, Kemper MJ, Burdelski M, et al. Long-term results of pre-emptive liver transplantation in primary hyperoxaluria type 1. Pediatr Transplant. 2000; 4(3): 177–181.

98. Holmes RP, Assimos DG, Leaf CD, Whalen JJ. The effects of (L)-2-oxothiazolidine-4-carboxylate on urinary oxalate excretion. J Urol. 1997; 158(1): 34–37.

99. Holmes RP, Assimos DG, Wilson DM, Milliner DS. (L)-2-oxothiazolidine-4-carboxylate in the treatment of primary hyperoxaluria type 1. BJU Int. 2001; 88(9): 858–862.

100. Grossman M, Wilson JM. Retroviruses: delivery vehicle to the liver. Curr Opin Genet Dev. 1993; 3(1): 110–114.

101. Ledley FD. Hepatic gene therapy: present and future. Hepatology. 1993; 18(5): 1263–1273.

102. Raper SE, Wilson JM. Cell transplantation in liver-directed gene therapy. Cell Transplant. 1993; 2(5): 381–400; discussion 407–410.

103. Chlebeck PT, Milliner DS, Smith LH. Long-term prognosis in primary hyperoxaluria type II (L-glyceric aciduria). Am J Kidney Dis. 1994; 23(2): 255–259.

104. Chalmers RA, Tracey BM, Mistry J, Griffiths KD, Green A, Winterborn MH. L-Glyceric aciduria (primary hyperoxaluria type 2) in siblings in two unrelated families. J Inherit Metab Dis. 1984; 7(Suppl 2): 133, 134.

105. Seargeant LE, deGroot GW, Dilling LA, Mallory CJ, Haworth JC. Primary oxaluria type 2 (L-glyceric aciduria): a rare cause of nephrolithiasis in children. J Pediatr. 1991; 118(6): 912–914.

106. Williams HE, Smith LH, Jr. L-glyceric aciduria. A new genetic variant of primary hyperoxaluria. N Engl J Med. 1968; 278(5): 233–238.

107. Cramer SD, Ferree PM, Lin K, Milliner DS, Holmes RP. The gene encoding hydroxypyruvate reductase (GRHPR) is mutated in patients with primary hyperoxaluria type II. Hum Mol Genet. 1999; 8(11): 2063–2069.

108. Webster KE, Ferree PM, Holmes RP, Cramer SD. Identification of missense, nonsense, and deletion mutations in the GRHPR gene in patients with primary hyperoxaluria type II (PH2). Hum Genet. 2000; 107(2): 176–185.

109. Milliner DS, Wilson DM, Smith LH. Phenotypic expression of primary hyperoxaluria: comparative features of types I and II. Kidney Int. 2001; 59(1): 31–36.

110. Monico CG, Persson M, Ford GC, Rumsby G, Milliner DS. Potential mechanisms of marked hyperoxaluria not due to primary hyperoxaluria I or II. Kidney Int. 2002; 62(2): 392–400.

111. Breslau NA, Brinkley L, Hill KD, Pak CY. Relationship of animal protein-rich diet to kidney stone formation and calcium metabolism. J Clin Endocrinol Metab. 1988; 66(1): 140–146.

112. Nguyen QV, Kalin A, Drouve U, Casez JP, Jaeger P. Sensitivity to meat protein intake and hyperoxaluria in idiopathic calcium stone formers. Kidney Int. 2001; 59(6): 2273–2281.

113. Edwards P, Nemat S, Rose GA. Effects of oral pyridoxine upon plasma and 24-hour urinary oxalate levels in normal subjects and stone formers with idiopathic hypercalciuria. Urol Res. 1990; 18(6): 393–396.

114. Balcke P, Schmidt P, Zazgornik J, Kopsa H, Minar E. Pyridoxine therapy in patients with renal calcium oxalate calculi. Proc Eur Dial Transplant Assoc. 1983; 20: 417–421.

115. Curhan GC, Willett WC, Rimm EB, Stampfer MJ. A prospective study of the intake of vitamins C and B6, and the risk of kidney stones in men. J Urol. 1996; 155(6): 1847–1851.

116. Mitwalli A, Ayiomamitis A, Grass L, Oreopoulos DG. Control of hyperoxaluria with large doses of pyridoxine in patients with kidney stones. Int Urol Nephrol. 1988; 20(4): 353–359.

117. Prien EL, Sr., Gershoff SF. Magnesium oxide-pyridoxine therapy for recurrent calcium oxalate calculi. J Urol. 1974; 112(4): 509–512.

118. Rattan V, Sidhu H, Vaidyanathan S, Thind SK, Nath R. Effect of combined supplementation of magnesium oxide and pyridoxine in calcium-oxalate stone formers. Urol Res. 1994; 22(3): 161–165.

119. Campieri C, Campieri M, Bertuzzi V, et al. Reduction of oxaluria after an oral course of lactic acid bacteria at high concentration. Kidney Int. 2001; 60(3): 1097–1105.

120. Kumar R, Mukherjee M, Bhandari M, Kumar A, Sidhu H, Mittal RD. Role of Oxalobacter formigenes in calcium oxalate stone disease: a study from north India. Eur Urol. 2002; 41(3): 318–322.

121. Sidhu H, Schmidt ME, Cornelius JG, et al. Direct correlation between hyperoxaluria/oxalate stone disease and the absence of the gastrointestinal tract-dwelling bacterium Oxalobacter formigenes: possible prevention by gut recolonization or enzyme replacement therapy. J Am Soc Nephrol. 1999; 10 Suppl 14: S334–S340.

122. Sidhu H, Allison MJ, Chow JM, Clark A, Peck AB. Rapid reversal of hyperoxaluria in a rat model after probiotic administration of Oxalobacter formigenes. J Urol. 2001; 166(4): 1487–1491.

123. Duncan SH, Richardson AJ, Kaul P, Holmes RP, Allison MJ, Stewart CS. Oxalobacter formigenes and its potential role in human health. Appl Environ Microbiol. 2002; 68(8): 3841–3847.

124. Brandle E, Bernt U, Kleinschmidt K. EO8: a specific inhibitor of the renal tubular oxalate secretion - a new concept in the medical treatment of calcium oxalate stones. In: Urolithiasis 2000 Book of Proceedings. Vol. 2., (Rodgers AL, Hibbert BE, Hess B, Khan SR, Preminger GM, eds.). University of Cape Town, Cape Town, 2000; p. 480.

125. Kothari S, Verma N, Barjatiya MK. Antioxidants have adjuvant therapeutic value in the management of hyperoxaluria. In: Urolithiasis 2000 Book of Proceedings. Vol. 2., (Rodgers AL, Hibbert BE, Hess B, Khan SR, Preminger GM, eds.). University of Cape Town, Cape Town, Africa, 2000; p. 482.

126. Poonguzhali PK, Chegu H. The influence of banana stem extract on urinary risk factors for stones in normal and hyperoxaluric rats. Br J Urol. 1994; 74(1): 23–25.

127. Ramakrishnan V, Lathika KM, D'Souza SJ, Singh BB, Raghavan KG. Investigation with chitosan-oxalate oxidase-catalase conjugate for degrading oxalate from hyperoxaluric rat chyme. Indian J Biochem Biophys. 1997; 34(4): 373–378.

128. Buck AC, Lote CJ, Sampson WF. The influence of renal prostaglandins on urinary calcium excretion in idiopathic urolithiasis. J Urol. 1983; 129(2): 421–426.

129. Naya Y, Ito H, Masai M, Yamaguchi K. Association of dietary fatty acids with urinary oxalate excretion in calcium oxalate stone-formers in their fourth decade. BJU Int. 2002; 89(9): 842–846.

130. Buck AC, Davies RL, Harrison T. The protective role of eicosapentaenoic acid [EPA] in the pathogenesis of nephrolithiasis. J Urol. 1991; 146(1): 188–194.

131. Baggio B, Budakovic A, Nassuato MA, et al. Plasma phospholipid arachidonic acid content and calcium metabolism in idiopathic calcium nephrolithiasis. Kidney Int. 2000; 58(3): 1278–1284.

8

Renal Acid–Base Balance and Renal Tubular Acidosis

Andrew I. Chin, MD

Key Words: Nephrolithiasis; pH; renal physiology.

INTRODUCTION

Renal stone disease is frequently associated with abnormal urinary acid–base balance. Renal tubular defects may influence urinary pH and alter urinary excretion of various substances, predisposing to stone formation. This chapter provides a background for the understanding of acid–base disorders, mainly from a renal perspective. Most of the concepts of pulmonary and renal acid–base regulation are well established. The concepts of renal tubular acidosis, however, are still being refined. In the past several years, the developments of microbiological and genetic research have added new insights to the pathophysiology of renal tubular disorders. The topics in this section will touch on basic renal and nonrenal acid–base regulation, systemic and urinary buffering, and focus on regulation of urinary pH, and renal tubular acidosis.

ACID–BASE CHEMISTRY

pH

A substance that donates a free hydrogen ion or proton (H$^+$) in solution is termed an acid, whereas a substance that binds a free proton in solution is termed a base. The

From: Current Clinical Urology, *Urinary Stone Disease:*
A Practical Guide to Medical and Surgical Management
Edited by: M. L. Stoller and M. V. Meng © Humana Press Inc., Totowa, NJ

concentration of free protons in a heterogeneous solution of various acids and bases can be measured. By convention, the resulting number of free protons is stated as a pH value, simply the negative logarithm of the concentration of free hydrogen ion: $pH = -\log [H^+]$ (where the concentration of H^+ is in units of moles per liter). Normal physiologic arterial serum pH of 7.40 ± 0.02 indicates a free proton concentration around 40 nanomol per L (4×10^{-8} mol/L). Values of pH greater than 7.42 indicate an alkalemia and values less than 7.38 indicate an acidemia.

Buffering

Despite the constant bombardment of acid and alkali, the body maintains a remarkably stable pH. Both the serum and the urine contain buffers to minimize the degree of shift in pH when acid or alkali is added to the solution. A buffer is essentially a weak acid and its conjugate base:

$$HA \leftrightarrow H^+ + A^- \tag{1}$$

The rates of association and dissociation in Eq. 1 depend on the particular type of buffer, as well as the temperature of the solution. The rate of dissociation is given as the ionization constant, Ka, for a particular acid–base pair. The negative logarithm of this constant is termed pKa. For all weak acids, the law of mass action relates pH to the concentrations of the acid and conjugate base:

$$pH = pKa + \log \{[A^-]/[HA]\} \tag{2}$$

When the solution pH is less than the pKa, more protons are bound. When the solution pH is greater than the pKa, more of the acid will be dissociated yielding more free protons.

The predominant serum buffer system is represented by carbonic acid (H_2CO_3) and its conjugate base, bicarbonate (HCO_3^-):

$$H^+ + HCO_3^- \leftrightarrow H_2CO_3 \tag{3}$$

Most individuals accumulate acid in the course of a day through regular metabolic activities, developing a net acid load (see next section) of 50–100 mmol. Without a buffering system, the addition of this daily acid load to an average-sized individual would drop the pH to around 3.0. This does not occur, as the produced H^+ is buffered by binding to HCO_3^-, forming the weak acid H_2CO_3 and maintaining the $[H^+]$ close to physiologic levels. The H_2CO_3 does not accumulate to any large extent because of the action of carbonic anhydrase (CA) to produce water and carbon dioxide:

$$H_2CO_3 \leftrightarrow H_2O + CO_2 \tag{4}$$

The constant removal of CO_2 by the pulmonary system is the other crucial step in maintaining a pH of 7.40 during this buffering process, discussed in a later section.

Equations 3 and 4 can be combined to give the familiar expression:

$$H^+ + HCO_3^- \leftrightarrow H_2O + CO_2 \tag{5}$$

If we use (Eq. 2) in the above relationship, and knowing the pKa_1 of carbonic acid to be about 6.10 (at 37°C), we get the following:

$$pH = 6.10 + \log \{[HCO_3^-]/[CO_2]\} \tag{6}$$

The dissolved concentration of CO_2 is very low and is related to the partial pressure of CO_2 (pCO_2) by a factor of 0.03 to give the Henderson–Hasselbalch equation:

$$pH = 6.10 + \log \{[HCO_3^-]/(0.03 \times pCO_2)\} \tag{7}$$

Now, not only can the pH be calculated by knowing the serum HCO_3^- and the serum pCO_2, but also any single unknown in this relationship can be calculated when the other two variables are known. This formula is the basis for most of the clinical charts and tables relating pCO_2, pH, and HCO_3^- found in almost all acid–base texts and handbooks.

Other important serum buffers include phosphates and sulfates, derived from phosphoproteins and sulfur-containing amino acids, respectively. These buffers are found at much lower concentrations than bicarbonate but play an important role as urinary buffers. Anionic serum proteins, such as albumin, also buffer H^+ to a limited extent. Another major serum buffer is the skeletal system (1). Phosphates in mineralized bone can take up free protons in exchange for other bone cations such as sodium and calcium. Chronic acidosis can lead to decreased bone mineral content (2,3).

ENDOGENOUS ACID PRODUCTION

Inorganic Acids

For the most part, normal physiologic activities result in acid production. Daily endogenous noncarbonic acid production or the "acid load" is derived from dietary protein metabolism, predominantly those containing the amino acids cystine, methionine and arginine. Cystine and methionine result in the production of sulfuric acid, and arginine (also lysine and histinine) produces hydrochloric acid. The resulting acids (sulfuric and hydrochloric) are termed "fixed" or "inorganic" acids. As these are relatively strong acids with low pKa, they are mostly found in dissociated form at physiologic conditions. This implies that the dissociated H^+ will bind to the serum buffer HCO_3^-, consuming one molecule of bicarbonate for each molecule of inorganic acid formed. The carbonic acid (H_2CO_3) created by the reaction is broken down to H_2O and CO_2. The lungs normally exhale the CO_2. The average Western diet, which is quite high in protein, contributes about 50–100 mmol of H^+ (approx 1 mmol/kg of body weight) to the endogenous daily acid load.

Organic Acid and Carbonic Acid

Organic acids, including ketoacids, acetoacids, lactic acid, and uric acid, accumulate from normal metabolic activities and from the diet. The organic acids (or organic anions) differ from the inorganic acids, in that many organic anions can be further metabolized to a neutral end product plus HCO_3^-. Organic anions, therefore, represent a potential bicarbonate source, if the appropriate metabolic pathways are intact. When these pathways are disrupted, the organic anions may accumulate and result in an anion gap metabolic acidosis. On the other hand, if organic anions are lost, for example through abnormal renal proximal tubular handling, a mild nonanion gap metabolic acidosis may result from the loss of a potential bicarbonate source. Some investigators believe that organic ion metabolism may actually account for an important fraction of the bicarbonate regenerated in maintaining homeostasis (4).

The metabolism of carbohydrates and fats produces upwards of 15,000 mmol of CO_2, which has the potential to form carbonic acid (H_2CO_3) when combined with H_2O (Eq. 4). The constant removal of CO_2 via the pulmonary system prevents H_2CO_3 from accumulating, and the actual serum concentration of H_2CO_3 is insignificant. H_2CO_3 is often termed a "volatile" acid and does not contribute to the usual daily endogenous acid load in a healthy individual. With impaired ventilation, a respiratory acidosis will occur with build up of CO_2 and subsequently H_2CO_3. By measuring arterial pCO_2 and serum bicarbonate, the resultant pH can be predicted by the Henderson–Hasselbalch equation (Eq. 7).

The amino acids aspartate and glutamate are metabolized to a neutral end product plus bicarbonate molecules. Individuals on very strict vegetarian diets can consume proportionately more proteins containing these amino acids than proteins with acidic metabolic products, resulting in a lesser degree of acidosis than nonvegetarians (5).

With the endogenous acid load from protein breakdown, each H^+ consumes an equal amount of HCO_3^-. The body is left with a deficit of HCO_3^-. To maintain homeostasis, new bicarbonate must be formed. In regenerating bicarbonate, acid is excreted, a process commonly referred to as renal net acid excretion (NAE). The contributions of nonrenal mechanisms of acid–base regulation are also significant.

PULMONARY AND OTHER NONRENAL ACID–BASE REGULATION
Pulmonary

The pulmonary system provides two important processes in the regulation of acid–base balance: removal of carbon dioxide and maintaining oxygenation for aerobic metabolism. The production of CO_2 in the metabolism of carbohydrates and fats leads to production of carbonic acid (H_2CO_3) via the enzyme carbonic anhydrase, which is found in numerous cell types. The buildup of carbonic acid is a potentially enormous acid burden. However, there is constant removal of CO_2 with pulmonary ventilation, keeping the $[H_2CO_3]$ extremely low. Even a small rise in the partial pressure of CO_2 (pCO_2) is a powerful stimulant for increased minute ventilation. When ventilation becomes inadequate, the pCO_2 rises quickly with a drop in pH: $\downarrow pH = 6.10 + \log \{[HCO_3^-]/(0.03 \times \uparrow pCO_2)\}$ as predicted by the Henderson–Hasselbalch equation. With long-standing elevations of pCO_2, the renal system will increase the production of HCO_3^- to a higher baseline steady-state level to bring the pH closer to 7.40. Renal adjustments of HCO_3^- serve as adaptive mechanisms to compensate for nonrenal disturbances in acid–base balance and will not be further discussed.

The other important, although indirect, role of the pulmonary system in maintaining acid–base homeostasis is the oxygenation of tissues to allow aerobic metabolism. Anaerobic cellular metabolism from lack of intracellular oxygen produces lactic acid, an organic acid. With return of aerobic metabolism, lactic acid is usually quickly and efficiently metabolized, consuming a proton (and thus regenerating HCO_3^-) in the process: lactate + H^+ = glucose + CO_2. Because this anion represents potential bicarbonate, the loss of lactate before its metabolism by the liver and muscles can result in a nongap acidosis.

Hepatic

Hepatic function is indirectly tied to acid–base regulation by its processing of amino acids, as well as by its processing of organic anions such as lactate, citrate, and ketones. Conversion of nitrogen-containing substances, such as amino acids, to urea is the job of the liver. Urea formation, however, consumes bicarbonate. The alteration of the urea cycle in different states of acid–base balance is well described, but whether or not this represents true adaptability to acid–base disturbances remains controversial. Nonetheless, hepatic uptake of amino acids is decreased in the setting of metabolic acidosis, allowing a greater availability of amino acids for renal ammonium production and enhanced acid excretion (6,7). In addition, the liver plays a major role in the metabo-

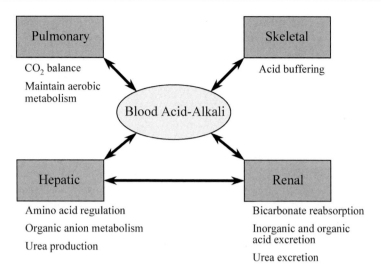

Fig. 1. Contributions of renal and nonrenal organs to acid homeostasis.

lism of organic anions. The breakdown of some organic anions results in the utilization of protons, and thus formation of bicarbonate. Other anions such as citrate are metabolized to more that one bicarbonate molecule, and its processing by the liver is important in converting this potential bicarbonate source into usable buffer. Conversely, the liver is the primary organ for urea formation, and in doing so bicarbonate is consumed. In the setting of liver function abnormalities, either acute or chronic, the handling of these anions can be significantly impaired, leading to a metabolic acidosis.

Bone

The skeletal system serves as a large buffer for acids. The ability of phosphates in the bone to buffer protons allows pH to be regulated at the expense of bone minerals such as calcium. The short-term consequences of acidosis on the skeletal system are unclear, but chronic acidosis may play a role in the development of bone disease *(3)*. The destructive effect of acidosis on bone formation is most commonly seen in children with chronic acidemia. Long-term acidosis inhibits both matrix formation as well as bone mineralization, and correction of the acidosis usually leads to dramatically improved skeletal growth in these children *(8)*. The contribution of various organ systems is illustrated in Fig. 1.

RENAL ACID–BASE REGULATION

The role of the kidneys in acid–base regulation can be simplified to two basic tasks: the reclamation of filtered bicarbonate, and the excretion of accumulated, endogenous noncarbonic acid. The two processes are frequently described as functionally separate, but there is substantial overlap in the physiology.

Reclamation of Filtered Bicarbonate

One of the first, and arguably most crucial, functions of the kidneys in acid–base regulation is the reclamation of the filtered bicarbonate, which is freely filtered by the glomeruli. Assuming a normal glomerular filtration rate of 100 mL/min and a serum bicarbonate concentration of 24 mmol/L, approx 3500 mmol of bicarbonate are filtered in a day ($100\, mL/min \times 1440\, min/d \times 1L/1000\, mL \times 24\, mmol/L = 3456\, mmol/d$). This filtered bicarbonate needs to be actively transported back into the serum. The reclamation process does not generate any new bicarbonate, yet defects in this vital function can lead to profound buffer losses and a resulting metabolic acidosis.

PROXIMAL TUBULE

The proximal tubule, ascending limb of the loop of Henle and collecting tubules are all involved in this task. The proximal tubule is responsible for the bulk (80–85%) of the reabsorption. In normal circumstances, essentially all of the filtered bicarbonate is recovered by the time the urine leaves the collecting tubules, with normal fractional excretion of bicarbonate (FE_{HCO3}) <0.1%. In all segments, the reclamation of bicarbonate involves a proton-secreting event rather than the direct removal of an intact bicarbonate molecule from the filtrate.

The proximal tubule performs the vast majority of the bicarbonate reclamation. Carbonic anhydrase found on the luminal side of the tubular cell, specific luminal surface Na^+/H^+ exchangers, H^+-ATPase and basolateral Na^+/HCO_3^- cotransporters give this tubular segment the ability to remove large amounts of bicarbonate from the filtrate (Fig. 2). The driving force for this process is the electrochemical gradient produced by the basolateral Na^+/K^+-ATPase, which produces a relatively electronegative, low $[Na^+]$ environment within the proximal tubular cell. This favors the movement of Na^+ from the filtrate into the cell via the antiporter, with subsequent transport of H^+ out of the cell into the luminal space. Energy-requiring ATPase also pumps H^+ out of the cell. H^+ combines with the HCO_3^- in the filtrate, forming H_2CO_3. Because carbonic anhydrase (isoform 4) is present on the luminal surface of the proximal tubule (9,10), the H_2CO_3 is rapidly converted to H_2O and CO_2, which pass easily into the cell. Once inside, the two are combined again to form H_2CO_3 via another isoform (isoform 2) of carbonic anhydrase (9–11), and then dissociates to H^+ and HCO_3^-. The proton goes back out into the luminal space via the Na^+/H^+ exchanger for the next cycle. Finally, the HCO_3^- remaining in the cell is transported out by the basolateral Na^+/HCO_3^- cotransporter, into the peritubular fluid, and eventually into the serum as one molecule of reclaimed bicarbonate. This mechanism in the proximal tubule reclaims about 85% of the filtered HCO_3^- load in normal conditions.

The molecular biology of the proximal tubule transporters has been recently elucidated. Two important channels have been described in detail: the luminal Na^+/H^+ exchanger (NHE) and the basolateral Na^+/HCO_3^- cotransporter (NBC). The proximal tubular Na^+/H^+ exchanger (NHE3) is in a family of transmembrane transporters found in various tissues, of which seven types have been identified so far. These transporters are important for cellular volume control as well as for intracellular pH regulation (12,13). The NHE3 channel function can be controlled by cytosolic C-terminal alterations, including phosphorylation and binding by other proteins (13). The gene for human NHE3 is now determined to be on chromosome 5p15.3 (14).

The Na^+/HCO_3^- cotransporter (NBC) is also in a family of transporters important for pH regulation. The kidney type of the cotransporter (kNBC1) is predominantly found in the basolateral side of proximal tubular cells and cotransports one Na^+ molecule with three HCO_3^- molecules. kNBC1 is mapped to chromosome 4p21 (15). Defects in these membrane channels are the basis for some forms of proximal renal tubular bicarbonate handling problems, discussed in the section on renal tubular acidosis.

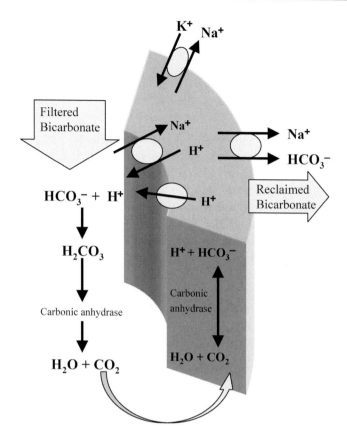

Fig. 2. Proximal tubular cell: basic mechanisms for bicarbonate reclamation.

LOOP OF HENLE AND COLLECTING DUCT

The thick ascending limb of Henle's loop (TALH), the distal tubule and the collecting duct are responsible for the remaining 15% of filtered bicarbonate not reclaimed by the proximal tubule. Recent evidence supports the TALH as being important in the reabsorption of the majority of the remaining bicarbonate coming out of the proximal segment. The mechanism, including luminal carbonic anhydrase, Na^+/H^+ exchangers, and basolateral Na^+/HCO_3^- cotransporters, is similar to that of the proximal tubule (16). Although proportionally not large, the actual amount of remaining bicarbonate in the filtrate is quite substantial, making the reclamation function of these distal segments important in maintaining acid–base homeostasis. The molecular biology of the ion transporters in the TALH is similar to that of the proximal tubule. NHE3 channels and kNBC1 are also sparingly found on the TALH (17).

Although the collecting duct is predominantly important for net acid excretion, this segment performs bicarbonate reabsorption to a small degree. Importantly, luminal carbonic anhydrase (isoform 4) is generally not found in this segment.

Acid Excretion

The second major task of the renal system in maintaining acid–base homeostasis is the excretion of accumulated noncarbonic acid. As discussed, the reclamation of bicarbonate from the filtrate does not regenerate any previously consumed HCO_3^- from the buffering of daily acid production. To maintain equilibrium, bicarbonate regeneration must be equivalent to the net amount of endogenous acid produced, approx 50–100 mmol for someone eating an average Western diet. Net acid excretion (NAE) essentially results in bicarbonate formation.

URINARY BUFFERS

As in the serum, buffering in the urine, mainly by phosphates and ammonia, maintains the urine pH within a specific physiologic range. Although bicarbonate is found in large amounts in the filtrate, the bicarbonate reclamation process usually removes the vast majority of this buffer by the time the urine reaches the distal tubular segments. Thus, bicarbonate is usually not a major urinary buffer. The H^+ from acid production cannot be excreted as free protons; the number of free protons—which determines urinary pH—is trivial compared with the number excreted bound to urinary buffers. NAE requires an adequate amount of nonbicarbonate urinary buffers to bind the secreted protons. The amount of phosphate, or "titrateable" acid, can increase a few-fold if increased acid excretion is required (18). However, the amount of H^+ that can be excreted in the form of ammonium can be increased dramatically when more acid excretion is required (19). Each proton excreted with a nonbicarbonate urinary buffer represents a regenerated bicarbonate molecule.

AMMONIAGENESIS AND THE AMMONIA CYCLE

Ammonia (NH_3) production begins within the proximal tubular cells. The amino acid glutamine is broken down to ammonium (NH_4^+) and glutamate by glutaminase within the cell: Glutamine $\rightarrow NH_4^+$ + Glutamate. Subsequently, the glutamate is broken down by glutamate dehydrogenase in the reaction: Glutamate $\rightarrow NH_4^+ + \alpha$-ketoglutarate. The α-ketoglutarate is eventually metabolized within both the tubular cell as well as the liver to form two molecules of HCO_3^-. Thus, the net result of one mole of glutamine is 2 mol of NH_4^+ and 2 mol of HCO_3^- (19). Some of the ammonium is transported back into the blood and metabolized to urea via the liver. In this process, H^+ is produced, consuming HCO_3^-, resulting in no net gain or loss of acid. However, when the ammonium produced by the proximal tubule is excreted, there a net loss of acid.

The route of ammonium excretion is quite circuitous and demands contributions from various tubular segments. The movement of NH_4^+ from within the proximal tubule to the collecting tubule is commonly referred to as the "ammonia cycle" (Fig. 3). Ammonium produced by the proximal tubule moves out of the proximal tubular cell by substituting for H^+ in the Na^+/H^+ antiporter. The pKa of $NH_4^+ \leftrightarrow H^+ + NH_3$ is approx 9.0. Therefore, at usual urine pH of 5.0–6.0, most of the H^+ remains bound to NH_3 in the tubular lumen. The ammonium then moves with the filtrate to the thick ascending limb of the loop of Henle (TALH) where approx 50% of the ammonium is reabsorbed. Some of the ammonium moves by way of paracellular channels, whereas the majority substitutes for potassium on the $Na^+/K^+/2$ Cl^- pump, moving into the cell reliant on the energy consuming effort of the basolateral Na^+/K^+-ATPase (20,21). At this point, some of the ammonium is reabsorbed by the capillaries, and in doing so, effectively cancels any net acid–base change; urea formation from ammonium by the liver consumes bicarbonate. The remaining ammonium dissociates to NH_3 and H^+ in the renal medulla.

This transport by the TALH is the primary method of medullary concentration of ammonia. Some to the ammonia diffuses back into more proximal segments where it is

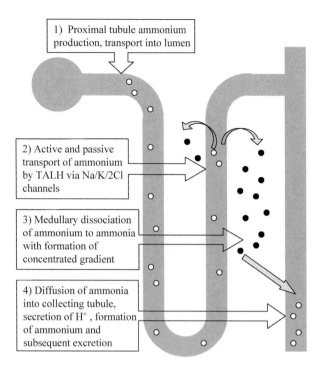

Fig. 3. The ammonia cycle.

again converted to ammonium and "cycles" through to the TALH. The medullary concentration gradient provides the driving force for ammonia diffusion into the cortical collecting duct. Once in the distal luminal nephron segment, free H^+, if present, can bind to the ammonia, given the favorable pKa of the reaction, forming ammonium again. The NH_4^+ is now "trapped" in the tubule because of the molecule's polarity and lack of luminal transport channels in the collecting duct. Excretion into the urine, along with chloride or other anions to maintain electro negativity, is the final step in this aspect of NAE.

Collecting Duct in Net Acid Excretion

The collecting ducts are responsible for the secretion of H^+, and if ammonia is present, will allow the formation of ammonium. In doing so, one new bicarbonate molecule is effectively added back into the circulation. Bicarbonate, consumed by previous serum buffering of endogenously produced acids, is now regenerated.

Collecting duct cellular mechanisms are highly specialized for this purpose and involve a few important types of cells. There is varied distribution of these cell types among the cortical collecting duct and the inner and outer medullary collecting ducts. However, for purposes here, the collecting duct cell types will be generalized. Type A intercalated cells (Fig. 4) have apical energy-requiring H^+-ATPase as well as H^+/K^+-ATPase. These pumps push intracellular protons out into the lumen to create an H^+ gradient. Intracellular carbonic anhydrase (CA2) is necessary for supplying these protons, and defects or deficiencies in this enzyme may lead to acidification defects to be

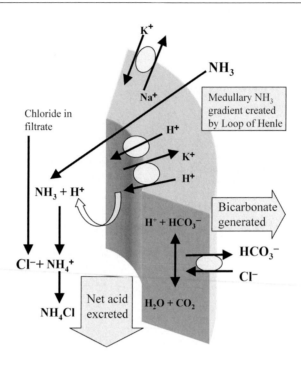

Fig. 4. α-Intercalated cell in the cortical collecting duct: ammonium excretion.

discussed later. The formation of an H^+ gradient also requires an intact luminal membrane to keep the protons from leaking back into the cell. The basolateral HCO_3^-/Cl^- exchanger (AE1 or band 3 protein) is important for the transport of the bicarbonate out of the cell and into the capillaries. Recent discoveries have implicated defects in both the proton pump and the AE1 as causes of inherited forms of distal renal tubular acidosis (22,23). The importance of the H^+/K^+-ATPase is also being recognized as a potential pathologic defect in some cases of distal renal tubular acidosis (RTA).

The β-intercalated cell is found in the collecting ducts as well. The arrangement of transporters is inverse to that found on the α-intercalated cell, with mechanisms for pumping HCO_3^- out of the cell and H^+ into the circulation (Fig. 5). Currently there is not a known pathologic defect in this cell to account for renal acidosis. Theoretically, over-activity in the β-intercalated cell can create a RTA.

The principal cell is the second cell type found adjacent to intercalated cells in the collecting ducts (Fig. 6). Although mainly responsible for sodium reabsorption and potassium excretion, the principal cell influences proton secretion by its active sodium reabsorption, which provides the electronegative luminal environment favoring H^+ secretion by the type-A intercalated cells. In other words, increased rates of distal sodium absorption will facilitate distal proton secretion.

In summary NAE requires: (1) functional distal H^+ secretion, including an appropriate lumen electronegativity; (2) functional CA2; (3) adequate urinary buffer (i.e., ammonia) to bind the protons; and (4) intact distal luminal membrane to allow formation of a H^+ gradient. Defects in one or more of these steps result in either deficient NAE or problems with distal urine acidification.

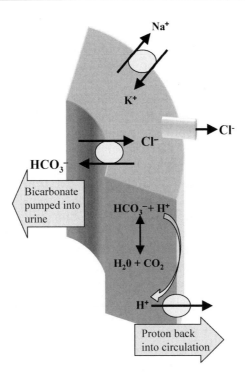

Fig. 5. β-Intercalated cell in the cortical collecting duct: bicarbonate secretion.

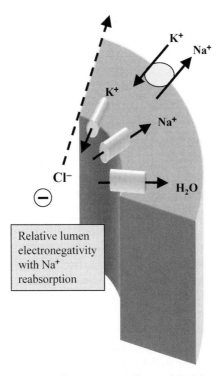

Fig. 6. Principal cell in the collecting duct: sodium chloride reabsorption with luminal electronegativity.

CONTROL OF NET ACID EXCRETION

Net acid excretion relies on the workings of many tubular segments: proximal tubule for ammonia production, the TALH for medullary concentration of ammonia, and the collecting tubule for H^+ secretion. Regulation of this process involves local, hormonal, and neurological controls at each of these tubular segments.

Intracellular pH and potassium levels regulate proximal tubular ammoniagenesis. A metabolic acidosis (but not a respiratory acidosis) with decreased intracellular pH will stimulate ammonium production (24). Hypokalemia is a potent stimulator for proximal ammonium production (25,26). On the other hand, hyperkalemia may not reduce ammonium production, but may decrease ammonium transport from the proximal tubule to the collecting duct (19,27). Increased dietary protein intake, which increases the amount of acid to be excreted, will stimulate proximal tubule ammonium production (28). Aldosterone also plays a role in its positive control of ammoniagenesis. In addition, chronic acidosis also increases the synthesis of transporters, such as Na^+/H^+ exchangers in the proximal tubule (29).

Intracellular pH and aldosterone levels influence distal regulation of proton secretion. This is accomplished through mechanisms that affect transport kinetics, modulate membrane transporters, and alter the number of transporters by inserting or removing them from the membranes. First, the optimum environment for proton secretion is partially reliant on the luminal electronegativity provided by sodium reabsorption in the principal cells; this is under the control of aldosterone. Second, aldosterone can increase both apical H^+ secretion as well as basolateral Cl^-/HCO_3^- exchange (30,31).

Intracellular pH of the cortical collecting ducts influences the pattern and number of H^+-ATPase in the membrane. Experimentally, there is an increase in intracellular calcium with acidosis, causing increased exocytosis of intracellular vesicles containing preformed H^+-ATPase channels, via a calmodulin/microtubule system (32). In addition, basolateral AE1 (Cl^-/HCO_3^- exchanger) protein synthesis may increase during acidemia, as evidenced by animal studies showing increased transporter mRNA in the intercalated cells (33).

Other hormonal modulators of collecting duct acid–base control include vasopressin, glucagon, prostaglandin E_2, and calcitonin (34). There is also evidence that locally produced mediators, such as nitric oxide (NO), may play a role in acid regulation by affecting H^+-ATPase activity (35).

URINARY PH AND ASSESSMENT OF ACID EXCRETION

Determinants of Urinary pH

Urinary buffers in normal conditions consist predominantly of inorganic anions and ammonia. The inorganic anions, often referred to as titrateable acids, consist predominantly of phosphates. Under situations of increased acidemia, the inorganic anion availability can increase by about twofold. Ammonia production, on the other hand, can increase 10-fold if needed to excrete a large acid lead.

Physiologic urinary pH ranges from 4.5 to 7.5, implying urinary $[H^+]$ ranging from $32 \mu mol/L$ to 32 nanomol/L. Urinary pH provides information only about the availability of free protons in the urine. This amount of free H^+, even at the lowest physiologic urine pH, represents a trivial fraction of the total number of protons excreted to maintain acid–base balance. The bulk of daily H^+ excretion occurs when protons are bound to the excreted urinary buffers. An isolated urine pH does not give information about the adequacy of acid excretion or the availability of urinary buffers.

To illustrate this point, take the example of an alkaline urine pH (pH >6.0) with an underlying metabolic acidosis. This scenario can be seen when excessive buffers are delivered to the distal tubules and relatively more H^+ is bound to the buffer. This results in a more alkaline urine pH even with intact distal tubular proton secretion. Clinically, bicarbonaturia during the bicarbonate-losing stage of proximal tubular renal tubular acidosis will give this set of findings. On the other hand, a defect in distal nephron proton secretion with adequate buffer formation, as in classic or type I distal renal tubular acidosis, will provide the same disturbances of acidosis and elevated urine pH, but through a completely different set of defects. Conversely, an acidic urine pH (pH <5.5) with a metabolic acidosis may be owing to inadequate urinary buffer formation and delivery to the distal nephron, despite adequate distal nephron acidification. Here, net acid excretion is impaired because of a lack of buffer. The various causes of type 4 RTA with decreased ammoniagenesis are examples of this process. Thus, urinary pH in isolation provides useful but limited information in discerning the underlying cause of renal acid–base disturbance.

Assessment of Net Acid Excretion

Measurement of net acid excretion (NAE) relies on additional information beyond the urine pH. NAE, which must be equal to net acid production to maintain homeostasis, can be theoretically viewed as the difference between urinary excretion of acids and bases: NAE = (phosphate + ammonium) – (bicarbonate + organic anions). Organic anions are potentially important factors in NAE because the loss of these anions, such as β-hydroxybutyrate and citrate, is a loss of a potential bicarbonate source. Additionally, there is evidence that the kidney will preferentially excrete nonorganic acids and limit organic acid losses, such as citrate, when an acid load is placed on the system, in an attempt to save these potential bicarbonate substrates *(36)*. Therefore, some investigators include the organic anion variable in their evaluation of NAE *(4)*. In normal circumstances, bicarbonate and organic anion losses are minimal, so the term can be simplified to: NAE = phosphate + ammonium. The ability to increase phosphate in the urine is limited, and with a large acid burden, it is the large increase in ammonium excretion that permits the increased acid excretion. Therefore, measurement of urinary ammonium excretion would be the most important assessment of NAE. Ammonium measurement is, unfortunately, not conveniently available. Alternative methods must be used to indirectly estimate NAE.

URINARY ANION GAP

One method of indirectly determining the adequacy of NAE is to calculate a Urinary Anion Gap (UAG) using the concentrations of the primary urinary electrolytes: UAG = $[Na^+] + [K^+] - [Cl^-]$. The usual UAG is a negative number (usually < –10), indicating that there is the presence of unmeasured cations, presumably ammonium. Conversely, a positive UAG would signify inadequate ammonium excretion. This is illustrated in Fig. 7.

There are limitations to the use of the UAG. In some situations, the finding of a positive UAG does not indicate a decreased amount of ammonium being excreted. For example, when other nonchloride anions, such as bicarbonate, ketoacids or some an-

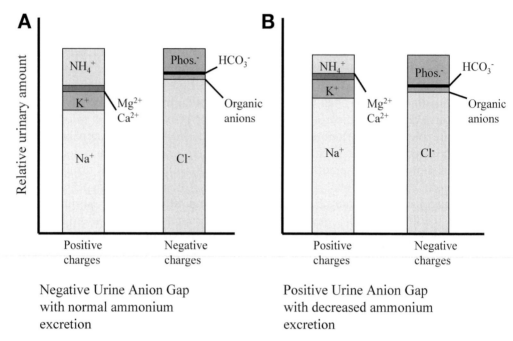

Fig. 7. Urine anion gap with **(A)** normal ammonium excretion and **(B)** decreased ammonium excretion.

tibiotics, are excreted in large concentrations in the urine, the calculated UAG will often be positive. In addition, other urinary electrolytes such as calcium and magnesium are generally not part of the calculation, although technically they do make up a small part of the cation content, and excretion of these ions can be quite variable. Nonetheless, the calculated UAG, although best viewed as a semiquantitative tool, is clinically useful in the evaluation of renal-mediated metabolic acidosis.

URINARY OSMOLAR GAP

A second method of estimating NAE involves calculation of a urine osmolar gap (UOG). Because the urine osmolarity should be the sum of the major charged particles and the major uncharged particles, the following should hold true: urine osmolarity = (positive charged) + (negative charged) + (uncharged). We can assume the number of positively charged particles to be equal to the number of negatively charged ones because urine is not a charged substance, and the major uncharged particles are urea and glucose. This brings the relationship to: urine osmolarity = $2(Na^+ + K^+ + NH_4^+)$ + urea +glucose (in mmol/L). Solving for ammonium results in: $NH_4^+ = 0.5$ {urine osmolarity $- [2(Na^+ + K^+) -$ urea $-$ glucose]} (in mmol/L). If the daily urinary volume is known, 24-h ammonium excretion can be estimated. The correlation of this method of urinary ammonium estimation to measured urinary ammonium is quite good, and may be more precise and accurate than the UAG (*37*).

The limitations of using the UOG are similar to that of using the UAG; if there are other unmeasured substances, the calculation may inaccurately predict the urine ammonium content. In using the UOG, other osmotically active substances such as glucose, mannitol, or glycerol must not be present in large quantities.

Additional Tests

Evaluation of renal tubular acidification sometimes involves additional provocative tests to challenge the function of tubular segments. These include bicarbonate loading, acid loading, urine-to-blood carbon dioxide gradient determination, and urine pH measurement after furosemide challenge (Table 1). The table is meant only as a guideline and to explain the rationale behind each test.

The bicarbonate-loading test evaluates proximal tubular reabsorption capability. If significant bicarbonaturia occurs when the serum bicarbonate is brought closer to normal levels, proximal RTA is diagnosed. It should be noted that complete correction or over correction of the metabolic acidosis with sodium bicarbonate will lead to increased bicarbonaturia, regardless of the underlying condition, and some investigators believe that evaluation for proximal RTA is better when plasma bicarbonate levels are kept below normal *(38)*. Proximal RTA usually results in fractional excretion of bicarbonate >15% with this challenge, as well as an increase in urine pH levels from <5.5 to >6.0.

When bicarbonate loading is performed, measuring the urine-to-blood partial pressure of carbon dioxide (U-B pCO_2) gradient may be helpful in evaluating the function of H^+ secretion in the collecting tubule. Essentially, bicarbonaturia is induced with a rise in the urine pH >7.5. This ensures that there is enough bicarbonate in the distal segments to bind most of the secreted protons. If proton delivery is intact, there should be a rise in urine CO_2 levels ($H^+ + HCO_3^- \leftrightarrow H_2O + CO_2$). The simultaneous blood pCO_2 value is measured and subtracted from the urinary value, giving a gradient expressed in units of mmHg. The normal value is >20 mmHg gradient. The value should be interpreted only when the urine pH is elevated to >7.5 where urinary bicarbonate is elevated.

The results of acid loading determine whether or not there is a defect in distal acidification. In many instances, the underlying RTA disorder already gives an acidemia, with serum pH of <7.35 and a significant metabolic acidosis. In such a circumstance, the use of an acid stress test is probably unnecessary. In addition, the formulation commonly causes gastrointestinal upset. Nonetheless, in cases where the diagnosis is unclear, where there is suspected distal acidification defects in addition to a known proximal defect, or where there is a suspected incomplete RTA, the use of an acid load can be very informative. Acid loading is usually accomplished by administering oral NH_4Cl, 0.1 g/kg body weight per day in divided doses *(39)*, given orally for 3 d. Numerous variations of this protocol are available, including shorter ones for children *(40)*, but the goals are the same: to induce a degree of acidemia and acidosis large enough to evaluate the appropriateness of acid excretion. This, in effect, tests the entire NAE process, including the availability of ammonia, the distal ability to secrete H^+, and the membrane integrity. Of course, if the result of the NH_4Cl test is abnormal, other tests may be necessary to determine the exact mechanism of decreased NAE.

The normal response to a noncarbonic acid load is increased NAE. Urine pH should be <5.5 and the urine titrateable acidity and ammonium content should be increased. Because the latter two are difficult or inconvenient to measure, the urine anion gap or urine osmolar gap may be used to estimate ammonium excretion. After NH_4Cl loading, a serum pH of <7.35 and a decrease in bicarbonate of >3 meq/L general indicates an adequate load was given. Urine pH and the UAG should be measured at regular intervals, often hourly, after an acidemia and acidosis are clearly established. A persistent urine pH of >5.5 indicates abnormal distal acidification. Usually, NAE is also decreased. A possible exception is in one form of incomplete RTA, where an exaggerated proximal ammonium production is felt to be the underlying defect (see section on incomplete

Table 1
Tests of Renal Tubular Function

Test	Goal	Method	Result
Bicarbonate loading	• To determine defect in bicarbonate reclamation	• Sodium bicarbonate usually given orally to correct bicarbonate to near-normal levels	• Fractional excretion of bicarbonate >15% in proximal RTA
Urine to blood partial pressure of CO_2 gradient measurement	• To determine if there is a distal acidification defect	• With bicarbonate loading, ensure urine pH is > 7.0–7.5 and measure simultaneous blood and urine pCO_2	• Gradient (urine–blood) is normally >20 mmHg. Abnormal value of <20 mmHg found in classic distal RTA, some forms of hyperkalemic, rate-dependent and incomplete RTA
NH_4Cl loading	• To determine if there is a distal acidification defect	• Oral NH_4Cl loading of 0.1 g/kg/d for 1–3 d and measuring serum and urine pH; consider urinary ammonium or urine anion gap measures	• Failure to acidify urine (pH >5.5) with inadequate ammonium formation suggests distal acidification defect. Usually abnormal in distal RTAs. Incomplete RTA may give pH >5.5 with normal ammonium
Furosemide testing	• To determine if there is a distal acidification defect owing to inadequate sodium delivery	• Furosemide is given at 40–80 mg orally, or an as intravenous dose; measure urine pH when there is a documented naturesis	• Failure to acidify urine (pH >5.5) when sodium delivery is increased suggests a secretory defect in the distal tubule. Usually normal in proximal RTA, some rate-dependent RTA, type 4 RTA

RTA, renal tubular acidosis.

136

RTA) *(41)*. In this case, the ammonium excretion and UAG would theoretically be appropriate for the degree of acidemia, but the urine pH remains high because of a large amount of nonbicarbonate buffer delivery to the distal segments.

The inadequate delivery and reabsorption of sodium in the collecting tubules can lead to an acidosis due a lesser degree of luminal electronegativity. The furosemide test attempts to provide an adequate sodium load to the distal segment of the nephron with subsequent measurement of urine pH to see if acidification can take place. Sometimes, a mineralocorticoid is given before the administration of furosemide to ensure that a deficiency in hormone is not the underlying problem as opposed to a true defect in the distal tubular segments. Furosemide can be given orally at 40 or 80 mg as a single dose. Other protocols give larger, intravenous doses at 1 mg/kg *(42)*. Urinary sodium concentrations of >20 meq/dl indicate a good level of sodium delivery. Urine pH is then measured. The normal response is a urine pH of <5.5, which is also seen in proximal RTA, type 4 RTA, and some dRTAs with a voltage-dependent defect. Those with a true secretory or permeability defect usually maintain the urine pH >5.5.

RENAL TUBULAR ACIDOSIS

The term renal tubular acidosis (RTA), first coined in the 1950s, refers to a varied collection of disorders characterized by hyperchloremic metabolic acidosis (HCMA) initiated and maintained by a renal defect in acid–base handling. In addition, RTA should be diagnosed only when glomerular filtration is not significantly impaired; acidosis associated with decreased renal mass may be difficult to separate from true tubular defects. Determining that a HCMA exists requires a basic work-up, including arterial blood gas analysis, chemistries and thorough review of systems. The findings of: (1) a mild to moderate acidemia; (2) a decreased pCO_2; (3) a decreased serum HCO_3^-; (4) a normal serum anion gap; and (5) no obvious gastrointestinal causes for acidosis, hint that an RTA exists. In other situations, such as in "incomplete RTA," the acidemia and metabolic acidosis may be mild or absent altogether. These cases require additional testing to demonstrate a renal tubular pathology.

The pathophysiology of RTAs can be broadly divided into two defects: (1) defects in reclamation of filtered bicarbonate and (2) defects in distal nephron acid excretion. Although this dichotomy aids in the evaluation and treatment of RTAs, the pathologic mechanisms oftentimes overlap with this simplified classification. The development of more intricate assays has led to new insights into this rather complicated spectrum of disease. The following sections on renal tubular acidosis will be divided based on the underlying pathophysiology of the defect, and not exclusively on the laboratory findings, such as potassium levels or urine pH. Nonetheless, a proposed algorithm based on common laboratory tests is provided in Fig. 8.

Proximal Renal Tubular Acidosis

The proximal tubule performs two major tasks in acid–base homeostasis: the reclamation of the vast majority of filtered bicarbonate and the production of ammonium necessary for acid excretion in the collecting tubule. A defect in the bicarbonate reclamation process is the primary cause of a proximal renal tubular acidosis (pRTA), also termed a type II, RTA. This results in a lowered serum bicarbonate threshold for renal bicarbonate wasting. When the serum bicarbonate drops below this threshold, acidification of the urine can be established, because there is no defect in the distal segments (Fig. 9A–C).

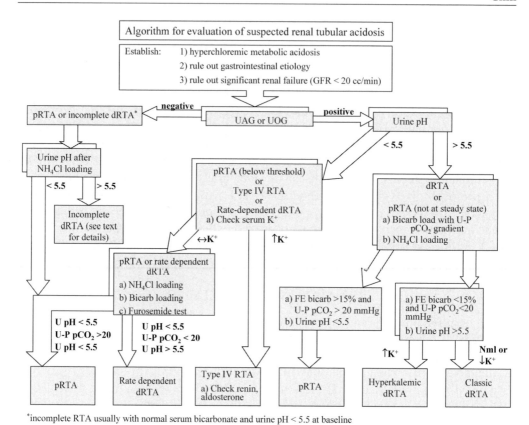

Fig. 8. Differentiating the types of renal tubular acidoses.

Causes of Proximal RTA

Proximal RTA is a rare entity. It is often seen in association with other proximal tubular abnormalities including urinary leakage of amino acids, phosphates, glucose, and variable amounts of protein. The combination of pRTA with other proximal tubular problems is termed the renal Fanconi syndrome. The causes of pRTA, with or without Fanconi syndrome, are listed in Table 2. Isolated pRTA, without renal Fanconi syndrome, can be found in hereditary form, both as an autosomal dominant and an autosomal recessive type, and as a spontaneous, sporadic process *(17)*.

As discussed in the section on proximal tubular bicarbonate handling, HCO_3^- reclamation involves a Na^+/H^+ exchanger (NHE3) as well as an H^+-ATPase to secrete protons into the lumen, and a basolateral Na^+/HCO_3^- cotransporter (kNBC1) to move intracellular bicarbonate out into the capillary circulation. Mutations in these ion transporters are the pathologic defects in some cases of isolated pRTA. In addition, carbonic anhydrases (CA2, isoform 2 located intracellular and CA4, isoform 4 on the luminal surface) are critical enzymes in the function of this tubular segment. Abnormalities in CA2 have been found in patients with a combined proximal and distal renal tubular acidosis.

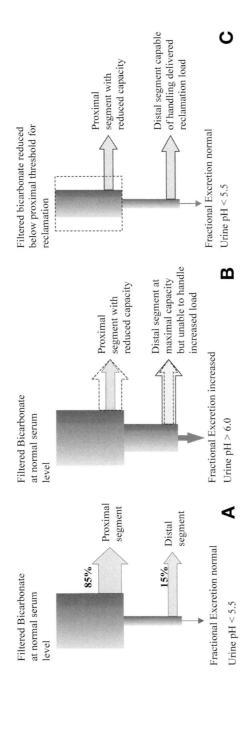

Fig. 9. (**A**) Normal bicarbonate reabsorption with minimal urinary bicarbonate loss. (**B**) Proximal RTA: serum bicarbonate above lowered "threshold" for proximal reabsorption, resulting in active bicarbonaturia. (**C**) Proximal RTA: serum bicarbonate below lowered "threshold" for proximal reabsorption with cessation of bicarbonaturia.

Table 2
Classification and Causes of Proximal
Renal Tubular Acidosis (Type 2 RTA)

Primary disorder
- Isolated
  - Hereditary
    - Autosomal recessive
    - Autosomal dominant
    - Carbonic anhydrase II deficiency
  - Sporadic/transient
- With generalized tubular abnormalities (Fanconi syndrome)
  - Hereditary
  - Sporadic
  - Inborn errors of metabolism
    - Tyrosinemia
    - Cystinosis
    - Wilson's disease
    - Lowe's disease
    - Galactosemia
    - Glycogen storage disease type I

Secondary/acquired disorder
- Toxin/Drug (oftentimes with Fanconi Syndrome)
  - Heavy metals
    - Lead
    - Cadmiun
    - Mercury
  - Prescribed medications
    - Cisplatin
    - Gentamicin
    - Streptozocin
    - Cyclosporine
    - Ifosfamide
    - Tetracycline
    - Valproic acid
    - Acetazolamide
- Systemic diseases
  - Multiple myeloma
  - Amyloidosis
  - Light-chain disease
  - Sjogren's syndrome
  - Hyperparathyroidism
- Others conditions
  - Renal transplantation
  - Medullary cystic kidney disease

CLINICAL PRESENTATION

Children with pRTA usually present for initial evaluation based on growth or growth velocity retardation. In autosomal recessive types, children may also present with mental retardation or ocular problems *(38)*. When pRTA is found with other transport defects, as in cystinuria or Fanconi syndrome, the presenting problems may be varied.

Many autosomal recessive cases have, as the primary defect, a mutation in the gene coding for the kNBC1 cotransporter. Because this protein is also found in corneal endothelial cells (43,44), ocular findings may be presenting symptoms as well. An mRNA splice variant of the same gene codes for a similar transporter in the brain and spinal cord, and possibly accounts for the mental retardation seen in some cases (15).

Autosomal dominant pRTA has been found in only one described pedigree (45). The molecular aspects have not been clarified, but there is speculation of a mutation in the NHE3-coding gene for the Na^+/H^+ exchanger. Sporadic cases in children are felt to be caused by immaturity of the NHE3 exchanger (46). In infants, the proximal tubular bicarbonate threshold is lower than that of older children or adults (46). Maturation of the NHE3 exchanger may be just slower in these children identified as having spontaneous, sporadic pRTA.

The acquired forms of pRTA, often in association with Fanconi syndrome, involve various tubular transport abnormalities, some caused by medications and toxins. Amino acid and phosphate transport require Na^+-dependent transporters. Therefore, transporter abnormalities or disruption of sodium gradients would impair absorption of many substances handled normally by the proximal tubule. Theories of membrane co-transporter defects, Na^+ gradient defects and energy depletion problems have all been proposed (47,48).

LABORATORY FINDINGS AND TESTING IN pRTA

The lowered proximal tubular cell threshold for bicarbonate wasting in pRTA results in large amounts of bicarbonate excretion when the serum bicarbonate level is above this threshold; distal mechanisms for bicarbonate reclamation are overwhelmed by the amount of bicarbonate coming out of the proximal segment in the bicarbonate losing stages. Consequently, urine pH is elevated during active bicarbonaturia. Cations must be excreted with the bicarbonate to maintain electroneutrality. As a result, sodium, potassium and magnesium are lost during this phase. Hypokalemia is often a useful diagnostic criterion for pRTA during bicarbonate loading tests.

Once serum bicarbonate concentrations drop below the threshold of bicarbonate reclamation capacity, typically around 10–15 meq/L, bicarbonaturia returns to normal low levels and urine pH can be acidified to <5.5, because distal acidification and NAE are intact. Active potassium and sodium losses will cease at this point. Studies have demonstrated intact sodium, phosphorous and calcium handling in patients with isolated pRTA (49). Acid homeostasis is maintained, albeit at a lower serum bicarbonate level. Therefore, calculations to estimate NAE, such as urinary anion gap and urinary osmolar gap, are in the normal range assuming they are measured at steady state. Certainly if there is a significant Fanconi syndrome, abnormal urinary levels of anionic molecules, such as phosphates and organic anions, may make the UAG abnormal.

Confirmation of pRTA involves looking at baseline potassium levels (usually normal at steady state in pRTA), urine pH measurement, evaluation for glucosuria, phosphaturia, and aminoaciduria (presence or absence of Fanconi syndrome), and bicarbonate loading. As serum bicarbonate approaches normal levels with alkali loading, finding a fractional excretion of bicarbonate of >15% suggests a pRTA.

Additional provocative testing includes bicarbonate loading with measurement of urine to blood partial pressure of CO_2 (U-B pCO_2) gradient. Theoretically, if bicarbonaturia is present and distal delivery of H^+ is intact, there should be a build up of H_2CO_3 within the distal nephron with some slow dehydration of H_2CO_3 to form CO_2. The CO_2 builds up in the urine, and the resulting gradient with blood pCO_2 levels is measured. In suspected pRTA, a gradient of >20 mmHg is consistent with intact distal H^+ secretion *(38,50)*. Urine must be carefully collected to prevent equilibration of urine pCO_2 with atmospheric conditions.

Acid loading in isolated pRTA should theoretically result in appropriate acid excretion. Interestingly, partially impaired ammoniagenesis has been found in some individuals with pRTA. Usually, net endogenous acid excretion is normal in pRTA as evidenced by the ability to acidify urine to pH <5.5 and to maintain a constant, although lower, serum bicarbonate level under average dietary conditions. Laboratory findings and results of provocative testing are summarized in Table 3.

A recent investigation suggested that under an exaggerated acid "stress" as in exogenous NH_4Cl loading, ammonium excretion was significantly less in patients with pRTA than in controls *(51)*. In this same study, pRTA patients at baseline relied on a higher percentage of titrateable acid excretion than ammonium excretion when compared with normal controls; ammoniagenesis was inappropriately low given the degree of acidemia.

Although the reasoning for this finding is unclear, it has been suggested that perhaps the intracellular pH in the proximal tubular cells is higher than that of normal individuals *(24,51)*. Because bicarbonate reabsorption and ammoniagenesis would both be down regulated if intracellular pH were elevated, this explanation would fit the laboratory findings. In addition, citrate excretion is normal in isolated pRTA. In a chronic acidotic state, proximal tubule reabsorption of this anion would be predictably higher than normal (because citrate is a potential bicarbonate source) with resulting hypocitraturia. However, it is well documented that citraturia in pRTA is essentially normal at steady state *(49)*. An elevated intracellular pH in the proximal tubular cell could also explain why the proximal tubular segment does not more avidly retain citrate in pRTA.

TREATMENT OF pRTA

Alkali replacement remains the mainstay of treatment for pRTA of any cause. Treating children with alkali gives the best chance at improving growth and avoiding co-morbidity *(50)*. In adults with acquired forms of pRTA, the chronic acidosis may cause problems with protein catabolism *(52–54)* and bone disease *(49,55)*. Oftentimes adults are asymptomatic with the degree of acidosis, and there is always debate as to how aggressively to treat adults with only moderate degrees of pRTA.

Alkali can be given in the form of a bicarbonate salt or as an organic anion salt such as citrate. The amounts needed to correct the acidosis are usually very high, sometimes in the range of 15–20 meq/kg for children *(38)*. Even at these high doses, the acidosis may not be fully corrected. The resulting bicarbonaturia will lead to increased urine cation losses. Hypokalemia, probably caused by both the bicarbonate loss and the increased distal tubular sodium delivery, requires replacement; a combination sodium and potassium citrate salt is often appropriate. Although urinary calcium loss is not a finding of pRTA in steady state, the increased distal tubular flows from alkaline salt replacement can increase calciuria. In individuals with renal Fanconi syndrome, replacement of phosphorous and amino acids may also be required. The rickets of Fanconi syndrome in children can be improved with phosphorous and vitamin D to promote gastrointestinal absorption of the phosphorous.

Distal Renal Tubular Acidosis

Distal tubular function is important for excretion of endogenously accumulated acid and the acidification of urine. Distal renal tubular acidosis (dRTA) is characterized by

Table 3
Guideline for Renal Tubular Acidosis

	pRTA	Classic dRTA	Hyperkalemic dRTA	Rate-limited dRTA	Incomplete RTA	Type 4 RTA
Presence of HCMA	Y	Y	Y	Y	N	Y
Serum K$^+$	↔ or ↓	↔ or ↓	↑	↔	↔	↑
Urine pH (baseline)	<5.5	>5.5	>5.5	<5.5	>5.5	<5.5
UAG or UOG	−	+	+	+	−	+
NH4 excretion	↔	→	→	→	←	→
Citrate excretion	↔	→	→	→	→	↔ or ↓
Bicarbonate load with FE Bicarb >15%	Y	N	N	N	N	N
U-B pCO$_2$ after bicarbonate load	>20 mmHg	<20 mmHg	<20 mmHg	<20 mmHg	>20 mmHg	>20 mmHg
NH$_4$Cl load urine pH	<5.5	>5.5	>5.5	<5.5	>5.5	<5.5
Furosemide challenge urine pH	<5.5	>5.5	>5.5	>5.5	<5.5	<5.5
Renal stones	N	Y	N?	Y	Y	N

Y, yes; N, no; HCMA, hyperchloremic metabolic acidosis; UAG, urinary anion gap; UOG, urinary osmolar gap; U-B pCO2, urine to blood partial pressure carbon dioxide gradient.

143

Table 4
Classification and Causes of Distal Renal Tubular Acidosis

Secretory defect
- Primary
  - Autosomal dominant
  - Autosomal recessive
  - Carbonic anhydrase deficiency
- Secondary
  - Obstructive uropathy
  - Renal transplant rejection
  - Autoimmune disorder
    - Sjogren's syndrome
    - SLE
    - Rheumatoid arthritis
    - Primary biliary cirrhosis
- Genetic diseases
  - Ehler-Danlos syndrome
  - Wilson's disease
  - Fabry's disease
- Toxin/drug
  - Toluene
  - Vanadate
  - Lithium

Voltage/rate dependent defect
- Decreased distal sodium delivery
- Drugs
  - Amiloride
  - Triamterene

Permeability defect
- Drugs
  - Amphotericin B
- Spontaneous

Combined ammonia ± distal secretion defect
- Incomplete RTA
  - Increase ammonium production
  - Partial secretory defect
- Chronic interstitial disease
- Obstructive uropathy
- Hyperkalemia

a decreased ability to acidify urine and to excrete acid in the setting of a chronic nongap metabolic acidosis. This clinical entity is found both as primary defects (usually in children) and as secondary to multisystem disease processes (more often in adults).

Causes of Distal Renal Tubular Acidosis

The primary forms and secondary causes of dRTA are listed in Table 4. When first described, the pathophysiology of dRTA was felt to be the inability of the luminal membrane to maintain a proton gradient. Microbiological and laboratory information from the past three decades has demonstrated that the underlying cause of dRTA often involves a H^+ secretion problem, either through a direct H^+-ATPase defect or a secondary defect resulting in decreased proton secretion. The pathophysiology of dRTA can be better understood by recollecting that acidification of the urine requires: (1) appropriate distal tubular proton secreting mechanism; (2) functional intracellular carbonic anhydrase; (3) adequate luminal electronegativity to allow H^+ secretion; and 4) intact luminal membrane to prevent back diffusion of H^+. Although some genetic mutations have been discovered for a subset of the primary, inherited forms of dRTA, the mechanisms of secondary dRTA are not finalized. Figure 10 points out a few of the proposed mechanisms of dRTA and where in the collecting ducts the defects reside.

Proton Secretion Defect

An inability to move H^+ from the intracellular space of the intercalated cell out into the luminal space would impair NAE and urinary acidification. An autosomal recessive

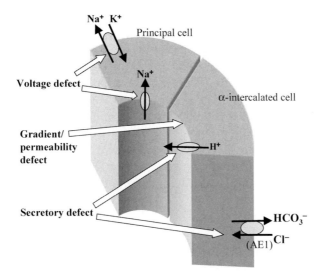

Fig. 10. Mechanisms of distal renal tubular acidosis and the associated membrane structural/functional defect.

mutation in the gene coding for a subunit (B1) of the H^+-ATPase apical pump is found in many patients with a form of inherited dRTA, which is also associated with neurosensory deafness *(56,57)*. A mutation in a different gene also coding for a subunit of the H^+-ATPase is implicated in other cases of sporadic and autosomal recessive dRTA *(58)*.

One form of autosomal dominant dRTA is now believed to be caused by a mutation in the gene coding for the basolateral HCO_3^-/Cl^- exchanger (AE1 or band 3 protein) *(59,60)*. The dysfunction of this transporter would lead to an inability to remove bicarbonate from the intracellular space of the collecting duct, decrease the $H_2O + CO_2 \rightarrow H^+ + HCO_3^-$ reaction, and would secondarily limit the ability to generate protons for apical secretion. The same mutation in this AE1 exchanger can also lead to red blood cell abnormalities, including hereditary spherocytosis and ovalocytosis *(61,62)*. However, there must be more to this condition because only a small number of patients with autosomal dominant dRTA have a red cell abnormality and only a small number of patients with the red cell defect have dRTA *(46)*.

Other nongenetic causes of dRTA related to proton secretory defects include medullary sponge kidney disease and chronic renal transplant rejection *(63)*. In addition, autoimmune diseases such as Sjogren syndrome are associated with dRTA. Obstructive nephropathy related dRTA is also mentioned as a secretory defect in some classifications *(63)* and borne out by some studies showing altered distribution of vacuoles containing H^+-ATPase *(64)*. However, the etiology of the tubular defect in obstruction is probably more complicated than this because hyperkalemia is a frequent finding. Experimentally, defective salt handling (leading to a voltage defect) secondary to impaired basolateral Na^+/K^+-ATPase is also touted as a cause of dRTA in obstructive nephropathy.

Carbonic Anhydrase Defect

Carbonic anhydrase is intricately involved in the proper function of the intercalated cell by providing the substrate for the apical H^+-ATPase. Defects or deficiencies in this enzyme lead to findings consistent with a dRTA. Some mutations in the gene for this enzyme, located on chromosome 8q22 *(65)* will also cause significant bone, central nervous system and mental development problems *(66)*. The majority of the cases (72%) are found in individuals of Arabic descent *(67)*. Defects in CA2 can lead to findings of pRTA or dRTA or both *(68–70)*. This is not surprising because CA2 is just as important for normal proximal tubular bicarbonate reabsorption as it is for distal proton secretion. The use of the carbonic anhydrase inhibitor acetazolamide provides a similar finding of proximal and distal acidification problems.

A combined proximal and distal defect in acid handing was originally termed type 3 RTA. The term has fallen out of favor, and the initial use of this term probably referred to pediatric cases where immature channels or a high salt intake were the etiology of the combined defect *(38)*.

Gradient Defect

A proton gradient or membrane permeability defect is well documented for amphotericin B induced dRTA. This polyene antibiotic is arguably one of the most powerful antifungal agents available and has been in clinical use for over 35 yrs. The antifungal effects of this medication are due to its high affinity to ergosterol found in fungal cell membranes. The binding of Amphotericin B to the fungal membrane forms pores and increases permeability to ions, which leads to cell destruction *(71,72)*. A similar process occurs in the collecting tubular cells *(73)*, with ion "holes" being punched into the cells. The back leak of H^+ prevents adequate proton gradient formation. Urine acidification and net acid excretion is then impaired. Interestingly, there has been one report of a sporadic, pediatric case of dRTA where a gradient defect is demonstrated to be the probable etiology *(74)*.

Voltage Dependent Defect

A voltage dependent defect resulting in decreased luminal electronegativity in the collecting ducts would decrease transmembrane potential for secretion of positively charged particles. Sodium absorption in the principal cells leaves a relatively negative-charged environment consisting of Cl^- molecules. Although chloride moves passively out of the urine through cellular and paracellular channels, its movement is slower than that of sodium. In effect, the lag in Cl^- uptake provides a negative luminal environment. The prototypical defect of this process is observed with the use of amiloride and trimethoprin, which block the Na^+ channels in the principal cells (Fig. 6). This decrease in sodium absorption makes for a relatively more positive lumen than usual, which impedes the secretion of both H^+ and K^+. The result is a nongap metabolic acidosis often with elevated serum K^+, hence the term hyperkalemic dRTA.

Hyperkalemic dRTA from obstructive nephropathy is felt, at least in part, to be caused by such a voltage defect by some investigators. The impaired sodium handling may be secondary to an underlying problem with decreased function of the basolateral Na^+/K^+-ATPase from the obstruction *(75,76)*. Na^+/K^+-ATPase dysfunction would certainly also disrupt K^+ excretion leading to hyperkalemia. However, abnormal proton secretion may also be part of the pathophysiology of obstructive nephropathy as mentioned previously *(63,64)*. Chronic tubulointerstitial diseases and autoimmune diseases (systemic lupus erythematosus in particular), often with mild renal insufficiency, may manifest a hyperkalemic dRTA possibly caused by a voltage defect with variable degrees of cellular resistance to the mineralocorticoids *(77)*. Hyperkalemic dRTA may involve a combination of voltage defect and H^+-ATPase defect, as investigators have found mixed findings with testing of patients with this form of RTA (78,79).

Aldosterone deficiency can lead to a salt wasting state with a similar pathophysiology of acidosis and hyperkalemic dRTA. Mineralocorticoid deficiencies, especially with underlying mild renal insufficiency, are often associated with other proximal tubular abnormalities such as impaired ammoniagenesis with clinical findings consistent with the definition of a type 4 RTA. Therefore, the line between hyperkalemic dRTA and type 4 RTA is not always clear. Indeed, some classification schemes do not make the distinction between hyperkalemic dRTA and type 4 RTA, and essentially group both disorders under type 4 RTA. Nonetheless, subtle differences such as in baseline urine pH values may substantiate the delineation of these two entities.

Other Disease States

The cause of dRTA in various autoimmune diseases has been investigated and deserves mention. Systemic lupus erythematosus (SLE) and Sjogren syndrome are two of many autoimmune diseases clearly associated with dRTA (80–82). Immunochemical staining has demonstrated a decrease or absence of H^+-ATPase in many but not all of these patients (83,84). One theory proposes that autoantibodies from these diseases destroy or impair the apical proton pumps in the intercalated cells. Autoantibodies to the intracellular carbonic anhydrase (CA2) have also been demonstrated in SLE (85,86). A recent case report of IgE-related vasculitis and dRTA (87) found antibodies binding to CA2 and other membrane proteins on the intercalated cell, giving this antibody-mediated mechanism of tubular dysfunction some additional support.

CLINICAL PRESENTATION

Children with underlying dRTA present for evaluation of growth retardation (88). Unlike pRTA, dRTA is associated with hypocitraturia, hypercalciuria and nephrocalcinosis. Combined with a mildly alkaline urine pH, nephrolithiasis can be the presenting issue in many cases. An additional presenting symptom may include deafness (for many autosomal recessive forms). Bone abnormalities are seen in dRTA, especially with CA2 mutations. This defect, however, probably involves the proximal tubule as well (69,70).

Secondary forms of dRTA usually involve a fairly obvious systemic disease. The symptoms related to the tubular abnormalities may include weakness if hypokalemia is a prominent finding. Because dRTA is not a self-limiting condition (as is the case in pRTA), the metabolic acidosis can progress to dangerous levels.

LABORATORY FINDINGS AND TESTING IN dRTA

The primary initial laboratory findings in dRTA include a hyperchloremic metabolic acidosis and an inappropriately elevated (>5.5) urinary pH in light of the acidemia. Net acid excretion is impaired and should be reflected by a positive urine anion gap or urine osmolar gap. Despite acid loading in dRTA, urine pH remains >5.5. Serum potassium is also useful in further defining the probable defective mechanism. Hypocitraturia and hypercalciuria are two additional findings, at least for the classic type of dRTA.

Provocative testing is sometimes used to prove a distal acidification defect. These tests have already been discussed; the bicarbonate load test and furosemide test are particularly useful in examining distal nephron acidification. Bicarbonate loading in

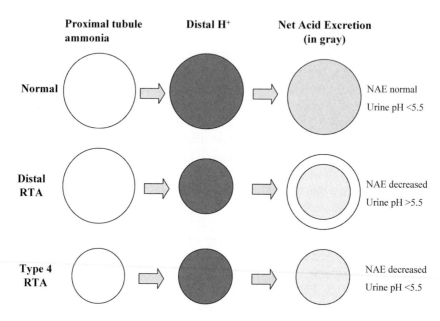

Fig. 11. Balance of ammonia availability and distal proton availability determines net acid excretion (NAE) and the urine pH. Type 4 RTA and distal RTA both have decreased NAE but, typically, have differing urine pH because of this mismatch of buffer to proton.

dRTA would reveal a fractional excretion of bicarbonate of <15% and U-P pCO_2 gradient of <20 mmHg.

Measurement of renin and aldosterone levels may prove useful in differentiating the hyperkalemic dRTA from type 4 RTA. However, the aldosterone level in hyperkalemic dRTA from tubulointerstitial diseases can be quite variable *(79)*. Typically, the urine pH in hyperkalemic dRTA is >5.5, implying a distal acidification problem. The urine pH in type 4 RTA, however, is usually <5.5 despite impaired NAE, suggesting that the decreased capability to distally acidify the urine is matched by a decrease in supplied ammonia (Fig. 11). Table 3 provides some basic laboratory differences among the RTAs.

TREATMENT OF DISTAL RTA

Provision of alkali and citrate represents the primary treatment of dRTA. The alkali required is usually substantially less than that required to treat pRTA. Because endogenous acid production is about 1 meq/kg body weight, a similar replacement of alkali should provide the amount of buffer needed to maintain acid–base homeostasis in adults. Children and infants require substantially higher doses (4–10 meq/kg) as a result of ongoing bone growth and, especially in infants, a decreased bicarbonate reabsorptive capacity *(89)*. If there is significantly decreased serum bicarbonate to begin with, not uncommon with dRTA, the initial replacement dose may need to be larger to replace this deficit. Sodium bicarbonate can be used, in two or three divided doses per day. Children treated with alkali for dRTA can resume normal growth, minimize nephrolithiasis and nephrocalcinosis, and possibly preserve kidney function *(8)*.

Hypokalemia is often seen with classic dRTA, and the use of potassium containing salts may be necessary or preferable. The combination sodium and potassium citrate salts are commonly used to not only replace alkali and potassium, but also to supply citrate to treat the hypocitraturia.

In secondary forms of dRTA, treatment of the underlying disorder, such as SLE, may improve the RTA (90). Individuals with hyperkalemic forms of dRTA may require the discontinuation of medications that suppress the renin–aldosterone axis. This includes many of the medications that can cause a type 4 RTA. Mineralocorticoid replacement can sometimes help this form of dRTA if other measures fail. Although loop diuretics may help with the hyperkalemia, the increased calciuria may be counterproductive if nephrolithiasis is an issue.

With treatment of the acidosis, hypercalciuria in dRTA can lessen. The hypocitraturia, on the other hand, may persist (38,91). Caution must be taken to avoid overly aggressive sodium bicarbonate replacement, because excess sodium excretion will cause hypercalciuria as well.

Rate-Dependent RTA

The term "rate dependent" RTA is a vague term in the classification of RTA. In general, the term applies to those situations where there is a mild defect in urine acidification with perhaps a milder degree of metabolic acidosis; this may imply a non-H^+ pump related defect of dRTA. This would encompass all causes of dRTA owing to voltage dependent defects as well as aldosterone deficiency or resistance. More specifically, the term has also been used to designate individuals who have impaired distal H^+ capacity based on measurement of U-B pCO_2 (<20 mmHg), but appropriate urine acidification (<5.5) when an acid load is given (92).

Although the pathophysiology is probably varied and overlaps the various mechanisms outlined previously, a partial distal tubular defect in the availability of protons, from any cause, can give this constellation of findings. At baseline mild acidosis, the H^+ defect would theoretically lead to an elevated urine pH. The tests of the distal tubule would be abnormal (U-P pCO_2 <20 mmHg after bicarbonate load, and urine pH >5.5 with furosemide challenge). When an acid load is provided, and thus a greater acidemic stimulus, distal acidification takes place with urine pH of <5.5. Whether there is further progression of these rate-dependent RTAs to a complete dRTA is unclear. Rate-dependent RTA is sometimes categorized as a subset of incomplete RTA. Mechanistically, though, the above definition of rate-dependent RTA differs from at least one theory of incomplete RTA.

Incomplete RTA

Incomplete RTA is usually discovered in the metabolic evaluation of nephrolithiasis or osteoporosis. Osteopenia and osteoporosis may also be associated with an underlying incomplete RTA (93). This entity is characterized by normal serum electrolytes and normal serum bicarbonate levels (41,93) implying appropriate net acid excretion under normal acid loads. Hence, abnormalities of acid regulation are often initially overlooked. More thorough investigation, however, usually reveals a mildly elevated urine pH, decreased urine citrate excretion and elevated urine calcium excretion (91,94). The "gold standard" for evaluation of incomplete RTA remains the acid load test. The lack of a renal acid excretory reserve characterizes this problem. At this point, two different mechanisms for incomplete RTA have been described. These two theories have substantially different findings with careful, formal testing of tubular function.

The first theory of the mechanism of incomplete RTA speculates that there is a mild H^+ secretion defect. This, in effect, describes a milder form of the classic type I RTA, characterized by distal tubular secretion defects not severe enough to give an obvious metabolic acidosis. As would be expected, the findings on U-P pCO_2 gradient measure and furosemide challenge would be abnormal. This condition is sometimes included in the "rate-dependent" form of dRTA—the acidification defect is mild and brought out only with acid loading or testing of the distal segments.

The second theory of incomplete RTA demonstrates a vastly different mechanism. The elevated urine pH in this form of incomplete RTA is felt to be caused by a greatly exaggerated increase in ammonia production and distal delivery, not caused by impaired distal H^+ secretion. The increased ammonia delivery to the distal nephron is felt to be so large, that the majority of the H^+ is bound, leaving relatively fewer free protons; a high urine pH is the result. Evidence of an exaggerated ammonia production rate despite normal serum pH and bicarbonate levels hint that a proximal tubular cell abnormality may be the basis of incomplete RTA (41). This theory contrasts with the mechanism described earlier, where urine pH remains elevated because of a distal tubular secretory defect despite normal ammoniagenesis. Net acid excretion is theoretically different between the two entities; incomplete RTA caused by a mild secretory defect would have slightly decreased NAE, whereas incomplete dRTA caused by ammonia overproduction would have normal or even elevated NAE.

Overall, the etiology of incomplete RTA is not well described, and the diagnosis may encompass various defects, ranging from AE1 (basolateral HCO_3^-/Cl^- exchanger on intercalated cells) mutations (95) to decreased intracellular pH in the proximal tubular cells. The findings of provocative tests are summarized in Table 3. In addition, whereas incomplete RTA is usually discussed in the context of distal RTAs because of the elevated urine pH, a proximal tubular abnormality may be the primary defect based on some evidence. One proposed mechanism of incomplete RTA mentioned previously suggests that the proximal tubule may have a chronically decreased intracellular pH as a reason for the increased ammonia production (41). This would also prompt hypocitraturia despite the absence of overt systemic acidosis, typical for incomplete RTA. The chronic increased ammonia production and cycling may stimulate inflammation, eventually leading to chronic interstitial disease and possibly complete dRTA with a distal acidification problem (96–98). The development of complete dRTA from incomplete RTA is speculative but noted in some case reports.

There are numerous diseases associated with incomplete RTA, including vitamin D or lithium use, sickle cell, medullary sponge kidney, and glycogen storage diseases. Autoimmune disorders, more commonly associated with complete dRTA or hyperkalemic RTA, can be associated with incomplete RTA (99,100). Treatment of incomplete RTA is directed predominantly at the nephrolithiasis and osteoporosis. This entails correction of hypocitraturia and maneuvers to decrease calcium excretion. Because metabolic acidosis is not a finding in this form of RTA, the use of alkali has questionable benefit.

Type 4 Renal Tubular Acidosis

Type 4 RTA is the most common form of RTA in adults (63). The disorder is characterized by distal tubular findings consistent with a combination of a "rate-limited" H^+

Table 5
Causes of Type 4 RTA

Mineralocorticoid deficiency
- Normal renal function
  - Addison's Disease
  - Congenital adrenal hyperplasia
  - Hereditary
- Chronic renal disease
  - Diabetic nephropathy
  - HIV associated nephropathy

Mineralocorticoid resistance
- Genetic
  - Pseudohypoaldosteronism type I
  - Pseudohypoaldosteronism type II (Gordon's syndrome)
- Chronic renal disease
  - Obstructive uropathy
  - Renal transplant rejection
  - Medullary cystic kidney disease

Medications
- Spironolactone/eplerenone
- Angiotensin converting enzyme receptor blocker
- Long-term heparin
- Cyclosporine

secretory defect and a voltage dependent defect. The hyperkalemia that is usually associated with type 4 RTA contributes to impairment in proximal tubular ammoniagenesis. In addition, a level of aldosterone deficiency characterizes this type of RTA and probably also leads to decreased ammoniagenesis *(101)*. The combination of these defects results in a hyperchloremic metabolic acidosis with hyperkalemia, a positive urine anion gap (impaired NAE), and an acidified urine (<5.5) at baseline. Many patients also have some mild renal insufficiency.

CAUSES OF TYPE 4 RTA

Aldosterone deficiency or resistance is the underlying issue in many of the causes of type 4 RTA. As aldosterone is important in the sodium absorption in the principal cells of the collecting tubule, a low aldosterone state would decrease the voltage gradient for H^+ secretion (voltage defect). In addition, aldosterone deficiency would impair distal tubular proton secretory capability (secretory defect). The hyperkalemia seen in type 4 RTA can also be attributed to low aldosterone, to some degree. Ammoniagenesis is decreased, perhaps as a result of the hyperkalemia *(101)*. Table 5 lists disease states and medications associated with these conditions.

Many commonly used medications can cause aldosterone resistance and induce a type 4 RTA. Oftentimes this is clinically evident in patients who are predisposed to developing this form of RTA. Individuals with diabetes mellitus or mild chronic interstitial renal disease are especially prone to this condition when ACE inhibitors, nonsteroidal anti-inflammatory medications or spironolactone is used.

Clinical Findings and Laboratory Findings

The clinical findings in type 4 RTA are usually not very remarkable. The hyperkalemia is usually silent unless there is severe dietary indiscretion or the use of antagonizing medications. Renal stones are usually not associated with this form of RTA. Although urine citrate excretion may be decreased, there is commonly a mild degree of renal insufficiency, which decreases calcium excretion and may protect from nephrolithiasis *(102)*.

The baseline urine pH is usually acidic in type 4 RTA despite an underlying mild distal acidification defect, which can be detected by U-P pCO_2 measurement after bicarbonate loading. The decreased ammoniagenesis may account for the low urine pH, because buffer delivery is low, and the matched decrease in urine proton availability is enough to provide a urine pH of <5.5. Overall, NAE is decreased (Fig. 11).

Treatment

Treatment for type 4 RTA includes mineralocorticoids to correct the underlying low aldosterone state, loop diuretics to manage the hyperkalemia, and dietary restrictions to limit potassium intake. Mineralocorticoids such as fludrocortisone may increase distal nephron tubular sodium absorption and provide a more favorable electronegative lumen for both H^+ and K^+ secretion *(103)*. The increased sodium absorption, however, may lead to edema and hypertension, especially in those with some renal insufficiency to begin with. Loop diuretics are especially useful for type 4 RTA *(104)*. The K^+ wasting effect not only treats the hyperkalemia, but in doing so may also stimulate ammoniagenesis in the proximal tubules to aid in NAE. The increase in distal sodium delivery also favors distal proton secretion. If the acidosis remains severe despite these measures, alkali is often provided at about 1–2 meq/kg *(104)*. Dietary restriction of potassium by itself has been found to ameliorate the acidosis of type 4 RTA by the mechanisms mentioned previously *(105)*.

REFERENCES

1. Lemann J, Jr., Litzow JR, Lennon EJ. The effects of chronic acid loads in normal man: further evidence for the participation of bone mineral in the defense against chronic metabolic acidosis. J Clin Invest 1966; 45(10): 1608–1614.
2. Bushinsky DA. Net proton influx into bone during metabolic, but not respiratory, acidosis. Am J Physiol 1988; 254(3 Pt 2): F306–310.
3. Bushinsky DA. Stimulated osteoclastic and suppressed osteoblastic activity in metabolic but not respiratory acidosis. Am J Physiol 1995; 268(1 Pt 1): C80–88.
4. Kamel KS, Briceno LF, Sanchez MI, et al. A new classification for renal defects in net acid excretion. Am J Kidney Dis 1997; 29(1): 136–146.
5. Reddi AS. Essentials of renal physiology. College Book Publishers. East Hanover, NJ 1999: 337.
6. Nissim I, Cattano C, Lin Z. Acid-base regulation of hepatic glutamine metabolism and ureagenesis: study with 15N. J Am Soc Nephrol 1993; 3(7): 1416–1427.
7. Boon L, Blommaart PJ, Meijer AJ, et al. Acute acidosis inhibits liver amino acid transport: no primary role for the urea cycle in acid-base balance. Am J Physiol 1994; 267(6 Pt 2): F1015–1020.
8. Caldas A, Broyer M, Dechaux M, et al. Primary distal tubular acidosis in childhood: clinical study and long-term follow-up of 28 patients. J Pediatr 1992; 121(2): 233–241.
9. Tashian RE. The carbonic anhydrases: widening perspectives on their evolution, expression and function. Bioessays 1989; 10(6): 186–192.
10. Breton S. The cellular physiology of carbonic anhydrases. JOP 2001; 2(4 Suppl): 159–164.
11. Dobyan DC, Bulger RE. Renal carbonic anhydrase. Am J Physiol 1982; 243(4): F311–324.

12. Wakabayashi S, Shigekawa M, Pouyssegur J. Molecular physiology of vertebrate Na+/H+ exchangers. Physiol Rev 1997; 77(1): 51–74.

13. Putney LK, Denker SP, Barber DL. The changing face of the Na+/H+ exchanger, NHE1: structure, regulation, and cellular actions. Annu Rev Pharmacol Toxicol 2002; 42:527–552.

14. Ghishan FK, Knobel SM, Summar M. Molecular cloning, sequencing, chromosomal localization, and tissue distribution of the human Na+/H+ exchanger (SLC9A2). Genomics 1995; 30(1): 25–30.

15. Abuladze N, Lee I, Newman D, et al. Molecular cloning, chromosomal localization, tissue distribution, and functional expression of the human pancreatic sodium bicarbonate cotransporter. J Biol Chem 1998; 273(28): 17,689–17,695.

16. DuBose TD, Jr., Good DW. Role of the thick ascending limb and inner medullary collecting duct in the regulation of urinary acidification. Semin Nephrol 1991; 11(2): 120–128.

17. Igarashi T, Sekine T, Inatomi J, et al. Unraveling the molecular pathogenesis of isolated proximal renal tubular acidosis. J Am Soc Nephrol 2002; 13(8): 2171–2177.

18. Smulders YM, Frissen PH, Slaats EH, et al. Renal tubular acidosis. Pathophysiology and diagnosis. Arch Intern Med 1996; 156(15): 1629–1636.

19. DuBose TD, Jr., Good DW, Hamm LL, et al. Ammonium transport in the kidney: new physiological concepts and their clinical implications. J Am Soc Nephrol 1991; 1(11): 1193–1203.

20. Wall SM. Ammonium transport and the role of the Na,K-ATPase. Miner Electrolyte Metab 1996; 22(5–6): 311–317.

21. Hamm LL, Simon EE. Ammonia transport in the proximal tubule. Miner Electrolyte Metab 1990; 16(5): 283–290.

22. Tanner MJ. Band 3 anion exchanger and its involvement in erythrocyte and kidney disorders. Curr Opin Hematol 2002; 9(2): 133–139.

23. Karet FE, Finberg KE, Nelson RD, et al. Mutations in the gene encoding B1 subunit of H+-ATPase cause renal tubular acidosis with sensorineural deafness. Nat Genet 1999; 21(1): 84–90.

24. Halperin ML, Kamel KS, Ethier JH, et al. What is the underlying defect in patients with isolated, proximal renal tubular acidosis? Am J Nephrol 1989; 9(4): 265–268.

25. Kurtz I. Role of ammonia in the induction of renal hypertrophy. Am J Kidney Dis 1991; 17(6): 650–653.

26. Sastrasinh S, Tannen RL. Effect of potassium on renal NH3 production. Am J Physiol 1983; 244(4): F383–391.

27. Halperin ML, Ethier JH, Kamel KS. Ammonium excretion in chronic metabolic acidosis: benefits and risks. Am J Kidney Dis 1989; 14(4): 267–271.

28. Remer T. Influence of nutrition on acid-base balance–metabolic aspects. Eur J Nutr 2001; 40(5): 214–220.

29. Krapf R, Pearce D, Lynch C, et al. Expression of rat renal Na/H antiporter mRNA levels in response to respiratory and metabolic acidosis. J Clin Invest 1991; 87(2): 747–751.

30. Kuwahara M, Sasaki S, Marumo F. Mineralocorticoids and acidosis regulate H+/HCO3– transport of intercalated cells. J Clin Invest 1992; 89(5): 1388–1394.

31. Hays SR. Mineralocorticoid modulation of apical and basolateral membrane H+/OH–/HCO3– transport processes in the rabbit inner stripe of outer medullary collecting duct. J Clin Invest 1992; 90(1): 180–187.

32. Schwartz GJ, Al-Awqati Q. Regulation of transepithelial H+ transport by exocytosis and endocytosis. Annu Rev Physiol 1986; 48:153–161.

33. Da Silva Junior JC, Perrone RD, Johns CA, et al. Rat kidney band 3 mRNA modulation in chronic respiratory acidosis. Am J Physiol 1991; 260(2 Pt 2): F204–209.

34. Hamm LL, Hering-Smith KS. Acid-base transport in the collecting duct. Semin Nephrol 1993; 13(2): 246–255.

35. Ortiz PA, Garvin JL. Role of nitric oxide in the regulation of nephron transport. Am J Physiol Renal Physiol 2002; 282(5): F777–784.

36. Simpson DP. Citrate excretion: a window on renal metabolism. Am J Physiol 1983; 244(3): F223–234.

37. Dyck RF, Asthana S, Kalra J, et al. A modification of the urine osmolal gap: an improved method for estimating urine ammonium. Am J Nephrol 1990; 10(5): 359–362.

38. Rodriguez Soriano J. Renal tubular acidosis: the clinical entity. J Am Soc Nephrol 2002; 13(8): 2160–2170.

39. Fry ID, Cusick PE, Alston WC, et al. The acidification response of normal subjects to ammonium chloride using a 3-day loading test. Ann Clin Biochem 1988; 25 (Pt 4):403–407.

40. Monnens L. A modification of the short ammonium chloride loading test in children. Nephron 1974; 12(2): 129–132.

41. Donnelly S, Kamel KS, Vasuvattakul S, et al. Might distal renal tubular acidosis be a proximal tubular cell disorder? Am J Kidney Dis 1992; 19(3): 272–281.

42. Rodriguez-Soriano J, Vallo A, Castillo G, et al. Defect in urinary acidification in nephrotic syndrome and its correction by furosemide. Nephron 1982; 32(4): 308–313.

43. Jentsch TJ, Keller SK, Koch M, et al. Evidence for coupled transport of bicarbonate and sodium in cultured bovine corneal endothelial cells. J Membr Biol 1984; 81(3): 189–204.

44. Lepple-Wienhues A, Rauch R, Clark AF, et al. Electrophysiological properties of cultured human trabecular meshwork cells. Exp Eye Res 1994; 59(3): 305–311.

45. Brenes LG, Brenes JN, Hernandez MM. Familial proximal renal tubular acidosis. A distinct clinical entity. Am J Med 1977; 63(2): 244–252.

46. Rodriguez-Soriano J. New insights into the pathogenesis of renal tubular acidosis–from functional to molecular studies. Pediatr Nephrol 2000; 14(12): 1121–1136.

47. Yanase M, Orita Y, Okada N, et al. Decreased Na+-gradient-dependent D-glucose transport in brush-border membrane vesicles from rabbits with experimental Fanconi syndrome. Biochim Biophys Acta 1983; 733(1): 95–101.

48. Bergeron M, Dubord L, Hausser C, et al. Membrane permeability as a cause of transport defects in experimental Fanconi syndrome. A new hypothesis. J Clin Invest 1976; 57(5): 1181–1189.

49. Lemann J, Jr., Adams ND, Wilz DR, et al. Acid and mineral balances and bone in familial proximal renal tubular acidosis. Kidney Int 2000; 58(3): 1267–1277.

50. Gregory MJ, Schwartz GJ. Diagnosis and treatment of renal tubular disorders. Semin Nephrol 1998; 18(3): 317–329.

51. Brenes LG, Sanchez MI. Impaired urinary ammonium excretion in patients with isolated proximal renal tubular acidosis. J Am Soc Nephrol 1993; 4(4): 1073–1078.

52. Reaich D, Channon SM, Scrimgeour CM, et al. Correction of acidosis in humans with CRF decreases protein degradation and amino acid oxidation. Am J Physiol 1993; 265(2 Pt 1): E230–235.

53. Ballmer PE, Imoberdorf R. Influence of acidosis on protein metabolism. Nutrition 1995; 11(5): 462–468; discussion 470.

54. Ballmer PE, McNurlan MA, Hulter HN, et al. Chronic metabolic acidosis decreases albumin synthesis and induces negative nitrogen balance in humans. J Clin Invest 1995; 95(1): 39–45.

55. Ahmed A, Sims RV. Proximal renal tubular acidosis associated with osteomalacia. South Med J 2001; 94(5): 536–539.

56. Stoll C, Gentine A, Geisert J. Siblings with congenital renal tubular acidosis and nerve deafness. Clin Genet 1996; 50(4): 235–239.

57. Karet FE, Finberg KE, Nayir A, et al. Localization of a gene for autosomal recessive distal renal tubular acidosis with normal hearing (rdRTA2) to 7q33-34. Am J Hum Genet 1999; 65(6): 1656–1665.

58. Smith AN, Skaug J, Choate KA, et al. Mutations in ATP6N1B, encoding a new kidney vacuolar proton pump 116-kD subunit, cause recessive distal renal tubular acidosis with preserved hearing. Nat Genet 2000; 26(1): 71–75.

59. Bruce LJ, Cope DL, Jones GK, et al. Familial distal renal tubular acidosis is associated with mutations in the red cell anion exchanger (Band 3, AE1) gene. J Clin Invest 1997; 100(7): 1693–1707.

60. Karet FE, Gainza FJ, Gyory AZ, et al. Mutations in the chloride-bicarbonate exchanger gene AE1 cause autosomal dominant but not autosomal recessive distal renal tubular acidosis. Proc Natl Acad Sci USA 1998; 95(11): 6337–6342.

61. Lima PR, Sales TS, Costa FF, et al. Arginine 490 is a hot spot for mutation in the band 3 gene in hereditary spherocytosis. Eur J Haematol 1999; 63(5): 360–361.

62. Ribeiro ML, Alloisio N, Almeida H, et al. Severe hereditary spherocytosis and distal renal tubular acidosis associated with the total absence of band 3. Blood 2000; 96(4): 1602–1604.

63. Batlle D, Flores G. Underlying defects in distal renal tubular acidosis: new understandings. Am J Kidney Dis 1996; 27(6): 896–915.
64. Purcell H, Bastani B, Harris KP, et al. Cellular distribution of H(+)-ATPase following acute unilateral ureteral obstruction in rats. Am J Physiol 1991; 261(3 Pt 2): F365–376.
65. Nakai H, Byers MG, Venta PJ, et al. The gene for human carbonic anhydrase II (CA2) is located at chromosome 8q22. Cytogenet Cell Genet 1987; 44(4): 234–235.
66. Sly WS, Hewett-Emmett D, Whyte MP, et al. Carbonic anhydrase II deficiency identified as the primary defect in the autosomal recessive syndrome of osteopetrosis with renal tubular acidosis and cerebral calcification. Proc Natl Acad Sci USA 1983; 80(9): 2752–2756.
67. Hu PY, Roth DE, Skaggs LA, et al. A splice junction mutation in intron 2 of the carbonic anhydrase II gene of osteopetrosis patients from Arabic countries. Hum Mutat 1992; 1(4): 288–292.
68. Ohlsson A, Cumming WA, Paul A, et al. Carbonic anhydrase II deficiency syndrome: recessive osteopetrosis with renal tubular acidosis and cerebral calcification. Pediatrics 1986; 77(3): 371–381.
69. Bregman H, Brown J, Rogers A, et al. Osteopetrosis with combined proximal and distal renal tubular acidosis. Am J Kidney Dis 1982; 2(3): 357–362.
70. Nagai R, Kooh SW, Balfe JW, et al. Renal tubular acidosis and osteopetrosis with carbonic anhydrase II deficiency: pathogenesis of impaired acidification. Pediatr Nephrol 1997; 11(5): 633–636.
71. Warnock DW. Amphotericin B: an introduction. J Antimicrob Chemother 1991; 28 (Suppl B): 27–38.
72. Andreoli TE, Monahan M. The interaction of polyene antibiotics with thin lipid membranes. J Gen Physiol 1968; 52(2): 300–325.
73. Capasso G, Schuetz H, Vickermann B, et al. Amphotericin B and amphotericin B methylester: effect on brush border membrane permeability. Kidney Int 1986; 30(3): 311–317.
74. Bonilla-Felix M. Primary distal renal tubular acidosis as a result of a gradient defect. Am J Kidney Dis 1996; 27(3): 428–430.
75. Kimura H, Mujais SK. Cortical collecting duct Na-K pump in obstructive nephropathy. Am J Physiol 1990; 258(5 Pt 2): F1320–1327.
76. Sabatini S, Kurtzman NA. Enzyme activity in obstructive uropathy: basis for salt wastage and the acidification defect. Kidney Int 1990; 37(1): 79–84.
77. Arruda JA, Batlle DC, Sehy JT, et al. Hyperkalemia and renal insufficiency: role of selective aldosterone deficiency and tubular unresponsiveness to aldosterone. Am J Nephrol 1981; 1(3–4): 160–167.
78. Schlueter W, Keilani T, Hizon M, et al. On the mechanism of impaired distal acidification in hyperkalemic renal tubular acidosis: evaluation with amiloride and bumetanide. J Am Soc Nephrol 1992; 3(4): 953–964.
79. Rastogi S, Bayliss JM, Nascimento L, et al. Hyperkalemic renal tubular acidosis: effect of furosemide in humans and in rats. Kidney Int 1985; 28(5): 801–807.
80. Fortenberry JD, Kenney RD. Distal renal tubular acidosis as the initial manifestation of systemic lupus erythematosus in an adolescent. J Adolesc Health 1991; 12(2): 148–151.
81. Caruana RJ, Barish CF, Buckalew VM, Jr. Complete distal renal tubular acidosis in systemic lupus: clinical and laboratory findings. Am J Kidney Dis 1985; 6(1): 59–63.
82. Bossini N, Savoldi S, Franceschini F, et al. Clinical and morphological features of kidney involvement in primary Sjogren's syndrome. Nephrol Dial Transplant 2001; 16(12): 2328–2336.
83. Cohen EP, Bastani B, Cohen MR, et al. Absence of H(+)-ATPase in cortical collecting tubules of a patient with Sjogren's syndrome and distal renal tubular acidosis. J Am Soc Nephrol 1992; 3(2): 264–271.
84. DeFranco PE, Haragsim L, Schmitz PG, et al. Absence of vacuolar H(+)-ATPase pump in the collecting duct of a patient with hypokalemic distal renal tubular acidosis and Sjogren's syndrome. J Am Soc Nephrol 1995; 6(2): 295–301.
85. Itoh Y, Reichlin M. Antibodies to carbonic anhydrase in systemic lupus erythematosus and other rheumatic diseases. Arthritis Rheum 1992; 35(1): 73–82.
86. Inagaki Y, Jinno-Yoshida Y, Hamasaki Y, et al. A novel autoantibody reactive with carbonic anhydrase in sera from patients with systemic lupus erythematosus and Sjogren's syndrome. J Dermatol Sci 1991; 2(3): 147–154.

87. Juncos LI, Muino JC, Garcia NH, et al. Renal tubular acidosis and vasculitis associated with IgE deposits in the kidney and small vessels. Am J Kidney Dis 2000; 35(5): 941–949.
88. Domrongkitchaiporn S, Pongsakul C, Stitchantrakul W, et al. Bone mineral density and histology in distal renal tubular acidosis. Kidney Int 2001; 59(3): 1086–1093.
89. Rodriguez-Soriano J, Vallo A, Castillo G, et al. Natural history of primary distal renal tubular acidosis treated since infancy. J Pediatr 1982; 101(5): 669–676.
90. Fang JT, Chan YC. Systemic lupus erythematosus presenting initially as hydrogen ATPase pump defects of distal renal tubular acidosis. Ren Fail 2000; 22(4): 517–521.
91. Norman ME, Feldman NI, Cohn RM, et al. Urinary citrate excretion in the diagnosis of distal renal tubular acidosis. J Pediatr 1978; 92(3): 394–400.
92. Batlle D, Grupp M, Gaviria M, et al. Distal renal tubular acidosis with intact capacity to lower urinary pH. Am J Med 1982; 72(5): 751–758.
93. Weger W, Kotanko P, Weger M, et al. Prevalence and characterization of renal tubular acidosis in patients with osteopenia and osteoporosis and in non-porotic controls. Nephrol Dial Transplant 2000; 15(7): 975–980.
94. Nicar MJ, Skurla C, Sakhaee K, et al. Low urinary citrate excretion in nephrolithiasis. Urology 1983; 21(1): 8–14.
95. Rysava R, Tesar V, Jirsa M, Jr., et al. Incomplete distal renal tubular acidosis coinherited with a mutation in the band 3 (AE1) gene. Nephrol Dial Transplant 1997; 12(9): 1869–1873.
96. Tolins JP, Hostetter MK, Hostetter TH. Hypokalemic nephropathy in the rat. Role of ammonia in chronic tubular injury. J Clin Invest 1987; 79(5): 1447–1458.
97. Clark EC, Nath KA, Hostetter MK, et al. Role of ammonia in progressive interstitial nephritis. Am J Kidney Dis 1991; 17(5 Suppl 1): 15–19.
98. Nath KA, Hostetter MK, Hostetter TH. Increased ammoniagenesis as a determinant of progressive renal injury. Am J Kidney Dis 1991; 17(6): 654–657.
99. Shiozawa S, Shiozawa K, Shimizu S, et al. Clinical studies of renal disease in Sjogren's syndrome. Ann Rheum Dis 1987; 46(10): 768–772.
100. Viergever PP, Swaak TJ. Renal tubular dysfunction in primary Sjogren's syndrome: clinical studies in 27 patients. Clin Rheumatol 1991; 10(1): 23–27.
101. DuBose TD, Jr. Hyperkalemic hyperchloremic metabolic acidosis: pathophysiologic insights. Kidney Int 1997; 51(2): 591–602.
102. Uribarri J, Oh MS, Pak CY. Renal stone risk factors in patients with type IV renal tubular acidosis. Am J Kidney Dis 1994; 23(6): 784–787.
103. Sebastian A, Schambelan M, Lindenfeld S, et al. Amelioration of metabolic acidosis with fludrocortisone therapy in hyporeninemic hypoaldosteronism. N Engl J Med 1977; 297(11): 576–583.
104. Sebastian A, Schambelan M, Sutton JM. Amelioration of hyperchloremic acidosis with furosemide therapy in patients with chronic renal insufficiency and type 4 renal tubular acidosis. Am J Nephrol 1984; 4(5): 287–300.
105. Maher T, Schambelan M, Kurtz I, et al. Amelioration of metabolic acidosis by dietary potassium restriction in hyperkalemic patients with chronic renal insufficiency. J Lab Clin Med 1984; 103(3): 432–445.

9 Urinary Stone Inhibitors

Citrate and Magnesium

Harrison M. Abrahams, MD, Maxwell V. Meng, MD, and Marshall L. Stoller, MD

CONTENTS

Key Words: Nephrolithiasis; stone inhibition.

INTRODUCTION

It is intriguing that despite marked abnormal urinary factors, most humans will not form stones. Alternatively, some patients develop stones despite normal urinary composition. The key element, therefore, appears to be inhibition of the steps in calculogenesis (nucleation, crystal growth, aggregation, and crystal/stone retention). Urolithiasis will not develop if any one of these steps is blocked. Despite this simple fact, it is unclear exactly why many people form stones. Numerous molecules have been identified that inhibit crystallization in vitro but many stone formers have normal levels of these substances; others will continue to develop stones despite replacement of these known inhibitors. The formation of urinary calculi requires a complex combination of factors, both promoting and inhibiting stone formation. Fortunately, there are many patients who can be helped because of our existing knowledge about two specific urinary inhibitors: citrate and magnesium. This chapter will discuss the in vitro and in vivo evidence regarding citrate and magnesium as inhibitors of urinary stone disease.

From: Current Clinical Urology, *Urinary Stone Disease:*
A Practical Guide to Medical and Surgical Management
Edited by: M. L. Stoller and M. V. Meng © Humana Press Inc., Totowa, NJ

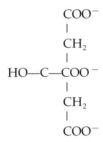

Fig. 1. Chemical composition of citrate.

CITRATE

Background

Citrate is the most well-studied inhibitor of calcium-based stones. It is therefore appropriate to detail the investigations leading to this discovery and outline the proof of its use in the treatment and prevention of urolithiasis.

Sabatini is credited as first discovering the ability of citrate to bind to calcium in the 1930s *(1)*. Hypocitraturia was noted in two patients with urinary stones by Boothby and Adams in 1934 but the significance of this report was not fully appreciated *(2)*. Hypocitraturia was again noted by Kissin and Locks in 1941 who first postulated that citrate replacement might treat and/or prevent calcium-based calculi *(3)*. Howard first described the clinical use of citrate as an alkalinizing agent for the treatment of noncalcium stones in 1954 *(4)*.

Scientific interest in urinary citrate was rekindled in the early 1980s as numerous studies verified hypocitraturia in stone patients *(5–7)*. Citrate replacement therapy for prevention of calcium-based nephrolithiasis was introduced in 1981 by Butz and Dulce *(8)*. They noted that a combination of sodium citrate and potassium citrate lowered urinary calcium levels and raised urinary citrate concentrations. Dissolution of existing calcium-based stones with potassium citrate was reported by Pak and colleagues in 1983 *(9)*. These reports spurred countless investigations and led to the approval of potassium citrate by the United States Food and Drug Administration in 1985.

Chemistry

Citrate is a tricarboxylic acid (Fig.1) and is entirely ionized above a pH of 6.5 at 37°C *(10,11)*. Citrate is almost entirely absorbed by the gastrointestinal tract *(12)*. Plasma concentrations range from 0.05 to 0.3 mM *(13)*. Assuming a normal glomerular filtration rate of 125 mL/min, citrate is filtered at rates ranging from 6.25 to 37.5 µmol/min. Approximately 75% is reabsorbed by the proximal convoluted tubule (Fig. 2) *(14)*. Ten to 35% (by volume) of oral citrate is excreted in the urine unchanged and is dependent on the renal acid/base status. Renal tubular cells can additionally extract citrate from the peritubular fluid at a rate of 0.5 to 3 µmol/min *(11)*. Therefore, the citrate concentration in the renal cortex can exceed that of peripheral serum.

Urinary citrate excretion is strongly dependent on the acid-base status of renal tubular cells. When the cells are in an acidotic state, as much as 95% of the filtered citrate is sequestered by proximal tubular mitochondria as an additional source of energy in the Krebs cycle (also known as citric acid cycle and tricarboxylic acid cycle) *(11,15)*.

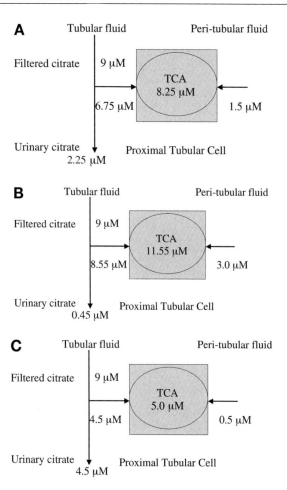

Fig. 2. Citrate handling under normal, acidotic, and alkalotic states. **(A)** Normal state: approx 75% of filtered citrate is reabsorbed. **(B)** Acidotic state: to preserve citrate for the citric acid cycle, the proximal tubular cells increase reabsorption from the filtrate and from the peritubular fluid. Overall, as much as 95% of filtered citrate is reabsorbed. **(C)** Alkalotic state: when the cells have an excess of alkali, reabsorption is reduced, thereby increasing urinary citrate levels.

This is the common pathway that cells use to liberate energy from the final steps of oxidation, generating carbon dioxide (CO_2) and water. Citrate extraction from the peritubular fluid is also increased via a sodium-citrate co-transporter which is activated in an acidotic state *(15,16)*. This results in significantly lower urinary citrate levels as the citrate is sequestered in the proximal tubular cell. Conversely, in an alkalotic state, up to 50% of filtered citrate may be excreted in the urine as the reabsorption of citrate into the proximal tubular cells is dramatically reduced.

Any condition that results in intracellular acidosis, including hypokalemia, high protein diet, and exercise, will cause a decrease in urinary citrate concentrations (Table 1). Androgens, acetozolamide, angiotensin converting enzyme inhibitors, volume expansion and starvation are thought to lower urinary citrate levels through similar mechanisms *(14,17,18)*.

Table 1

Conditions and Compounds Known to Decrease Urinary Citrate

- Intracellular acidosis
- Renal tubular acidosis
- High protein diet
- Exercise
- Acetozolamide
- Thiazides
- Starvation

- Hypokalemia
- Chronic diarrhea
- High sodium diet
- Androgens
- Angiotension converting enzyme inhibitors
- Volume expansion
- Active urinary tract infection

(Adapted from refs. *11,14,17,18, and 34.*)

Table 2

Conditions and Compounds Known to Increase Urinary Citrate

- Organic acids
  (malate, succinate, and fumarate)
- Pregnancy
- Parathormone (PTH)
- Lithium
- Vitamin D

- Tamarind/Tartaric acid
  (spice)
- Last portion of the menstrual cycle
- Magnesium
- Calcitonin

(Adapted from refs. *11,14,19–21.*)

Other clinical states may result in decreased urinary citrate levels (Table 2). For example, organic acids such as malate, succinate, and fumarate provide an alkali load and therefore stimulate intrarenal citrate synthesis and decrease sequestration from both the filtrate and the peritubular fluid *(19,20)*. The spice tamarind may also increase urinary citrate levels through its high levels of tartaric acid *(20)*. Increases in urinary citrate concentration have been documented during pregnancy and during the latter half of the menstrual cycle *(21)*. These increases are likely related to the elevated estrogen and progesterone levels. The hypercalciuria of pregnancy may be offset by the concomitant increase in urinary citrate excretion. This may protect pregnant women from developing urinary stones despite the marked increased urinary calcium. Parathormone (PTH), magnesium, lithium, calcitonin, and vitamin D also have been found to increase urinary citrate levels *(14)*.

Citrate: "Normal" Levels

Urinary citrate levels vary substantially throughout the day, and from day to day. "Normal" levels, therefore, are difficult to define. Pak has created a "functional" definition of hypocitraturia based on 24-h urinary citrate levels of patients with renal tubular acidosis *(22)*. These patients had urinary citrate levels less than 320 mg/d. He concluded, therefore, that normal patients should have a urinary citrate level greater than 320 mg/d. Parks and Coe found a urinary citrate level of 729 ± 47 mg/24 h in a group of normal females and 547 ± 31 mg/24 h in normal males. Others have used a cutoff of 115 mg in males and 200 mg in females as a cutoff for hypocitraturia *(23)*. A recent comparison of male and female stone patients shows no difference in urinary citrate levels until the seventh decade when citrate levels fell in women *(24)*. Premenopausal and postmenopausal women had similar levels. In another study, 28 postmenopausal women taking estrogen replacement had higher urinary citrate levels than 41 postmenopausal women that were not taking estrogen therapy (576.6 ± 237.9 vs 306.2 ± 209.9 mg./24 h, $p < 0.001$) *(25)*. Litholink®, a commercial laboratory evaluating 24-h urine collections, suggests that "normal" urinary citrate levels are 450 mg/d for men and 550 mg/d for women *(26)*. Obviously, this dramatic range of "normal" values demonstrates that an optimal level remains ill-defined. Therapeutic citrate supplementation may be warranted in more patients than previously thought owing to the ambiguity of "normal" urinary citrate levels.

Hypocitraturia: Incidence

Seventeen to 63% of stone patients have hypocitraturia as a risk factor, depending on its definition *(27–31)*. Gentle et al evaluated 24-h urine collections from 5942 patients. Hypocitraturia (<320 mg/24 h) was found as an isolated abnormality in 18.6% of the patients whereas another 9.3% of the patients had hypocitraturia in conjunction with another urinary abnormality (hypocitraturia with hyperoxaluria, 2.9%; hypocitraturia with hypercalciuria, 1.9%; hypocitraturia with hyperuricosuria, 2.3%; hypocitraturia with multiple other defects, 2.2%) *(32)*. Among patients younger than 65 years of age, 17% were found to have hypocitraturia as the sole metabolic defect. Hypocitraturia was associated with other metabolic defects in an additional 10% of these patients. In contrast, there was a higher incidence of hypocitraturia as a sole urinary abnormality in stone patients older than 65 (29%). An additional 7% of these geriatric patients had hypocitraturia in conjunction with other urinary defects. In a smaller study, 8.5% of 31 stone patients with no other demonstrable metabolic abnormality had hypocitraturia (<322 mg/24 h) *(30)*. More than 50% of 194 patients with other metabolic abnormalities had urinary citrate levels below the lowest level for controls (320 mg/24 h).

The incidence of hypocitraturia in children with calcium-based renal stones has recently been investigated *(33)*. Seventy-eight stone forming children (age 1–15 yr) were examined and compared with 24 controls. Median urinary citrate levels for the stone forming children was 261 ± 256 mg/24 h compared with 491 ± 490 mg/24 h in the control group ($p = 0.002$). Sixty-four percent (64%) of the stone forming children had urinary citrate levels less than 320 mg/24 h compared with 29% of the controls.

Hypocitraturia: Disease Associations

Hypocitraturia is associated with many clinical entities, most commonly renal tubular acidosis (RTA) type I (distal). In this disorder, impaired hydrogen excretion causes intracellular acidosis and reduced urinary citrate by the mechanisms described above (*see* Chapter 8). Clinically, patients with calcium-based stones and a quantitative urinary citrate of less than 50 mg/24 h can be assumed to have type I RTA. These patients require aggressive citrate supplementation to help prevent future calculi. Although hypocitraturia may be seen in other forms of RTA, it is not clinically important, as stones do not typically form in these patients. Patients taking acetazolamide may have an RTA-like pattern, with hypocitraturia caused by the blockade of proximal tubule bicarbonate reabsorption.

Other common entities associated with hypocitraturia include chronic diarrheal syndromes, thiazide induced hypocitraturia and idiopathic hypocitraturia *(11)*. Chronic diarrheal syndromes result in intestinal loss of alkali leading to a metabolic acidosis and therefore hypocitraturia. These include patients who have undergone gastrectomy, bowel resection, intestinal bypass, or those with inflammatory bowel diseases. Thiazide diuretics can result in hypocitraturia from the renal loss of potassium and the resultant intracellular acidosis. Some "idiopathic" stone formers may have hypocitraturia caused by a high sodium diet (34), rigorous exercise (35) or active urinary tract infection (11). In the latter situation, bacteria may use citrate to augment their energy needs, thus effectively consuming urinary citrate. Pak reported that a small subset of patients will show a blunted response to citrate replacement. Such patients have hypocitraturia without acidosis, leading to the proposition of a rare genetic alteration in the sodium-citrate transport gene (36). Impaired gastrointestinal uptake is no longer considered a probable cause of hypocitraturia (37).

Citrate: Mechanism of Action?

Citrate inhibits many of the steps in calculogenesis. One mechanism of action is the binding of urinary calcium in solution, thus effectively lowering ionic calcium concentrations. This leads to lower saturations of calcium oxalate and calcium phosphate (38). Dissolution of calcium salts may theoretically occur once the urine concentration of these salts is lower than the saturation level (11). However, this mechanism of complexing calcium may be minimal (39). Ashby and Sleet mixed equal concentrations of citrate and oxalate and added calcium oxalate crystals until a steady state was reached (40). The supersaturation of calcium oxalate in the solution only varied by less than 1% despite varied citrate concentrations. This study suggests that inhibition of calcium oxalate by citrate is mainly caused by mechanisms other than calcium complexation.

Citrate lowers the spontaneous nucleation of calcium oxalate (41) and prevents the heterogeneous nucleation of calcium oxalate by urate crystals (42,43). By this mechanism, the generation of a stone nidus may be inhibited. However, if calcium phosphate crystals precipitate as a result of over-alkalinization, calcium phosphate nucleation may occur. Aggregation of calcium oxalate and calcium phosphate crystals is diminished at normal physiologic citrate concentrations (44–46). Citrate reduces crystal growth rates of calcium oxalate by 33% in a seeded metastable in vitro growth system (38) and when tested in urine from stone formers (47–49). Calcium phosphate (apatite) crystal growth rates are decreased in the presence of citrate in a similar manner (50). These effects are independent of the urinary pH changes brought about by potassium citrate supplementation. Citrate inhibits multiple steps in stone formation including nucleation, aggregation, and crystal growth.

There is debate as to which inhibitory mechanism is most important in the prevention of calcium-based stones. Citrate is likely most powerful because of its high urinary concentration, and is actually less powerful on a molar basis than other potential urinary inhibitors (51).

Citrate: Supplementation

Potassium citrate is the most common formulation of citrate supplementation studied. Other forms of citrate replacement include sodium citrate, sodium potassium citrate, calcium citrate, citrus juices, potassium magnesium citrate, and combination preparations. These formulations will be discussed separately.

Potassium citrate is used for both the treatment and prevention of urinary stone disease. Barcelo and colleagues performed a randomized, placebo controlled prevention trial of potassium citrate therapy in patients with hypocitraturic calcium nephrolithiasis (52). Fifty-seven patients with moderately severe urinary stone disease (two or more stones in the last 2 yr) and low (<342 mg/24 h) or low normal (<642 mg/24 h) urinary citrate levels were randomized. Sixteen patients were noncompliant and two discontinued therapy secondary to gastrointestinal side effects. Eighteen patients received potassium citrate tablets (30–60 meq/d) for 3 yr. Urinary citrate levels increased from 1.9 ± 0.5 mmol/d (359 ± 95 mg/d) to 2.8-3.5 mmol/d (529–661 mg/d). Urinary pH levels increased from 5.4 ± 0.5 to 6.1–6.7. Stone formation rates dropped dramatically from 1.2 ± 0.6 before treatment to 0.1 ± 0.2 per patient year ($p < 0.0001$) after treatment. Thirteen (72%) of these patients did not form any stones during the trial period. No patient with existing renal stones showed significant stone growth while on potassium citrate therapy. In contrast, the 20 patients taking placebo for 3 yr showed no significant change in stone formation rate ($1.1 \pm 0.4 – 1.1 \pm 0.3$ per patient year). Twenty percent (20%) of controls showed remission of stone production during the trial. Three patients demonstrated significant stone growth in the placebo arm. There was no comment regarding potassium citrate and stone dissolution. There are multiple anecdotal reports regarding potassium citrate therapy but this remains the only randomized, placebo-controlled trial.

The use of potassium citrate for hyperuricosuric calcium oxalate nephrolithiasis was validated by Pak and Peterson in 1986. Nineteen patients were treated with 60–80 meq of potassium citrate per day (43). The treatment raised urinary pH by 0.55–0.85 and increased urinary citrate levels by 249–402 mg/d to a mean of 643 mg/d. It also decreased stone formation from 1.55 ± 2.70 per patient-year to 0.38 ± 1.22 per patient-year during the 2.4-yr average treatment period. This study documents the use of potassium citrate in patients with nonhypocitraturic forms of calcium nephrolithiasis.

Potassium citrate is also beneficial in uric acid stone disease as first reported by Pak and colleagues in 1986. Eighteen patients with uric acid stones were treated with potassium citrate for an average of 2.8 yr (53). Urinary citrate levels rose from 503 ± 225 mg/d to 852–998 mg/d, urinary pH increased from 5.30 ± 0.31 to 6.19–6.46, and new stone formation rate declined from 1.20 ± 1.68 stones/yr to 0.01 ± 0.04 stones/yr ($p < 0.001$). Potassium citrate has become the hallmark method of urinary alkalinization. Treatment of uric acid stone formers is centered on increasing urinary pH. Potassium citrate, therefore, is effective therapy to dissolve and prevent uric acid nephrolithiasis.

The use of potassium citrate for the prevention of cystine stone formation was reviewed by Hess in 1990 (54). The solubility of cystine increases dramatically above a pH of 7.0, reaching 1000 mg/L at a urine pH of 8.0. Although sodium bicarbonate could be used for alkalinization, potassium citrate is preferred because the sodium load will raise urinary calcium and may actually increase the urinary cystine levels (53). A recent comparison of potassium citrate and sodium bicarbonate therapy for patients with homozygous cystinuria demonstrated equal alkalinization with the two therapies (55). Average urinary cystine and urinary citrate levels were similar with both medications. Urinary sodium increased significantly with sodium bicarbonate but not with potassium citrate. There was a linear correlation between urinary sodium and urinary cystine excretion, thereby making potassium citrate the recommended medication. This correlation is likely caused by the presence of sodium dependent cystine pumps (56).

Potassium citrate has been used more recently to dissolve fragments remaining after shockwave lithotripsy (SWL). In one study, specific medical therapy (allopurinol or potassium citrate) was given to 80 patients after SWL. Medical therapy reduced the stone formation rate by 91% in patients who were stone free and by 81% in those with residual fragments after SWL *(57)*. This was compared to a 35% and 17% reduction in those who discontinued their medical therapy, respectively. In another study, 40 patients with residual calcium stone fragments received sodium potassium citrate therapy. Seventy-five percent (75%) cleared their residual stones compared to only 32% of controls *(58)*. Citrate decreased the rate of stone growth and fragment reaggregation (5% in citrate group vs 47% in the control group). Residual fragments grew in 16% in those that were compliant with potassium citrate as opposed to 55% in patients not taking their pre-scribed medication. A third recent study evaluated the use of potassium citrate to prevent recurrence and aid in stabilization of lower pole fragments after SWL *(59)*. Patients who were stone free after lower pole SWL had lower recurrence rates with potassium citrate than those without treatment (0 vs 28.5%, $p < 0.05$). Patients with residual lower pole fragments after SWL had higher remission rates with therapy (44.5 vs 12.5%) than untreated patients ($p < 0.05$). These studies demonstrate the use of potassium citrate to help dissolve, clear and prevent recurrent nephrolithiasis.

Tekin et al documented the use of potassium citrate for children with hypocitraturic (<320 mg/1.73 m^2/24 h), calcium-based stones. Sixty-four hypocitraturic children (ages 1–15, median 7.2 yr), including 20 that had recurrent nephrolithiasis, were treated with potassium citrate tablets or liquid (1meq/kg in 3 divided doses) for an average of 22 mos*(60)*. No adverse reactions were observed. Daily urinary citrate levels increased from 197 ± 72 to 632 ± 218 mg/1.73 m^2 ($p < 0.01$). Mean urinary calcium levels decreased from 3.5 ± 2.7 to 2.5 ± 2.7 mg/kg ($p < 0.05$). The children with recurrent stone disease experienced a decrease in stone recurrence from 0.32 to 0.17 stones per patient-year. The overall recurrence rate was 0.07 per patient-year and none of the 44 first-time stone formers recurred. Although no control group was included in this study, the authors concluded that potassium citrate therapy was beneficial and safe in children with hypocitraturic calcium-based stones.

The efficacy of potassium citrate is mainly related to the alkali load presented to the proximal renal tubular cells. This alkali load invokes changes in the cells that result in decreased reabsorption of citrate from the filtrate and peritubular fluid, thus increasing urinary citrate concentrations. Potassium citrate is almost entirely absorbed from the gastrointestinal tract *(11)*. The citrate component is largely oxidized through the citric acid cycle to carbon dioxide and water, although Pak suggests that up to 20% of the citraturic response to citrate therapy may be caused by direct excretion in the urine *(61)*. Potassium citrate therapy causes sustained increases in urinary pH and urinary citrate levels *(61)*, which lead to a lower level of ionized calcium and therefore lower urinary saturation levels of calcium oxalate and uric acid. Crystallization is therefore inhibited by numerous mechanisms. The increase in urinary pH can induce precipitation of cal-cium phosphate crystals *(62)* but does not cause precipitation of magnesium ammonium phosphate *(63)*.

Potassium citrate is available in liquid, crystal and wax matrix tablet formulations (Table 3). Most clinicians use three divided daily doses for wax matrix tablets and liquid preparations; crystal preparations are typically given twice per day. Single evening dosing of sodium potassium citrate has been tested and might be applicable to potassium citrate (*see* Sodium Potassium Citrate Section) *(64)*. The crystal form may encourage increased fluid intake caused by the need to dissolve the crystals in fluid. Many formu-lations have a bitter taste and this may further increase fluid intake *(64)*.

The tablet preparation, however, is more convenient for many, raises urinary citrate levels and pH for a longer time *(65)*, and may offer less gastrointestinal upset *(66)*. The

Table 3
Potassium Citrate Preparations Available in the United States

Drug	Trade name
Potassium citrate/sodium citrate	Citrolith Tablets
Potassium citrate/citric acid	K Liquid
Potassium citrate/citric acid	Cytra Polycitra K Liquid
Potassium citrate/citric acid/sodium citrate	Polycitra LC Liquid
Potassium citrate/citric acid/sodium citrate	Polycitra Syrup
Potassium citrate/citric acid/sodium citrate	Cytra 3 Syrup
Potassium citrate	Polycitra Crystals
Potassium citrate	Urocit-K (wax matrix tablet)
Sodium citrate/citric acid	Bicitra

(Source: Internet search, June, 2006.)

tablet is large and therefore may not be effective in children or adults who have difficulty swallowing. The wax matrix tablet passes through the gastrointestinal tract and therefore is typically seen in the stool. Patients should be informed that the potassium citrate is fully absorbed despite the remaining wax matrix appearing as an intact tablet. Rarely, in patients with rapid intestinal transit times, the potassium citrate may not be adequately absorbed. These rare patients should be changed to the liquid or crystal preparation.

Dosing regimens of potassium citrate are typically 30–60 meq/d, depending on pre-treatment citrate levels and clinical response. Some recommend increasing the dosage (up to 1 meq/kg) until urinary pH and/or urinary citrate concentrations reach the desired level (66). The most common side effect of potassium citrate therapy is gastrointestinal irritation (diarrhea, dyspepsia, nausea). Potassium citrate efficacy is considered to be equal when taken on an empty stomach or with meals (65), but is probably tolerated better when taken with meals (66). Potential complications associated with potassium citrate include hyperkalemia, especially in those patients on potassium-sparing diuretics and those with renal insufficiency, and gastric erosions or rarely intestinal obstruction in those taking the wax matrix tablet. Potassium citrate can be used as an alternative to potassium chloride supplementation in patients taking potassium-wasting diuretics. Patients with renal failure should be started on one-third or one-half the usual dose and monitored with serial serum electrolytes. Aluminum absorption has been reported to increase secondary to oral citrate therapy (67,68). However, Sakhaee and colleagues showed no increase in total body aluminum retention in those with normal renal function (69).

The role of intermittent alkali therapy has been reviewed recently. The rationale is that one may be able to replicate the body's normal urinary pH fluctuations by giving three to seven doses per week (70,71). Potential indications for intermittent therapy are asymptomatic large stones and prophylaxis regimens. Potential advantages include fewer side effects, avoidance of systemic alkalosis, lower risk of calcium phosphate crystallization, and improved compliance (70). There are no prospective trials regarding intermittent potassium citrate therapy. One retrospective study comparing regular medical prophylaxis (64 patients, mean duration of therapy 27.8 ± 4.8 mo), intermittent medical therapy (80 patients, mean duration of treatment 7.9 ± 4.9 mo) and no medical therapy (169 patients) demonstrated that regular medical treatment with potassium citrate markedly reduced the stone recurrence rate compared to the intermittent group (7.8% vs 30%) *(71)*. Kaplan–Meier curves and log-rank tests revealed that patients on intermittent therapy had statistically similar recurrence rates to those patients who refused therapy altogether. This study, therefore, suggests that patients who occasionally are compliant with their potassium citrate likely will recur as often as those without any therapy. The findings do not suggest, however, that a standardized intermittent regimen of potassium citrate would be ineffective. Theoretically, if urinary pH and citrate were occasionally elevated, calculogenesis may be inhibited. Prospective standardized trials are necessary to adequately ascertain whether intermittent therapy is efficacious.

Sodium citrate and sodium potassium citrate supplementation are more commonly used in Europe than in North America *(72)*. Potassium citrate has many advantages over sodium citrate. Potassium replacement is a necessary treatment for patients with RTA, diarrheal syndromes and thiazide-induced hypocitraturia. Correcting the hypokalemia reduces the acidosis and leads to a less pronounced hypocitraturic state. In contrast, sodium citrate does not treat the underlying potassium deficit. In addition, potassium citrate lowers urinary calcium levels in patients with RTA and may temporarily reduce urinary calcium in other diseases *(73,74)*. Conversely, sodium citrate may increase urinary calcium and cause sodium-urate crystallization of calcium oxalate *(53)*. A global dietary recommendation for patients with calcium-based stones is a decreased sodium intake in order to reduce urinary calcium excretion via the sodium dependent calcium pumps *(75)*. Therefore, a nonsodium-based alkali supplement is advantageous. The sodium load is also a central issue in patients with cardiac failure, renal failure, hypertension, or pulmonary edema in relation to their overall fluid homeostasis.

A single daily dose of sodium potassium citrate (1 g = 3.6 mmol citrate, 4.4 mmol potassium, and 4.4 mmol sodium) was tested in healthy volunteers and calcium stone forming patients *(64)*. The volunteer group was given a single dose (men 5 g and women 3.5 g) at 8 PM. Urinary pH remained elevated until 10 AM the following morning but urinary citrate levels did not increase. In the stone formers, a single evening dose at 8 pm (3.75 g, 5 g, or 7.5 g) raised the urinary citrate levels from 1.7 ± 1.2 mmol/24 h to 3.0 ± 1.3 mmol/24 h ($p < 0.001$). Urinary calcium decreased from 6.6 ± 3.2 mmol/24 h to 5.6 ± 2.5 mmol/24 h ($p < 0.001$). Stone formation rates decreased from 0.35 ± 1.14 to 0.16 ± 0.36 over the mean treatment length of 3.5 ± 1.7 yr, but this decrease was not statistically significant. Stone occurrence rates before treatment were lower in this study than other similar studies and this might account for the lack of statistical significance.

In a prospective randomized trial of 50 patients with calcium oxalate stone disease treated with either sodium potassium citrate or dietary changes, stone recurrence rates were the same with or without medical treatment *(76)*. In the control group, stone rates decreased from 1.8/yr to 0.7. In the treatment group, stone rates were 2.1 and 0.9/yr before and after treatment, respectively. An objective benefit of alkali citrate could not be established. This study had a substantial decrease in stone rates in the control group and this dramatic "clinic effect" may explain the lack of difference between the treatment and control groups.

Calcium citrate has not been investigated as a therapy for urolithiasis. Long term use of calcium citrate raises urinary citrate levels marginally and raises urinary calcium but does not alkalinize the urine *(77,78)*. As a calcium supplement, calcium absorption may be higher than with calcium carbonate preparations *(79)*. Calcium citrate is therefore not recommended for a citrate supplement in patients with hypocitraturic calcium-based nephrolithiasis.

Urinary citrate can be elevated with the use of natural citrus juices. Lemons, grapefruit, pineapples, and oranges all have a high concentration of citrate. Seltzer and colleagues showed the use of drinking 2 L/d of reconstituted lemonade *(80)*. Of the 12 patients, 11 had increased urinary citrate levels (average increase of 204 mg/d). Average levels increased from 142 mg daily (range <10–293) at baseline to 346 mg daily (range 89–814) after treatment (*p* <.001). Urinary oxalate was unchanged and urinary calcium decreased, although not in a significant amount. Patients were compliant with this nonpharmacologic mode of citrate supplementation. In a similar study, Wabner and Pak compared the effect of ingesting 1.2 L of orange juice per day with standard potassium citrate supplementation *(81)*. Urinary citrate levels and pH increased with orange juice to the same degree as with potassium citrate. However, urinary oxalate levels also increased, either because of the oxalate content of orange juice or the conversion of ascorbic acid (vitamin C) to oxalate. The saturation of calcium oxalate was unchanged with orange juice but decreased significantly with potassium citrate therapy. Similar effects were seen in a recent study detailing the effect of grapefruit juice on urine chemistries *(82)*. An acute load of grapefruit juice was given to 7 healthy volunteers. Three hours after ingestion, urinary citrate increased from 18.7 mg/h to 25.8 mg/h and urinary calcium increased from 3.3 mg/h to 6.7 mg/h. No long-term studies are available detailing the urinary effects of citrus juice therapy.

MAGNESIUM

The significance of urinary magnesium in preventing stone formation has been debated for decades. Most data evaluating urinary magnesium is based on older animal studies *(83)*. In 1962, Gersoff and Andrus first noted that diets low in magnesium increased calcium oxalate deposits in rat kidneys in their ethylene glycol rat model *(84)*. Lyon followed with the finding that high magnesium diets prevented calcium oxalate encrustation of zinc disks implanted into rat bladders *(85)*. Robertson demonstrated that magnesium binds oxalate in human urine *(86)*. In superphysiologic concentrations, magnesium can inhibit nucleation and growth of calcium oxalate crystals *(84,87)*. A more recent animal study involving rats on an ethylene glycol induced hyperoxaluric diet showed no change in renal calcifications with the addition of magnesium oxide *(88)*. Some studies have shown increased urinary calcium when magnesium is supplemented. The overall importance of urinary magnesium may relate to its enhancement of urinary citrate concentrations *(83,89,90)*.

One reason why magnesium has not been considered an important inhibitor is the low incidence of hypomagnesuria in stone formers (4.3–11%) *(91)*. Normal urinary magnesium levels according to Litholink® laboratory are 30–120 mg/24 h *(26)*. Parks and Coe documented urinary magnesium levels of 84 ± 5 mg in 27 nonstone forming females and 99 ± 6 mg in 33 nonstone forming males *(92)*. Mean urinary magnesium levels in stone formers older than 65 years of age were 77 mg/24 h (standard deviation, SD, 39) and 83 mg/24 h (SD, 39) in stone patients younger than 65 yr *(32)*. Urinary magnesium levels in 78 calcium stone forming children were the same as control children, using a definition of hypomagnesuria of less than 1.2 mg/kg in 24 h *(33)*.

Most patients with low urinary magnesium also have hypocitraturia, thereby confusing the significance of magnesium levels *(91)*. It has been suggested that the magnesium-to-calcium ratio may be more important *(93)*. Melnick sited a low urinary magnesium level in patients of the "stone belt," and related this to low soil magnesium content in this region *(94)*.

Magnesium replacement therapy for prophylaxis in urinary stone patients was first introduced by Moore and Bunce in 1964 *(95)*. Gershoff and Prien reported that magnesium oxide reduced stone rates from 1.3/patient year to 0.1 *(96)*. Melnick also found similar results over a 4-yr trial *(94)*. Selikowitz and Olsson compared the efficacy of magnesium oxide, hydrochlorothiazide, methylene blue, and sodium phosphate to prevent and treat CaOx stones in a rat model *(97)*. Magnesium oxide prevented renal stone formation entirely and limited the area of parenchymal calcification. Randomized trials by Wilson (1984) *(98)* and Ettinger (1988) *(99)* found no difference in stone formation between patients treated with magnesium hydroxide and those without treatment. Lindburg documented only a minimal increase in urinary magnesium with magnesium citrate and magnesium oxide unless taken with food *(100)*. The latter produced a decrease in the supersaturation of calcium oxalate and brushite. Urinary citrate levels did increase with magnesium citrate and magnesium oxide. This study included only 11 patients, making conclusions unreliable. Preminger has documented the use of oral magnesium citrate in those patients with hypomagnesuric calcium stones *(91)*. Intravenous magnesium sulfate was given to stone formers and controls in another recent study from Thailand. Urinary citrate increased with supplementation, leading to the idea that magnesium's effect on stone formation may be indirect *(89)*.

The combined use of potassium, magnesium and citrate has gained much attention in the last decade *(11,101,102)*. In a comparison study of potassium citrate and potassium magnesium citrate including five normal volunteers and five calcium stone formers, urinary pH, urinary magnesium and urinary citrate rose higher with potassium magnesium citrate therapy *(102)*. Calcium oxalate saturation and agglomeration declined and calcium phosphate inhibition rose to a greater extent with the potassium magnesium citrate preparation. Both treatment regimens had the same dose of potassium but the magnesium potassium citrate preparation contained 50% more citrate. Another comparison study demonstrated equal potassium delivery with potassium citrate, potassium chloride and potassium magnesium citrate and equal magnesium delivery with magnesium citrate and potassium magnesium citrate *(103)*. Of these four preparations, potassium magnesium citrate produced the largest citraturic response (125 mg/d increase). Potassium magnesium citrate also may be useful for correcting thiazide-induced hypokalemia *(101,104)*, hypomagesuric calcium oxalate nephrolithiasis *(91)*, and chronic diarrheal states in which patients are often hypocitraturic, hypomagnesuric and hypokalemic. The major side effect of magnesium replacement is gastrointestinal symptoms.

CONCLUSIONS

This chapter has focused on two inhibitors of urinary stone formation: citrate and magnesium. The former is of true clinical importance whereas the latter is potentially of historic interest only. From a clinical standpoint, citrate is the most important inhibitor. There is limited prospective data regarding the use of citrate replacement. It is clear, however, that citrate supplementation will decrease stone recurrence. Multiple preparations are available, allowing the therapy to be tailored to the patient. Any patient with acidosis will likely have hypocitraturia and correction of the acidosis will increase urinary citrate levels. Magnesium may act indirectly by increasing urinary citrate levels.

REFERENCES

1. Scott WW, Huggins C, Selman B C. Metabolism of citric acid in urolithiasis. J Urol 1943; 50: 202.
2. Boothby WM, Adams, M. The occurrence of citric acid in urine and body fluids. Am J Physiol 1934; 107: 47.
3. Kissin B, Locks MO. Urinary citrates in calcium urolithiasis. Proc Soc Exp Biol Med 1941; 46: 216.
4. Howard JE. Clinical and laboratory research concerning mechanisms of formation and control of caclulous disease of the kidney. J Urol 1954; 72: 999.
5. Rudman D, Dedonis JL, Fountain MT, et al. Hypocitraturia in patients with gastrointestinal malabsorption. N Engl J Med 1980; 303: 657.
6. Menon M, Mahle CJ. Urinary citrate excretion in patients with renal calculi. J Urol 1983; 129: 1158.
7. Nicar MJ, Skurla C, Sakhaee K, Pak CY. Low urinary citrate excretion in nephrolithiasis. Urology 1983; 21: 8.
8. Butz M, Dulce HJ. Enhancement of urinary citrate in oxalate stone formers by the intake of alkaline salts. In: Urolithiasis: Clinical and Basic Research, (Smith L, Robertson WG, Finlayson B. eds.). Plenum Press, New York, NY, 1981; pp. 881–884.
9. Pak CY, Sakhaee K, Fuller CJ. Physiological and physiochemical correction and prevention of calcium stone formation by potassium citrate therapy. Trans Assoc Am Physicians 1983; 96: 294.
10. Jenkins AD. Calculus formation. In: Adult and Pediatric Urology, 4th Ed., (Gillenwater, JY, Grayhack, JT, Howards SS, Mitchell ME. eds.). Lippincott Williams & Wilkins, Baltimore, MD, 2002; pp. 355–392.
11. Pak CY. Hypocitraturic Calcium Nephrolithiasisin: Urolithiasis: A Medical and Surgical Reference, (Resnick MI, Pak CY. eds..) WB Saunders, Philadelphia, PA, 1990; pp. 89–103.
12. Fegan J, Khan R, Poindexter J, Pak CY. Gastrointestinal citrate absorption in nephrolithiasis. J Urol, 1992; 147: 1212.
13. Menon M, Resnick, MI. Urinary lithiasis: etiology, diagnosis, and medical management. In: Campbell's Urology, 8th Ed., (Walsh, PC, Retik, AB, Vaughan, ED, Wein, AJ. eds.). WB Saunders Company, Philadelphia, PA, 2002; pp. 3242–3305.
14. Simpson DP. Citrate excretion: a window on renal metabolism. Am J Physiol 1983; 244: F223-34.
15. Jenkins AD, Dousa TP, Smith LH. Transport of citrate across renal brush border membrane: effects of dietary acid and alkali loading. Am J Physiol 1985; 249: F590.
16. Kippen I, Hirayama B, Klinenberg JR, Wright EM. Transport of tricarboxylic acid cycle intermediates by membrane vesicles from renal brush border. Proc Natl Acad Sci 1979; 76: 3397.
17. Costello LC, Stracey R, Franklin R. Parathyroid hormone effects on soft-tissue citrate levels. Horm Metab Res 1970; 2: 242.
18. Melnick JZ, Preisig PA, Haynes S, Pak CY, Sakhaee K, Alpern RJ. Converting enzyme inhibition causes hypocitraturia independent of acidosis or hypokalemia. Kidney Int 1998; 54: 1670.
19. Baruch SB, Burich RL, Eun CK, King VF. Renal metabolism of citrate. Med Clin North Am 1975; 59: 569.
20. Down WH, Sacharin RM, Chasseaud LF, Kirkpatrick D, Franklin ER. Renal and bone uptake of tartaric acid in rats: comparison of L(+) and DL-forms. Toxicology 1977; 8: 333.
21. Shorr E, Bernheim AR, Taussky H. The relation of urinary citric acid excretion to the menstrual cycle and the steroidal reproductive hormones. Science 1942; 95: 606.
22. Preminger GM, Sakhaee K, Skurla C, Pak CY: Prevention of recurrent calcium stone formation with potassium citrate therapy in patients with distal renal tubular acidosis. J Urol 1985; 134: 20.
23. Menon M, Mahle CJ. Urinary citrate excretion in patients with renal calculi. J Urol 1983; 129: 1158.
24. Heller HJ, Sakhaee K, Moe OW, Pak CY. Etiological role of estrogen status in renal stone formation. J Urol 2002; 168: 1923.
25. Dey J, Creighton A, Lindberg JS, Fuselier HA, Kok DJ, Cole F.E, et al. Estrogen replacement increased the citrate and calcium excretion rates in postmenopausal women with recurrent urolithiasis. J Urol 2002; 167:169.
26. Litholink.com website. Accessed 1/15/2003.

27. Menon M, Mahle CJ. Prevalence of hyperoxaluria in "idiopathic" calcium oxalate urolithiasis: relationship to other metabolic abnormalities. Presented at American Urological Association, Las Vegas, NV, 1983.

28. Pak CY. Citrate and renal calculi. Miner Electrolyte Metab 1987; 13: 257.

29. Francois B, Cahen R, Pascal B. Inhibitors of urinary stone formation in 40 recurrent stone formers. Br J Urol 1986; 58: 479.

30. Nicar MJ, Skurla C, Sakhaee K, Pak CY. Low urinary citrate excretion in nephrolithiasis. Urology 1983; 21: 8.

31. Hosking DH, Wilson JW, Liedtke RR, Smith LH, Wilson DM. Urinary citrate excretion in normal persons and patients with idiopathic calcium urolithiasis. J Lab Clin Med 1985; 106: 682.

32. Gentle DL, Stoller ML, Bruce JE, Leslie SW Geriatric urolithiasis. J Urol 1997; 158: 2221.

33. Tekin A, Tekgul S, Atsu N, Sahin A, Ozen H, Bakkaloglu M. A study of the etiology of idiopathic calcium urolithiasis in children: hypocitraturia is the most important risk factor. J Urol 2000; 164: 162.

34. Sakhaee K, Harvey JA, Padalino PK, Whitson P, Pak CY. The potential role of salt abuse on the risk for kidney stone formation. J Urol 1993; 150: 310.

35. Sakhaee K, Nigam S, Snell P, Hsu MC, Pak CY. Assessment of the pathogenetic role of physical exercise in renal stone formation. J Clin Endocrinol Metab 1987; 65: 974.

36. Pak CY. Citrate and renal calculi: an update. Miner Electrolyte Metab 1994, 20: 371.

37. Fegan J, Khan R, Poindexter J, Pak CY. Gastrointestinal citrate absorption in nephrolithiasis. J Urol 1992; 147: 1212.

38. Meyer JL, Smith LH. Growth of calcium oxalate crystals II Inhibition by natural urinary crystal growth inhibitors. Invest Urol 1975; 13: 36.

39. Lieske, JC, Coe, FL. Urinary inhibitors and renal stone formation. In: Kidney Stones: Medical and Surgical Management, (Coe, FL, Favus, MJ, Pak, CY, Parks, JH, Preminger, GM, eds.). Lippincott-Raven, Philadelphia, PA, 1996; pp. 65–113.

40. Ashby RA, Sleet RJ. The role of citrate complexes in preventing urolithiasis. Clin Chim Acta 1992; 210: 157.

41. Nicar MJ, Hill K, Pak CY. Inhibition by citrate of spontaneous precipitation of calcium oxalate in vitro. J Bone Miner Res 1987; 2: 215.

42. Tiselius HG, Berg C, Fornander AM, Nilsson MA. Effects of citrate on the different phases of calcium oxalate crystallization. Scanning Microsc 1993; 7: 381.

43. Pak CY, Peterson R. Successful treatment of hyperuricosuric calcium oxalate nephrolithiasis with potassium citrate. Arch Intern Med 1986; 146: 863.

44. Tiselius HG, Fornander AM, Nilsson MA. The effects of citrate and urine on calcium oxalate crystal aggregation. Urol Res 1993; 21: 363.

45. Kok DJ, Papapoulos SE, Bijvoet OL. Excessive crystal agglomeration with low citrate excretion in recurrent stone-formers. Lancet 1986; 10: 1056.

46. Kok DJ, Papapoulos SE, Blomen LJ, Bijvoet OL. Modulation of calcium oxalate monohydrate crystallization kinetics in vitro. Kidney Int 1988; 34: 346.

47. Grases F, Genestar C, March P, Conte A. Variations in the activity of urinary inhibitors in calcium oxalate urolithiasis. Br J Urol 1988; 62: 515.

48. Grases F, Genestar C, Conte A, March P, Costa-Bauza A. Inhibitory effect of pyrophosphate, citrate, magnesium and chondroitin sulfate in calcium oxalate urolithiasis. Br J Urol 1989; 64: 235.

49. Grases F, Gil J.J, Conte A. Urolithiasis inhibitors and calculus nucleation. Urol Res 1989; 17: 163.

50. Bisaz S, Felix R, Neuman WF, Fleisch HQ uantitative determination of inhibitors of calcium phosphate precipitation in whole urine. Miner Electrolyte Metab 1978; 1: 74.

51. Menon M, Parulkar BG, Drach G.W. Urinary lithiasis: etiology, diagnosis and medical management. In: Campbell's Urology, 7th Ed., (Walsh, PC, Retik, AB, Vaughan, ED, Wein, AJ, eds.). WB Saunders, Philadelphia, PA, 1998; pp. 2661–2733.

52. Barcelo P, Wuhl O, Servitge E, Rousaud A, Pak CY. Randomized double-blind study of potassium citrate in idiopathic hypocitraturic calcium nephrolithiasis. J Urol 1993; 150: 1761.

53. Pak CY, Sakhaee K, Fuller C. Successful management of uric acid nephrolithiasis with potassium citrate. Kidney Int 1986; 30: 422.

54. Hess B. Prophylaxis of uric acid and cystine stones. Urol Res 1990; 18: S41.

55. Fjellstedt E, Denneberg T, Jeppsson JO, Tiselius HG. A comparison of the effects of potassium citrate and sodium bicarbonate in the alkalinization of urine in homozygous cystinuria. Urol Res 2001; 29: 295.

56. Shekarriz Band Stoller ML. Cystinuria and other noncalcareous calculi. Endocrinil Metab Clin N Am 2002; 31: 951.

57. Fine JK, Pak CY, Preminger GM. Effect of medical management and residual fragments on recurrent stone formation following shock wave lithotripsy. J Urol 1995; 153: 27.

58. Cicerello E, Merlo F, Gambaro G, et al. Effect of alkaline citrate therapy on clearance of residual renal stone fragments after extracorporeal shock wave lithotripsy in sterile calcium and infection nephrolithiasis patients. J Urol 1994; 151: 5.

59. Soygur T, Akbay A, Kupeli S. Effect of potassium citrate therapy on stone recurrence and residual fragments after shockwave lithotripsy in lower caliceal calcium oxalate urolithiasis: a randomized controlled trial. J Endourol 2002; 16: 149.

60. Tekin A, Tekgul S, Atsu N, Bakkaloglu M, Kendi S. Oral potassium citrate treatment for idiopathic hypocitraturia in children with calcium urolithiasis. J Urol 2002; 168: 2572.

61. Pak CYCitrate and renal calculi: new insights and future directions. Am J Kidney Dis 1991; 17: 420.

62. Shekarriz B, Stoller ML. Uric acid nephrolithiasis: current concepts and controversies. J Urol 2002; 168: 1307.

63. Ogawa Y, Sugaya K, Koyama Y, Hatano T. Impact of citrate therapy on the circadian rhythm of urinary magnesium ammonium phosphate saturation in normal individuals. Int J Urol 2000; 7: 287.

64. Berg C, Larsson L, Tiselius HG. The effects of a single evening dose of alkaline citrate on urine composition and calcium stone formation. J Urol 1992; 148: 979.

66. Moran ME, Abrahams HM, Burday DE, Greene TD. Utility of oral dissolution therapy in the management of referred patients with secondarily treated uric acid stones. Urology 2002; 59: 206.

65. Pak CY, Oh MS, Baker S, Morris JS. Effect of meal on the physiological and physicochemical actions of potassium citrate. J Urol 1991; 146: 803.

67. Molitoris BA, Froment DH, Mackenzie TA, Huffer WH, Alfrey AC. Citrate: a major factor in the toxicity of orally administered aluminum compounds. Kidney Int 1989; 36: 949.

68. Slanina P, Frech W, Ekstrom LG, Loof L, Slorach S, Cedergren A. Dietary citric acid enhances absorption of aluminum in antacids. Clin Chem 1986; 32: 539.

69. Sakhaee K, Ruml L, Padalino P, Haynes S, Pak CY. The lack of influence of long-term potassium citrate and calcium citrate treatment in total body aluminum burden in patients with functioning kidneys. J Am Coll Nutr, 1996; 15: 102.

70.. Rodman JS. Intermittent versus continuous alkaline therapy for uric acid stones and ureteral stones of uncertain composition. Urology 2002; 60: 378.

71. Lee YH, Huang WC, Tsai JY, Huang JK. The efficacy of potassium citrate based medical prophylaxis for preventing upper urinary tract calculi: a midterm follow-up study. J Urol 1999; 161: 1453.

72. Herrmann U, Schwille PO, Schwarzlaender H, Berger I, Hoffmann G. Citrate and recurrent idiopathic calcium urolithiasisA longitudinal pilot study on the metabolic effects of oral potassium sodium citrate administered as short-, medium- and long-term to male stone patients. Urol Res 1992; 20: 347.

73. Preminger GM, Sakhaee K, Pak CY. Alkali action on the urinary crystallization of calcium salts: contrasting responses to sodium citrate and potassium citrate. J Urol 1988; 139: 240.

74. Sakhaee K, Nicar M, Hill K, Pak CY. Contrasting effects of potassium citrate and sodium citrate therapies on urinary chemistries and crystallization of stone-forming salts. Kidney Int 1983; 24: 348.

75. Borghi L, Schianchi T, Meschi T, et alComparison of two diets for the prevention of recurrent stones in idiopathic hypercalciuria. N Engl J Med 2002; 346: 77.

76. Hofbauer J, Hobarth K, Szabo N, Marberger MAlkali citrate prophylaxis in idiopathic recurrent calcium oxalate urolithiasis—a prospective randomized study. Br J Urol 1994; 73: 362.

77. Sakhaee K, Baker S, Zerwekh J, Poindexter J, Garcia-Hernandez PA, Pak CY. Limited risk of kidney stone formation during long-term calcium citrate supplementation in non-stone forming subjects. J Urol 1994; 152: 324.

78. Harvey JA, Zobitz MM, Pak CY. Calcium citrate: reduced propensity for the crystallization of calcium oxalate in urine resulting from induced hypercalciuria of calcium supplementation. J Clin Endocrinol Metab 1985; 61: 1223.

79. Sakhaee K, Bhuket T, Adams-Huet B, Rao DS. Meta-analysis of calcium bioavailability: a comparison of calcium citrate with calcium carbonate. Am J Ther 1999; 6: 313.

80. Seltzer MA, Low RK, McDonald M, Shami GS, Stoller ML. Dietary manipulation with lemonade to treat hypocitraturic calcium nephrolithiasis. J Urol 1996; 156: 907.

81. Wabner CL, Pak CY. Effect of orange juice consumption on urinary stone risk factors. J Urol 1993; 149: 1405.

82. Trinchieri A, Lizzano R, Bernardini P, et al. Effect of acute load of grapefruit juice on urinary excretion of citrate and urinary risk factors for renal stone formation. Dig Liver Dis 2002; 34: S160.

83. Schwartz BF, Bruce J, Leslie S, Stoller MLRethinking the role of urinary magnesium in calcium urolithiasis. J Endourol 2001; 15: 233.

84. Gershoff SN, Andrus SB. Effect of vitamin B6 and magnesium on deposition of calcium oxalate induced by ethylene glycol administration. Proc Soc Exp Biol Med 1962; 109: 99.

85. Lyon ES, Borden TA, Ellis JE, Vermeulen CW. Calcium oxalate lithiasis produced by pyridoxine deficiency and inhibition with high magnesium diets. Invest Urol 1966; 4: 133.

86. Robertson WG, Hambleton J, Hodgkinson A. Peptide inhibitors of calcium phosphate precipitation in the urine of normal and stone-forming men. Clin Chim Acta 1969; 25: 247.

87. Desmars JF, Tawashi R. Dissolution and growth of calcium oxalate monohydrateIEffect of magnesium and pH. Biochim Biophys Acta 1973; 313: 256.

88. Su CJ, Shevock PN, Khan SR, Hackett RL. Effect of magnesium on calcium oxalate urolithiasis. J Urol 1991; 145: 1092.

89. Reungjui S, Prasongwatana V, Premgamone A, Tosukhowong P, Jirakulsomchok S, Sriboonlue P. Magnesium status of patients with renal stones and its effect on urinary citrate excretion. BJU Int 2002; 90: 635.

90. Schwille PO, Schmiedl A, Herrmann U, et alMagnesium, citrate, magnesium citrate and magnesium-alkali citrate as modulators of calcium oxalate crystallization in urine: observations in patients with recurrent idiopathic calcium urolithiasis. Urol Res 1999; 27: 117.

91. Preminger GM, Baker S, Peterson R, Poindexter J, Pak CY. Hypomagnesiuric hypocitraturia: an apparent new entity for calcium nephrolithiasis. J Lith Stone Dis 1989; 1: 22.

92. Parks JH, Coe FL. A urinary calcium-citrate index for the evaluation of nephrolithiasis. Kidney Int 1986; 30: 85.

93. King JS Jr, O'Connor FJ Jr, Smith MJ, Crouse L. The urinary calcium-magnesium ratio in calcerous stone formers. Invest Urol 1968; 6: 60.

94. Melnick I, Landes RR, Hoffman AA, Burch JF. Magnesium therapy for recurring calcium oxalate urinary calculi. J Urol 1971; 105: 119.

95. Moore CA, Bunce GE. Reduction in frequency of renal calculus formation by oral magnesium administration: A preliminary report. Invest Urol 1964; 2: 4.

96. Gersoff SN, Prien EL. Effects of daily Mg and vitamin b6 administration to patients with recurring calcium oxalate kidney stones. Am J Clin Nutr 1967; 20: 393.

97. Selikowitz SM, Olsson CA. Comparative effects of anticalculous management in the rat. Invest. Urol, 1976; 14: 120.

98. Wilson DR, Strauss AL, Manuel MA. Comparison of medical treatments for the prevention of recurrent calcium nephrolithiasis. Urol Res 1984; 12: 39.

99. Ettinger B, Citron JT, Livermore B, Dolman LI. Chlorthalidone reduces calcium oxalate calculous recurrence but magnesium hydroxide does not. J Urol 1988; 139: 679.

100. Lindberg J, Harvey J, Pak CY. Effect of magnesium citrate and magnesium oxide on the crystallization of calcium salts in urine: changes produced by food-magnesium interaction. J Urol 1990; 143: 248.

101. Ruml LA, Pak CYEffect of potassium magnesium citrate on thiazide-induced hypokalemia and magnesium loss. Am J Kidney Dis 1999; 34: 107.

102. Pak CY, Koenig K, Khan R, Haynes S, Padalino P. Physicochemical action of potassium-magnesium citrate in nephrolithiasis. J Bone Miner Res 1992; 7: 281.

103. Koenig K, Padalino P, Alexandrides G, Pak CY. Bioavailability of potassium and magnesium, and citraturic response from potassium-magnesium citrate. J Urol 1991; 145: 330.

104. Wuermser LA, Reilly C, Poindexter JR, Sakhaee K, Pak CY. Potassium-magnesium citrate vs potassium chloride in thiazide-induced hypokalemia. Kidney Int 2000; 57: 607.

10 Modulators of Crystallization of Stone Salts

Saeed R. Khan, PhD and Dirk J. Kok, PhD

Key Words: Nephrolithiasis; crystallization; saturation.

INTRODUCTION

As a direct consequence of the renal function of water preservation urine becomes supersaturated with slightly soluble salts like calcium oxalates and calcium phosphates *(1)*. When the supersaturation is high enough and lasts long enough, crystals will form. Crystallization involves crystal nucleation, growth, and aggregation *(2–5)*. Most crystals are, however, discharged during urination without causing any discomfort *(6,7)*. But in some individuals, a number of crystals remain in the urinary space either by adhering to the urothelium or by accreting mass through aggregation *(8,9)*. Under appropriate conditions, retained crystals evolve into stone nidi thus establishing a base for stone growth *(10)*. Apparently there are mechanisms to ensure crystals can be passed harmlessly. It has become clear that defense mechanisms act at all levels, from supersaturation to nucleation, crystal growth, crystal aggregation, crystal structure, crystal habit, crystal surface properties, and crystal interactions with the epithelial lining of the renal tubules and urinary tract. In fact there also appears to be a mechanism for removal of material that passed the previous defenses. Crystals that are retained in the renal tubules can enter the renal interstitium where they are attacked by macrophages *(11–13)* that are attracted

From: Current Clinical Urology, *Urinary Stone Disease:*
A Practical Guide to Medical and Surgical Management
Edited by: M. L. Stoller and M. V. Meng © Humana Press Inc., Totowa, NJ

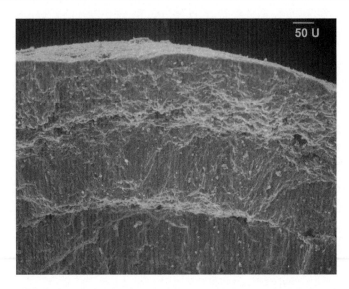

Fig. 1. SEM of the fractured surface of calcium oxalate monohydrate stone. The stone is compact and shows distinct concentric laminations and radial striations. Concentric laminations are the result of outward growth of the stone. Radial striations are the result of a plate-like habit of calcium oxalate monohyydrate crystals.

by the chemokines such as MCP-1 *(14)* produced by renal epithelial cells as well as the crystal-associated compounds like osteopontin *(11,15)*.

Urinary compounds that can associate with the crystals mediate these mechanisms in several ways. First, urine supersaturation can be decreased by lowering the salt ion concentrations or by making them unavailable for crystallization. For example, citrate will bind calcium, magnesium binds oxalate, and increasing total urine ionic strength directly increases the amount of calcium oxalate or -phosphate that can be held in solution. Thus a mainstay of therapy has been to reduce the supersaturation by dilution (drinking advice), by decreasing excretion of stone ions (e.g., restricted oxalate intake), or by increasing excretion of chelators (alkali therapy to increase citrate excretion). However, the fact that people who do not form stones also periodically have supersaturated urine and crystalluria has prompted investigators to look at the processes beyond supersaturation and at the role these compounds play in urine.

The stones can contain a variety of crystals including calcium oxalate (CaOx), calcium phosphate (CaP), uric acid, struvite, and cystine *(2–4,16)*. CaP is the most common crystal in both the urine and stones whereas CaOx is the major crystal in most stones. The stones, particularly those containing CaOx or uric acid, have a highly compacted structure (Fig. 1). Their outer surfaces appear smooth at low magnification but reveal the presence of individual tabular or platelike CaOx monohydrate (COM) crystals at higher magnifications (Fig. 2). Crystal habits are generally not evident on surfaces exposed by cutting or fragmenting the stone. Such surfaces are typically stratified with radial striations and concentric laminations or layers, with radial striations being the predominant feature. Some of the striations run through many laminations whereas the others are limited to only one. Many of them converge to a point at the base of a lamination mimicking the arrangement of petals in a flower. These points are suggested to be the nucleation

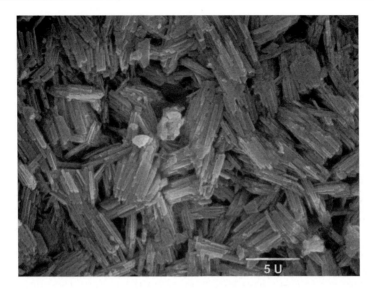

Fig. 2. Outer surface of calcium oxalate monohydrate stone. Edges of tabular crystals are clearly visible.

sites of crystals. The laminations are approx 50–60 µm thick and in many stones can be easily separated from each other exposing the underlying surfaces. These surfaces show the same structure as the outer surface of the stone with protruding tips of the tabular crystals of COM frequently covered with amorphous to flaky matrix material. Many stones have a well-defined nucleus. The stone nucleus appears granular and nonstratified and is generally occupied by spherulitic or amorphous CaP and/or aggregates of dumb-bell-shaped twinned COM crystals. CaP is frequently seen filling the space between CaOx crystals as well as the concentric laminations.

Like other products of crystallization in biological systems *(17)*, stones are a composite of crystals and organic materials *(18–22)*. The latter are often referred to as matrix and comprise macromolecules generally present in the urine. These macromolecules play a significant role in the development of kidney stones. Some promote crystal formation, growth, and aggregation whereas others inhibit these processes. Still others promote or inhibit crystal retention within the urinary space. Activity of a macromolecule is often controlled by conditions prevalent in the urine at the time of crystallization. The same macromolecule can promote or inhibit a process. For example macromolecules in solution behave differently than when they are attached or adsorbed to a surface. This chapter will summarize our current understanding of the involvement of urinary macromolecules in various phases of crystallization in the urine and the development of urinary stones. Special emphasis will be given to crystallization of CaOx, because it is the major crystal in most stones and, as such, has been investigated extensively. We will start with a discussion of the stone matrix, emphasizing crystal/matrix associations in urinary crystals and stones, and then examine some of the urinary macromolecules and other compounds that constitute stone matrix and are known to influence crystallization events in the urinary tract. Although these compounds can both stimulate and inhibit several crystallization processes, they are usually referred to as crystallization inhibitors or modulators.

STONE MATRIX

The organic matrix of most urinary stones accounts for 2–3% of their total dry weight, the rare matrix stones with 65% matrix contents notwithstanding. Boyce and co-workers defined and established the importance of stone matrix in the formation of kidney stones postulating an active architectonic role for matrix *(18–20)*. In their view the matrix acts as a ground substance and controls crystallization within its bounds. An opposite hypothesis was advanced by Vermeulen and co-workers, who viewed matrix and its ubiquitous presence as a mere coincidence because stones form as a result of crystallization in urine in the presence of large macromolecules *(23,24)*. According to them the matrix is adventitiously acquired primarily by physical adsorption of urinary mucoproteins on crystal surfaces. The theory of physical adsorption of urinary proteins on surfaces of CaOx crystals was tested by solution depletion method *(25)* and examination of crystals by transmission electron microscopy after incubation in protein solutions *(26)*. Results showed proteins have a strong affinity for CaOx crystals. Adsorption of anionic proteins was found sensitive to calcium ion concentration, whereas cationic protein adsorption depended on the oxalate ion concentration with temperature and pH playing only a minor role. Proteins formed a discontinuous coat around the crystals ranging in thickness from 10 to 20 nm. It has been suggested that newly formed crystals with a macromolecular coat are less likely to dissolve during the routine urinary ionic and pH changes and therein may lie the importance of matrix in stone formation *(22)*.

MORPHOLOGY

Stone matrix is extremely insoluble. As a result, chemical identification of all the constituent macromolecules has been difficult. However this property has provided the opportunity to microscopically examine the mostly EDTA-insoluble matrix and identify matrix components using a variety of stains and more recently specific antibodies. Morphological examination of decalcified as well as intact stones has provided evidence that their matrix is pervasive (Fig. 3), distributed throughout the stones, and has both amorphous as well as fibrous components *(20–22)*. The crystal matrix association is so intimate that dipyramidal habit of CaOx dihydrate (COD), monoclinic, or plate-like habit of COM and spherulitic habit of CaP stayed intact even after the total removal of their mineral contents *(22,27)*. Scanning electron microscopic examination of the decalcified COM stone revealed the matrix to be organized in concentrically arranged layers. Individual layers were 2–5 µm thick, much thinner than the laminations seen in an intact stone, and had a uniform thickness throughout the circumference. Successive layers appeared as leaves or rings of an onion bulb with very little or no space between them. The layers were made of loosely or tightly matted fibers and contained empty columns representing crystal ghosts, which were presumably formed by dissolution of tabular COM crystals. These crystal ghosts were often arranged radially in relation to the stone center reminiscent of the radially arranged crystals in the intact stones. Examination of these concentrically arranged layers by transmission electron microscopy confirmed that they contained radially arranged columnar crystal ghosts surrounded by an amorphous electron dense coat and embedded in a fibrous matrix. An electron dense material was also present inside the crystal ghosts. Cellular degradation products including degenerating nuclei, mitochondria, endoplasmic reticulum, and membrane fragments as well as vesicles occupied the intercrystalline spaces *(22)*.

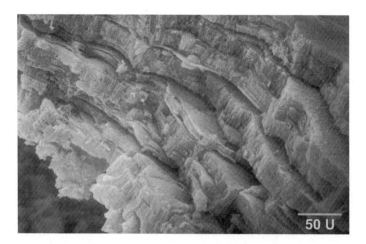

Fig. 3. Fractured surface of demineralized calcium oxalate monohydrate stone. Demineralization was accomplished by treating the stone pieces with EDTA. Once the stone became translucent, it was dried and fractured to expose the interior. Microanalysis of the stones showed no calcium. A comparison with Fig. 1 indicates the ubiquitous nature of the organic matrix. Increase in concentric laminations and loss of radial striations suggests that the organic matrix became incorporated during the outward growth of the stones.

Histochemically the layered matrix was sudanophilic *(28)*, and stained positive with periodic acid schiff (PAS) and colloidal iron *(29–31)* indicating the presence of lipids, proteins and glycosaminoglycans (GAG). Immunohistochemical examination of decalcified stones using antibodies against osteopontin (OPN) and calprotectin showed them to stain both the stone center and concentric laminations *(32)*. Ultrastructural immunodetection using specific antibodies showed the OPN and osteocalcin as major components of the matrix of human kidney stones as well as CaOx crystals and stones experimentally induced in male rats *(11)*. OPN was detected both inside the crystals as well as on their surfaces. Ultrastructural examination of decalcified stones also showed the crystal associated matrix to stain positive with malachite green indicating the presence of phospholipids *(33)*.

Chemical Composition

Organic matrix of urinary stones contains lipids, GAG carbohydrates, and proteins, with proteins comprising approx 64% of the matrix. Table 1 lists the compounds identified in the stone matrices; and as to be expected most of them are proteinaceous in nature. Many other proteins have also been detected but not identified. Initially lipids were not recognized as constituent of stone matrix *(20)* even though detected as an osmiophilic substance during histochemical examination of decalcified stones. As discussed later in the chapter, recent studies have provided compelling evidence that lipids are an important component of stone matrix and play a significant role in stone formation.

It is now generally understood that matrix components play a significant role in stone formation and that stone matrix is derived from the incorporation of urinary macromolecules in the growing stones. All macromolecules present in the urine can become part

Table 1
Macromolecules Detected in CaOx/CaP Stones and/or Crystals

Macromolecules	References
• Proteins	
Albumin	18, 42
α-1-microglobulin	34
α-1-acid glycoprotein	260
α and γ-globulins	18, 42
α-1-antitrypsin	299
Apolipoprotein A1	260
β-2-microglobulin	260
Calprotectin (Calgranulin)	32, 300
Haemoglobin	298
Inter-α-inhibitor	43, 192, 193
Nephrocalcin	156–158
Neutrophil elastase	298
Osteopontin (Uropontin)	218
Porin	40
Renal lithostatin	260
Retinol binding protein	260
Superoxide dismutase	40
Tamm-Horsfall protein	42
Transferin	257
Urinary prothrombin fragment-1	237–239
• Glycosaminoglycans	
Heparan sulfate	36–39
Hyaluronic acid	
• Lipids	
Phospholipids, cholesterol, glycolipids	28, 33, 280

of the stone matrix but only some of them are there because they participated in crystallization and stone formation. This appreciation has led investigators to study crystallization in vitro, using freshly collected urine and determine the macromolecules that become a part of the crystal matrix (34,35). As we discuss later, crystal matrix also contains lipids, GAGs, and proteins.

GLYCOSAMINOGLYCANS (GAGS)

GAGs can account for up to 20% of the stone matrix (36). Heparan sulfate (HS) and hyaluronic acid (HA) are the two major GAGs in the matrix of both stones and CaOx crystals precipitated in the urine (37,38). The most abundant urinary GAG, chondroitin sulfate (CS) has not been detected in the matrices of CaOx crystals or stones indicating selectivity in incorporation (39). Keratan sulfate and dermatan sulfate are occasionally present in trace amounts.

PROTEINS

More than twenty individual proteins have been detected in the matrix of various types of stones. Although most of them have been identified (Table 1), some still remain nameless (40) and a few await confirmation of their identification (41). Here we will discuss in greater details some of the proteins investigated for their perceived importance in stone formation. Human serum albumin (HAS), α and γ globulins and Tamm-Horsfall protein (THP) were the first proteins identified in stone matrix *(42)*. Albumin is a major component of the matrix of all type of stones including CaOx, uric acid, struvite, and cystine. Albumin is also found in the matrix of CaOx and CaP crystals precipitated from the human urine and it is more pronounced in crystals induced in stone formers urine *(43,44)*. Both CaOx and CaP crystals are known to adsorb HAS.

THP is not always detected in stones and even then in only minor quantities, 0.002–1.04 mg/g (w/w) of stone *(45)*. We found THP in matrices of both the CaOx and CaP crystals induced in human urine and as a major component of CaP crystal matrix. We also discovered that THP associated with CaOx crystals could be easily removed by washing the crystals with sodium hydroxide solution *(43,44,46)*, indicating that THP interacts with crystal surfaces. Ultrastructural investigations of human CaOx urinary stones (unpublished results) and CaOx nephroliths induced in an animal model also demonstrated that THP interacts primarily with the crystal surfaces and does not appear to be occluded in the crystalline mass *(47,48)*. This may explain THP's scanty presence in the stone matrix.

Of the other stone matrix proteins listed in Table 1, OPN, α-1-microglobulin, urinary prothrombin fragment-1 (UPFT-1), and light and heavy chains of inter-α-inhibitor have been identified in the matrix of CaOx and CaP crystals precipitated from the urine of normal and stone forming individuals *(43,44)*. Ultrastructurally OPN is the major component of the matrix of CaOx stones *(11,49)*. More OPN is present in CaOx monohydrate stones (800 µg /100 mg stone) than in COD stones (10 µg /100 mg stone).

LIPIDS

Lipids are an integral part of the organic matrices of all mineralized tissues and pathological calcifications *(50–52)*. Even though they account for a relatively small proportion of the matrix; 7–14% in bone, 2–6% in dentin, 12–22% in newly mineralized enamel, approx 9.6% in submandibular salivary gland calculi, and 10.2% in supragingival calculi *(50–55)*, lipids play a significant role in the calcification process. They promote crystal nucleation, modulate growth and aggregation and become incorporated in the growing calcifications.

The matrix of all stones investigated to date including struvite, uric acid, CaOx, and CaP contains lipids *(28,33)*. The protein to lipid ratio is, however, higher in the matrix of struvite and uric acid stones than the matrix of CaOx and CaP stones (Table 2). Even though there are no significant differences in various types of lipids determined, matrix of struvite stones contain more cholesterol, cholesterol ester, and triglycerides than the other three types of stones. Analysis by one dimensional thin layer chromatography separated and identified various phospholipids and glycolipids including sphingomyelin (SM), phosphatidyl choline (PC), phosphatidyl ethanolamine (PE), and cardiolipin (CL) and trace amounts of phosphatidylserine (PS) in matrices of all stones. Occasionally stone matrix also contains phosphatidyl inositol (PI), lyso-PC, lyso-phosphatidic acid (PA) and lyso-PE. Glycolipids detected in all stones include gangliosides, D-sphingosine, and glucocerebrosides. In addition, struvite stone matrix contains sulfatides and digalacto diglycerides whereas matrices of CaOx and CaP stones contain cerebrosides 1 and 2 and digalacto-diglycerides.

The matrices of all stones comprise both complexed and noncomplexed lipids. The amount of complexed lipids is highest in CaP stones and lowest in the uric acid stones.

Table 2
Stone Matrix Composition (% of EDTA Soluble Matrix) and Lipid Constituents (mg/g stone)

Stone type	Protein	Lipid	Total cholesterol	Triglycerides	Glycolipids	Phospholipid
Struvite ($n = 5$)	74%	26%	1.53 ± 0.72	10.71 ± 9.17	0.13 ± 0.05	0.06 ± 0.04
Calcium oxalate ($n = 5$)	20%	80%	0.64 ± 0.27	1.64 ± 0.60	0.16 ± 0.06	0.05 ± 0.03
Calcium phosphate ($n = 3$)	33%	67%	0.76 ± 0.50	1.45 ± 0.13	0.17 ± 0.10	0.05 ± 0.02
Uric acid ($n = 5$)	75%	25%	0.20 ± 0.07	1.60 ± 0.34	0.09 ± 0.03	0.03 ± 0.01

Table 3
Lipids Present in the Matrix of Crystals Produced
in Normal Human Urine (mg/total crystal/24 h)

Crystal type	Cholesterol	Triglycerides	Glycolipids	Phospholipids
Calcium oxalate	0.37 ± 0.09	3.11 ± 2.9	1.15 ± 1.20	0.09 ± 0.04
Calcium phosphate	0.27 ± 0.10	2.51 ± 2.4	1.35 ± 1.04	0.02 ± 0.01

Both complexed and noncomplexed lipids contain cholesterol, triglycerides, phospholipids and gangliosides.

Both CaOx and CaP crystals induced in the urine contain lipids *(33)*. However, there are no significant differences in either the nature of lipid constituents or the lipid amounts per gram of crystals between the two types of calcific crystals (Table 3). Glucocerebrosides are the most common glycolipids, whereas SM is the most common phospholipid. Gangliosides are the second most common glycolipid and PC and PE the most common phospholipids. Determinations of lipids in the urine before and after experimental induction of CaOx crystals show that the formation of crystals depletes the urine of its phospholipids indicating its incorporation in the crystal matrix. Almost all urinary phospholipids become incorporated in the formation of crystals *(33)*.

CRYSTALLIZATION MODULATORS IN URINE

In urine, three classes of crystallization modulators can be recognized; low-molecular weight (MW) compounds like citrate and pyrophosphate; (glyco)-proteins; and high-MW nonprotein compounds such as glycosaminoglycans, acid mucopolysaccharides, and various types of lipids. All have some influence on crystallization and urolithiasis, either through direct involvement in the various processes such as crystal nucleation, growth, aggregation, and retention or by influencing the urinary environment. From crystallization experiments with diluted and undiluted whole urine, it appears that in nonstone formers the concerted actions of these compound ensure that: (1) the crystals formed remain unaggregated and small enough to be excreted *(56,57)*, (2) the crystals have a reduced affinity for epithelial cells *(58,60)*, and (3) the crystals if needed are easily recognized and removed by macrophages *(61)*.

Which inhibitors play a major role in this? The first approach to answering this question has been to identify individual compounds in the urine and test their "inhibitory" effectiveness in crystallization and cell-culture systems. The next problem has been to translate these data to the whole urine situation where singular inhibitors may also co-operate or compete with each other and where restrictions posed by the kidney and urinary tract itself (flow-rates, residence time, and changing urine composition) affect their inhibitory and stimulatory powers. We will discuss the actions of individual modulators in inorganic solutions as well as in the urinary conditions.

Low-MW Compounds

Pyrophosphate and Its Analogs

Citrate and pyrophosphate are two major representatives of the low MW compounds that have an effect on crystallization. Pyrophosphate is present in urine at micromolar concentrations (Table 4) and effective as inhibitor at those same concentrations. When

Table 4
Inhibitor Characteristics

| Compound | MW | Urinary excretion, mg/24-h avg (range) | |
		Control	Stone former
Total GAGs, mg/24 h		23–28 (0–50)	23 (0–53)
Chondroitin sulfate A, C [a]	5–20 kDa	14 (8–18)	14 (4–19)
Chondroitin sulfate C [a]			
Keratan sulfate [a]	5 kDa	2 (0.5–7)	2 (0.5–7)
Dermatan sulfate (Chs-B) [a]		1 (0.5–2)	1 (0.5–2)
Heparan sulfate [a]		5 (2–14)	5 (3–14)
Hyaluronic acid [a]	up to 10^6 Da [b]	3 (1.8–7.5)	3 (1–8)
Pentosanpoly sulfate [c]	4–7 kDa		1–16
Pyrophosphate (μM)	178 Da	30–70 (15–100)	36–50 (8–94)

[a] Based on measurements of separate GAGs and on reported percentages of the total GAGs.
[b] 12% >100 kDa, 64% 10–100, 24% <10 kDa
[c] Excretion rate at a 400 mg/24-h oral dose.
(Data from References 62, 71–75, 97, 107, 108, 124, 126, 128, 130, 301–308.)

tested as a single compound in a seeded crystal growth system, it inhibits CaOx crystal growth by 50% at a concentration of 16–20 μM (62–65), (Table 5) which is within its urine concentration range (Table 6). In addition, pyrophosphate under nonurine conditions inhibits the growth of CaPs (66,67) and causes preferential formation of COD (68). The effectiveness of pyrophosphate suggested that it may significantly contribute to the crystal growth inhibitory potential of urine. At its urine concentration range (15–100 μM) pyrophosphate inhibits CaOx monohydrate crystal growth up to 80% when it is tested in vitro. These data also prompted interest in the effect of nonbiodegradable pyrophosphate analogs, bisphosphonates on crystallization, as these can be given therapeutically. It was found that bisphosphonates yield 50% COM crystal growth inhibition at concentrations ranging from 1 to 20 μM (69). Some bisphosphonates inhibit crystal growth at lower concentrations then pyrophosphate.

Pyrophosphate and several analogs inhibit crystallization of hydroxyapatite and brushite. Pyrophosphate was most effective in inhibiting hydroxyapatite precipitation whereas phytate most effectively blocked brushite precipitation (66). COD is preferentially formed in the presence of citrate 1.0×10^{-3} mol/L and pyrophosphate 2.0×10^{-4} mol/L. Nearly pure COD produced with pyrophosphate was stable over 7 d, whereas that with citrate underwent partial transformation within 48 h. An additive effect of citrate and pyrophosphate was found on the stability of COD. It was concluded that a pyrophosphate concentration above a critical point was sufficient to prevent solution-mediated transformation of COD, and this critical point might be lowered to the physiological range with the presence of citrate (68).

Further studies revealed that the effectivity of the bisphosphonates depends on how well they can bind to the calcium ions on the crystal surface. This is regulated by the concerted action of the two phosphonate groups and the rest group attached to the same carbon atom of the molecule. A hydroxyl group or amino-group as rest group yields the best inhibitors (69). The growth inhibitory power further depends on the protonation state of the bisphosphonate, thus on the pH and the pKa-values of the bisphosphon-

Table 5
Inhibitor Activity

Concentration (M) for:	50% GI[a]	%G.I. in urine[b]	AggI[c]	Crystal-cell binding[d]	
				MDCK, mg/L	BSC-1, mM
RNA	3×10^{-9}				
Chondroitin sulfate A, C[a]	$40\text{–}50 \times 10^{-6}$	15–20	No to small effect	>100	0.6
Chondroitin sulfate C[a]	10^{-6}			>100	—
Keratan sulfate[a]	10^{-6}				—
Dermatan sulfate (Chs-B)[a]	10^{-6}			>100	0.1
Heparin	$3\text{–}20 \times 10^{-9}$		No effect	3.1	0.002–0.015
Heparan sulfate[a]	6×10^{-9}	30–40	Strong inhibition	>100	0.1
Hyaluronic acid[a]	10^{-6}	No to small effect	>100	0.02	
Pentosan polysulfate[c]	$2\text{–}6 \times 10^{-6}$	35[e]	No effect	2	0.02
Pyrophosphate	$2\text{–}20 \times 10^{-6}$	50–60	Strong inhibition		
Bisphosphonates	$1\text{–}50 \times 10^{-6}$		Variable		

[a] As % reduction of growth rate in inhibitor-free control experiment.

[b] The % GI excerted in an in vitro experiment by the average concentration present in urine.

[c] Techniques employed in literature are too diverse to allow for quantitation.

[d] The dose needed for 50% reduction in the binding of COM crystals to quiescent layers of renal epithelial cell cultures of MDCk (16) and BSC-1 (18).

[e] Expected concentration at 400 mg/d dose is 16 mg/L. Addition to urine at 10 mg/L increased % GI from 45 to 59% (73).

(Data from References 58, 60, 63–65, 93, 111, 112.)

Table 6
Distribution of Individual GAGs as % of Total GAGs Population

| Compound | Urine | | Crystals semiquantitative | Stone semiquantitative |
	Control	SF		
Chondroitin sulfate	30–68	14–70	0 [a]	0
Heparan sulfate	8–51	9–50	+++	+++
Hyaluronic acid	3–23	5–32		++
Keratan sulfate	2–27	2–21		+
Dermatan sulfate	1–8	1–6		

[a] When HS is absent from urine, Chs can become included into crystal matrix.
(Data from references *36–38*.)

ate molecule. The more of the triply deprotonated form is present, the more effectively crystal growth is inhibited. This pH-dependency is also encountered for pyrophosphate. In the urine pH range the ionic species of pyrophosphate are PP^{4-}, HPP^{3-}, and H_2PP^{2-}. The first two adsorb onto CaOx monohydrate crystals *(70)*. As the urine pH approaches 7 these inhibitors will thus become more effective.

The effects of pyrophosphate and bisphosphonates on crystal aggregation are more complex. Pyrophosphate increasingly inhibits crystal aggregation at increasing concentrations *(63)*. Although some bisphosphonates have a comparable effect, others show no effect, a stimulatory effect on aggregation or even a biphasic effect, inhibiting aggregation at low concentrations and stimulating it at higher concentrations. This variation relates to the way the bisphosphonate molecules bind to the crystal surface and to their tendency to form large polynuclear complexes with calcium. Although single bisphosphonate molecules may cover the CaOx crystal surface to form a layer that prevents their aggregation, the large polynuclear complexes actually bridge from one crystal surface to another and stimulate the formation of large aggregates *(69)*.

Thus pyrophosphate and bisphosphonates can be very potent inhibitors of crystal growth and in some cases also of crystal aggregation. Both inhibitory actions of bisphosphonates can be increased by changing their structure. Although variation of the bisphosphonate part of the molecule affects its crystal growth inhibitory power, variation of the side chains of the bisphosphonate molecule can disturb the tendency to form polynuclear complexes with calcium. Adding a large cyclic structure to the backbone of the bisphosphonate abolishes its tendency to form large polynuclear complexes (by steric hindrance), and makes it more effective in inhibiting crystal aggregation. Variation of the pKa3 value of the bisphosphonate part furthermore may take away the problem of its anti bone resorptive capacity. Overall it is possible to construct a bisphosphonate that strongly inhibits CaOx crystal growth and crystal aggregation at the urine pH levels and does not interfere with bone resorption activity at the low pH levels existing under active osteoclasts. Development and application of such compounds are possible future projects.

PYROPHOSPHATE AND BISPHOSPHONATE, EXCRETION AND THERAPY

Because pyrophosphate is such an effective inhibitor under nonurine conditions, several groups have investigated if stoneformers excrete different amounts of pyrophosphate in their urine. Pyrophosphate enters the urine in the glomerular filtrate. The plasma concentration is 2–3 μM, of which 70–80% is ultrafilterable. The urine excretion rate is extremely variable. In male nonstone formers the average concentration is 20–40 μM, and the average 24 h excretion rate is 30–60 μmoles (range 15–98 μmoles) (Table 4). Some investigators have found that the 24 h pyrophosphate excretion was unchanged in stone formers, 36 μmoles/24 h (range 8–94), although they noted some variation with types of hypercalciuria (62). Other groups reported a decreased average excretion (51 in stone formers vs 71 in controls) (71), a decreased average pyrophosphate/ creatinine ratio in stone formers (72), or a decreased pyrophosphate excretion as single abnormality in 12% of the stoneformers (73). Invariably, however the range of excretion rates was comparable to that of controls. Women tended to have a higher average pyrophosphate excretion, but this was not significant (4.23 ± 3.34 vs 1.98 ± 1.0). In female stone formers and male stone formers the ppi/creat ratio was comparable, 2.16 ± 2.27 (73). Overall the findings do not conclusively show a lower pyrophosphate excretion in stone-formers. In view of its inhibitory power in inorganic solutions it is nevertheless possible that increasing pyrophosphate excretion may increase the growth inhibitory power of the urine and thus be beneficial. Two problems then must be addressed: can urine pyrophosphate excretion be manipulated and does pyrophosphate also contribute to the inhibitory power in the whole urine situation?

Pyrophosphate excretion can be increased by oral orthophosphate therapy (74) but oral orthophosphate therapies in general have not proven to be effective for preventing stone formation. Controlled trials have not been performed. Treatment with neutral potassium phosphate (75) and with diclofenac sodium (71) (a nonsteroidal anti-inflammatory drug) also increased pyrophosphate excretion. The first also increases citrate excretion and this combination increased the ability of whole urine (diluted 1:5 to mimic the situation in the renal collecting ducts) to inhibit crystal agglomeration and reduced the propensity for spontaneous nucleation of brushite (75). All these data suggest that an increase in urine pyrophosphate concentration will raise its inhibitory power, especially with regard to crystal formation and aggregation. However, it has not been shown that they increase the inhibition of crystal growth in urine, despite their actions in nonurine conditions. Finally, it is not known whether pyrophosphate and bisphosphonates have an effect on crystal–cell interactions. To put their potential in perspective, at a concentration of 0.2 mM citrate decreased the binding of COM crystals to cultures of the renal epithelial cell line BSC-1 by 50% (60). In view of the normal urine concentration range of citrate, >1.5 mM, small molecules like citrate might help prevent negative impact of crystal–cell interaction.

Whether or not these activities actually help prevent stone formation has not been answered. In fact therapies that increase pyrophosphate excretion also increase phosphate excretion and thereby will increase the propensity for CaP precipitation in the loop of Henle, which may precede CaOx crystallization further downstream in the nephron (76).

Bisphosphonates have been applied with the aim of preventing stone formation by increasing the inhibitory power of urine. The results with etidronate, however, were not positive and severe renal side-effects were noted (77). In addition, the effect of bisphosphonates on bone turnover may also be unwanted. In later studies it was shown that etidronate is one of the bisphosphonates with a tendency to form very large polynuclear complexes with calcium (78).

High MW Compounds

GLYCOSAMINOGLYCANS

In 1684 Anton von Heyde discovered the presence of a mucoprotein matrix in stone *(79)*. Later, urine was found to contain many different anionic proteins and nonprotein anions, including GAGs, RNA, and acid mucopolysaccharides. The most prominent are the GAGs; polyanionic compounds with varying MW of usually 18–40 kDa but may be up to 10^6 Da. They may enter the urine in several ways, by filtration, by release from the glomerular basement membrane, from the surface of the tubular epithelial lining, and from the urothelium downstream in the urinary tract. Well known GAGs include heparin (not present in urine) and the urinary GAGs HS, chondroitin sulfate A, B, and C (CS-A, CS-B, and CS-C), dermatan sulfate (DS), keratan sulfate (KS), and nonsulfated HA.

Some, but not all urinary GAGS are found in crystals and stones *(35–39)*. This selective inclusion suggests that some GAGs interact more actively with CaOx crystals than others. Is this selectivity related to differences in excretion rate and/or differences in affinity for calcium salt crystals? Several research groups have investigated GAGs excretion in stone formation. Exact determination of the excretion rate of polyanions has however been a problem. Total GAGs excretion can be measured with several methods *(80)*. The often-used Alcian blue generally precipitates all polyanionic macromolecules including GAGs, THP, acid mucopolysaccharides plus anionic (glyco)-proteins, and RNA. In early studies recurrent stone formers were found to excrete less of this mixture *(81–94)*. Precipitation by the cation cetylpyridinium chloride produces a similar precipitate. When the isolation procedure involves determination of the total hexuronic acid content using a colometric assay *(85)*, an indication of the total amount of free GAGs plus protein bound GAGs is obtained, expressed as µmoles of glucuronic acid. A drawback of this method is that DS is missed because it contains iduronate instead of glucuronate. Many studies have been performed using a combination of anion isolation and determination of glucuronic acid content. In nonstone formers total GAGs excretion varies between 0 and 50 µmoles glucuronic acid/24h. Several studies show a decreased excretion of GAGs in stone formers *(81–84,86–92)*. However, at least equal number of studies find comparable GAGs excretion by stone formers and nonstone formers *(72,93–102)*. The differences in results may relate to differences in the techniques, differences in the patient populations, epithelial damage, or the contribution of bladder excretions to the total GAG pool *(103)*. One study showed no change for the total group of stone formers but decreased GAGs excretion in recurrent stone formers *(72)*. Total GAGs excretion for instance is considerably increased in interstitial cystitis owing to increased excretion of nonsulfated GAGs (HA) *(103)*. The finding that excretion of uronic acid containing compounds (mainly GAGs) increases with age (from 0 to 15 yr) *(105,106)* may well be related to the increase of bladder epithelial surface area with age. Epithelial damage may explain why the GAGs excretion increased on ESWL treatment *(107)*. Of course it may just as well be that the stone present before ESWL acted as a sink for GAGs. A decreased GAGs excretion would then reflect the presence of a stone. Overall there is no conclusive evidence that differences in total GAGs excretion exist and play a role in stone formation.

Another approach has been to look at individual GAGs. This can be done by a combination of gel electrophoresis and enzymes that cleave specific GAGs, antibodies for specific GAGs or binding proteins (e.g., HA binding protein). When pure reference GAGs are available, quantitation is also possible. The data can then be expressed as mg or µmoles of the specific reference GAG. It must be noted, however, that GAGSs have variable MW. They can be found in a free state or bound to a protein. Same GAGs from different sources differ in MW. Thus the choice of which GAG to use as a reference will affect the result.

Overall, the studies that have looked at the excretion of individual GAGs do not show consistent changes in GAGs patterns in stone patients (87,97,108,109). The limitations of the methods make it difficult to compare excretion data from one publication to another or to establish general reference ranges for excretion of GAGs. The numbers given in Table 4 are combined data from the literature and are meant as a tool for placing the concentrations used in vitro experiments in an in vivo perspective. Unless some gold standard is developed, it is recommended to include the correct controls for measuring GAGs in urine and not to rely on historic reference ranges.

INHIBITORY ACTIONS OF GAGS

Some data indicate that there are structural and functional differences in GAGs. Urinary macromolecules and urine from children inhibit crystal aggregation better than urine of adults. The pediatric macromolecule fraction contained more GAGs (110). GAGs from stone formers had an increased nucleation promoting activity but similar crystal growth inhibitory activity (71). The first appeared related to a changed action of HA in stone formers (111). However CS of healthy individuals also shows a basal crystallization-promoting property (112).

To put such data in perspective you must first know how the several GAG species effect crystallization in inorganic solutions and under urine conditions. Table 5 summarizes data from the literature on the effect of GAGs on crystal growth, aggregation and nucleation when tested in inorganic solutions. Under these conditions the nonurine GAG heparin is the most effective on a molar basis. Of the GAGs present in urine HS is most effective followed at a distance by CS and HA. The heparin analog pentosan polysulfate has effectiveness between heparin and CS. As was shown for pentosan polysulfate, the inhibition of crystal growth does not change when pH is varied from 5 to 7 (113).

With respect to crystal–cell interactions, coating of crystals by GAGs decreased the binding of crystals to renal epithelial cells in culture (58,60).

Putting these data in perspective of urine concentration of those compounds, HS should contribute the most to the crystallization inhibitory power of urine. CS should have some effect as it is the GAG with the highest concentration. If the GAGs would act synergistically their contribution to the overall inhibitory power of urine should be significant. However, how do GAGs perform in urine?

Inhibitor Action in Whole Undiluted Urine

Undiluted whole urine strongly affects calcium salt nucleation, crystal growth and crystal aggregation. When preformed CaOx crystals were added to supersaturated whole undiluted urine their growth was almost completely stopped. Crystal growth only occurred when the supersaturation was drastically increased by adding extra oxalate (76). Urine has an overabundance of inhibitors. Tested in vitro as single compounds some are clearly more effective than the others, however experimental data suggest that when the most efficient compounds are lacking, others readily take over. For instance, the low MW compound citrate can inhibit crystal growth very effectively at concentrations between 0.1 and 1 mM. When citrate was added at these concentrations to urine, however, it did not change the growth inhibitory action of that urine (56).

In studies of large groups of stone formers and healthy controls where urine was tested in a 1:5 dilution, approximating the degree of dilution existing in the collecting ducts, both urine from stone formers and normal subjects strongly inhibited CaOx crystal growth (56,57,114). When all macromolecules were removed from urine by ultrafiltration, the degree of crystal growth inhibition was only slightly reduced (115). In vitro tests have however shown that macromolecules are most effective inhibitors of crystal growth. Apparently the low MW compounds take over the inhibitory function when the high MW compounds are gone.

An additional effect of growth inhibition may be that the supersaturation will persist longer and the process of nucleation will have more time to proceed (116). How relevant this is, in view of the short transit times of urine through the nephron (a few minutes) (9), is not clear.

Normal urine can also strongly inhibit crystal aggregation. This function is reduced in single-case stone former urine and severely reduced in recurrent stone former urine (56,57). Aggregation is important as it can lead to particle retention, just like crystal cell interactions and disturbed flow conditions (9). The inhibition of aggregation in urine is correlated to the citrate concentration (57). However, in ultrafiltered urine this relationship is gone (114). Apparently citrate modulates the effect that high MW compounds have on crystal aggregation. In addition it was found that the urinary macromolecular fraction (>10.000 D MW) of single-case stone formers inhibited crystal aggregation less than that of normals. The fraction from recurrent stone formers was even less efficient (116). In this study 70–90% of the inhibitory activity was destroyed by proteinase treatment. Citrate has been shown to improve the inhibitory effect of THP on crystal aggregation (117).

Overall it appears that urine contains numerous components, both small and large, which compete and co-operate in inhibiting stone formation. What is the role of GAGs in this?

The Effects of GAGs on Crystallization in Urine

The effect of 1% urine on crystal growth and aggregation was only slightly related to the uronic acid content and overall the contribution of GAGs (95,102,116,117). Apparently the effects of GAGs in an inorganic solution cannot predict their actions in the urine situation. Overall it appears that CS is not active as inhibitor in urine. In fact, it might even stimulate nucleation and stone-formation. HS has some effect in urine on crystal growth and aggregation and in addition may also promote nucleation. The synthetic GAG pentosan polysulfate also can inhibit crystal growth under urine conditions and reduces renal crystal deposition in rat models for stone formation.

These data agree with the change in relative distribution of GAGs going from urine to crystals and stones (Table 6). Although in urine CS is by far the most abundant GAG, crystals produced from whole urine ordinarily contain HS and none to some HA and no CS (36–38). Crystals produced in absence of HS do contain CS, thus the changed distribution is a competition effect. In stone matrix: 8–20% of total dry weight are GAGs. These stone GAGs include no CS, a large amount of HS and some HA (36,37).

Overall it appears that GAGs can have an "inhibitory" action in urine, but their contribution to the actual activity in urine seems small at best. Nevertheless, increasing the urine excretion of GAGs might add to the inhibitory power of urine.

Another reason to try to increase GAG excretion may lie in their ability to influence Band-3 protein governed oxalate exchange, as shown in red blood cells (118). The oxalate self exchange is decreased in stone patient red blood cells and this can be corrected in vitro by adding HS. When patients received short term oral GAGS treatment, the RBC oxalate self exchange also normalized *(119)*.

Furthermore GAGs may interfere with crystal cell interactions. In cell-culture studies, preformed CaOx crystals do not bind to well developed MDCK cells (distal tubule/collecting duct origin). However the same cells during migration and proliferation do bind crystals, where HA appears to act as a crystal binding molecule *(120)*. Adhesion of COM crystals to these cells was reduced by heparin, CS-A or B, HS, and HA, the nonsulfated polyglutamic acid and polyaspartic acid, nephrocalcin, uropontin, pentosan polysulfate, and citrate but not CS-C and THP *(58,60)*. Of the GAGs heparin and pentosan polysulfate were most effective at the lowest concentrations (Table 5). Also, coating of stents with heparin prevents encrustation of the stents when placed in a bladder for up to 120 d *(121)*. Thus, under nonurine conditions GAGs appear capable of preventing crystal adhesion to cells and other surfaces. When crystals are preincubated in whole urine and then added to cell cultures in an inorganic solution, this reduced their binding to immobilized HA, confirming the crystal binding action of the latter. However, it did not significantly reduce the crystal–cell attachment *(59)*. Just as was the case for crystallization inhibition, effects on crystal–cell attachment differ from inorganic solutions to semi-urine conditions.

These combined data raise the question: can long term GAGs therapy decrease stone formation by decreasing the propensity for crystallization and crystal attachment to renal cells?

Glycosaminoglycans in Therapy

During GAGs therapy oxalate excretion decreased on a short-term basis *(119)*. The long-term effect on oxalate excretion has not been studied.

The only long-term study with administration of a GAG to stone formers was with pentosan polysulfate (PPS, Elmiron). In this study the stone formation rate in stone formers receiving 400 mg Elmiron daily was followed, first in an open study, later compared to a control group receiving standard advice. From studies with radioactive labeled Elmiron it is known that only 8% of an intravenous 40 mg pentosan polysulfate dose reaches the urine. After an oral dose of 400 mg/d, plasma levels reached 0.02 to 0.05 μg/mL. The urinary excretion in a 24 h period was 0.05–0.1% (1–2 mg). In rats 4% of a dose of 10 mg/kg/d of PPS reached the urine *(123)*. In man 1–4% reaches the urine *(124)*. Thus of the 400 mg/d dose given in the clinical trial 4–16 mg may reach the daily urine. All of this will not be intact. In comparison, 50% of heparin is desulfated in the liver *(125)*. If the same occurs with Elmiron, 2–8 mg will reach the urine of the daily dose of 400 mg. When we assume a MW of 5000 Dalton and a daily urine volume of 1.5 L this means a concentration of 0.4–1.6 μM. Under nonurine conditions this is approximately the concentration that gives 50% inhibition of crystals growth. In the first report from 1986, 100 patients were started on 400 mg Elmiron/d. A report was given on 70 patients who received Elmiron for a period of at least 12 mo *(126)*. Long-term trials with Elmiron given for other indications show some side effects at doses of 150 to 450 mg/d *(122)*. In this interim report six patients stopped because of gastrointestinal side effects and a trend was suggested that stone formation was reduced. In a second report from 1988, 100 patients were treated for a period of 12–56 mo, with 16 patients withdrawing. After this period 85% remained stone free. The results were however, obtained without a proper control group and thus contaminated by the stone clinic effect. The results encouraged an open study in which 121 patients were followed for 3 yr. Data collected showed that 48% of the patients remained stone free, whereas 52 % continued to form stones. The stone formation rate was not statistically different from that in patients without treatment *(127)*. The conclusion seems to be that although pentosan polysulfate shows potential when tested in the laboratory, when used in therapy at the dose of 400 mg/d it does not prevent stone formation. Possibly a higher dose is required but this may have the risk of considerable drop-out owing to side effects.

GAGs affect the morphology of COM crystals differently depending on the species. Chondroitin-6-sulfate produces elongated less wide crystals. Dermatan sulfate and heparin are incorporated into the crystals, CS-C is not. Experiments using dicarboxylates, a simple model of GAG molecules, showed that the distance between the side groups was important for their morphological effects *(128)*.

In male rats a vitamin A-deficient diet caused a decrease in the concentration of urinary GAGs and lesions of the cuboidal epithelium that covers the papillae *(129)*. The plasma vitamin A levels in urolithiasic humans did not significantly differ from those in a control group. Nevertheless a significant increase in vitamin E and in the vitamin E/ vitamin A ratio was observed. These results could be related to a possible deficit of vitamin A in kidneys of stone formers, this being one of the diverse factors that can contribute to urolith development. Moreover, the deficit of important urinary crystallization inhibitors normally found in stone-formers, such as pyrophosphate and phytate, can also be related to the presence of low levels of renal vitamin A, which prevents the enzymatic degradation of such inhibitors *(130)*.

Proteins

Table 7 lists major urinary proteins with known potential to influence crystallization of CaOx and/or CaP. Renal epithelial cells normally produce many of these whereas others are currently considered as plasma proteins. However, recent animal model and tissue culture studies demonstrate that the renal epithelial cells in the presence of hyperoxaluria and CaOx crystals can also produce many of the so-called plasma proteins.

TAMM-HORSFALL PROTEIN

A number of excellent reviews have been written on Tamm-Horsfall protein (THP) involvement in nephrolithiasis *(131–133)*. THP is one of the most abundant proteins in normal human urine and the major constituent of urinary casts. It was first isolated from the urine by Tamm and Horsfall and characterized as a glycoprotein that inhibits viral hemagglutination *(134)*. Muchmore and Decker isolated a protein called uromodulin from the urine of pregnant women *(135)*. Based on amino acid and carbohydrate analysis THP and uromodulin were shown to be identical *(136)*. There is a considerable variation in daily urinary excretion of THP by both humans and rats. In humans it ranges between 20 and 100 mg/d with a daily urinary volume of 1.5 L and in rats it ranges between 552 and 2865 µg/d with a daily urinary volume of 16.5 mL *(137)*. When converted to mg/l rats excrete 34.5 ± 38.6 to 180 ± 38.6 mg/L THP in their urine. THP has a molecular weight of approx 80 kDa with a tendency to aggregate to polymeric form. Polymerization is increased in the presence of free calcium ions, at high ionic strength and osmolality, and at low pH. Sialylated, sulfated and GalNac containing carbohydrates make up 30% of its weight. It contains 616 amino acid residues including approx 50 half-cysteine molecules, which can be involved in disulfide bridge formation.

Table 7
Some Urinary Proteins With Potential to Modulate Crystallization [a]

Protein name	MW (kDa)	Origin (normal/hyperoxaluria)	Unique features	Role in crystallization	Presence in urine
• Tamm-Horsfall	80–100	TAL of the kidney	12% ASP	Promotor; inhibitor of aggregation	20–200 mg/d
• Nephrocalcin	14	PT, TAL of the kidney	2–3 Gla residues	Inhibitor of nucleation, growth, aggregation	5–16 mg/L
• Osteopontin	42–80	TDL, TAL of the kidney	RGD sequence	Inhibitor of nucleation, growth, aggregation	2.4–3.7 mg/L
• α-1 Microglobulin	31	Plasma/REC	5.34 mg/L		
• Calprotectin	36.5	Granulocytes/REC	Calcium-binding domain		<50 µg/L
• Human serum albumin	68	Plasma	Binds to crystals	Facilitates binding of other proteins to crystals	1.6–34.2 mg/d
• Urinary prothrombin fragment 1	31	Plasma/TAL of the kidney	10 GLA residues	Inhibitor of aggregation	13.4 nM/d
• Inter-α-inhibitor		Plasma/REC	Sulfated GAGs	Inhibitor of nucleation, growth, and aggregation	2–10mg/d
— H1 (Heavy Chain 1)	78				Yes
— H2 (Heavy Chain 2)	85				Yes
— HI-30 (Bikunin)	30–35				Yes

[a] Location in kidneys based on studies in rats; urinary excretion rate in normal humans; role in crystallization based mostly on CaOx crystal studies. ASP, Aspartic acid; GLA, γ-carboxyglutamic acid; REC, renal epithelial cells; RGD, arginine–glycine–aspartic acid; PT, proximal tubule; TAL, thin ascending limb of the loop of Henle; TDL; thick descending limb of the loop of Henle.

THP has been the subject of extensive research for its implication in stone formation. However, its exact contribution to urolithiasis remains unclear and the results of various studies have been controversial *(131)*. Results of some studies indicated that THP promoted CaOx and CaP crystallization *(138,139)*, whereas other studies demonstrated that the macromolecule does not support CaOx crystallization and has no effect on spontaneous precipitation *(140)*. Still other studies indicated that THP has no effect on nucleation or growth, but is a potent inhibitor of CaOx crystal aggregation *(141–143)*. Hess et al. found that the addition of citrate reduced CaOx crystal aggregation by reducing the self-aggregation of THP isolated from stone formers urine *(142)*. It is important to point out that low citrate or hypocitraturia is common in stone formers and can contribute to crystal aggregation and stone formation in this fashion. THP activity is controlled by its concentration, urinary osmolality and physicochemical environment of the urine *(144)*. For example, at low concentrations, THP has a minor effect on CaOx crystallization yet promotes it at higher concentrations. Also, when ionic strength was increased or the pH lowered the inhibition of CaOx monohydrate crystal aggregation by THP was decreased *(141)*. Apparently, at high ionic strength, high THP concentration and low pH, the viscosity of THP increases owing to its polymerization.

Several studies have shown that there is no significant difference in the daily urinary excretion of THP between normal subjects and CaOx stone formers *(145)*. This fact led Hess et al. to hypothesize that THP of stone formers is structurally different from that of the healthy subjects *(141)*. They showed that THP isolated from the urine of stone formers contained less carbohydrate (mainly sialic acid) than the THP obtained from control subjects *(146)*. It has been suggested that the abnormality may be inherited, but sufficient evidence to support this concept is not available at this time. Studies have also shown differences in sialic acid contents and surface charge between THP from stone formers and normal individuals. Isoelectric focussing (IEF) studies have shown that THP from healthy individuals has a pI value of approx 3.5, whereas THP from recurrent stone formers has pI values between 4.5 and 6 and the two exhibit completely different IEF patterns *(147)*.

THP is exclusively produced in the kidneys. Based primarily on studies in rat kidneys, it is agreed that THP is specifically localized in epithelial cells of the thick ascending limbs of the loops of Henle *(133,148)* and is generally not seen in the papillary tubules. When CaOx crystal deposits, the nephroliths, are experimentally induced in rat kidneys, THP is seen in close association with the crystals, both in the renal cortex as well as papillae *(47,48)*. However, THP is not seen occluded inside the crystals nor produced by cells other than those lining the limbs of the Henle's loop *(149)*. There are no significant biochemical differences in the THP between one secreted by normal rats or rats with CaOx nephroliths. They have similar amino acid composition, carbohydrate contents, molecular weights and rates of urinary excretion. However, THP from nephrolithic rats has slightly less sialic acid contents, 20% of the total carbohydrate in nephrolithic rats vs 26% in normal rats. In an aggregation assay, both the normal rat THP and nephrolithic rat THP reduced CaOx crystal aggregation in vitro by approx 47%. Results of these rat model studies led to the conclusions that THP is most likely involved in controlling aggregation and that the major difference between normal and stone formers THP may be their sialic acid contents. However animal studies can not rule out THP's role in modulating crystal nucleation or growth.

Another rat model study has shown increased expression of THP in kidneys following unilateral ureteric ligation, which caused tubular dilatation *(150)*. The results indicate that THP expression in kidneys may be increased without crystal deposition and that increased expression in nephrolithic kidneys may be a result of crystal associated injury to the renal epithelial cells. Even rat model studies have provided controversial results for THP. One study shows decreased renal expression of THP during CaOx crystal deposition *(151)* whereas results of another study show upregulation of the THP gene *(152)*.

Nephrocalcin

Nephrocalcin (NC) has been the subject of many reviews *(153,154)*. NC is a glycoprotein with a monomeric molecular weight of approx 14 kDa and has a tendency to self aggregate into a larger macromolecule and thus can exist as a dimer, trimer, or tetramer with molecular weights of 23–30, 45–48, or 60–68 kDa respectively *(156–160)*. NC can also bind to THP in the presence of calcium and magnesium ions. NC can be reversibly dissociated into its monomeric form with incubation in ethylenediaminetetraacetic acid (EDTA) for several days. NC is composed of 110 amino acid residues of which 25% are glutamic and aspartic acid. It contains two cysteine and two or three γ-carboxyglutamic acid (Gla) residues which are suggested to play a significant part in its ability to inhibit CaOx crystallization. Carbohydrate content represents about 10.3% of its weight, with no glucuronic acid and 0.4% sialic acid.

Originally purified from human urine, NC has subsequently been isolated from human kidney tissue culture medium, human renal cell carcinoma, kidneys of many vertebrates, mouse renal proximal tubular cells in culture and rat kidney and urine *(153,155)*. Immunohistochemical techniques have localized NC in the renal epithelial cells of proximal tubules and thick ascending limb of Henle's loop *(161)*. The site of its synthesis has not yet been confirmed by localization of NC mRNA. Daily excretion of NC in human urine is about 5–16 mg *(156,157)*.

NC was originally regarded as the principal inhibitor of COM crystallization in the urine, accounting for approx 90% of the total urinary crystallization inhibitory activity *(156)*. According to the recent results however, the contribution of this inhibitor is suggested to be limited to only 16% *(162)*. NC is suggested to inhibit nucleation, growth, and aggregation of COM crystals. The fractional inhibition of nucleation owing to the presence of NC was shown to be equal to that of urine *(163)*, suggesting that this inhibitor accounts for the total nucleation inhibitory activity of urine. In an aggregation assay determined spectrophotometrically, NC exhibited inhibition of aggregation similar to THP when tested at 5×10^{-7} M or more *(164)*. If used at a lower concentration, NC showed less aggregation inhibitory activity than THP. The inhibitory activity of NC appeared to be reduced when ionic strength was increased, but diminished only slightly when the pH was lowered. Moreover, it was reported that this inhibitor may aggregate or bind to THP when calcium and magnesium ions were present in the milieu. NC is also suggested to participate in crystal retention by inhibiting the adhesion of COM crystals to renal epithelial cells *(168)*.

NC isolated from the urine of stone formers was structurally abnormal, and lacked Gla residues *(157)*. Similarly the NC isolated from kidney stones also did not contain Gla residues and showed less inhibitory activity toward COM crystal formation *(158)*. However, the amino acid composition and carbohydrate contents of NCs from both the stone formers and normals appeared similar.

Although considerable information is available regarding its pathophysiology, the amino acid sequence of NC has not yet been described and thus its identity remains to be authenticated. In this regard, Desbois et al. hypothesized a relationship between NC and osteocalcin *(166)*, the most abundant noncollagenous bone protein. The osteocalcin gene cluster is composed of three genes: osteocalcin gene 1 *(OG1)*, osteocalcin gene 2 *(OG2)*, and osteocalcin related gene *(ORG)*. *OG1* and *OG2* were expressed only in bone, whereas *ORG* is transcribed in kidney, but not in bone. Because *ORG* has a similar expression pattern and identical structure features to NC, Desbois et al. proposed that *ORG* is the gene coding for NC in the kidney. Recently *(41)*, NC was recognized as a fragment (HI-14) of the light chain of IαI, the bikunin, on the basis of SDS-PAGE, inhibitory, and gel filtration properties and amino acid sequence of its two peptides. However the hypothesis that bikunin is NC requires confirmation owing to the fact that bikunin is a part of IαI which does not contain γ-carboxyglutamic acid (Gla) whereas normal NC contains two or three Gla residues. Obviously there is considerable uncertainty about the identity of NC and its contribution to crystallization inhibition, which needs to be resolved. As discussed above, NC occurs in many polymeric forms with molecular weights from 14 to 68, and it elutes from DEAE-cellulose in at least four forms.

INTER-α-INHIBITOR

Inter alpha inhibitor (IαI) and related molecules, collectively referred to as the IαI family, are a group of plasma protease inhibitors *(167–171)*. These molecules are normally synthesized in the liver and are common in plasma. They are composed of a combination of heavy chains, H1 (60 kDa), H2 (70 kDa), and H3 (90 kDa) covalently linked via a CS bridge to a light chain called bikunin (35–45 kDa). Separate genes located on three different chromosomes encode these chains. Bikunin originates from a precursor that also codes for α1-microglobulin (α1-m). The heavy and light chains also exist independently as single molecules. IαI (180–240 kDa) is a heterotrimer consisting of bikunin linked to heavy chains H1and H2. Pre-α-inhibitor (PαI, 125 kDa) is composed of bikunin and heavy chain H3. The macromolecule consisting of bikunin linked to heavy chain H2 is called IαI like inhibitor (IαLI). Bikunin is a broad-spectrum protease inhibitor and an acute-phase reactant. IαI and related proteins have been linked to various pathological conditions such as inflammatory diseases *(172,173)*, cancer *(174–176)*, renal failure *(177)*, and more recently the urinary stone disease, which we will discuss later.

In normal rat kidneys, staining for the IαI related proteins is mostly limited to the proximal tubules and generally to their luminal contents *(178)*. We investigated renal and urinary expression of various members of the IαI family in male rats with or without experimentally induced hyperoxaluria and CaOx crystal deposition. The expression of bikunin mRNA increased in renal epithelial cells exposed to oxalate and CaOx crystals *(178,179)*. Eight weeks after induction of hyperoxaluria, various sections of renal tubules stained positive for IαI, bikunin as well as H3. Positive staining was observed in both the tubular lumina as well as cytoplasm of the epithelial cells. Crystal associated material was heavily stained. Western blot analysis of urinary proteins recognized 7 bands. Urinary expression of H1, H3, and pre-α-inhibitor was significantly increased. Tissue culture studies have shown that human renal proximal tubular epithelial cells constitutively express genes for bikunin and H3 components *(180)*. Bikunin gene is also expressed in MDCK cells and was upregulated when they were exposed to oxalate *(181)*.

Both heavy and light chains have been identified in the urine *(182–194)*. The average concentration of IαI in the plasma of healthy human subjects is approx 450 mg/L *(194)*. Urinary excretion is 2–10 mg/d but can increase to 50–100-fold or more in certain pathological conditions such as cancer. Plasma concentration of IαI is on the other hand reduced during various pathological conditions including renal failure. Several investigators have determined the concentration of bikunin in the normal human urine. Some of the published values are: 0.225–0.650 μg/mL *(189)*, 5.01 ± 0.91 μg/mL *(188)*, 10.13 ± 1.13 μg/mL, and 6.72 ± 0.93 μg/mL in normal men and women respectively *(190)*, 4.82 ± 2.46 mg/d and 3.86 ± 1.35 mg/d in normal men and women respectively *(191)*, and 17.5 mg/d *(195)*. It has been suggested that most of these values are overestimations because quantification employed immunoassays using polyclonal antibodies against bikunin. Such antibodies will cross react with all bikunin containing members of IαI family and thus actually overestimate the concentration of free bikunin in the samples.

As we mentioned above, bikunin excretion is generally increased in the urine of patients with renal disease. As a result an increase in CaOx inhibitory activity is anticipated. However, this was not the case, suggesting that bikunin obtained from stone formers may be structurally abnormal. It was shown that bikunin isolated from the patients, contained less sialic acid and exhibited less crystallization inhibitory activity than that purified from the urine of healthy subject *(186)*. In a separate study mean urinary bikunin to creatinine ratio was found to be significantly higher in stone formers than in nonstone forming healthy male and female controls *(187)*. Western analysis showed that a significantly higher proportion of stone patients had a 25 kDa bikunin in their urine in addition to the normal 40 kDa species. The 25 kDa bikunin was similar to the deglycosylated bikunin and was less inhibitory. Yet another study found decreased urinary excretion of bikunin by stone forming patients. Mean urinary excretion of bikunin in 18 healthy individuals was 5.01 ± 0.91 μg/mL and 2.54 ± 0.42 μg/mL ($p = 0.007$) in 31 stone patients *(188)*.

With respect to kidney stone formation, Atmani et al. isolated a 35 kDa urinary protein, which inhibited growth of CaOx crystals. They named the protein uronic acid rich protein (UAP), because of the high uronic acid content: D-glucuronic and L-iduronic acids being major constituents *(182)*. Amino acid composition revealed it to be rich in aspartic and glutamic acid residues, which account for 24% of the total amino acids. No Gla residues were detected. Basic and aromatic amino acids represented 10% and 13%. Carbohydrates accounted for 8.5% of its weight. N-terminal amino acid sequence analysis of human protein demonstrated the homology with IαI, specifically with bikunin *(183)*. Later we isolated the UAP from the rat urine *(184)* and showed it to have characteristics similar to the human UAP in molecular weight, amino acid composition as well as the crystallization inhibitory activity. In addition, on Western blot analysis, both reacted with an inter-α-trypsin inhibitor antibody. Later on the basis of bikunin antibody reaction with the UAP in Western blot analysis and similarity of the sequence of first 25 N-terminal amino acid residues of UAP being identical to that of bikunin we identified the UAP as bikunin *(185)*.

IαI proteins have been shown to inhibit CaOx crystallization in vitro *(182–185,188, 189,193,195)*. The inhibitory activity is confined to the carboxy terminal of the bikunin fragment of IαI *(195)*. Both rat and human urinary bikunin inhibited nucleation and growth of CaOx crystals. Treatment with chondroitinase AC had no effect on this inhibitory activity, which was destroyed by pronase treatment indicating that the activity lies not with the chondroitin chain but with the peptide. In an in vitro experiment nucleation and aggregation of CaOx crystals were studied by measuring turbidity at 620 nm *(196)*. Crystallization was induced by mixing calcium chloride and sodium oxalate at final concentrations of 3 and 0.5 m*M*, respectively. Both solutions were buffered with 0.05 *M*

Tris, 0.15 M NaCl, pH 6.5. Nucleation measurements were performed at 37°C, with stirring at 800 rpm. Inhibition of nucleation was estimated by comparing the induction time in the presence or absence of the inhibitor. In the aggregation assay, the optical density of the solution containing CaOx monohydrate crystals was monitored. Inhibition of aggregation was evaluated by comparing the turbidity slope in the presence of the inhibitor with control values. The data showed that urinary bikunin, at concentrations of 2.5–20 µg/mL, retarded crystal nucleation by 67–58% and inhibited crystal aggregation by 59–80%. These results were confirmed later when inhibition of CaOx crystal growth and aggregation by IαI, its heavy chains, light chain (bikunin) with or without chondroitinase treatment, and bikunin's carboxy terminal domain (HI 8) was tested in an in vitro crystallization assay (195). IαI was a weak inhibitor whereas heavy chains showed no discernable activity. Bikunin and HI 8 effectively inhibited the crystallization. Chondroitinase treatment had no effect on the inhibitory activity of bikunin. IαI molecule itself is also an effective inhibitor of CaOx crystal growth (185) and in a recent study was shown to be more efficient than another crystal growth inhibitor, prothrombin fragment-1 (189).

Bikunin has also been implicated in modulating adhesion of CaOx crystals to the renal epithelial cells (197). MDCK cells were exposed in culture to CaOx monohydrate crystals in the presence or absence of various protein fractions isolated from normal human urine. A single fraction with a molecular weight of 35 kDa was found to be most inhibitory of crystal adhesion. This protein inhibited crystal adhesion at the minimum concentration of 10 ng/mL and completely blocked it at 200 ng/mL. Amino acid sequence of the first 20 amino acids of the N-terminal was structurally homologous with bikunin.

α1-Microglobulin (α1-m) is also an inhibitor of CaOx crystallization in vitro (198). α1-M was isolated from human urine. Two species of 30 and 60 kDa, recognized by the antibody against α1-m, were isolated. Both inhibited CaOx crystallization in a dose dependent manner. Using an ELISA assay, urinary concentration of α1-m was found to be significantly lower in 31 CaOx stone formers than in 18 healthy subjects (2.95 ± 0.29 vs 5.34 ± 1.08 mg/L respectively, $p = 0.01$).

Recent studies have provided evidence that CaOx stone-forming men excrete significantly more IαI and IαLI in their urine than age and race matched nonstone-forming men (199). The increased expression was not limited to CaOx stone forming males. Uric acid stone formers demonstrated similar tendencies. In contrast high molecular weight IαI related proteins were common in both stone forming and nonstone-forming women. When urinary proteins were resolved by SDS-PAGE, the relative density of IαI was approx threefold greater in females than in males (200). Male children ($\leq$10 yr) excreted two- to sevenfold higher amounts of the high molecular weight IαI than the adult males (201). Because stones are much more common in adult males than in females, it was argued that perhaps urinary excretion of these high molecular weight IαI macromolecules was somehow responsible for the difference and that it was influenced by the sex hormones. However a comparison between normal male adults, male adults undergoing androgen deprivation, and/or postmenopausal females on estrogen therapy showed that there were no differences in the relative levels of urinary IαI among various groups of age and sex matched individuals (201).

OSTEOPONTIN

Diverse functions and widespread distribution of OPN have recently been reviewed (14,202,203). OPN is a noncollagenous phosphoprotein originally isolated from mineralized bone matrix where it is made by osteoblasts. Its apparent molecular weight has been estimated from 44 to 75 kDa depending on the percentage of polyacrylamide gel used. This anomalous migration is assumed to be owing to differences in glycosylation and phosphorylation. In addition to its existence as a monomeric form, the protein may also aggregate to form a higher molecular weight entity.

Amino acid analysis of rat OP revealed that it contains 319 residues of which 36% are aspartic and glutamic acid *(202,204)*. It also contains 30 serine, 12 phosphoserine, and 1 phosphothreonine residues. None of the glutamic acid residues are γ-carboxylated. The carbohydrate content represents 16.6% with the presence of 10 sialic acid residues per molecule. The presence of mannose and *N*-acetylgalactose suggests an N and O-linked oligosaccharides respectively. One interesting part in the structure of OPN is the identification of the sequence Arg-Gly-Asp (RGD), which is presumed to be involved in cell attachment via $\alpha_v\beta_3$ integrin receptors. In close proximity to the RGD region is a thrombin cleavage site. Thrombin cleaves OPN into two fragments, an amino (N)-terminal fragment with RGD sequence and a carboxyl (C)-terminal fragment. OPN affects cell functions through its receptors, the members of integrin and CD 44 families *(205,206)*. The thrombin cleavage of OPN allows for greater access of the RGD domain to the receptor sites. Osteopontin from all species has high aspartate/asparagine contents accounting for as much as 16–20% of all amino acid residues in the molecule. This highly negatively charged molecule can chelate 50 calcium ions/molecule of protein *(207)*.

In addition to bone cells, OPN is present in many epithelial tissues in kidneys, gastrointestinal tract, gall bladder, pancreas, lung, salivary gland, and inner ear *(203)*. It is also expressed in a variety of other cell types including macrophages *(208,209)*, activated T cells, smooth muscle cells and endothelial cells. Regulation of OPN expression, synthesis and production is incompletely understood but is considered to be controlled by a variety of factors such as parathyroid hormone, vitamin D, CaP, various growth factors, cytokines, sex hormones, and a variety of drugs *(14,202,203)*. For example mediators of acute inflammation such as tumor necrosis factor-α (TNFα) *(210)* and interleuken-1β *(211)* induce OPN expression. Other mediators that can induce OPN expression are angiotensin-II and transforming growth factor-β (TGF-β). OPN expression is enhanced in the injury and recovery processes including inflammation, fibrosis, mineralization and regeneration.

Localization studies in mouse kidney by immunohistochemistry and *in situ* hybridization have shown that the expression of OPN is somewhat heterogeneous *(212,213)*. OPN was detected in thick and thin ascending limb of the loop of Henle and distal convoluted tubules and macula densa. It was prominent along the apical surface of the cells lining the lumen. The expression of the protein becomes stronger in pregnant or lactating female mice *(213)*. In aging mice this expression was extended from its normal distal locations to proximal locations including glomeruli. The expression of OPN mRNA was not detected in proximal tubules, thin descending limbs, collecting ducts or glomeruli. Recent studies in rats have shown that OPN is localized to thin limbs of the loop of Henle as well as the papillary surface epithelium in the calyceal fornix *(47,214)*. In normal human kidneys OPN is localized primarily to the thick ascending limb of the Henle's Loop and distal convoluted tubules *(215)*. Apparently the expression of OPN in normal kidneys is species, age and gender dependent.

The mean OPN excretion for normal humans varies between 2.4 and 3.7 mg/d *(216)* or 1.9 µg/mL *(217)*, is inversely related to urinary volume and is not affected by urinary excretion of calcium. Urinary OPN was originally isolated as a glycoprotein with a molecular weight of approx 50 kDa on 16% SDS-polyacrylamide gel. It showed a structural homology with OPN and was named uropontin based on its origin from kidney and presence in the urine *(218)*. Stone formers excrete less OPN than nonstone formers, presumably because of the incorporation of OPN in crystals of the growing stone *(219)*. The significantly higher incidence of a single base mutation in the OPN gene has been found in the patients with recurrent or familial nephrolithiasis *(220)*.

OPN is intimately involved in both the physiological and pathological mineralization processes including crystallization in the urine and development of calcific kidney stones. Experiments with hyperoxaluric rats have provided convincing evidence for an association between CaOx crystal deposition and OPN expression. Experimentally induced hyperoxaluria is almost always associated with increased epithelial expression of OPN *(47,152,221)*, which co-localizes with CaOx crystal deposits *(47,221)*. In a recent study hyperoxaluria and CaOx crystal deposition was induced in male Sprague-Dawley rats. Immunohistochemical localization, *in situ* hybridization and reverse transcriptase quantitative competitive polymerase chain reaction (RTPCR) were employed to examine OPN expression in the kidneys. Urinary excretion of OPN was investigated by sodium dodecyl sulfate-polyacrylamide gel electrophoresis (SDS-PAGE), western blotting and densitometric analysis of the Western blots. OPN expression increased significantly after hyperoxaluria and increased even further after crystal deposition *(222)*. Urinary excretion concomitantly increased. Although there was an increase in the expression of OPN during hyperoxaluria, it was primarily limited to cells of the thin loops of Henle and the papillary surface epithelium. However after crystal deposition OPN was expressed throughout the kidneys including segments of the proximal tubules. A number of compounds such as citrate *(223)*, allopurinol *(224)*, and female sex hormones *(225)* have been shown to reduce CaOx crystal deposition in kidneys of hyperoxaluric rats. Administration of these compounds also reduced OPN expression in the hyperoxaluric rats leading the authors to conclude that reduction in crystal deposition may also be a result of down regulation of OPN synthesis and secretion.

Support for the concept of oxalate and CaOx crystal induced up regulation of OPN is also derived from tissue culture studies. Exposure of MDCK or BSC-1 cells to CaOx monohydrate crystals stimulated the production of OPN *(226)*. Similarly when human renal proximal tubular epithelial cells were exposed to 1mM total oxalate there was a significant increase in OPN mRNA *(227)*.

OPN is a potent inhibitor of nucleation *(228,229)*, growth and aggregation of CaOx crystals *(230)*. OPN is also a regulator of crystal adherence to cell surfaces, which may lead to crystal retention within the kidneys, an important aspect of stone formation. Recently it was demonstrated that OPN also inhibits the adhesion of CaOx monohydrate as well brushite crystals to BSC-1 renal epithelial cells in culture *(60)*. Adhesion inhibition was accomplished by coating the crystal surfaces and not the cell surfaces. Interestingly OPN has no effect on adhesion of uric acid crystals in similar assays using BSC-1 renal epithelial cell line. Other studies have however, shown that OPN promotes adhesion of CaOx crystals to the renal epithelial cells. Exposure of MDCK cells to CaOx crystals in the presence of added OPN promoted crystal adherence to the cells *(231)*. On the other hand removal of OPN from the culture medium by adding OPN polyclonal antibody, thrombin, cyclic Arg-Gly-Asp peptides, or tunicamycin-inhibited crystal adherence by 80%, 50–80%, 60–80%, or 50–60% respectively. Inhibition of OPN synthesis by NRK-52E cells transfected with antisense OPN expression vector resulted in decreased adherence of CaOx crystals *(232)*. Similarly inhibition of OPN production by MDCK cells by introducing antisense oligonucleotide also resulted in decreased crystal adherence *(233)*.

Support for the CaOx crystallization inhibitory actions of OPN is further strengthened by studies in OPN knockout mice *(234)*. When comparable hyperoxaluria is induced in OPN knockout and wild-type mice, knockout mice developed significant intratubular deposition of CaOx crystals whereas wild-type remained free of any crystals. In addition wild-type hyperoxaluric mice showed significant increase in OPN expression in their kidneys, indicating a reno-protective role for OPN.

Results of one study show OPN favoring crystallization of COD over COM *(235)*, which may influence the development of kidney stones because renal epithelium is more likely to bind COM crystals than the COD crystals.

It appears that structural defects, and various post-translational modifications, such as glycosylation and phosphorylation may influence the effect of OPN on crystallization in urine.

URINARY PROTHROMBIN FRAGMENT-1(UPTF-1)

A protein with a molecular weight of 31 kDa was found selectively associated with CaOx crystals experimentally induced in human urine *(236)*. This protein was called crystal matrix protein (CMP). The amino acid sequence analysis of CMP showed an identity with prothrombin *(237–239)*, a plasma protein involved in coagulation cascade. In the presence of different activation factors, prothrombin (PT) is subjected to a series of cleavages releasing small fragments including fragment 1 (F1) and F1+2. Prothrombin as well as fragments 1 and 2 has been detected in the urine. Suzuki et al. proposed that CMP is the activation peptide of human prothrombin *(239)*. By using specific antibodies for prothrombin and F1+2 fragment, Stapleton and Ryall demonstrated *(238)* that CMP is prothrombin fragment F1 (UPTF-1). The mean value of daily urinary fragment F1 excretion is 13.4 nM/d as estimated by using radioimmunoassay technique *(240)*. Excretion is increased in pregnant women to 47.2 nM/d. F1 fragment contains about 154 amino acids of which 23% are glutamic and aspartic acids *(241)*. In the first 34 amino acid residues, 10 of the glutamic acids are γ-carboxylated. The carbohydrate contents represent 17% of its molecular weight.

Anderson and coworker reported the localization of PT exclusively in the liver *(242)*. Stapleton et al. using a polyclonal antibody found a positive reaction in the kidneys *(243)*. The staining was localized in cytoplasm of the epithelial cells of thick ascending limb of the loop of Henle and the distal convoluted tubules including the macula densa. The amount of F1 was significantly increased in the kidneys of stone patients compared to those in healthy subjects *(244)*. Recent studies have provided evidence that PT gene is expressed in both the human and rat kidneys indicating the possibility of PT biosynthesis in both human and rat kidneys *(245–247)*.

Recent studies using purified urinary proteins have confirmed earlier results and have demonstrated UPTF-1 to be an inhibitor of both crystal growth and aggregation *(248)*. Results of another study where a comparison was made between the white and black South Africans with regard to urinary crystallization inhibition showed that UPTF-1 is a strong inhibitor of crystal nucleation *(249)*. UPTF-1 from normal black males reduced crystal nucleation by 63.6% as compared to the protein from normal white males that reduced the nucleation by 23.4%. When crystallization inhibitory potential of all the prothrombin related peptides, the PT, thrombin (T), and fragments

1 and 2 was tested using a simple inorganic solution, both prothrombin and fragment 1 were found to inhibit crystal aggregation *(250)*. Various peptides reduced the size of aggregates in the order F1>PT>F2>T. However when similar experiments were conducted using undiluted, centrifuged and ultrafiltered human urine *(251)*, crystal aggregation was inhibited only by PT fragment-1.

The crystallization inhibitory activity depends on the Gla domain, which is absent from thrombin and F2, but both PT as well as F1 fragments include *(251)*. Why is F1 more potent than PT? Probably as a result of F1's greater charge to mass ratio. Prothrombin has the same number of Gla residues as F1 but a molecular weight of 72 kDa, which is more than double that of F1 at approx 31 kDa. Prothrombin's isoelectric point is also higher.

CALGRANULIN (CALPROTECTIN)

Calgranulin is a 28 kDa member of S100 family of calcium binding proteins, which are small, ubiquitous, and acidic proteins involved in normal developmental and structural activities *(252)*. However they are also implicated in a number of diseases *(253)*. The protein was recently isolated from human urine *(254)* at a concentration of 3.5–10 n*M*. Purified urinary calgranulin inhibited both CaOx crystal growth (44%) and aggregation (50%) in nanomolar range. A 28 kDa calgranulin was cloned from the human kidney expression library. Western analysis of rat and human kidneys as well as renal epithelial cell lines, BSC-1 and MDCK confirmed its renal presence. Calgranulin is also known as leukocyte antigen L1 and has been identified in circulating neutrophils and monocytes and has bacteriostatic antifungal activity *(255)*. It has also been identified in matrix of infectious or struvite stones *(256)*.

ALBUMIN

Albumin is a one of the most abundant proteins in the urine *(19,46,257)* and has been detected in the matrix of both urinary stones *(18,19,257)* as well as crystals *(43,44, 258)* made in the whole human urine. It is known to bind to CaOx as well as uric acid crystals *(259,260)* but does not inhibit their growth *(143,259)*. However it has been shown to inhibit CaOx crystal aggregation in concentration dependent manner *(261– 263)*. When immobilized to surfaces and exposed to metastable solutions albumin promotes crystal nucleation *(264,265)*. When dissolved in solution albumin exists either in monomeric or and polymeric form *(264)*. In metastable CaOx solutions both monomeric and polymeric forms promote nucleation of CaOx. In addition, nucleation by albumin leads exclusively to the formation of COD crystals. Urinary albumin purified from healthy subjects contained significantly more polymeric forms and was a stronger promoter of CaOx nucleation than albumin from idiopathic calcium stone formers. Promotion of CaOx nucleation and formation of large number of COD crystals might be protective. Nucleation of large number of small crystals would allow their easy elimination and decrease CaOx saturation preventing crystal growth and aggregation and subsequent stone formation. COD crystals are more common than COM crystals in nonstone formers urine and are generally found in lesser quantities in stones than COM crystals. In addition crystals present in the urine from nonstone formers are significantly smaller than those in stone formers urine. Albumin also exhibits the capacity to bind some of the urinary proteins. Interestingly, urinary proteins that show great affinity for albumin are also those that are included in the stone matrix. It is suggested that proteins become a part of stone matrix by binding to the albumin coating CaOx crystals.

It is also suggested that unlike other calcium binding urinary proteins, albumin promotes nucleation by interacting with calcium through the carboxyl group. Strong nucleation activity was observed at pH 7 but was totally eliminated at pH 4 when carboxyl groups are no longer ionized. In addition, morphological studies showed CaOx crystals to nucleate through calcium rich face *(264)*.

MODEL PEPTIDES

A number of studies have been carried out investigating the effect of model peptides on crystallization in vitro. Polyaspartic acid (PolyD) with molecular weights of 8, 12, 15, and 37.6 and ployglutamic acids (PolyE) with molecular weight of 13 have been examined. A clear understanding of the crystallization inhibitory mechanisms of various glycoproteins has been the main purpose of these studies. Crystallization of CaOx was induced in vitro in a buffered salt solution containing calcium and oxalate in different ratios and at various supersaturations, in the absence or presence of the polypeptides with pH and ionic strength in the range of normal human urine *(235,266,267)*. In the absence of proteins, CaOx monohydrate was the preferred crystalline form for all Ca to Ox ratios *(266,267)*. The number of CaOx monohydrate crystals increased with increasing oxalate concentrations. The presence of either the Poly D or E produced COD crystals. PolyE was less effective at producing COD than PolyD *(267)*. At a concentration of 800 nM and equimolar Ca and Ox concentrations only 20% of the crystals were CODs. It did however have an effect on COM crystal morphology by producing dumbbell shaped crystals, a morphology common in human and rat urine. Under similar conditions of supersaturation and Ca and Ox concentrations PolyD, however, favored the formation of COD requiring very low concentrations <200 nM. A 12, 15, and 37.6 molecular weight PolyD were able to exclusively produce almost all CODs. Higher CaOx supersaturations required higher amounts of PolyD to cause COD formation. It is concluded that change from COM to COD is the result of inhibition of COM nucleation by protein adsorption onto nascent nuclei. COD is formed to relieve the chemical potential favoring crystallization. The importance of these results with regard to nephrolithiasis lies in the observations that COD crystals are less likely to adhere to the renal epithelium than COM crystals and thus less likely to be retained in the kidneys and promote the formation of kidney stones *(267)*.

Both PolyD and PolyE have also been tested for their effect on COM crystal growth and adherence to renal epithelial cells in culture. Both proved potent inhibitors of the growth of COM crystals and also blocked the adhesion of COM to BSC-1 cells *(60)*.

Lipids and Cellular Membranes

The role of cellular membranes and their lipids in both physiological and pathological calcification is well-established *(268–270)*. According to current concepts, initial CaP deposition in a number of calcific diseases occurs on cellular membranes, which are present at the calcification sites either as a limiting membrane of the so called matrix vesicles *(269,270)* or as cellular degradation products *(268)*. One of the main reasons that cellular membranes act as specific nucleators of CaP is proposed to be the presence of lipids and in particular the acidic phospholipids. Lipids have been demonstrated both histochemically and biochemically at physiological as well as pathological calcification sites. In vitro, membranes, acidic phospholipids, lipid extracts from various calcified tissues, as well as lipid containing liposomes have been shown to initiate CaP formation from metastable solutions.

Small amounts of lipids appear in urine under normal circumstances, whereas urinary excretion of cholesterol, phospholipids, triglycerides and free fatty acids is increased in many diseases *(271)*. Many of the lipids may be of membrane origin because epithelial cells are continuously sloughed and excreted by both normal human males and females *(272)*. Biochemical analysis discloses that urine from stone formers contain more and different phospholipids than that from normal humans *(273)*. Human urine is metastable with respect to the common calcific crystals, CaOx and CaP, i.e. urine would require a substrate or a nucleation platform for crystallization to occur. Membrane vesicles and fragments with their lipids provide a suitable site for crystal nucleation. Membranous vesicles obtained from the brush border of the rat renal tubular epithelium *(274)* and lipid components of the human stone matrix are good nucleators of CaOx from an inorganic metastable solution *(275)*. When CaOx crystallization was induced in whole human urine by the addition of oxalate, CaOx crystals appeared in association with the cellular membranes and almost all phospholipids present in the urine became a part of the crystal matrix *(33)*. To verify that cellular membranes present in the urine promote nucleation of CaOx we removed these urinary constituents by filtration or centrifugation and induced crystallization by adding oxalate before and after filtration or centrifugation *(276)*. We also performed reconstitution studies in which substances such as total retentate, proteins, total lipids, neutral lipids, and phospholipids, which are removed during filtration, were added back into the filtered urine before induction of nucleation. In addition, we examined CaOx crystallization after membrane vesicles isolated from rat renal tubular brush border were introduced into the filtered or centrifuged urine. We also determined urinary metastable limit with respect to CaOx. Both filtration and centrifugation resulted in a significant increase in metastable limit, which was reduced by the addition of membrane vesicles. Filtration resulted in a significant reduction in the number of crystals formed. A highly significant increase occurred when various components were added back into the filtered urine. The highest and most significant increase occurred when phospholipids were added back into the filtered urine.

To understand crystallization in the kidneys one has to appreciate the following. (1) Urine spends only a few minutes (approx 3 min) in the renal tubules *(9,277)* and only seconds in various segments *(76)*. (2) Urinary composition, pH, and supersaturation with regard to CaOx and CaP changes as urine courses through the renal tubules *(277–279)*. Urine in the loop of Henle can support nucleation of CaP whereas in the distal tubules and collecting ducts urine is susceptible to nucleation of CaOx. With this in mind, we studied crystallization of CaOx in vitro *(278)*. Nucleation was allowed to occur in vitro in solutions with ionic concentrations simulating urine in various segments of the renal tubules namely proximal tubules, descending and ascending limbs of the loop of Henle, distal tubules and collecting ducts. A constant composition system was used and experiments were run for 2 h with or without the added renal brush border membrane vesicles (BBM). The addition of BBM significantly reduced the nucleation lag time and increased the rate of crystallization. The average nucleation lag time decreased from 84.6 ± 43.4 min to 24.5 ± 19 min in proximal tubule urine, from 143.6 ± 29 to $70.2 + 53.4$ min in descending limb of the loop of Henle urine, from 17.6 ± 8.6 min to 0.625 ± 0.65 min in distal tubules urine, and from 9.54 ± 3.03 min to 0.625 ± 0.65 min in collecting duct urine. There was no nucleation without BBM in the urine from ascending limb of the Henle's loop. COD was common in most solutions. CaP also nucleated in the urine in descending limb of the loop and collecting duct. In the absence of BBM there was no crystallization in any of the solutions within the time frame that urine generally spends in the renal tubules indicating the unlikelihood of homogeneous crystal nucleation in the renal tubules. In addition, whole urine contains many crystallization inhibitors which should make it even more difficult. However BBM-supported nucleation is likely in both distal tubules and collecting ducts because in these segments nucleation lag time for CaOx was much shorter than the urine residence time.

It is suggested that anionic head groups of membrane lipids when exposed to urine attract Ca^{2+} ions. A cluster of sufficient number of properly aligned Ca^{2+} ions can then interact with oxalate or phosphate leading to nucleation of CaOx or CaP crystals (280,281). In vitro crystallization studies with Langmuir monolayers of phospholipids have demonstrated selective nucleation of CaOx monohydrate crystals with the (10–1) calcium rich face towards the monolayer (282–285). Normal membranes do not expose many anionic head groups on their surfaces. Catastrophic events can however, induce both lateral and transpremembrane migration of phospholipids and sequester them in specific domains (286). Exposure to high levels of calcium and oxalate, a most likely event because increased urinary excretion of oxalate and calcium is common in stone formers, induces several changes in the renal epithelial cell membrane. Oxalate and CaOx crystals induce redistribution of PS from the inner leaflet of the membrane to the outside (287–289) and high levels of calcium (290) partition them in specific domains. Vesicles derived from these membranes would be capable of supporting crystallization in the urine metastable for CaP and CaOx.

Altered membrane properties that support crystal nucleation can also provide for crystal attachment to the renal epithelium (286) as well as crystal aggregation (8,281). Crystal binding to membrane fragments flowing in the urine would promote crystal aggregation. This is evident in vivo from the observations that urine from hyperoxaluric rat shows crystals aggregating around and associated with membrane fragments (8). Binding of crystals with their calcium rich face to negatively charged cell membrane of the renal epithelium would possibly promote crystal adhesion and retention within the renal tubules. PS has been thoroughly studied as a crystal adhesion molecule on cell surfaces. There was a dose dependent increase in the cell surface PS when continuous cultures of the inner medullary collecting duct were exposed to oxalate (286,287). Increased surface expression of PS correlated with a corresponding increase in CaOx monohydrate crystal attachment to the cells. Crystal attachment was inhibited by treatment with Annexin V, a protein that specifically binds to PS. In addition insertion of PS into the cell membranes promoted crystal attachment. The possibility of PS associated attachment of CaOx crystals is highly feasible in the kidneys of stone formers. Renal epithelial cells exposed to high levels of oxalate and/or CaOx crystals undergo apoptosis (288) in which PS moves from inside to outside of the membrane and thus becomes exposed to the urinary environment.

Further evidence of the role of cellular membrane constituents in urolithiasis is provided by investigations of human and experimental nephrolithiasis. Experimental studies of CaOx urolithiasis induced in laboratory rats have shown that irrespective of the nature of the hyperoxaluria inducing agent used, the administration protocol used, or the location of crystal deposition within the urinary system, CaOx crystals were always found associated with cellular degradation products consisting mostly of membrane bound vesicles (8,291,292). Even when a foreign body was implanted in the urinary bladder of hyperoxaluric rats, crystals did not nucleate on the native foreign body but on the membranous organic material that coated the foreign body surface (293).

Intranephronic calculosis in the laboratory rat caused by feeding a purified diet is membrane mediated *(294,295)*. Vesicles derived from the microvillus brush border of the proximal tubules provide the nidus for intratubular deposition of CaP. The deposits start in the lumens of segment I of the proximal tubule and travel down the nephron while at the same time accrued mass by laminar growth in which both membranous vesicles and mineral are involved. Finally these microliths become large enough to be retained at the junction of the proximal tubule and the loop of Henle. The mineral content of the microliths increases with the result that they become much more compact and the laminated structure is finally lost.

In the case of human nephrolithiasis, a number of renal stones start at the tips of renal papillae on sites called Randall's plaques *(30,296)*. These plaques contain cellular degradation products and crystals of CaP. Stones formed on such plaques, were once thought to be rare but a study of five hundred spontaneously passed small stones, collected in Spain by Cifuentes-Delatte, has shown that 142 (28.4%) of them contained nidi of necrotic material identifiable as calcified tips of the renal papillae *(297)*. The results indicate that at least in these cases the stones could have originated by heterogeneous nucleation of crystals on the membranous cellular degradation products.

SUMMARY

Urine contains compounds that modulate the nucleation, growth and aggregation of crystals as well as their attachment to renal epithelial cells. These compounds may function to protect the kidneys against; (1) the possibility of crystallization in tubular fluid and urine, which are generally metastable with respect to calcium salts, and (2) crystal retention within the kidneys thereby preventing stone formation. Because oxalate is the most common stone type, effect of various modulators on CaOx crystallization has been examined in greater details. Most of the inhibitory activity resides in macromolecules such as glycoproteins and glycosaminoglycans whereas nucleation promotion activity is most likely sustained by membrane lipids. Nephrocalcin, Tamm-Horsfall protein, osteopontin, urinary prothrombin fragment 1, and bikunin are the best studied inhibitory proteins, whereas CS, HS, and HA are the best studied glycosaminoglycans. Most of the inhibitory molecules are anionic, with many acidic amino acid residues, frequently contain post-translational modifications such as phosphorylation and glycosylation, and appear to exert their effects by binding to CaOx surface. In a number of cases, stone patients exhibit abnormalities of protein structure or function. It is not yet known what proportion of stone formers have an abnormality of inhibitor function. The specific structural motifs that favor crystal nucleation, binding and inhibition are not yet fully understood. Lipid head groups appear to be involved in crystal nucleation.

A number of the proteins and glycosaminoglycans are produced in the kidneys. Some glycosaminoglycans are added to the urine in the bladder. Still others gain access by glomerular filtration. Recent tissue culture and animal model studies demonstrate that exposure of renal epithelial cells to high levels of oxalate and CaOx crystals upregulates the expression and production of many glycoproteins such as bikunin, osteopontin, and Tamm-Horsfall protein. The presence of lipids in the urine is an outcome of death and degradation of renal epithelial cells caused by exposure to high levels of urinary oxalate and CaOx crystals.

Further information on regulation of expression of these macromolecules and their activities in the specific microenvironment may provide new avenues for the prevention and recurrence of stone formation.

REFERENCES

1. Kok DJ. Clinical implications of physicochemistry of stone formation. Endocrinol Metab Clin N Am 2002; 31: 1–13.
2. Coe FL, Parks JH. Pathophysiology of kidney stones and strategies for treatment. Hospital Practice 1988; 23: 185–216.
3. Finlayson B. Physicochemical aspects of urolithiasis. Kid Intl 1978; 13: 344–360.
4. Finlayson B. Calcium Stones: Some physical and clinical aspects. In: Calcium Metabolism in Renal Failure and Nephrolithiasis, (David DS, ed.). Wiley, New York, NY, 1977; pp. 337–382.
5. Finlayson B, Khan SR, Hackett RL. Theoretical chemical models of urinary stone. In: Renal Tract Stone - Metabolic Basis and Clinical Practice, (Wickham JEA, Colin Buck A, eds.). Churchill Livingston, New York, NY, 1990; pp. 133–147.
6. Robertson WG, Peacock M. Calcium oxalate crystalluria and inhibitors of crystallisation in recurrent renal stone-formers. Clin Sci 1972; 43: 499–506.
7. Hallson PC, Rose GA. Crystalluria in normal subjects and stone formers with and without thiazide and cellulose phosphate treatment. Br J Urol 1976; 48: 515–524.
8. Khan SR Experimental calcium oxalate nephrolithiasis and the formation of human urinary stones. Scann Microsc 1995; 9(1): 89–101.
9. Kok DJ. Khan, S.R.:Calcium oxalate nephrolithiasis, a free or fixed particle disease. Kid Intl 1994; 46: 847–854.
10. Randall A. The etiology of primary renal calculus. Intl Abst Surg 1940; 71: 209–240.
11. Mckee MD. Nanci, A., Khan, S.R.: Ultrastructural immunodetection of osteopontin and osteocalcin as major matrix components of renal calculi. J Bone Mineral Res 1994; 10: 1913–1929.
12. de Water R, Noordermeer C, Kok DJ, et al. Calcium oxalate nephrolithiasis: Effect of renal crystal deposition on the cellular composition of the renal interstitium. Am J Kidney Dis 1999; 33: 761–771.
13. de Water R, Noordermeer C, Houtsmuller AB, Kok DJ, Nizze H, Schröder FH. The role of macrophages in Nephrolithiasis in rats: An analysis of the renal interstitium. Am J Kidney Dis 2000; 36: 615–625.
14. Umekawa T, Chegini N, Khan SR. Oxalate ions and calcium oxalate crystals stimulate MCP-1 expression by renal epothelial cells. Kid Intl 2002; 61: 105–112.
15. Xie YS, Sakatsume M, Nishi S, Narita I, Arakawa M, Gejyo F. Expression, roles, receptors, and regulation of osteopontin in the kidney. Kidney Int 2001; 60: 1645–1657.
16. Khan SR, Hackett RL. Identification of urinary stone and sediment crystals by scanning microscopy and x-ray microanalysis, J Urol 1987; 135: 818–825.
17. Lowenstam HA, Weiner S. On Biomineralization. Oxford University Press, New York, Oxford, 1989.
18. Boyce WH, Garvey FK. The amount and nature of the organic matrix in urinary calculi: a review. J Urol 1956; 76: 213–227.
19. Boyce WH. Organic matrix of human urinary concretions. Am J Med 1968; 45, 673–683.
20. Boyce WH. Some observations on the ultrastructure of idiopathic human renal calculi. In: Urolithiasis: Physical Aspects, (Finlayson B, Hench LL, Smith LH, eds.). National Academy of Sciences, Washington, DC, 1972; pp. 97–130.
21. Iwata H, Kamei O, Abe Y, et al. The organic matrix of urinary uric acid crystals. J Urol 1988; 139: 607–610.
22. Khan SR, Hackett RL. Role of organic matrix in urinary stone formation; an ultrastructural study of crystal matrix interface of calcium oxalate monohydrate stones. J Urol 1993; 15: 239–245.
23. Vermeulen CW, Lyon ES. Mechanisms of genesis and growth of calculi. Am J Med 1956; 45: 684–691.
24. Finlayson B, Vermeulen CW, Stewart EJ. Stone matrix and mucoprotein in urine. J Urol 1961; 86: 355–362.
25. Leal JJ, Finlayson B. Adsorption of naturally occurring polymers onto calcium oxalate crystal surfaces. Invest Urol 1977; 14: 278–281.
26. Khan SR, Finalyson B, Hackett RL. Stone matrix as proteins adsorbed on crystal surfaces: a microscopic study. Scanning Electron Microsc 1983; 1, 379–184.

27. Khan SR, Finalyson B, Hackett RL. Agar-embedded urinary stones: a technique useful for studying microscopic architecture. J Urol 1983; 130: 992–995.

28. Khan SR, Shevock PN, Hackett RL. Presence of lipids in urinary stones: results of preliminary studies. Calcified Tissue Intl 1988; 42: 91–95.

29. Khan SR, Hackett RL. Hitochemistry of colloidal iron stained crystal assicyted material in urinary stones and experimentally induced intrarenal deposits in rats. Scanning Electron Microsc 1986; II: 761–765.

30. Khan SR, Finalyson B, Hackett RL. Renal papillary changes in a patient with calcium oxalate lithiasis. Urology 1984; 13: 194–199.

31. Watanabe T. Histochemical studies on mucosubstances in urinary stones. Tohuku J Exp Med 1972; 107: 345–357.

32. Tawada T, Fujite K, Sakakura T, et al. Distributionof oetopontin and calcprotectin as matrix protein in calcium containing stone. 1999; Urol Res 27:238–242.

33. Khan SR, Atmani F, Glenton P, Hou ZC, Talham DR, Khurshid M. Lipids and membranes in the organic matrix of urinary calcific crystals and stones. Calcif. Tissue Int 1996; 59, 357–365.

34. Morse RM, Resnick MI. A new approach to the sudy of urinary macromlecules as a participant in calcium oxalate crystallization. J Urol 1988; 139: 869–872.

35. Morse RM, Resnick MI A study of the incorporation of urinary macromolecule onto crystals of different mineral composition. J Urol 1989; 141: 641–645.

36. Nishio S, Abe Y, Wakatsuki A, et al. Matrxi glycosaminoglycans in urinary stones. J Urol 1985; 134: 503–505.

37. Roberts SD, Resnick MI. Glycosaminoglycans content of stone matrix. J Urol 1986; 135: 1078–1083.

38. Yamaguchi S, Yoshioka T, Utsonomiya M, et al. Heparan sulfate in the stone matrix and its inhibitory effect on calcium oxalate crystallization. Urol Res 1993; 21: 187–192.

39. Suzuki K, Mayne K, Doyle IR, Ryall RL. Urinary glycosaminoglycans are selectively included into calcium oxalate crystals precipitated from whole human urine. Scan Microsc 1994; 8: 523–530.

40. Binette JP, Binette MB, Gawinowicz MA, Kendrick N. Urinary stone proteins: an update. Scanning Microsc 1996; 10: 509–518.

41. Tang Y, Grover PK, Moritz RL, Simpson RJ, Ryall RL. Is nephrocalcin related to the urinary derivative (bikunin) of inter-a-trypsin inhibitor? Br J Urol 1995; 75, 425–430.

42. Boyce WH, King J, Fielden M. Total non-dialyzable solids in human urine. XIII. Immunological detection of a component peculiar to renal calculus matrix and to urine of calculus patients. J Clin Invest 1962; 41: 1180–1189.

43. Atmani F, Glenton PA, Khan SR. Identification of proteins extracted from calcium oxalate and calcium phosphate crystals induced in the urine of healthy and stone forming subjects. Urol Res 1998; 26: 201–207.

44. Atmani F, Khan SR. Quantification of proteins extracted from calcium oxalate and calcium phosphate crystals induced in vitro in the urine of healthy controls and stone-forming patients. Urol Int 2002; 68: 54–59.

45. Grant AMS, Baker LRI, Neuberger A. Urinary Tamm-Horsfall glycoprotein in certain kidney disease and its content in renal and bladder calculi. Clin Sci 1973; 44: 377–384.

46. Maslamani S, Glenton PA, Khan SR. Changes in urine macromolecular composition during processing. J Urol 2000; 164: 230–236.

47. Gokhale JA, Glenton PA, Khan SR. Localization of Tamm-Horsfall protein and osteopontin in a rat nephrolithiasis model. Nephron 1996; 73: 456–461,

48. Gokhale JA, McKee MD, Khan SR. Immunocytochemical localization of Tamm-Horsfall protein in the kidneys of normal and nephrolithic rats. Urol Res 1996; 24:201–209.

49. Hoyer JR. Uropontin in urinary calcium stone formation. Miner Electrolyte Metab 1994; 20: 385–392.

50. Wuthier RE. Lipids of mineralizing epiphyseal tissues in the bovine fetus. J. Lipid Research 1968; 9: 68–79.

51. Boskey AL. Current concepts of physiology and biochemistry of calcification. Clin Orthop 1981; 157:225–257.

52. Anderson HC. Calcific diseases. Arch Pathol Lab Med 1983; 107: 341–348.

53. Slomiany BL, Murty VLN, Aono M, Sarosiek J, Slomiany A, Mandel ID. Lipid composition of the matrix of human submandibular salivary gland stones. Archs Oral Biol 1982; 27: 673–677.

54. Boskey AL, Burstein LS, Mandel ID. Phospholipids associated with human parotid gland sialoliths. Archs. Oral Biol 1983; 28: 655–657.

55. Boskey AL, Boyan-Salyers BD, Burnstein LS, Mandel ID. Lipids associated with mineralization of human submandibular gland sialoliths. Archs Oral Biol 1981; 26: 779–785.

56. Kok DJ, Papapoulos SE, Bijvoet OLM. Excessive crystal agglomeration with low citrate excretion in recurrent stone formers. Lancet 1986; i: 1056–1058.

57. Kok DJ, Papapoulos SE, Bijvoet OLM. Crystal agglomeration is a major element in calcium oxalate urinary stone formation. Kidney Int 1990; 37: 51–56.

58. Verkoelen CF, Romijn JC, Cao LC, Boeve ER, DeBruijn WC, Schröder FH. Crystal-cell interaction inhibition by polysaccharides. J Urol 1996; 155: 749–752.

59. Schepers MSJ, van der Boom BG, Romijn JC, Schröder FH, Verkoelen CF. Urinary crystallization inhibitors do not prevent crystal binding. J Urol 2002; 167: 1844–1847.

60. Lieske JC, Leonard R, Toback FG. Adhesion of calcium-oxalate monohydrate crystals to renal epithelial-cells is inhibited by specific anions. Am J Physiol-Renal Physiol 1995; 268: F604–F612.

61. de Water R, Leenen PJM, Noordermeer C, et al. Macrophages in nephrolithiasis: cytokine production induced by binding and processing of calcium oxalate crystals. Am J Kidney Dis 2001; 38: 331–338.

62. Schwille PO, Rumenapf G, Wolfel G, Kohler R. Urinary pyrophosphate in patients with recurrent urolithiasis and in healthy controls: a reevaluation. J Urol 1988; 140: 239–245.

63. Kok DJ, Papapoulos SE, Blomen LJMJ, Bijvoet OLM. Modulation of Calcium-Oxalate Monohydrate crystallization kinetics in vitro. Kidney Int 1988; 34: 346–350.

64. Ryall RL, Harnett RM, Marshall VR. The effect of urine, pyrophosphate, citrate, magnesium and glycosaminoglycans on the growth and aggregation of calcium oxalate crystals in vitro. Clin Chim Acta 1988; 112: 349–356.

65. Sidhu H, Gupta R, Thind SK, Nath R. Inhibition of calcium oxalate monohydrate crystal growth. Urol Res 1986; 14: 299–303.

66. Grases F, Ramis M, Costa-Bauza A. Effects of phytate and pyrophosphate on brushite and hydroxyapatite crystallization - Comparison with the action of other polyphosphates. Urol Res 2000; 28: 136–140.

67. Robertson WG. Factors affecting the precipitation of calcium phosphate in vitro. Calcif Tissu Res 1973; 11: 311–322.

68. Yuzawa M, Tozuka K, Tokue A. Effect of citrate and pyrophosphate on the stability of calcium oxalate dihydrate. Urol Res 1998; 26: 83–88.

69. Kok DJ. Inhibitors of calcium oxalate crystallization. In: Calcium Oxalate in Biological Systems, Chapter 2, (Khan S.R., ed.). CRC, Boca Raton, FL, 1995; pp. 23–36.

70. Wagner M, Finlayson B. The characteristics of adsorption of pyrophosphate and citrate onto whewellite. Invest Urol 1978; 15: 456–458.

71. Sharma S, Vaidyanathan S, Thind SK, Nath R. Urinary-excretion of inorganic pyrophosphate by normal subjects and patients with renal calculi in north-western India and the effect on Diclodenac sodium upon urinary-excretion of pyrophosphate in stone formers. Urol Int 1992; 48: 404–408.

72. Erturk E, Kiernan M, Schoen SR. Clinical association with urinary glycosaminoglycans and urolithiasis. Urology 2002; 59: 495–499.

73. Laminski NA, Meyers AM, Sonnekus MI, Smyth AE. Prevalence of hypocitraturia and hypopyrophosphaturia in recurrent calcium stone formers: as isolated defects or associated with other metabolic abnormalities. Nephron 1990; 56: 379–386.

74. Russell RGG, Bisaz S, Fleisch H. The influence of orthophosphate on the renal handling of inorganic pyrophosphate in man and dog. Clin Sci Mol Med 1976; 51: 435–443.

75. Breslau NA, Padalino P, Kok DJ, Kim YG, Pak CYC. Physicochemical effects of a new slow-release potassium phosphate preparation (Urophos-K) in absorptive hypercalciuria. J Bone Min Res 1995; 10: 394–400.

76. Kok DJ. Free and fixed particle mechanism, a review. Scanning Electron Microsc 1996; 10: 471–486.

77. Baumann JM, Bisaz S, Fleisch H, Wocker M. Biochemical and clinical effects of EHDP in calcium nephrolithiasis. Clin Sci Mol Med 1978; 54: 509–516.

78. Bone HG III, Zerwekh JE, Britton F, Pak CYC. Treatment of calcium urolithiasis with diphosphonate, efficacy and hazards. J Urol 1979; 121: 568–571.

79. Gruber GB. Harnsteine. In: Handlung der Speziellen Pathologischen Anatomie und Histologie, 1–2. Springer Verlag, Berlin, Germany, 1934; pp. 221–332.

80. Cao LC, Kok DJ, et al. Gags and semisynthetic sulfated polysaccharides: An overview of their potential application in treatment of patients with uro- thiasis. Urology 1997; 50: 173–183.

81. Scurr DS, Latif AB, Sergeant V, Robertson WG. Polyanionic inhibitors of calcium oxalate crystal agglomeration in urine. Proc Eur Dial Transplant Assoc 1983; 136: 128–131.

82. Baggio B, Gambaro G, Cicerello E. Urinary excretion of glycosaminoglycans in urological disease. Clin Biochem 1987; 20: 449, 450.

83. Nikkila MT. Urinary glycosaminoglycan excretion in normal and stone-forming subjects: significant disturbance in recurrent stone formers. Urol Int 1989; 44: 157–159.

84. Gianotti M, Genestar C, Palou A, Pons A, Conte A, Grases F. Investigation of GAGS on 24-hour and 2-hour urines from calcium oxalate stone formers and healthy subjects. Int Urol Nephrol 1989; 21: 281–288.

85. Blumenkrantz N, Asboe-Hansen G. New method for quantitative determination of uronic acid. Anal Biochem 1973; 54: 484–489.

86. Sidhu H, Hemal AK, Thind SK, Nath R, Vaidyanathan S. Comparative study of 24-hour urinary excretion of glycosaminoglycans by renal stone formers and healthy adults. Eur Urol. 1989; 16: 45–47.

87. Nesse A, Garbossa G, Romero MC, Bogado CE, Zanchetta JR. Glycosaninoglycans in urolithiasis. Nephron 1992; 62: 36–39.

88. Michelacci YM, Glashan RQ, Schor N. Urinary excretion of glycosaminoglycans in normal and stone forming subjects. Kidney Int 1989; 36: 1022–1028.

89. Conte A, Roca P, Genestar C, Grases F. Uric acid and its relationship with glycosaminoglycans in normal and stoneformer subjects. Nephron 1989; 52: 162–165.

90. Shum DKY, Gohel MDI. Separate effects of urinary chondrotiinsulphate and heparan sulphate on the crystallization of urinary calcium oxalate: differences between stone formers and normal control subjects. Clin Sci 1993; 85: 33–39.

91. Akcay T, Konukoglu D, Dincer Y. Urinary glycosaminoglycan excretion in urolithiasis. Arch Dis in Childhood, 1999; 80: 271, 272.

92. Robertson WG, Peacock M, Heyburn PJ, Marshall DH, Clark PB. Risk factors in calcium stone disease of the urinary tract. Br J Urol 1978; 50: 449–454.

93. Hesse A, Wuzel H, Vahlensieck W. The excretion of glycosaminoglycans in the urine of calciumoxalate stone patients and healthy persons. Urol Int 1986; 41: 81–87.

94. Caudarella R, Stefani F, Rizzoli E, Malavolta N, D'Antuono G. Preliminary results of glycosaminoglycans excretion in normal and stone forming subjects: relationship with uric acid excretion. J Urol 1983; 129: 665–667.

95. Ryall RL, Marshall VR. The relationship between urinary inhibitory activity and endogenous concentrations of glycosaminoglycans and uric acid: comparison of urines from stone-formers and normal subjects. Clin Chim Acta 1984; 141: 197–204.

96. Ryall RL, Marshall VR. The value of the 23 hour urine analysis in male stone-formers attending a general hospital outpatients clinic. Br J Urol 1983; 55: 1–5.

97. Samuell CT. A study of glycosaminoglycan excretion in normal and stone forming subjects using a modified cetylpyridinium chloride technique. Clin Chim Acta 1981; 117: 63–73.

98. Harangi F, Gyorke Z, Melegh B. Urinary glycosaminoglycan excretion in healthy and stone-forming children. Ped Nephrol 1996; 10: 555–558.

99. Akinci M, Esen T, Kocak T, Ozsoy C, Tellaloglu S. Role of inhibitor deficiency in urolithiasis. I. Rationale of urinary magnesium, citrate, pyrophosphate and glycosaminoglycan determinations. Eur Urol 1991; 19: 240–243.

100. Fellström B, Lindsjö M, Danielson BG, Ljunghall S, Wikström B. Binding of glycosaminoglycans to sodium urate and uric acid crystals. Clin Sci 1986; 71: 61–64.

101. Trinchieri A, Mandressi A, Luongo P, Rovera F, Longo G. Urinary excretion of citrate, glycosaminoglycans, magnesium and zinc in relation to age and sex in normal subjects and in patients who form calcium stones. Scand J Urol Nephrol 1992; 26: 379–386.

102. Sallis JD, Bichler KH, Korn S, Haussman A. Urinary glycosaminoglycan excretion in patients with urolithiasis. In: Urolithiasis: Clinical and Basic Research, (Smith LH, Robertson WG, Finlayson B eds.). Plenum, New York, NY, 1981; pp. 619–622.

103. Edyvane KA, Ryall RL, Marshall VR. The contribution of bladder secretions to the crystal growth inhibitory activity of urine. In: Urinary Stone, (Ryall RL, Brockis JG, Marshall VR, Finlayson B, eds.). Churchill Livingstone, London, UK, 1983; pp. 198–201.

104. Wei DC, Politano VA, Selzer MG, Lokeshwar VB. The association of elevated urinary total to sulfated glycosaminoglycan ratio and high molecular mass hyaluronic acid with interstitial cystitis. J Urol 2000; 163: 1577–1583.

105. Teller WM, Burke EC, Rosevaer JW, McKenzie BF. Urinary excretion of acid mucopolysaccharides in normal children and patients with gargoylism. J Lab Clin Med 1962; 59: 95–101.

106. Rich C, DiFerrante N, Archibald RM. Acid mucopolysaccharide excretion in the urine of children. J Lab Clin Med 1957; 50: 686–695.

107. Winter P, Ganter K, Leppin U, Schoeneich G, Hesse A. Glycosaminoglycans in urine and extracorporeal shock wave lithotripsy. Urol Res 1995; 23: 401–405.

108. Goldberg JM, Cotlier E. Specific isolation and analysis of mucopolysaccharides (glycosaminoglycans) from human urine. Clin Chim Acta 1972; 41: 19–27.

109. Wessler E. The nature of non-ultrafiltrable glycosaminglycans of normal urine. Biochem J 1971; 122: 373–384.

110. Miyake O, Yoshimura K, Tsujihata M, et al. Possible causes for the low prevalence of pediatric urolithiasis. Urology 1999; 53: 1229–1234.

111. Gohel MD, Shum DKY, Li MK. The dual effect of urinary macromolecules on the crystallization of calcium oxalate endogenous in urine. Urol Res 1992; 20: 13–17.

112. Shum DKY, Gohel MDI, Tam PC. Hyaluronans: Crystallization-promoting activity and HPLC analysis of urinary excretion. J Am Soc Nephrol 1999; 10: S397–S403.

113. Martin X, Werness PG, Bergert JH, Smith LH. Pentosan polysulfate as an inhibitor of calcium oxalate crystal growth. J Urol 1984; 132: 786–788.

114. Erwin DT, Kok DJ, Alam J, Cole FE et al. Predicting Recurrent Renal Stone formation and Therapy using crystal agglomeration inhibition. Am J Kidney Dis 1994; 24: 893–900.

115. Drach GW, Thorson S, Randolph A. Effects of urinary organic macromolecules on crystallization of calcium oxalate; Enhancement of nucleation. Trans Am Assoc Genitourin Surg 1979; 16: 62.

116. Koide T, Takemoto M, Itatani H, Takaha M, Sonoda T. Urinary macromolecular substances as natural inhibitors of calcium oxalate crystal aggregation. Invest Urol 1981; 18: 382–386.

117. Hess B, Jordi S, Zipperle L, Ettinger E, Giovanoli R. Citrate determines calcium oxalate crystallization kinetics and crystal morphology - studies in the presence of Tamm-Horsfall protein of a healthy subject and a severely recurrent calcium stone former. Nephrol Dial Transplant 2000; 15: 366–374.

118. Baggio B, Marzaro G, Gambaro G, Marchini R, Williams HE, Borsatti A.: Glycosaminoglycan content, oxalate self-exchange and protein phosphorylation in erythrocytes of patients with "idiopathic" calcium oxalate nephrolithiasis. Clin Sci 1990; 79: 113–116.

119. Baggio B, Gambaro G, Marchini F, Marzaro G, Williams HE, Borsatti A. Correction of erythrocyte abnormalities in idiopathic calcium-oxalate nephrolithiasis and reduction of urinary oxalate by oral glycosaminoglycans. Lancet 1991; 338: 403–405.

120. Verkoelen, C.F., van der Boom, B.G., Romijn, J.C.:Identification of hyaluronan as a crystal-binding molecule at the surface of migrating and proliferating MDCK cells. Kidney Int 2000; 58: 1045–1054.

121. Hildebrandt, P, Sayyad M, Rzany A, Schaldach M, Seiter H. Prevention of surface encrustation of urological implants by coating with inhibitors. Biomaterials 2001; 22: 503–507.

122. Hammerl H, Kranzl Ch, Pichler O, Studlar M. Zur therapeutischen Indikationsstallung von SP54 anf Grund Klinisch-Experimenteller Untersuchungen. Med Welt 1967; 18: 638–642.

123. Taugner R, Karsunsky KP, Metz J. Zur Pharmakokinetik des "Heparinartigen"sulfatierten polyanions SP54. Arch int Pharmacodyn 1971; 189: 250–256.

124. Parsons CL, Schmidt JD, Polle JJ. Succesful treatment of interstitial cystitis with pentosanpolysulfate. J Urol 1983; 130: 51–53.

125. Mc Allister BM, Demis DJ. Heparin metabolism: isolation ad characterization of uroheparin. Nature 1966; 212: 293.

126. Danielson BG, Fellström B, Backman U, et al. Glycosaminoglycans and renal stone disease; clinical effects of pentosan polysulphate (Elmiron). Fortsschr Urol u Nephrol 1986; 25: 345, 346.

127. Fellström B, Backman U, Danielson BG, Wikström B. Treatment of renal calcium stone disease with the synthetic glycosaminoglycan pentosan polysulfate.World J Urol 1994; 12: 52–54.

128. Shirane Y, Kurokawa Y, Sumiyoshi Y, Kagawa S. Morphological effects of glycosaminoglycans on calcium oxalate monohydrate crystals. Scanning Microsc 1995; 9: 1081–1088.

129. Grases F, Garcia-Gonzalez R, Genestar C, Torres JJ, March JG.Vitamin A and urolithiasis. Clin Chim Acta 1998; 269: 147–157.

130. Werness PG, Bergert JH, Lee KE. Urinary crystal growth: effect of inhibitory mixtures. Clin Sci 1981; 61: 487–492.

131. Hess B. Tamm-Horsfall glycoprotein - inhibitor or promoter of calcium oxalate monohydrate crystallization processes? Urol Res 1992; 20: 83–86.

132. Hess B. Tamm-Horsfall glycoprotein and calcium nephrolithiasis. Miner Electrolyte Metab. 1994; 20: 393–398.

133. Hoyer JR, Seiler MW. Pathophysiology of Tamm-Horsfall protein. Kidney Int 1979; 16: 279–289.

134. Tamm I, Horsfall FL. Characterization and separation of an inhibitor of viral hemagglutination present in urine. Proc Soc Exp Biol Med 1950; 74: 108–114.

135. Muchmore AV, Decker SM: Uromodulin: A unique 85-kilodalton immunosupprssive glycoprotein isolated from urine of pregnant women. Science 1985; 229: 479–481.

136. Kumar S, Muchmore AL. Tamm-Horsfall protein-uromodulin (1950–1990). Kid Intl 1990; 37: 1395–1401.

137. Gokhale JA, Glenton PA, Khan SR. Biochemical and quantitative analysis of Tamm-Horsfall protein in rats. Urol Res 1997; 25: 347–352.

138. Hallson PC, Rose GA. Uromucoids and urinary stone formation. Lancet 1979; 1: 1000–1002.

139. Rose GA, Sulaiman S. Tamm-Horsfall mucoproteins promote calcium oxalate crystal formation in urine: quantitative studies. J Urol 1982; 127: 177–179.

140. Yoshioka T, Koide T, Utsunomiya M, Itatani H, Oka T, Sonoda T. Possible role of Tamm-Horsfall glycoprotein in calcium oxalate crystallization. Br J Urol 1989; 64:463–467.

141. Hess B, Nakagawa Y, Parks JH, Coe FL. Molecular abnormality of Tamm-Horsfall glycoprotein in calcium oxalate nephrolithiasis. Am J Physiol 1991; 260: F569–F578.

142. Hess B, Zipperle L, Jaeger P. Citrate and calcium effects on Tamm-Horsfall glycoprotein as a modifier of calcium oxalte crystal aggregation. Am J Physiol 1993; 265: F784–F791.

143. Ryall RL, Harnett RM, Hibberd CM, Edyvane KA, Marshall VR. Effects of chondroitin sulphate, human serum albumin and Tamm-Horsfall mucoprotein on oxalate crystallization in indiluted human urine. Urol Res 1991; 19: 181–188.

144. Scurr DS, Robertson WG. Modifiers of calcium oxalate crystallization found in urine. II. studies on their mode of action in artificial urine. J Urol 1986; 136: 128–131.

145. Bichler KH, Kirchner CH, Ideler V. Uromucoid excretion of normal individuals and stone formers. Brit J Urol 1976; 47: 733–738.

146. Hess B, Jaggi M, Zipperle L, Jaeger P. Reduced carbohydrate content of Tamm-Horsfall glycoprotein (THP) from severely recurrent renal calcium stone formers (RCSF). J Am Soc Nephrol 1995; 6: 949–952.

147. Schnierle P. A simple diagnostic method for the differentiation of Tamm-Horsfall glycoproteins from healthy probands and those from recurrent calcium oxalate renal stone formers. Experientia 1995; 51: 1068–1072.

148. Bachmann S, Metzger R, Bunnemann B. Tamm-Horsfall protein-mRNA synthesis is localized to the thick ascending limb of Henle's loop in rat kidney. Histochemistry 1990; 94: 517–523.

149. Gokhale JA, Glenton PA, Khan SR. Chracterization of Tamm-Horsfall protein in a rat nephrolithiasis model. J Urol 2001; 166: 1492–1497.

150. Miyake O, Yoshioka T, Yoshimora T, et al. Expression of Tamm-Horsfall protein in stone forming rat models. Br J Urol 1998; 81: 14–19.

151. Marengo SR, Chen DH-C, Kaung H-LC, Resnick MI, Yang L. Decreased renal expression of the putative calcium oxalate inhibitor Tamm-Horsfall protein in the ethylene glycol rat model of calcium oxalate urolithiasis. J Urol 2002; 167: 2192–2197.

152. Katsuma S, Shiojima S, Hirasawa A, et al. Global analysis of differentially expressed genes during progression of calcium oxalate nephrolithiasis. Biochem Biophys Res Commun 2002; 296: 544–552.

153. Coe FL, Nakagawa Y, Asplin J, Parks JH. Role of nephrocalcin in inhibiytion of calcium oxalate crystallization and nephrolithiasis. Miner Electrolyte Metab 1994; 20: 378–384.

154. Worcester EM, Nakagawa Y, Coe FL. Glycoprotein calcium oxalate crystal growth inhibitor in urine. Mineral Electrolyte Meta 1987; 13: 267–272.

155. Worcester EM, Blumenthal SS, Beshensky AM, Lewand DL. The calcium oxalate crystal growth inhibitor protein produced by mouse kidney cortical cells in culture is osteopontin. J Bone Mineral Res 1992; 7: 1029–1036.

156. Nakagawa Y, Abram V, Kezdy FJ, Kaiser ET, Coe FL. Purification and characterization of the principal inhibitor of calcium oxalate monohydrate crystal growth in human urine. J Biol Chem 1983; 258: 12,594–12,600.

157. Nakagawa Y, Abram V, Parks JH, Lau HSH, Kawooya JK, Coe FL. Urine glycoprotein crystal growth inhibitors. Evidence for a molecular abnormality in calcium oxalate nephrolithiasis. J Clin Invest 1985; 76: 1455–1462.

158. Nakagawa Y, Ahmed M, Hall SL, Deganello S, Coe FL. Isolation from human calcium oxalate renal stones of nephrocalcin, a glycoprotein inhibitor of calcium oxalate crystal growth. Evidence that nephrocalcin from patients with calcium oxalate nephrolithiasis is dificient in g-carboxy-glutamic acid. J Clin Invest 1987; 79: 1782–1787.

159. Nakagawa Y, Margolis HC, Yokoyama S, Kezdy FJ, Kaiser ET, Coe FL. Purification and characterization of calcium oxalate monohydrate crystal growth inhibitor from human kidney tissue culture medium. J Biol Chem 1981; 256: 3936–3644.

160. Nakagawa Y, Otsuki T, Coe FL. Elucidation of multiple forms of nephrocalcin by ^{31}P-NMR spectrometer. FEBS Letters 1989; 250: 187–190.

161. Nakagawa Y, Netzer M, Coe FL. Immunohistochemical localization of nephrocalcin (NC) to proximal tubule and thick ascending limb of Henle's loop of human and mouse kidney. Kid Intl 1990; 37: 474.

162. Worcester EM, Sebastian JL, Hiatt JG, Beshensky AM, Sadowski JA. The effect of warfarin on urine calcium oxalate crystal growth inhibition and urinary excretion of calcium and nephrocalcin. Calcif Tissue Int 1993; 53: 242–248.

163. Asplin J, DeGanello S, Nakagawa Y, Coe FL. Evidence that nephrocalcin and urine inhibit nucleation of calcium oxalate monhydrate crystals. Am. J. Physiol 1991; 261: F824–F830.

164. Hess B. The role of Tamm-Horsfall Glycoprotein and nephrocalcin in calcium oxalate monohydrate crystallization processess. Scanning Microsc 1991; 5: 689–696.

165. Lieske JC, Toback FG. Regulation of renal epithelial cell endocytosis of calcium oxalate monohydrate crystals. Am J Physiol 1995; 264: F604–F612.

166. Desbois C, Hogue DA, Karsenty G. The mouse osteocalcin gene cluster contains three genes with two separate spatial and temporal patterns of expression. J Biol Chem 1994; 269: 1183–1190.

167. Hochstrasser, K., Bretzel, G., Feuth, H., Hilla, W., Lempart, K.: The inter-α-trypsin inhibitor as precursor of the acid-stable protease inhibitors in human serum and urine. Hoppe-Seylers Z Physiol Chem 1976; 357: 153–162.

168. Enghild JJ, Thogersen IB, Pizzo SV, Salvesen G. Analysis of inter-α-trypsin inhibitor and a novel trypsin inhibitor, Pre-α-trypsin inhibitor from human plasma. Polypeptide chain stoichiometry and assembly by glycan. J Biol Chem 1989; 264: 15975.

169. Salier JP. Inter-α-trypsin inhibitor: emergence of a family within the Kunitz-type protease inhibitor superfamily, Trends Biochem Sci 1990; 15: 435.

170. Malki N, Balduyck M, Maes P, et al. The heavy chains of human plasma inter-α-trypsin inhibitor: their isolation, their identification by electrophoresis and partial sequencing. Biol Chem Hoppe-Seyler 1992; 373: 1009.

171. Salier J-P, Rouet P, Raguenez G, Daveau M. The inter-α-inhibitor family: from structure to regulation, Biochem J 1996; 315: 1.

172. Witte J, Jochum M, Scherer R, Schramm W, Hachstrasser K, Fritz F. Disturbances of selected plasma proteins in hyperdynamic septic shock. Intensive Care Med 1982; 8: 215.

173. Franck C, Pederson Z. Trypsin inhibitory activities of acid-stable fragments of the inter-alpha-trypsin inhibitor in inflammatory and uraemic conditions. Scand J Clin Lab Invest 1983; 43: 151.

174. Chawla RK, Rausch DJ, Miller FW, Vogler WR, Lawson DH. Abnormal profile of serum proteinase inhibitors in cancer patients. Cancer Res 1982; 44: 2718.

175. Yoshida E, Maruyama M, Sugiki M, Mohara H. Immunohistochemical demonstration of bikunin, light chain of inter-α-trypsin inhibitor in human brain tumours. Inflammation 1994; 18: 589.

176. Thogersen IB, Enghild JJ. Biosynthesis of bikunin protein in the human carcinoma cell line HepG2 and in primary human hepatocytes. J Biol Chem 1995; 270: 18,700.

177. Toki N, Sumi H. Urinary trypsin inhibitor and urokinase activities in renal diseases. Acta Haemat 1982; 67: 109.

178. Iida S, Peck AB, Johnson-Tardieu J, et al. Temporal changes in mRNA expressioin for bikunin in the kidneys of rats during calcium oxalate nephrolithiasis. J Am Soc Nephrol 1999; 10: 986.

179. Moriyama MT, Glenton PA, Khan SR. Expression of inter-α-inhibitor related proteins in kidneys and urine of hyperoxaluric rats. J Urol 2001; 165: 1687–1692.

180. Janssen U, Thomas G, Glant T, Phillips A. Expression of inter-α-trypsin inhibitor and tumor necrosis factor-stimulated gene 6 in renal proximal tubular epithelial cells. Kidney Int 2001; 60: 126–136.

181. Iida S, Peck AB, Byer KJ, Khan SR. Expression of bikunin mRNA in renal epithelial cells after oxalate exposure. J Urol 1999; 162: 1480.

182. Atmani F, Lacour B, Drueke T, Daudon M. Isolation and purification of a new glycoprotein from human urine inhibiting calcium oxalate crystallization. Urol Res 1993; 21: 61.

183. Atmani F, Lacour B, Strecker G, Parvy P, Drueke T, Daudon M. Molecular characteristics of uronic acid rich protein, a strong inhibitor of calcium oxalate crystallization in vitro. Biochem Biophys Res Commun 1993; 191: 1158–1165.

184. Atmani F, Khan S.R. Characterization of uronic-acid-rich inhibitor of calcium oxalate crystallization isolated from rat urine. Urol Res 1995; 23: 95.

185. Atmani F, Mizon J, Khan SR. Identification of uronic-acid-rich protein as urinary bikunin, the light chain of inter-α-inhibitor. Eur J Biochem 1996; 236: 984.

186. Atmani F, Lacour B, Jungers P, Drüeke T, Daudon M. Reduced inhibitory activity of uronic-acid-rich protein in urine of stone formers. Urol Res 1994; 22: 257–260.

187. Suzuki S, Kobayashi H, Kageyama S, Shibata K, Fujie M, Terao T. Excretion of bikunin and its fragments in he urine of patients with renal stones. J Urol 2001; 166: 268–274.

188. Medetognon-Benissan J, Tardivel S, Hennequin C, Daudon T, Drueke T, Lacour B. Inhibitory effect of bikunin on calcium oxalate crystallization in vitro and urinary bikunin decrease in renal stone formers. Urol Res 1999; 27: 69–75.

189. Dean C, Kanellos J, Pham H, et al. Effects of inter-alpha-inhibitor and several of its derivatives on calcium oxalate crystallization in vitro. Clin Science 2000; 98: 471.

190. Nishino N, Aoki K, Tokura Y, et al. Measurement of urinary trypsin inhibitor in urine, plasma and cancer tissues of patients with stomach cancer. Haemostasis 1989; 19: 112.

191. Usui T, Maehara S, Kawashita E, Ishibe T, Sumi H, Toki N. Radioimmunological quatitation of urinary trypsin inhibitor. Enzyme 1984; 31: 11–16.

192. Atmani F, Khan SR. Inter-alpha-inhibitor: another serum protein with potential involvement in calcium oxalate nephrolithiasis. J Am Soc Nephrol 1996; 7: 1798.

193. Dawson CJ, Grover PK, Ryall RL. Inter-alpha-inhibitor in urine and calcium oxalate crystals. Br J Urol 1998; 81: 20.

194. Steinbuch M. The inter-alpha-trypsin inhibitor. Methods Enzymol 1976; 45: 760–772.

195. Kobayashi H, Shibata K, Fujie M, Sugino D, Terao T. Identification of structural domains in inter-α-trypsin inhibitor involved in calcium oxalate crystallization. Kidney Int 1998; 53: 1727.

196. Atmani F, Khan SR. Role of urinary bikunin in the inhibition of calcium oxalate crystallization. J Am Soc Nephrol 1999; 10: S385.

197. Ebisuno S, Nishihata M, Inagaki T, Umehara M, Kohjimoto Y. Bikunin prevents adhesion of calcium oxalate crystals to renal tubular cells in human urine. J Am Soc Nephrol 1999; 10: S436.

198. Tardivel S, Medetognon J, Randoux C, et al. Alpha-1-microglobulin: inhibitory effect on calcium oxalate crystallization in vitro and decreased urinary concentration in calcium oxalate stone formers. Urol Res 1999; 27: 243–249.

199. Marengo SR, Resnick MI, Yang L, Chung J-C. Differential expression of urinary inter-α -trypsin inhibitor trimers and dimers in normal compared to active calcium oxalate stone forming men. J Urol 1998; 159: 1444.

200. Hedgepeth RC, Yang L, Resnick MI, Marengo SR. Expression of proteins that inhibit calcium oxalate crystallization in vitro in urine of normal and stone forming individuals. Am J Kid Dis 2001; 37: 104–112.

201. Ricchiuti V, Hartke DM, Yang LZ, et al. Lavels of urinary inter-α-trypsin inhibitoe as a function of age and sex-hormone status in males and females not forming stones. BJU Int 2002; 90: 513–517.

202. Denhardt DT, Guo X. Osteopontin: a protein with diverse functions. FASEB J 1993; 7: 1475–1482.

203. Brown LF, Berse B, Water LVD, et al. Expression and distribution of osteopontin in human tissues: widespread association with luminal epithelial surfaces. Mol Biol Cell 1992; 3: 1169–1180.

204. Prince CW, Oosawa W, Butler BT, et al. Isolation, characterization, and biosynthesis of a phosphorylated glycoprotein from rat bone. J Biol Chem 1992; 268: 15,180–15,184.

205. Ruoslahti E, Pierschbacher MD. New perspective in cell adhesion: RGD and integrins. Science 1987; 238: 491–497.

206. Weber GF, Ashkar S, Glimcher MJ. Cantor H: Receptor ligand interaction between CD44 and osteopontin (Eta-1). Science 1996; 271: 509–512.

207. Chen Y, Bal BS, Gorski JP. Calcium and collagen bnding properties of osteopontin, bone sialoprotein and bone acidic glycoprotein-75 from bone. J Biol Chem 1992; 267: 24,871–24,878.

208. Pollack SB, Linnemeyer PA, Gill S. induction og osteopontin mRNA expression during activation of murine NK cells. J Leukocyte Biol 1994; 55: 398–400.

209. Murry CE, Giachelli CM, Schwartz SM, Vracko R. Macrophages express osteopontin during repair of myocardial necrosis. Am J Pathol 1994; 145: 1450–1462.

210. Patarca R, Saavedra RA, Cantor H. Molecular and cellular basis of genetic resistance to bacterial infection: role of the early T-lymphocyte activation-1/osteopontingene. crit Rev Immunol 1993; 13: 225–246.

211. Yu XQ, Fan JM, Nikolic-Paterson DJ, et al. IL-1 up-regulates osteopontin expression in experimental crescentic glomerulonephriris in the rat. Am J Path 1999; 154: 833–841.

212. Kohri K, Nomura S, Kitamura Y, et al. Structure and expression of the mRNA encoding urinary stone protein (osteopontin). J Biol Chem 1993; 268(20): 15,180–15,184.

213. Lopez CA, Hoyer JR, Wilson PD, Waterhouse P, Denhardt DT. Heterogeneity of osteopontin expression among nephrons in mouse kidneys and enhanced expression in sclerotic glomeruli. Laboratory Invest 1993; 69: 355–363.

214. Kleinman JG, Beshensky A, Worcester EM, Brown D. Expression of osteopontin, a urinary inhibitor of stone mineral crystal growth in rat kidney. Kidney Int 1995; 47: 1585–1596.

215. Hudkins KL, Giachelli CM, Cui Y, Couser WG, Johnson RJ, Alpers CE. Osteopontin expression in fetal and mature human kidney. J Am Soc Nephrol 1999; 10: 447–457.

216. Chalko C, Krishna G, Hoyer JR, Goldfarb S. Characterization of urinary uropontin excretion in humans. J Am Soc Nephrol 1992; 3: 681.

217. Min W, Shiraga H, Chalko C, Goldfarb S, Hoyer JR. Quantitative studies of human urinary excretion of uropontin Kidney Int 1998; 53: 189–193.

218. Shiraga H, Min W, VanDusen WJ, et al. Inhibition of calcium oxalate crystal growth in vitro by uropontin: another member of the aspartic acid rich superfamily. Proc Net Acad Sci USA 1992; 89: 426–430.

219. Nishio S, Hatanaka M, Takeda H, et al. Calcium phosphate crystal-assiciated proteins: α-2-HS-glycoprotein, prothrombin fragment-1 and osteopontin. Intl J Urol 2001; 8: S58–S62.

220. Yamate T, Tsugi H, Amasaki N, Iguchi M, Kurita T, Kohri K. Analysis of osteopontin DNA in patients with urolithiasis. Urol Res 2000; 28: 159–166.

221. Yagisawa TM, Chandhoke PS, Fan J, Lucia S. Renal osteopontin expression in experimental urolithiasis. J Endourol 1998; 12: 171–176.

222. Khan SR, Johnson JH, Peck AB, Cornelius JG, Glenton PA. Expression of osteopontin in rat kidneys: induction during ethylene glycol induced calcium oxalate nephrolithiasis. J Urol 2002; 168: 1173–1181.

223. Yasui T, Sato M, Fujita K, Ito Y, Nomura S, Kohri K. Effects of citrate on renal stone formation and osteopontin expression in a rat urolithiasis model. Urol Res 2001; 29: 50–56.

224. Yasui T, Sato M, Fujita K, Tozawa K, Nomura S, Kohri K. Effects of allopurinol on renal stone formation and osteopontin expression in a rat urolithiasis model. Nephron 2001; 87: 171–176.

225. Iguchi M, Takamura C, Umekawa T, Kurita T, Kohro K. Inhibitory effects of female sex hormones on urinary stone formation in rats. Kidney Int 1999; 56: 479–485.

226. Lieske JC, Hammes MS, Hoyer JR, Toback FG. Renal cell osteopontin production is stimulated by calcium oxalate monohydrate crystals. Kidney Int 1997; 51: 679–683.

227. Jonassen JA, Cooney R, Kennington L, Gravel K, Honeyman T, Scheid CR. Oxalate-induced changes in the viability and growth of human renal epithelial cells. J Am Soc Nephrol 1999; 10: S446–451.

228. Asplin J, DeGanello S, Nakagawa Y, Coe FL. Evidence that nephrocalcin and urine inhibit nucleation of calcium oxalate monhydrate crystals. Am J Physiol 1991; 261: F824–F830.

229. Worcester EM, Snyder C, Beshensky AM. Osteopontin inhibits heterogeneous nucleation of calcium oxalate. J Am Soc Nephrol 1995; 6: 956.

230. Asplin JR, Hoyer J, Gillespie C, Coe FL. Uropontin (UP) inhibits aggregation of calcium oxalate monohydrate (COM) crystals. J Am Sci Nephrol 1995; 6: 941.

231. Yamate T, Kohri K, Umekawa T, et al. Interaction between osteopontin on Madin Darby canine kidney cell membrane and calcium oxalate crystals. Urol Int 1999; 62: 81–86.

232. Yasui T, Fujita K, Kiyofumi A, Kohri K. Osteopontin regulates adhesion of calcium oxalate crystals to renal epithelial cells. Int J Urol 2002; 9: 100–109.

233. Yamate T, Kohri K, Umekawa T, et al. Osteopontin antisense oligonucleotide inhibits adhesion of calcium oxalate crystals in Madin Darby canine kidney cell. J Urol 1998; 160: 1506–1512.

234. Mazzali M, Kipari T, Ophascharoensuk V, Wesson J, Johnson R, Hughes J. Osteopontin- amolecule for all seasons. QJMed 2002; 95: 3–13.

235. Wesson JA, Worcester EM, Wiessner JH, Mandel NS, Kleinman JG. Control of calcium oxalate crystal structure and cell adherence by urinary macromolecules. Kidney Int 1998; 53: 952–957.

236. Doyle IR, Ryall RL, Marshall VR. Inclusion of proteins into calcium oxalate crystals precipitated from human urine: a highly selective phenomenon. Clin Chem 1991; 37: 1589–1594.

237. Stapleton AMF, Simpson RJ, Ryall RL. Crystal matrix protein is related to human prothrombin. Biochem Biophys Res Comm 1993; 195: 1199–1203.

238. Stapleton AMF, Ryall RL. Crystal matrix protein-getting blood out of a stone. Miner Electrolyte Metab 1994; 20: 399–409.

239. Suzuki K, Moriyama M, Nakajima C, et al. Isolation and partial characterization of crystal matrix protein as a potent inhibitor of calcium oxalate crystal aggregation: evidence of activation peptide of human prothrombin. Urol Res 1994; 22: 45–50.

240. Bezeau A, Guillin MC. Quantitation of prothrombin activation products in human urine. Br J Haemetol 1984; 58: 579–606.

241. Aronson DL, Ball AP, Franza RP, Hugli TE, Fenton JW. Human prothrombin fragments F1 and F2: Preparation and characetrization of structural and biological properties. Thromb Res 1980; 20: 239–253.

242. Anderson GAF, Bardet MI. Prothrombin synthesis in the dog. Am J Physiol 1964; 206: 929–938.

243. Stapleton AMF, Seymour AE, Brennan JS, Doyle IR, Marshall VR, Ryall RL. Immunohistochemical distribution and quantification of crystal matrix protein. Kidney Int 1993; 44: 817–824.

244. Stapleton AMF, Timme TL, Ryall RL. Gene expression of prothrombin in the human kidney and its potential relevance to kidney stone formation. Br J Urol 1998; 81: 666–672.

245. Grover PK, Dogra SC, Davidson BP, Stapleton AMF, Ryall RL. The prothrombin gene is expressed in the rat kidney. Eur J Biochem 2000; 267: 61–67.

246. Suzuki K, Tanaka T, Miyazawa K, et al. Gene expression of prothrombin in human and rat kidneys: Implications for urolithiasis research. J Am Soc Nephrol 1999; 10: S408–S411.

247. Grover PK, Stapleton AMF, Ryall RL. Prothrombin gene expression in rat kdiensy provides an opportunity to examine its role in urinary stone pathogenesis. J Am Soc Nephrol 1999; 10: S404–S407.

248. Ryall RL, Grover PK, Stapleton AMF, et al. The urinary F1 activation peptide of human prothrombin is a potent inhibitor of calcium oxalate crystallization in undiluted human urine in vitro. Clin Sci 1989; 89: 533–541.

249. Durrbaum D, Rodgers AL, Sturrock ED. A study of crystal matrix extract and urinary prothrombin fragment 1 from a stone prone and stone free population. Urol Res 2001; 29: 83–88.

250. Grover PK, Ryall RL. Inhibition of calcium oxalate crystal growth and aggregation by prothrombin and its fragments in vitro, relationship between protein structure and inhibitory activity. Eur J Biochem 1999; 263: 50–56.

251. Grover PK, Ryall RL. Effect of prothrombin and its activation fragments on calcium oxalate crystal growth and aggregation in undiluted human urine in vitro: relationship between protein structure and inhibitory activity. Clin Sci 2002; 102: 425–434.

252. Zimmer D, Cornwall E, Landar A, Song W. The S100 protein family: history, function and expression. Brain Res Bull 1995; 37: 417–429.

253. Kahn H, Marks A, Thom H, Baumal R. Role of antibody to S100 protein in daignostic pathology. Am J Clin Pathol 1982; 79: 341–347.

254. Pillay SN, Asplin JR, Coe FL. Evidence that calgranulin is produced byt kidney cells and is an inhibitor of calcium oxalate crystallization. Am J Physiol 1998; 275: F255–F261.

255. Steinback M, Nasess-Anderson C, Lingass E, Dale I, Brandtzaeg P, Fagerhot M. Antibacterial acctions of calcium binding leucocyte L1 protein, calprotectin. Lancet 1990; 336: 763–765.

256. Bennett J, Dretler SP, Selengut J, Orme-Johnson WH. Identification of the calcum-binding protein calgranulin in the matrix of struvite stones. J Endourol 1994; 8: 95–98.

257. Fraij BM. Separation and identification of urinary proteins and stone matrix proteins by mini-slab sodium dodecyl sulfate polyacrylamide gel electrophoresis. Clin Chem 1989; 35: 658–662.

258. Atmani F, Opalko FJ, Khan SR. Association of urinary macromolecules with calcium oxalate crystals induced in vitro in normal human and rat urine. Urol Res 1996; 24: 45–50.

259. Worcester EM. Urinary calcium oxalate crystal growth inhibitors. J Am Soc Nephrol 1994; 5: S46–S53.

260. Dussol B, Geider S, Lilova A, et al. Analysis of the soluble organic matrix of five different kidney stones: Evidence for a specific role of albumin in the constitution of stone protein matrix. Urol Res 1995; 23: 45–51.

261. Edyvane KA, Ryall RL, Marshall VR. The influence of serum and serum proteins on calcium oxalate crystal growth and aggregation. Clin Chim Acta 1986; 157: 81–87.

262. Hess B, Meinhardt U, Zipperle L, Giovanoli R, Jaeger P. Simulataneous measurements of calcium oxalate crystal nucleation and aggregation: Impact of various modifiers. Urol Res 1995; 23: 231–238.

263. Grover PK, Moritz RL, Simpson RJ, Ryall RL. Inhibition of growth and aggregation of calcium oxalate crystals in vitro, a comparison of four human proteins. Eur J Biochem 1998; 253: 637–644.

264. Cerini C, Geider S, Dussol B, et al. Nucleation of calcium oxalate crystals by albumin: involvement in the prevention of stone formation. Kidney Intl 1999; 55: 1776–1786.

265. Ebrahimpour A, Perez L, Nancollas GH. Induced crystal growth of calcium oxalate monohydrate at hydroxyapatite surfaces. The influence of human serum albumin, citrate, and magnesium. Langmuir 1991; 7: 577–583.

266. Wesson JA, Worcester EM. Formation of hydrated calcium oxalates in the presence of poly-L-aspartic acid. Scanning Microsc 1996; 10: 415–424.

267. Wesson JA, Worcester EM, Kleinman JG. Role of anionic proteins in kidney stone formation: interaction between model anionic polypeptides and calcium oxalate crystals. J Urol 2000; 163: 1343–1348.

268. Anderson HC. Biology of disease; mechanism of mineral formation in bone. Lab Invest 1989; 60: 320–330.

269. Boskey AL. Current concepts of physiology and biochemistry of calcification. Clin Orthop 1981; 1527: 225–257.

270. Boskey AL. Phospholipids and calcification. In: Calcified Tissue, (Hukins DWL, ed.). CRC, Boca Raton, FL, 1989; pp. 215–243.

271. Martin RS, Small DM. Physicochemical characterization of the urinary lipid from humans with nephrotic syndrome. J Lab Clin Med 1984; 103: 798–810.

272. Prescott LF. The normal urinary excretion rates of renal tubular cells, leukocytes and red blood cells. Clin Sci 1966; 31: 425–435.

273. Khan SR, Glenton PA. Increased urinary excretion of lipids by patients with kidney stones. Br J Urol 1996; 77: 506–511.

274. Khan SR, Whalen PO, Glenton PA. Heterogeneous nucleation of calcium oxalate crystals in the presence of membrane vesicles. J Crystal Growth 1993; 134: 211–218.

275. Khan SR, Shevock PN, Hackett RL. In vitro precipitation of calcium oxalate in the presence of whole matrix or lipid components of the urinary stones. J Urol 1988; 139: 418–422.

276. Khan SR, Maslamani SA, Atmani F, et al. Membrane and their constituents as promoters of calcium oxalate crystal formation in human urine. Calcified Tissue Int 2000; 66: 90–96.

277. Finalyson B, Reid F. The expectation of free or fixed particles in urinary stone disease. Invest Urol 1978; 15: 442–448.

278. Fasano JM, Khan SR. Intratubular crystallization of calcium oxalate in the presence of membrane vesicles: an in vitro study. Kid Int 2001; 59: 169–178.

279. Hijgaard I, Tiselius H-G. Crystallization in the nephron. Urol Res 1999; 27: 397–403.

280. Khan SR, Glenton PA, Backov R, Talham DR. Presence of lipids in urine, crystals and stones: Implications for the formation of kidney stones. Kidney Int 2002; 62: 2062–2072.

281. Khan SR: Interactions between stone forming calcific crystals and macromolecules. Urologia Int 1997; 59: 59–71.

282. Whipps S, Khan SR, Opalko FJ, et al. Growth of calcium oxalate monohydrate at phospholipid Langmuir monolayers. J Cryst Growth 1998; 192: 243–249.

283. Letellier SR, Lochhead MJ, Cambell AA, Vogel V. Oriented growth of calcium oxalate monohydrate crystals beneath phospholipid monolayers. Biochim Biophys Acta—Gen Subjects, 1998; 1380, 31–45.

284. Backov R, Khan SR, Mingotaud C, Byer K, Lee CM, Talham DR. Precipitation of calcium oxalate monohydrate at phospholipid monolayers. J Am Soc Neph 1999; 10: S359–S363.

285. Backov R, Lee CM, Khan SR, Mingotad C, Fanucci GE, Talham DR. Calcium oxalate monohydrate precipitation at phosphatidylglycerol langmuir monolayers. Langmuir 2000; 16: 6013–6019.

286. Wiessner JH, Hasegawa AT, Hung LY, et al. Mechanisms of calcium oxalate crystal attachment to injured renal collecting duct cells. Kidney Int 2001; 59: 637–644.

287. Wiessner JH, Hasegawa AT, Hung LY, Mandel NS. Oxalate-induced exposure of PS on surface of renal epithelial cells in culture. J Am Soc Nephrol 1999; 10: S441–445.

288. Khan SR, Byer KJ, Thamilselvan S, et al. Crystal-cell interaction and apoptosis in oxalate-associated injury of renal epithelial cells. J Am Soc Nephrol 1999; 10: S457–463.

289. Cao L-C, Jonassen Honeyman TW, Scheid C. Oxalate-induced redistribution of phosphatidylserine in renal epithelial cells, implication for kidney stone disease. Am J Nephrol 2001; 21: 69–77.

290. Trump BF, Berezeski IK. Calcium-mediated cell injury and cell death. FASEB J 1995; 9:219–228.

291. Khan SR. Heterogeneous nucleation of calcium oxalate crystals in mammalian urine. Scanning Microsc 1995; 9: 597–616.

292. Khan SR, Finlasyon B, Hackett RL. Experimental calcium oxalate nephrolithiasis in rat: role of renal papilla. Am J Pathol 1982; 107: 59–69,

293. Khan SR, Hackett RL. Developmental morphology of calcium oxalate foreign body stones in rats. Calcif Tiss Int 1985; 37: 165–173.

294. Nguyen HT, Woodard J.C. Intranephronic calculosis in rats. Am J Pathol 1980; 100: 39–56.

295. Khan SR, Adair JH, Morrone AA, Hackett RL. Calcium phosphate deposition in rat kidneys. In: Hydroxyapatite and Related Materials, (Brown PW, Constanatz B, eds.). CRC, Boca Raton, FL, 1994; pp. 325–329.

296. Randall A. The etiology of primary renal calculus. Intl Abst Surg 1940; 71: 209–240.

297. Cifuentes-Delatte LD, Minon-Cifuentes J, Medina J. New studies on papillary calculli. J Urol 1987; 137: 1024–1029.

298. Petersen TE, Thorgesen I, Petersen SE. Identification of hemoglobin and two serine proteases in acid estracts of calcium containing kidney stones. J Urol 1989; 142: 176–180.

299. Umekawa T, Kohri K, Amasaki N, et al. Sequencing of a urinary stone protein identical to α-1-antitrypsin. Biochem Biophys Res Commun 1993; 193: 1049–1053,

300. Umekawa T, Kurita T. Calprotectin-like protein is related to soluble organic matrix in calcium oxalate urinary stone. Biochem Biophys Res Commun 1994; 34: 309–313.

301. March JG, Simonet BM, Grases F. Determination of pyrophosphate in renal calculi and urine by means of an enzymatic method. Clin Chim Acta, 2001; 314: 187–194.

302. Fellström B, Björklund U, Danielson BG, Eriksson H, Odlind B, Tengblad A. Pentosan polysulphate (Elmiron) pharmacokinetics and effects on the urinary inhibition of crystals growth. Fortsschr Urol U Nephrol 1986; 25: 340–344.

303. Wikström B, Danielson BG, Ljunghall S, McGuire M, Russell RGG. Urinary pyrophosphate excretion in renal stone formers with normal and impaired renal acidification. World J Urol 1983; 1: 150–154.

304. Fellström B, Danielson BG, Ljunghall S, Wikström B. Crystal inhibition: the effects of polyanions on calcium oxalate crystal growth. Clin Chim Acta 1986; 158: 229–235.

305. Suzuki K, Ryall RL. The effect of heparan sulfate on the crystallization of calcium oxalate in undiluted, ultrafiltered human urine. Br J Urol 1996; 78: 15–21.

306. Senthil D, Subha K, Saravanan N, Varalakshmi P. Influence of sodium pentosan polysulphate and certain inhibitors on calcium oxalate crystal growth. Mol Cell Biochem 1996; 56: 31–35.

307. Jappie D, Rodgers AL. Inhibition of calcium oxalate monohydrate crystal aggregation by chondroitinsulfate (CS), hyaluronic acid (HA) and Tamm Horsfall mucoprotein (THM). In: Eurolithiasis. (Kok DJ, Romijn HC, Verhagen PCMS, Verkoelen CF, eds.). Shaker Publishing, Maastricht, The Netherlands, 2001; pp. 64, 65.

308. Lama G, Carbone MG, Marrone N, et al. Promotors and inhibitors of calcium urolithiasis in children. Child Nephrol Urol 1990; 10: 81–85.

11 Hormonal Influences on Nephrolithiasis

Colonel Noah S. Schenkman, MD
and Major C. Gerry Henderson, MD

CONTENTS

Key Words: Nephrolithiasis; hormone; parathyroid; vitamin D.

INTRODUCTION

Urinary stone disease is a multifactorial disorder that is influenced by both intrinsic and environmental factors. Diet, climate, genetics, and metabolic processes may be involved in stone formation. Hormonal influences on stone disease have long been acknowledged and include disorders of calcium homeostasis, sex-related differences, and imbalances of other hormones that play a secondary role in calcium balance. Although the pathophysiologic mechanisms of some disorders, such as hyperparathyroidism, have been elucidated, the actions of other hormones on urolithiasis remain elusive.

PARATHYROID HORMONE

Parathyroid hormone (PTH) is an 84-amino acid single-chain polypeptide produced in the chief cells of the parathyroid glands. The N-terminal fragment, containing residues 1–34, is the biologically active component. PTH regulates serum calcium in three target organs: the kidney, bone, and indirectly, the intestinal mucosa. The most potent stimulus for PTH secretion is decreased serum calcium, especially the ionized fraction *(1)*.

From: Current Clinical Urology, *Urinary Stone Disease:*
A Practical Guide to Medical and Surgical Management
Edited by: M. L. Stoller and M. V. Meng © Humana Press Inc., Totowa, NJ

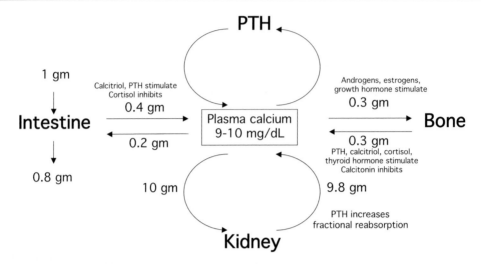

Fig. 1. Hormonal regulation of calcium balance. Parathyroid hormone (PTH), calcitonin, and other hormones regulate plasma levels of calcium by controlling GI absorption, renal excretion, and bone calcium flux.

In the kidney, PTH has three major effects: (1) stimulation of 1 α-hydroxylase in mitochondria of the proximal convoluted renal tubule that converts 25 hydroxyvitamin D_3 to 1,25 dihydroxyvitamin D_3 [1,25 $(OH)_2D_3$], (2) promotion of renal calcium reabsorption in the thick ascending loop of Henle, and (3) suppression of renal tubular reabsorption of inorganic phosphate in the proximal tubule *(1,2)*. The actions of PTH in the kidney are mediated by stimulating renal adenylate cyclase, leading to increased urinary cyclic adenosine monophosphate (cAMP). In addition, PTH decreases the reabsorption of bicarbonate in the kidney, which leads to a hyperchloremic acidosis. This acidosis aids in bone demineralization and decreases calcium binding to albumin, acutely increasing the serum ionized calcium concentration. In bone, PTH stimulates osteoclasts to breakdown apatite, releasing calcium and phosphorus into serum (Fig. 1).

Low serum calcium stimulates PTH secretion. PTH secretion is indirectly stimulated by increased serum phosphate levels, which decrease serum calcium. Hypomagnesemia stimulates PTH release; however severe magnesium depletion will decrease PTH because magnesium is necessary for parathyroid function. PTH is normally inhibited by increased serum calcium, elevated 1,25 $(OH)_2D_3$, and hypermagnesemia. The appropriate physiologic controls break down in primary and secondary hyperparathyroidism.

Hyperparathyroidism

Primary hyperparathyroidism (1HPT) is the most common endocrine disorder causing hypercalcemia. 1HPT usually results from a single parathyroid adenoma in 80% of patients. Fifteen percent of patients have hyperplasia; 5% have multiple adenomas; less than 0.5% will have cancer. Two to three percent of all calcium stone formers have 1HPT *(3–5)* with some sources noting rates as high as 8% *(3–6)*. 1HPT is two to four times more common in females than males, and patients usually present after the age of 50 *(7)*.

Table 1
Clinical Features of Hypercalcemia

Neurologic and psychiatric
- Lethargy, drowsiness
- Confusion, disorientation
- Disturbed sleep, nightmares
- Irritability, depression
- Hypotonia, decreased deep tendon reflexes
- Stupor, coma

Gastrointestinal
- Anorexia, vomiting
- Constipation
- Peptic ulceration
- Acute pancreatitis

Cardiovascular
- Arrhythmias
- Synergism with digoxin
- Hypertension

Renal
- Polyuria, polydipsia
- Hypercalciuria
- Nephrocalcinosis
- Impaired glomerular filtration

Most cases of hyperparathyroidism are sporadic; however the disorder can occur as part of the autosomal dominant multiple endocrine neoplasia (MEN) syndromes. MEN-1 (Wermer's syndrome) consists of tumors of the parathyroid, pancreatic islet cells, and the anterior pituitary. The genetic defect is at 11q13 *(8)*. HPT is present in 95% of MEN-1 patients and 90% of these patients present with hypercalcemia. MEN-2 (Sipple's syndrome) consists of tumors of the parathyroid glands and is associated with medullary thyroid carcinoma and pheochromocytomas. The genetic defect has been mapped to 10cen-10q11.2 *(9)*.

The mechanism for the elevated PTH in hyperparathyroidism is not clear. There appears to be an altered set point for the response to ionized calcium; a higher level of ionized calcium is required to turn off PTH production *(10,11)*. An absolute increase in the number of cells with a normal or near normal set point may cause excess production of PTH. This mechanism may be responsible for the changes seen in parathyroid hyperplasia *(12)*. In parathyroid adenomas, both mechanisms seem to be at work. In as many as 20% of parathyroid adenomas, genetically controlled clonal expansions of chief cells occur because of rearrangement of the PRAD1/cyclin D1 oncogene *(12–15)*.

Hypercalcemia is responsible for most of the clinical sequelae of the disease (Table 1). The hypercalcemia results from increased mobilization of calcium from bone, increased calcium absorption in the gut [from PTH-stimulated 1,25 $(OH)_2$ D_3 production], and

Stones
Stones
Renal stones
Nephrocalcinosis
Polyuria
Polydypsia
Uremia

Bones
Bones
Osteitis fibrosa with
Subperiosteal resorption
Osteoclastomas
Bone cysts
Radiological "osteoporosis"
Osteomalacia or rickets
Arthritis

Primary hyperparathyroidism
Signs and symptoms

Abdominal Groans	Psychic Overtones	Other
Abdominal Groans	**Psychic Overtones**	**Other**
Constipation	**Lethargy, fatigue**	**Proximal muscle weakness**
Indigestion, nausea, vomiting	**Depression**	**Keratitis, conjunctivitis**
Peptic ulcer	**Memory loss**	**? Hypertension**
Pancreatitis	**Psychoses-paranoia**	**Itching**
	Personality changes, neuroses	
	Confusion, stupor, coma	

Fig. 2. Mnemonic used for categorizing the signs and symptoms of hyperparathyroidism.

increased renal tubular reabsorption. In addition to hypercalcemia, 1HPT causes hypercalciuria, hypophosphatemia, bone disease, neuromuscular disease, peptic ulcer disease, pancreatitis and soft tissue calcifications (7) (Fig. 2).

There are many renal manifestations of 1HPT, including hypercalciuria, hyperphosphaturia, nephrolithiasis, nephrocalcinosis, hyperchloremic acidosis, hypertension, and distal renal tubular acidosis (16). The hypercalcemia leads to increased filtered load of calcium, which causes hypercalciuria despite the seemingly paradoxical effect of increased reabsorption of calcium in the proximal tubules (7). Stones are a result of hypercalciuria. Earlier series reported the incidence of stone disease in excess of 50%, but improved diagnostic schemes and earlier detection of disease have decreased the rate of renal calculi to 20% (16). Patients may have calcium oxalate kidney stones or calcium phosphate stones caused by alkaline urine and increased phosphaturia. In addition, increased urinary calcium and phosphate levels lead to precipitation of calcium phosphate salts in the soft tissues of the kidney which manifests as nephrocalcinosis. Medullary nephrocalcinosis may be present; occasionally cortical areas may be involved as well (16).

In addition to causing nephrolithiasis, 1HPT can cause chronic renal failure (17). The long-term effects on the kidneys may be insidious. First, loss of normal medullary concentrating ability occurs followed by impairment of glomerular filtration rate (18). Interstitial renal disease may cause urinary frequency, nocturia and mild dehydration impacting on the patient's quality of life.

Concomitant with the increased urinary excretion of calcium, the patient has increased intestinal absorption driven by increased serum levels of 1,25 $(OH)_2D_3$. Studies have shown patients with hyperparathytroidism and stones have serum levels of 1,25 $(OH)_2D_3$ that are no different from patients with hyperparathyroidism and no stones (19). Hypophosphatemia secondary to hyperphosphaturia provides another stimulus for 1,25 $(OH)_2D_3$ production. The elevated 1,25 $(OH)_2D_3$ caused by the elevated PTH also leads to increased intestinal absorption of calcium further increasing calcium serum concentration (7).

Diagnosis of 1HPT is made by finding an elevated PTH in the setting of serum calcium, greater than 11.5 ng/dL *(18)*. Often the serum calcium may be high normal or minimally elevated in asymptomatic patients with mild disease *(18,13)*. Detection of PTH in serum was initially performed with cross-reactive antibodies to bovine PTH recognizing the carboxy-terminal region of PTH. The next generation assays were antibodies to the amino-terminal and mid region of the hormone *(20,21)*. These assays were followed by measurements of intact hormone by double antibodies to both ends of PTH *(22)*. Currently, PTH is measured by immunoradiometric and/or immunochem-iluminometric assays providing greater specificity and sensitivity *(18,13)*.

The cure for primary hyperparathyroidism is parathyroidectomy; however, it is not clear that all patients need this operation. Complications from the operation may include hypoparathyroidism and recurrent laryngeal nerve injury. Injury to this nerve leads to vocal cord paralysis, resulting in hoarseness, or if bilateral, respiratory compromise. Identification of patients who will benefit from parathyroidectomy can be challenging *(18)*. Most patients with hyperparathyroidism have a single adenoma, are female and over 50 yr of age. Generally, hyperparathyroidism increases with age as do other comorbidities. The factors of age and comorbidities make some patients poor operative candidates. Risks and benefits must be carefully weighed as the sequelae of hypercalcemia may be disabling or life-threatening. High serum calcium causes neuromuscular irritability. This may result in fatigue, lethargy, depression, mental confusion, or even coma. Cardiac effects of high calcium levels include arrhythmias and cardiac arrest. Patients with hypercalcemia can have hypertension, peptic ulcer disease, acute pancreatitis, hypotonia, polyuria, and polydipsia (ref. *23*; Table 1).

A consensus development conference in 1991 established guidelines for surgical intervention *(24)*:

- Markedly elevated serum calcium.
- History of an episode of life-threatening hypercalcemia.
- Reduced creatinine clearance.
- Presence of kidney stone(s) detected by abdominal radiograph.
- Markedly elevated 24-h urinary calcium.
- Substantially reduced bone mass as determined by direct measurement.

Although 50% of the patients with 1HPT will meet these criteria for surgery, patients with nephrolithiasis should undergo parathyroidectomy. For other patients, Rodman and Mahler state, "because of the subtle ongoing effects of disordered calcium metabolism that are hard to measure, there must be a reason not to operate" *(18)*.

The experience of the surgeon may affect his willingness to operate. The learning curve is steep; 15 or more cases per year are needed, according to Sosa et al in their survey of parathyroid surgeons. Surgeons not performing the operation regularly should be wary of anatomic variations in the neck *(18)*.

Preoperative localization of the adenoma may be helpful. In 1991 the Consensus Development Conference concluded that preoperative imaging was not necessary because of low yield from existing technology *(24)*. During that time, 60% positive results and 15% false positive results were achieved with available imaging techniques. Since that time imaging techniques have improved. Nuclear scans, including technetium–99m sestamibi and technetium tetrofosmin, have greater than 95% accuracy *(18, 25–28)*. In centers where a high volume of parathyroid imaging is performed, standard computed tomography (CT) scan and ultrasound are reported to have 95% accuracy *(18)*.

Preoperative localization allows the surgeon to accurately plan the operation. Tumor localization may help prevent complications by allowing for a unilateral neck or chest exploration. Operating-room time and cost may be reduced. If diffuse hyperplasia is seen on localization studies, a more complex operation is planned involving exposure of all four parathyroid glands. This may dissuade the surgeon from operating in a frail patient with significant comorbidities (18,29). Despite improved localization studies, most parathyroid surgeons still insist on bilateral neck explorations. Mixed results are reported as to whether preoperative localization reduces operating room time (30,31). In borderline patients the localization may help in the decision to operate or not to operate. In patients with urolithiasis, a clear-cut indication to operate is almost always present (32). Therefore, the presence of urolithiasis in a patient with 1HPT should prompt the urologist to make the appropriate referral.

Secondary Hyperparathyroidism

The diagnosis of secondary hyperparathyroidism is made when normal serum calcium is found on serial examinations with an elevated PTH. Parathyroid hormone is appropriately elevated in this condition as a response to a low serum calcium from chronic renal failure, intestinal malabsorption (of vitamin D or calcium), or renal leak of calcium. In terms of nephrolithiasis, secondary hyperparathyroidism is most often seen with renal leak hypercalciuria. Serum calcium is normal and PTH levels are minimally elevated, or normal.

VITAMIN D

Both diet and synthesis in the skin are important sources of vitamin D_3. In the skin, ultraviolet light causes a photosynthetic conversion of 7-dehydrocholesterol to previtamin D_3 (Fig. 3). This heat labile previtamin is isomerized to vitamin D_3 (cholecalciferol). Vitamin D_3 is carried to the liver and is converted to 25-hydroxycholecalciferol [25-$(OH)_2D_3$] (33,34). In the kidney's proximal tubule, PTH stimulates 1 α-hydroxylase in the mitochondria to convert 25-$(OH)_2D_3$ to 1,25$(OH)_2D_3$ which is the active form of the vitamin. Decreased serum phosphate levels also activate the enzyme. Decreased serum calcium indirectly stimulates 1-α-hydroxylase production via stimulation of PTH production. 1,25 $(OH)_2D_3$ production is also stimulated by estrogen, growth hormone and prolactin (2).

Vitamin D functions to increase serum calcium and phosphorus levels to enhance bone mineralization. 1,25 $(OH)_2D_3$ stimulates absorption of calcium and phosphate from the brush border of the intestinal mucosa (33). The hormone increases calcium-binding protein synthesis in the kidney, which leads to renal calcium reabsorption.

Hypervitaminosis D

Hypercalcemia occurs in patients taking greater than 50,000 units of vitamin D daily (35). These patients may be self-administering excessive doses of vitamin D or are prescribed medical replacement for hypoparathyroidism. Infrequently, patients may develop urolithiasis and become symptomatic. Stones are typically calcium phosphate. More commonly, patients present with other signs and symptoms of hypercalcemia without nephrolithiasis (Table 1). Treatment is withdrawal of the vitamin D and calcium supplements, increased fluids and high-dose corticosteroid therapy (23).

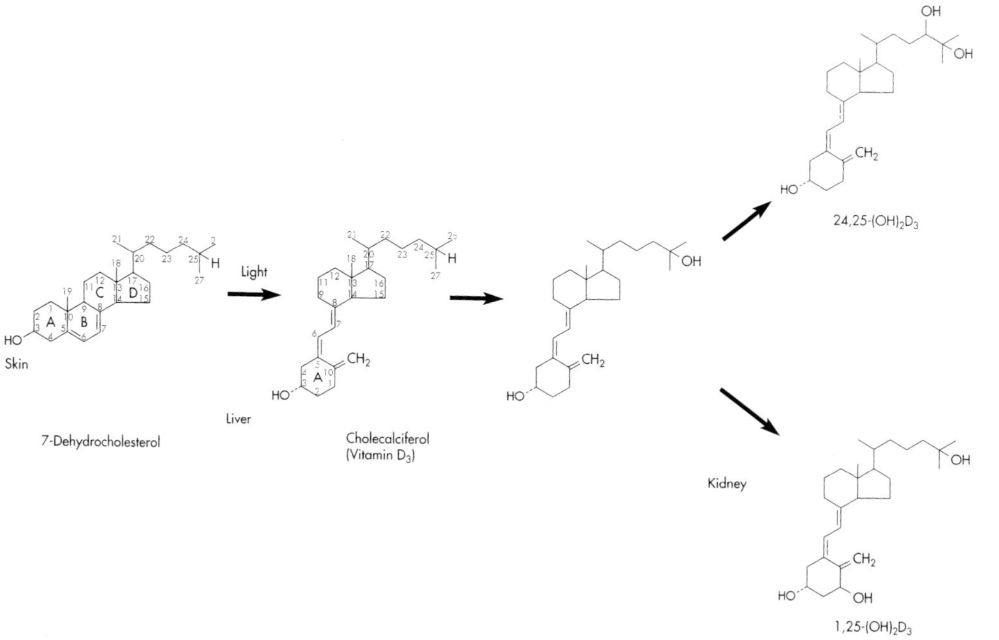

Fig. 3. Biosynthesis of 1,25-dihydroxycholecelciferol. (From ref. *2* with permission.)

CALCITONIN

Calcitonin is a 32-amino acid polypeptide produced by thyroid parafollicular cells. Its half-life in circulation is less than one hour, and it is inactivated in the kidney *(36)*. Calcitonin acts on bone and in the kidney to decrease serum calcium and phosphate. In bone, it inhibits bone resorption by blocking osteoclast activity and osteoclast precursor differentiation *(2)*. In the human kidney, calcitonin produces increased natriuresis and kaliuresis *(37)*. High dose infusion in humans acts to inhibit inorganic phosphate and calcium reabsorption *(2,19,37–39)*. The effects on calcium and phosphate handling at physiologic doses are controversial; some authors suggest a minimal role for this hormone in calcium homeostasis *(2,37)*. The actions of calcitonin are mediated by adenylate cyclase and c-AMP *(37)*. Calcitonin may stimulate 1α-hydroxylase activity in the proximal straight tubule of the kidney and have a role in vitamin D synthesis. Calcitonin secretion is stimulated by increased serum calcium. Gastrointestinal hormones such as gastrin, glicentin, secretin, and cholecystokinin-pancreozymin, may also stimulate calcitonin release.

There exists little objective evidence for a defined role for calcitonin in nephrolithiasis. Plasma concentration of calcitonin is significantly higher in children with idiopathic hypercalciuria *(40–42)*. D'Angelo et al. concluded that "calcitonin plays a contributory role in the pathogenesis of recurrent calcium nephrolithiasis that seems to be strictly correlated with dietary calcium intake; thus higher production and sensitivity to calcitonin could be related to persistent hypercalciuria" *(43)*.

SEX HORMONAL INFLUENCES

Significant sex-related differences exist in the rate of stone formation and types of stones formed. Soucie and associates determined the prevalence rate of all types of stone formation between men and women to be 2.64 to 1 *(44)*. Idiopathic calcium stones are even more common in men, with a 4–5 to 1 male to female ratio *(45,46)*. The risk in men peaks at age 35; women display a bimodal peak at ages 30 and 55 *(45)*. Men tend to have smaller stones made of pure calcium oxalate, whereas women have relatively larger stones with a higher relative percentage of calcium phosphate *(47)*. The risk of stone formation in men is influenced by testosterone. In adult women three different hormonal milieus exist: nonpregnant, pregnant, and postmenopausal.

Male Factors

The cause of the high rate of calcium oxalate stones in men has not been explained on the basis of limited clinical studies. Urinary oxalate levels have been implicated, and hyperoxaluria is up to three times more common among men than women *(48)*. Hammar et al. found no significant change in urinary citrate excretion or the calcium to citrate ratios of men before and after orchiectomy *(49)*. Van Aswegen et al. studied urinary testosterone in 14 calcium oxalate stone formers and 21 healthy subjects. Urinary testosterone levels in stone formers were lower than in the controls. They concluded that urinary testosterone was needed to help prevent calcium oxalate stone formation *(50)*. This finding seems counterintuitive, because it is assumed that testosterone is responsible for increased male calcium urolithiasis.

The clinical evidence does not affirm laboratory animal models investigating sex related differences in stone formation. The most practical and most commonly used animal model is ethylene glycol induced nephrolithiasis in the rat. Ethylene glycol (EG) consumption results in significant hyperoxaluria, which leads to stone formation in an animal that is not normally prone to renal stones. In the EG-induced rat model, a common trend is noted: calcium oxalate crystallization and stone formation are generally increased in the presence of testosterone and decreased in the presence of female hormones.

Many studies have focused on the effects of testosterone on oxalate excretion. Lee et al. fed EG to intact and castrated male and female rats and noted that intact male rats had the highest rates of hyperoxaluria, although urinary oxalate was increased in all rats fed EG. Furthermore, urolithiasis occurred most commonly among intact male rats and did not occur in female rats. Castrated males were noted to have a 14.3% rate of stone formation compared to 71.4% for intact males *(51)*.

A follow-up study showed that administration of testosterone to castrated males resulted in increased stone formation compared to castrated males without testosterone replacement. Castrated females given testosterone also exhibited urolithiasis much more frequently than intact females *(52)*. In another EG rat model, Fan et al. used a series of male and female rats, both intact and castrate, implanted with preparations of testosterone and estradiol. The groups with testosterone implants had much higher daily oxalate excretion than the groups with estradiol implants. No estradiol-implanted rats had calcium oxalate crystal deposition in the kidneys, whereas 15 of 22 rats implanted with testosterone had crystal deposition *(53)*.

Yagisawa et al. used an EG rat model to look in depth at sex hormone effects by focusing on osteopontin, a protein that plays a complex and incompletely elucidated role in stone formation. Osteopontin may act as a stone promoter by forming the matrix portion of stones; however it has also been shown to inhibit calcium oxalate crystallization in vitro. Twenty-four-hour urinalyses and osteopontin expression in renal tissue were studied in intact and castrated rats of both sexes. Testosterone promoted stone formation by suppressing osteopontin expression in the kidneys and increasing oxalate excretion. Estrogen appeared to inhibit stone formation by increasing osteopontin and decreasing urinary oxalate levels *(54)*.

In another EG induced urolithiasis rat model, the effects of castration and finasteride were investigated. Urinary oxalate levels were highest in EG-treated intact male rats and significantly lower in castrated rats and those treated with finasteride. The effect of finasteride led to the conclusion that some of the hyperoxaluria seen in the EG rat model was caused by the effect of dihydrotestosterone *(55)*.

Although vasectomy has no direct hormonal effects clinically, it has been associated with an increased incidence of urolithiasis. A study of over 11,000 men found an age-adjusted relative risk of urolithiasis of 1.67 in vasectomized men compared to men who did not undergo vasectomy. The highest relative risk was 2.6 for men age 30–34 *(56)*. To study the effect of vasectomy in the laboratory, Scherieber and Schwille divided rats into vasectomy, vasosvasotomy, and sham-operated groups. Two rats out of 12 in the vasectomy group developed nephrolithiasis, whereas no stones developed in the other two groups. Although serum and urinary testosterone levels were unchanged, serum magnesium was decreased and urine phosphate levels were increased in the vasectomy group. Tissue levels of phosphorus, calcium, and magnesium in the renal papillae were higher in the vasectomy group than the other groups. They concluded that vasectomy has subtle metabolic effects and hypothesized this may be related to a disturbance in autonomic tone resulting from vasectomy *(57)*.

Female Factors

Other than epidemiologic evidence, clinical evidence is scant concerning the low rate of calcium stone disease found in women. A survey of 1302 women in Scandinavia revealed a history of stone disease in 5% of all age groups, with the highest rate noted at 46 yr of age and the lowest at 62 yr of age. The incidence of stone disease in this study was 3.7 per 1000 women per year *(58)*.

The higher levels of urinary citrate in women compared to men have been cited as a likely cause of lower rates of calcium oxalate lithiasis. In a study of 173 stone formers, no differences could be found in urinary inhibitors (citrate, magnesium, pyrophosphate, and glycosaminoglycans) between men and women *(59)*. Another study focused on citrate, the most well characterized inhibitor of calcium lithiasis, in 24-h urine samples from three groups: pregnant women, postmenopausal women on hormonal replacement therapy, and castrated men. The urinary citrate levels were not altered significantly in any of these groups *(49)*.

A different study noted that postmenopausal women had significantly higher calcium excretion than groups of young women and groups of young and old men. Citrate levels were lowest in young men compared to either young women or old men. Older women had citrate levels not significantly different from young men. Magnesium excretion was higher in postmenopausal women than in young subjects of either sex *(60)*.

Iguchi et al. studied a female rat EG model to determine the effect of female hormones on stone formation. They noted that oophorectomized rats given EG had the highest rates of oxalate excretion and the highest rates of crystal deposition in the renal tissues. Osteopontin mRNA expression was highest in the oophorectomized group. Administration of female hormones reversed each of these elevated parameters. In contrast to the previously cited study by Yagisawa, et al., this study concluded that increased osteopontin levels were consistent with stone promotion. Citrate levels in the oophorectomized rats did not differ significantly from controls *(61)*.

MENOPAUSE

Menopause results in lower circulating levels of female hormones. Use of hormonal replacement therapy is variable and individualized. Many women in this stage of life are at risk for osteoporosis and are encouraged to take calcium supplements. This has raised concern among researchers about promotion of calcium urolithiasis in this group of women. Of added concern is that many stone formers have lower bone density than age matched controls, and thus, stone formers may be at greater risk for osteoporosis and more likely to require calcium supplementation *(61)*. Female stone formers age 36–68 placed on 1 gm/d calcium citrate were found to have increased urinary calcium excretion over a 6-mo study period. Citrate and oxalate excretion as well as calcium oxalate saturation were not significantly changed from baseline. Serum levels of parathyroid hormone and $1,25\,(OH_2)$ vitamin D concentration decreased significantly over the course of the study *(62)*.

A study of postmenopausal women given either calcium carbonate or calcium carbonate and calcitriol did not demonstrate increased calcium oxalate saturation *(63)*.

A study by the same team investigated the effects of calcium carbonate supplementation vs calcium carbonate plus estrogen replacement in healthy nonstone forming women. After 3 mo of treatment, no changes were noted in urinary excretion of calcium, citrate, or oxalate. Neither the calcium/creatinine ratio nor the calcium oxalate saturation in the urine was changed significantly from baseline *(64)*.

In 1454 adult calcium oxalate stone formers, Heller et al. compared outpatient metabolic evaluations of the men and postmenopausal women. Lower urinary calcium in women was noted until the age of 50 yr, whereas a reduction of urinary citrate below that observed in men occurred at the age of 60 yr. Postmenopausal women treated with estrogen had lower 24-h urinary calcium, 2-h fasting urinary calcium, and calcium oxalate saturation compared with untreated postmenopausal women. These data suggest that the lower risk of stones in women may be caused by lower urinary saturation and that estrogen replacement in postmenopausal women may reduce the risk of stone recurrence *(65)*.

PREGNANCY

Pregnancy induces anatomic and physiologic changes in the kidneys which have a bearing on urolithiasis. The kidney increases in weight and in length (about 1 cm) during pregnancy. These changes are caused by pregnancy related increases in renal interstitial and intravascular volume *(66)*. In the renal collecting system, the calices, pelvis, and ureters dilate and show hypertrophy of the ureteral smooth muscle and hyperplasia of connective tissue as well. Dilatation of the collecting system begins at 6–10 wk of gestation, is more prominent on the right renal unit, and occurs in 90% of women at term *(66–70)*. The etiology of this dilatation has not been fully elucidated but is related to anatomic obstruction of the distal ureter by the uterus as well as some effect from the hormone progesterone. Two findings give credence to the hormonal influence on pregnancy related hydronephrosis: (1) the ureters dilate before uterine enlargement; (2) prolonged ureteral catheterization does not reverse the collecting system dilatation during pregnancy *(66)*. Several factors argue for the influence of ureteral obstruction by the gravid uterus. The ureteral pressure when monitored in the third trimester of pregnancy is noted highest in the standing and supine positions; the pressure decreases in the lateral decubitus and knee–chest position. Ureteral pressures decrease immediately after caesarean section, and pressures are noted to decrease only above the pelvic brim *(66)*.

In addition to anatomic changes, the kidney undergoes functional changes that may influence the formation of urinary calculi. Both the glomerular filtration rate (GFR) and the renal plasma flow (RPF) increase markedly by 35–50% during pregnancy. The reasons may include increased cardiac output and increased extracellular volume. This is countered by a decrease in systemic vascular resistance and blood pressure. Pregnancy related changes in circulating hormones include increases in aldosterone, desoxycorticosterone, progesterone, prolactin, and chorionic gonadotropin, but these increases alone cannot explain the increase in GFR. GFR is increased because of an increase in RPF resulting from a decrease in renal vascular resistance. Values of plasma blood urea nitrogen and creatinine are also lower in pregnancy. The pregnant woman experiences an increase in glucosuria and aminoaciduria caused by increased filtered load of these substances. Uric acid excretion increases, and the serum levels of urate fall by 25%.

The incidence of urolithiasis in pregnancy has been estimated at 1 in 1500, with a range of 1 in 188 to 1 in 3821 pregnancies and an incidence rate of 0.026–0.53% *(71,72, 74)*. There is no increase in either the incidence of urolithiasis or numbers of recurrences of stones in pregnant women compared with nonpregnant women *(75)*. Pregnant women form the same types of stones same as nongravid stone formers *(75,76)* 80–90% of stones present clinically in the second or third trimester of pregnancy *(76,77)*.

Pregnant women have marked hypercalciuria and an increased urinary supersaturation ratio for calcium oxalate and brushite. Howarth et al. studied 1034 normal women in the third trimester and found 20% excreted >350 mg of calcium in 24 h, which exceeded the 95% limit for nonpregnant women *(78)*. These investigators felt increased calcium excretion was related to increased filtered load of calcium secondary to higher GFR *(78)*. In addition to increased GFR causing hypercalciuria, increases in levels of 1,25 vitamin D during gestation cause increases in the intestinal absorption of calcium, bone mobilization, and hypercalciuria.

Hypercalciuria and supersaturation of urinary salts is accompanied by an increase in inhibitors. Although the inhibitors citrate and magnesium are elevated in the urine during pregnancy, they are not elevated proportionally to the increase in supersaturation of stone constituents found in the urine *(79)*. This "inhibitor gap" has given investigators cause to search for other stone inhibiting substances. Pregnant women exhibit increased production of the inhibitory glycoprotein Tamm–Horsfall protein which decreases crystal aggregation and growth *(67,81–83)*. Another glycoprotein inhibitor of calcium oxalate lithiasis, nephrocalcin, has been found to increase significantly throughout pregnancy which may counterbalance the hypercalciuria *(82,83)*.

OTHER HORMONAL INFLUENCES

Other hormones not directly involved in calcium homeostasis or sexual function may also play a limited role in urolithiasis. These hormones may include insulin, growth hormone, thyroid hormone, glucocorticoids, and mineralocorticoids.

Insulin

Insulin acts at the proximal tubule of the kidney to increase urinary calcium excretion. Diabetes and glucose ingestion are associated with hypercalciuria *(37,85,86)*. Iguchi and associates showed that increases in plasma glucose levels following a glucose tolerance test were similar in stone formers and controls. Urinary calcium excretion increased in stone formers and controls in response to oral glucose, but the effect was greater in stone patients than in the control subjects *(86)*. Many investigators believe that diets high in refined sugars are partially responsible for the high rates of stone formation seen in Western countries *(87–89)*.

Growth Hormone

Urolithiasis may affect 12–39% of patients with acromegaly *(89–91)*. Animal studies show no acute effects of growth hormone on urinary excretion of calcium or phosphate; however patients with acromegaly and normal persons taking growth hormone exhibit increased levels of urinary calcium and magnesium. In one study 72% of the patients demonstrated hypercalciuria *(89)*. In addition, growth hormone may affect calcium balance by increasing renal calcitriol synthesis in a process mediated by insulin-like growth factor- I.

Thryoid Hormone

Thyroid hormone's renal effects include enhancing free water excretion, increasing urinary calcium and magnesium excretion and increasing renal tubular absorption of phosphate. Hyperthyroidism may cause hypercalcemia caused by a direct effect of thyroid hormone on bone resorption. Serum calcium may be elevated in 10–20% of patients with hyperthyroidism. Increased filtered load of calcium, resulting from increased GFR and mobilization of calcium from bones with suppression of PTH secretion, causes hypercalciuria. Nephrocalcinosis and nephrolithiasis may result from this abnormal calcium excretion *(16,37,93)*.

Adrenocortical Hormones

The long-term administration of exogenous mineralocorticoid results in increased levels of urinary calcium and magnesium in response to increased plasma volume. Serum calcium remains stable, possibly because of secondary parathyroid hormone secretion. Several case reports have documented nephrocalcinosis and nephrolithiasis associated with mineralocorticoid excess. Treatment with sprionolactone reverses the metabolic abnormalities and controls the nephrolithiasis *(93,94)*.

Glucocorticoid administration has been associated with hypercalciuria and hypermagnesiuria. The bone demineralizing effects of glucocorticoids may lead to nephrocalcinosis and calcium lithiasis *(16)*.

CONCLUSION

Hormonal effects play a role in most cases of stone disease. This role may range from a direct role in the case of hyperparathyroidism to a more subtle role in men and aging women. A significant amount of clinical and laboratory research will be needed to illuminate the specific contribution of hormonal influences on nephrolithiasis.

REFERENCES

1. Menon M, Resnik MI: Urinary lithiasis: etiology, diagnosis, and medical management. In: Campbell's Urology, 8th Ed., (Walsh PC, Retik AB, Vaughan ED, Jr, et al. eds.). Saunders, Philadelphia, PA, 2002; pp. 3243–3248.
2. Porterfield S. Endocrine Physiology, 2nd Ed., Mosby-YearBook, New York, NY, 2000; pp. 107–129.
3. Friedrichs R, Beherendt U, Graf K, et al. Primary hyperparathyroidism: Studies of 4000 urinary calculi patients treated with extracorporeal shock wave lithotripsy. Helvet Chir Acta 1991; 58: 327–330.
4. Fuss M, Pepersack T, Corvilain J, et al. Infrequency of primary hyperparathyroidism in renal stone formation. Br J Urol 1988; 62: 4–6.
5. Sedlack JD, Kenkel J, Czarapata BJ, et al. Primary hyperparathyroidism in patients with renal stone. Surg Gynecol Obstet 1990; 171: 206–208.
6. Peacock M, Marshall RW, Robertson WG, et al. Renal stone formation in primary hyperparathyroidism and idiopathic stone disease: diagnosis, etiology, and treatment. In: Colloquium on Renal Lithiasis. (Finlayson B, Thomas WD, Jr, eds.). University of Florida Press, Gainesville, FL, 1976.
7. Slatopolsky E, Hruska KA. Disorders of phosphorus, calcium, and magnesium metabolism. In: Diseases of the Kidney and Urinary Tract, 7th Ed., (Schrier RW, ed.) Lippincott Williams & Wilkins, Philadelphia, PA, 2001; pp. 2607–2660.
8. The BT, Farnedbo F, Phelan C. Mutation analysis of the MEN 1 gene in multiple endocrine neoplasia, type 1, familial acromegaly and familial isolated hyperparathyroidism. J Clin Endocrinol Metab 1998; 83: 2621–2626.
9. Thakker RV. Multiple endocrine neoplasia-syndrome of the twentieth century. J Clin Endocrinol Metab 1998; 883:2617–2620.
10. Brown EM, Broadus AE, Brennan MF, et al: Direct comparison in vivo and in vitro of suppressibility of parathyroid function by calcium in primary hyperparathyroidism. J Clin Endocrinol Metab 1979; 48: 604.
11. Khosla S, Ebeling PR, Firek AF, et al. Calcium infusion suggests a "set point" abnormality of parathyroid gland function if familial benign hypercalcemia and more complex disturbances in primary hyperparathyroidism. J Clin Endocrinol Metab. 1993; 76: 715.
12. Bilezikan JP. Primary hyperparathyroidism. In: Primer in the Metabolic Bone Diseases and Disorders of Mineral Metabolism, (Favis JM, ed.). Lippincott-Raven, Philadelphia, PA, 1996; pp. 181–186.
13. Silverberg SJ, Bilezikian JP. Primary hyperparathyroidism. In: Principles and Practice of Endocrinology and Metabolism, 3rd Ed, (Becker KL, ed.). 2001; pp. 564–574.
14. Rosenberg CL, Motokura T, Kronenberg HM, Arnold A. Coding sequence of the over expressed transcript of the putative oncogene PRADI/cyclin D1 in two primary human tumors. Oncogene 1993; 8: 519.
15. Hsi ED, Zukerberg LR, Yang W-I, Arnold A Cyclin D1/PRAD1 expression in parathyroid adenomas: an immunohistochemical study. J Clin Encdocrinol Metab 1996; 81: 1736.
16. Kelepouris E, Agus ZS, Effects of endocrine disease on the kidney. In: Principles and Practice of Endocrinology and Metabolism, 3rd Ed, (Becker KL, ed.). Lippincott Williams and Wilkins, Philadelphia, PA, 2001; pp. 1902–1908.
17. Benabe JE, Martinez-Maldonado M: Hypercalcemic nephropathy. Arch Intern Med 1978; 138: 777–779.
18. Rodman JS, Mahler RJ: Kidney stones as a manifestation of hypercalcemic disorders: hyperparathyroidism and sarcoidosis. Urol Clin North Am 2000; 27: 275–285.
19. Kurokawa K, Fukagawa M, Hayashi M, Saruta T. Renal receptors and cellular mechanisms of hormone action in the kidney. In: The Kidney: Physiology and Pathophysiology, 2nd Ed., (Seldin DW, Giebisch G, eds.). Raven Press, New York, NY, 1991; pp. 1339–1361.
20. Marx SJ, Sharp ME, Krudy A Radioimmunoassay for the middle region of human parathyroid hormone. J Clin Endocrinol Metab 1981; 53: 76–84.
21. Papapoulos SE, Manning RM, Handy CN. Studies of circulating parathyroid hormone in man using a homologous amino-terminal specific immunoradiometric assay. Clin Endocrinol 1980; 13: 57–67.

22. Nussbaum SR, Zahnadnik RJ, Labign JR. A highly sensitive two-site immunoradiometric assay of parathyroid hormone and its clinical utility in evaluating patients with hypercalcemia. Clin Chem 1987; 33: 1364–1367.

23. Bruder JM, Guise TA, Mundy GR. Mineral metabolism. In: Endocrinology & Metabolism, (Felig P, Frohman LA, eds.). McGraw-Hill, New York, NY, 2001; pp. 1079–1175.

24. Consensus development conference statement. J Bone Miner Res 1991; 6(suppl 2): 9–13.

25. Apostolopoulos DJ, Houstoulaki E, Giannakenas C, et al. Technetium-99m tetrofosmin for parathyroid scintigraphy. J Nucl Med 1998; 39: 1433–1441.

26. Hinde E, Melliere D, Jeanguillame C, et al. Parathyroid imaging using simultaneous double window recoding of technetium 99m sestamibi and iodine-123. J Nucl Med 1998; 39: 110–115.

27. Ishibashi M, Nishida H, Hiromatsu Y, et al. Comparison of technetium 99m MIBI, technetium 99m-tetrofosmin, ultrasound and MRI for localization of abnormal parathyroid glands. J Nucl Med 1998; 39: 320–324.

28. Ishibashi M, Nishida H, Strauss HW, et al. Localization of parathyroid glands using technetium 99m tetrofosmin imaging. J Nucl Med, 1997; 38: 706–711.

29. Salti GI, Fedorak I, Yashiro T, et al. Continuing evolution in the operative management of primary hyperparathyroidism. Arch Surg 1992; 127: 831–837.

30. Ryan JA, Eisenber B, Pado KM. Efficacy of selective unilateral exploration in hyperparathyroidism based on localization tests. Arch Surg 1997; 132: 886–891.

31. Serpell JW, Campbell PR, Young AE. Preoperative localization of parathyroid tumors does not reduce operating time. Br J Surg 1991; 78: 589–590.

32. Bilezikian JP. Surgery or no surgery for primary hyperparathyroidism. Ann Intern Med 1985; 102: 402.

33. Shoback D, Marcus R, Bikle D, Strewler G. Mineral metabolism and metabolic bone disease. In: Basic & Clinical Endocrinology, 6th Ed., (Greenspan FS, Gardner DG, eds.). Appleton & Lange, Stamford, CT, 2001; pp. 273–300.

34. Holick MF. The cutaneous photosynthesis of previtamin D_3: A unique photoendocrine system. J Invest Derm 1981; 76: 51–58.

35. Jacobus CH, Holick MF, Shao Q, et al. Hypervitaminosis D associated with drinking milk. N Engl J Med 1992; 326: 1173.

36. Ardaillou R, Paillard F. Metabolism of polypeptide hormones by the kidney. Adv Nephrol 1980; 9: 247–269.

37. Kimmel PL, Rivera A, Khatri P. Effects of nonrenal hormones on the normal kidney. In: Principles and Practice of Endocrinology and Metabolism, 3rd Ed., (Becker KL, ed.). Lippincott Williams and Wilkins, Philadelphia, PA, 2001; pp. 1885–1895.

38. Queener SF, Bell NH. Calcitonin: a general survey. Metabolism 1975; 24: 555.

39. Talmage RV, Wiel DV, Matthews JL. Calcitonin and phosphate. Mol Cell Endocrinol 1981; 24: 235–251.

40. Tieder M, Stark H, Shainkin–Kestenbaum R. Pathophysiologic studies in idiopathic hypercalciuria presenting in childhood. Int J Pediat Nephrol 1983; 4: 197–200

41. Tieder M, Stark H, Shainkin–Kestenbaum R. Idiopathic hypercalciuria in childhood. Chemical and Metabolic Studies. Ann Meet Europ Soc Pediatric Nephrology, September 1978.

42. Shainkin-Kestenbaum R, Winikoff Y, Lismer L. The role of calcitonin in calcium stone formation. Nephron 1984; 38: 154–155.

43. D'Angelo A, Calo L, Cantaro S, Giannini S. Calciotropic hormones and nephrolithiasis. Miner Electrolyte Metab 1997; 23: 269–272.

44. Soucie JM, Thun MJ, Coates RJ, McClellan W, Austin H. Demographic and geographic variability of kidney stones in the United States. Kidney Int 1994; 46: 893–899.

45. Robertson WG, Peacock M, Heyburn PJ, Hanes FA. Epidemiological risk factors in calcium stone disease. Scand J Urol and Nephrol 1980; 14: 15–27.

46. Otnes B. Sex differences in the crystalline composition of stones form the upper urinary tract. Scand J Urol Nephrol 1980; 14: 51–56.

47. Gaul MH, Chafe L, Palfrey P, Robertson. The kidney-ureter stone sexual paradox: a possible explanation. J Urol 1989; 141: 1104–1106.

48. Curhan GC, Willett WC, Speizer FE, Stampfer MJ. Twenty-four-hour urine chemistries and the risk of kidney stones among women and men. Kidney Int 2001; 59: 2290–2298.

49. Hammar ML, Berg GE, Larsson L, Tiselius H-G, Varenhorst E. Endocrine changes and urinary citrate excretion. Scand J Urol Nephrol 1987; 21: 51–53.
50. Van Aswengen CH, Hurter P, van der Merwe A, du Plessis DJ. The relationship between total urinary testosterone and renal calculi. Urol Res 1989; 17: 181–183.
51. Lee, YH, Huang WC, Hung C, Chen MT, Huang JK, Chang, LS. Determinant role of testosterone in the pathogenesis of urolithiasis in rats. J Urol 1992; 147: 1134–1138.
52. Lee YH, Huang WC, Huang JK, Chang LS. Testosterone enhances whereas estrogen inhibits calcium oxalate stone formation in ethylene glycol treated rats. J Urol 1996; 256: 502–505.
53. Fan J, Chandhoke PS, Grampsas SA. Role of sex hormones in experimental calcium oxalate nephrolithiasis. J Am Soc Nephrol 1999; 10: S376–S380.
54. Yagisawa T, Ito F, Osaka Y, Amano H, Kobayashi C, Toma H. The influence of sex hormones of renal osteopontin expression and urinary constituents in experimental urolithiasis. J Urol 2001; 166: 1078–1082.
55. Fan J, Glass MA, Chandhoke PS. Effect of castration and finasteride in urinary oxalate excretion in male rats. Urol Res 1998; 26: 71–75.
56. Kronmal RA, Krieger JN, Kennedy JW, et al. Vasectomy and urolithiasis. Lancet 1988; 2: 22–23.
57. Schreiber M, Schwille PO. Vasectomy in the rat—effects on mineral metabolism, with emphasis on renal tissue minerals and occurrence of urinary stones. J Urol 1995; 153: 1284–1290.
58. Bengtsson C, Lennartsson J, Lindquist O, and Noppa H. Renal stone disease – Experience from a population study of women in Gothenburg, Sweden. Scand J Urol Nephrol Suppl 1980; 53: 39–43.
59. Akinci M, Esen T, Kocak T, Ozsoy C, Tellaloglu S. Role of inhibitor deficiency in urolithiasis: I. Rationale of urinary magnesium, citrate, pyrophosphate and glycosaminoglycan determination. Eur Urol 1991; 19: 240–243.
60. Sarada B, Satyanarayana U. Influence of sex and age in the risk of urolithiasis- a biochemical evaluation in Indian subjects. Ann Clin Biochem 1991; 28: 365–367.
61. Iguchi M, Takamura C, Umekawa T, Jurita T, Kohri K. Inhibitory effects of female sex hormones on urinary stone formation in rats. Kidney Int 1999; 56: 479–485.
62. Levine BS, Rodman JS, Wienerman S, Bockman RS, Lane JM, Chapman DS. Effect of calcium citrate supplementation on urinary calcium oxalate saturation in female stone formers: implications for prevention of osteoporosis. Am J Clin Nutr 1994; 60: 592–596.
63. Domrongkitchaiporn S, Onghpiphadhanakul B, Stitchantrakul W, et al. Risk of calcium oxalate nephrolithiasis after calcium or combined calcium and calcitriol supplementation in postmenopausal women. Osteoporosis International 2000; 11: 486–492.
64. Domrongkitchaiporn S, Onghpiphadhanakul B, Stitchantrakul W, et al. Risk of calcium oxalate nephrolithiasis in postmenopausal women supplemented with calcium or combined calcium and estrogen. Maturitas 2002; 41: 149–156.
65. Heller HJ, Sakhaee K, Moe OW, Pak CY. Etiological role of estrogen status in renal stone formation. J Urol 2002; 168: 1923–1927.
66. Lindheimer MD, Katz AI. The normal and diseased kidney in pregnancy. In: Diseases of the Kidney and Urinary Tract, 7th Ed, (Schrier RW, ed.). Lippincott Williams and Wilkins, Philadelphia, PA, 2001; pp. 2129–2165.
67. Cietak KA, Newton JR. Serial qualitative maternal nephrosonography in pregnancy. Br J Radiol 1985; 58: 399–404.
68. Bailey RR, Rolleston GL. Kidney length and ureteric dilatation in the puerperium. J Obstet Gynaecol Br Commonw 1971; 78: 55–61.
69. Fried, AW, Woodring JH, Thompson DJ. Hydronephrosis of pregnancy: A prospective sequential study of the course of dilatation. J Ultrasound Med 1983; 2: 255–259.
70. Peake SL, Roxburgh HB, Langlois SLP. Ultrasonic assessment of hydronephrosis of pregnancy. Radiology 1983; 146: 167–170.
71. Maikranz P, Lindheimer MD, Coe FL. Nephrolithiasis and gestation. Clin Obstet Gynaecol (Baillière) 1994, 8: 375.
72. Drago JR, Rohner TJ, Chez RA. Management of urinary calculi in pregnancy. Urology 1982; 20: 587–581.
73. Harris RE, Donahue DE. The incidence and significance of urinary calculi in pregnancy. Am J Obstet & Gynecol 1967; 99: 237-241.

74. Hendricks SK, Ross SO, Krieger JN. An algorithm for diagnosis and therapy of management and complications of urolithiasis during pregnancy. Surg Gynecol Obstet 1991; 172: 49–54.
75. Coe FJ, Parks JH, Lindheimer MD. Nephrolithiasis during pregnancy. N Eng J Med 1978; 298: 324–326.
76. Horowitz E, Schmidt JD. Renal calculi in pregnancy. Clin Ob Gyn 1985; 28: 324–338.
77. Rodriquez PN, Klein AS. Management of urolithiasis during pregnancy. Surg Gynecol Obstet, 1988; 166: 103.
78. Howarth AT, Morgan DB, Payne RB. Urinary excretion of calcium in late pregnancy and its relation to creatinine clearance. Am J Obstet Gynecol 1977; 129: 499–502.
79. Maikranz P, Holley JL, Parks JH, et al. Gestational hypercalciuria causes pathological urine calcium oxalate supersaturations. Kidney Int 1989; 36: 108–113.
80. Swanson SK, Heilman RL, Eversman WG. Urinary tract stones in pregnancy. Surg Clin North Am 1995; 75: 123–142.
81. Maikranz P, Coe FL, Parks JH, et al. Nephrolithiasis and gestation. Baillieres Clin Ob Gyn 1987; 1: 909.
82. Wabner C, Sirivongs D, Maikranz P, et al. Evidence for increased excretion in pregnancy of nephrocalcin (NC), a urinary inhibitor of calcium oxalate (CaOx) crystal growth (abstract). Kidney Int 1987; 37: 359.
83. Wabner C, Sirivongs D, Maikranz P, Nakagawa Y, Coe F. Evidence for increased excretion in pregnancy of nephrocalcin, a urinary inhibitor of calcium oxalate crystal growth (abstract). Kidney Int 1987; 31: 359.
84. Davison JM, Nakagawa Y, Coe FL, and Lindheimer MD. Increases in urinary inhibitor activity and excretion of an inhibitor of crystalluria in pregnancy: a defense against the hypercalciuria of normal gestation. Hypertension in Pregnancy 1993; 12: 25–35.
85. Gambaro G, Cicerello E, Mastrosimone S, et al. Increased urinary excretion of glycosaminoglycans in pregnancy and in diabetes mellitus: A protective factor against Nephrolithiasis. Nephron 1988; 50: 62–63.
86. Iguchi M, Umekawa T, Takamura C, et al. Glucose metabolism in renal stone patients. Urol Int 1993; 51: 185–190.
87. Schwille PO, Rumenapf G, Kohler R. Blood levels of glucometalbolic hormones and urinary saturation with stone forming phases after an oral test meal in male patients with recurrent idiopathic calcium urolithiasis and in healthy controls. J Am Coll Nutr 1989; 8: 557–566.
88. Blacklock NJ. Sucrose and idiopathic renal stone. Nutr Health 1987; 5: 9–17.
89. Ieki Y, Miyakoshi H, Nagai Y, et al. The frequency and mechanisms of urolithiasis in acromegaly. Nippon Naibunpi Gakkai Zasshi 1991; 67: 755–763.
90. Heilberg IP, Czepielewski MA, Ajzen H, Ramos OL, Schor N. Metabolic factors for urolithiasis in acromegalic patients. Braz J Med Biol Res 1991; 24: 687–696.
91. Pines A, Olchovsky D. Urolithiasis in acromegaly. Urology 1985; 26: 240–242.
92. Kohri K, Kodama M, Umekawa T, et al. Calcium oxalate crystal formation in patients with hyperparathyroidism and hyperthyroidism and related metabolic disturbances. Bone Miner 1990; 8: 59–67.
93. Kabadi UM. Renal calculi in primary hyperaldosteronism. Postgrad Med J 1995; 71: 561–562.
94. Yasuda G, Zierer R, Maio A, et al. Ammonium urate nephrolithiasis in a variant of Barter's syndrome with intact renal tubular function. Clin Investig 1994; 72: 385–389.

12 Associated Systemic Diseases

Bowel and Bones

Michael E. Moran, MD

CONTENTS

Key Words: Nephrolithiasis; intestine; bone metabolism; vitamin D.

INTRODUCTION

Stone diseases have had known affinities to other systemic diseases for a large portion of written medical history. The first known stone to afflict a human was probably a metabolic product of uric acid metabolism in a boy of the predynastic Egyptian period, almost 7000 years ago. Galen (131–201 AD) proposed the concept that etiologic aspects of stone formation include heredity, climatic, and nutritional factors. Van Helmont (1577–1644) noted that kidney stones were products of undesirable minerals within the urine. Thomas Sydenham (1624–1689) suffered from gout and recurrent urolithiasis. He describes his own disease process with clarity and proposed three hypotheses for the pathophysiology of stone disease and other systemic illnesses. On his disquisition into gout he states:

"...the gout breeds the stone in the kidneys in many subjects, either (1) because the patient is obliged to lie long on his back, or (2) because the secretory organs have

From: Current Clinical Urology, *Urinary Stone Disease:*
A Practical Guide to Medical and Surgical Management
Edited by: M. L. Stoller and M. V. Meng © Humana Press Inc., Totowa, NJ

ceased performing their proper functions; else (3) because the stone is formed from a part of the same morbific matter…" (1).

Urolithiasis induced by systemic diseases such as inflammatory bowel disease is complicated and the management of these patients is difficult. The patients tend to be ill from other comorbid problems and the stone(s) must be dealt with in addition to other troubles. The long term risk for bone depletion comes from complex interactions by stimulation of vitamin D, parathyroid hormone, and calcium regulation. Bone resorption could be a final common pathway in these systemic diseases with calcium stone formation.

INFLAMMATORY BOWEL DISEASE

A correlation between stone formation with bowel disease, specifically chronic diarrheal syndromes has been known since Lindahl and Bargen published in 1941 *(2)*. Chronic diarrheal illnesses have been well investigated since the 1940s and the prevalence of stone disease has been reported. Each of the types of inflammatory bowel disease has a relative impact on stone formation. Worcester, in an extensive review of published series has tabulated the prevalence of stones for patients with Crohn's disease, ulcerative colitis, and in those patients requiring bowel and/or ileal resections *(3)*. There are many complicating issues in these patients including duration of disease, hydration, use of medications such as steroids and sulfasalazine, and disease-specific problems that directly impinge on the urinary tract (such as retroperitoneal abscess, ureteral obstruction, and vesicoenteric fistulae). Stone prevalence in Crohn's disease is about 6.3% (range 3–8%). In ulcerative colitis the rate is 4.4% (range 3–10%). Worcester found that these high risk patients have a threefold increase in stone formation by having bowel surgery *(3–7)*. In a modern large review of Crohn's disease patients, a survey of 7210 patients in Germany found a 19.6% return rate of questionnaires (1414 patients). Of these, it was noted that 17.2% had a urinary calculus dwarfing previous expectations *(4)*.

Stone Type

Most stones associated with inflammatory bowel disease are calcium oxalate. It has been estimated that 69–90% of stones associated with chronic diarrheal syndromes are calcium oxalate *(7–12)*. The incidence of uric acid stones is significantly higher than the normal population (5–10%), occurring in 20–30% of these patients. Surgery alters the relative distribution, and the presence of an ileostomy adversely affects the stone prevalence as well as the number of patients that form uric acid stones (as high as 50%). Other stones can be manifest in these complex patients. Struvite (magnesium ammonium phosphate hexahydrate) or infectious stones in the urinary tract, although infrequent, are associated with obstructive changes. Briefly highlighted previously has been the predisposition in patients with inflammatory bowel disease toward hydronephrosis. Multiple recurrent urinary tract infections in patients with known inflammatory bowel disease should be suspect for not only fistulae but also struvite stone formation. Another rare type of stone associated with chronic diarrhea, especially in patients with laxative abuse, are ammonium urate stones *(13)*. These stones are typically found as endemic bladder stones in developing countries and in impoverished regions. They are more common in patients with chronic diarrhea, especially accompanied by laxative abuse and in those patients with ileocolonic resection. Ammonium urate stones are typically lucent but can be mixed with calcium oxalate, calcium phosphate, and struvite. A final rare stone type deserves mention—acetylsulfapyradine stones. Sulfasalazine is a sulfonamide that has rarely been reported to cause crystalluria, stone formation, and acute renal failure *(14)*. These stones are also lucent and typically present in patients that are elderly, are under long-standing treatment with sulfasalazine, and have accompanying dehydration. The stone is usually a yellowish-brown color with a fine granular surface *(15)*. Acetylsulfapyridine is a metabolite of the drug sulfasalazine, which is metabolized by intestinal flora into sulfapyridine and 5-aminosalicylic acid. These are absorbed and acetylated by the liver before excretion in the urine. Acetylsulfapyridine is less soluble in acidic urine and can be treated by urinary alkalinization. The drug sulfasalazine should be discontinued and/or replaced with mesalamine (5-aminosalicylic acid) if these stones occur *(14)*.

Pathogenesis

The etiology of stone formation in patients with chronic diarrheal syndromes is multifactorial and complex. Numerous investigations have been conducted in patients and animal models. Of the inflammatory bowel disease patients, Crohn's disease and ulcerative colitis have been rigorously investigated. Both have tendencies toward chronic hypovolemia with subsequent low urinary volumes (<1.2 L/urine output/24 h). Both groups of patients tend to have chronic acid urine (pH <5.5). Both groups also tend to have lower urinary magnesium and citrate levels, which are thought to be important inhibitors of calcium oxalate stone formation in comparison to control groups and even compared to other stone forming patients.

A primary additional risk factor in these subgroups is ileal involvement by the primary disease, more common in Crohn's disease patients and in patients undergoing surgical interventions with small and large bowel resections. Ileal involvement by these disease processes promotes more diarrhea, greater loss of water and steatorrhea, which can complicate further the physiologic malabsorption leading to hyperoxaluria and hypocalciuria. All of these processes adversely alter the risk of urolithiasis in these patients. Add to that ileal and colonic resection and loss of greater lengths of small bowel and stone rates climb proportionally in these patients. In addition, the bowel flora itself have been altered by chronic antibiotic exposure. A gram-negative anaerobe, *Oxalobacter formigenes*, has been isolated from the feces of several animals and humans. This bacteria uses intestinal oxalate as a substrate for its metabolism and therefore may be important for the regulation of intestinal absorption of oxalate *(16)*. An overview of the pathophysiology of the intestinal derangements enhancing the lithogenic potential in these patients is necessary.

Ulcerative colitis was the initial inflammatory bowel disease (IBD) reported to have an increased incidence of urolithiasis from the Mayo Clinic *(17)*. Sixteen patients (eight males and eight females) followed for a prolonged period developed clinically significant urolithiasis (most requiring open surgical intervention). This same group followed-up on their original observations with a separate series clearly indicating that ileostomy diversion in these patients enhanced the risk of stone formation appreciably *(2)*. The risk factors in patients with chronic bowel disease are best evaluated by stone type.

As mentioned previously, uric acid stones are more common in patients with IBD than in the general population. The urine of these patients is low volume secondary to the gastrointestinal loss. Add an ileostomy and volume loss is even more pronounced. The average loss from pooled investigations of patients with an ileostomy is between 500 and 700 mL/d *(18,19)*. More than 90% of ileostomy fluid loss is water. Compared to the normal adult loss in feces of less than 150 mL per day, this loss is significant *(19)*. These same studies indicate that urine output is typically below 1 L/d.

In more detailed investigations, Clarke and colleagues noted total body water was depleted by 11% in patients with an ileostomy *(20)*. Additionally, sodium is lost accounting for a 7% decrease as well as significantly lowered urinary sodium concentrations *(21)*. Despite evidence for sodium conservation in these patients, plasma aldosterone concentrations have been controversial in most series *(22,23)*. Kennedy and coworkers noted in a group of 39 ileostomists with proctocolectomy and less than 10 cm of terminal ileum resected plus an ileostomy showed a significant rise in mean plasma aldosterone. Also, the plasma renin activity was increased, but not markedly so. They speculated that ileum adaptation might explain differences between studies *(18)*.

The second contributing factor increasing the risk of uric acid stone formation in patients with IBD is acidic urine. Because uric acid is a weak acid with its first dissociable hydrogen ion with a pKa of 5.35, the urine's pH plays a significant role in stone risk. At a urine pH of 5, only approx 100 mg/L of uric acid can be held in solution. Hydrogen ion excretion is known to be increased in IBD patients and markedly so in those with an ileostomy *(23)*. Unlike most uric acid stone formers without IBD, these patients have increased ammonium excretion in addition to titrateable acid. This is thought to be secondary to intestinal loss of bicarbonate. This again is intensified in patients with active ileal disease and with ileostomies because the pH of ileal fluid is 7.0 *(18)*.

There has been extensive investigation indicating that purine metabolism is not generally affected by IBD. The net excretion of uric acid is therefore not markedly higher than in normal patients. The water loss with subsequent lower urinary volume in addition to the lower pH drives the solubility product of uric acid into the high risk range. Ileostomy patients excrete significantly more urine supersaturated with uric acid than controls and even more than most patients with uric acid stone formation without IBD *(24)*.

The second and more common stone is calcium oxalate. In this association, far more complex physical chemistry is associated with the heightened risk of urolithiasis. The low urine volumes and fixed, acidic pH still apply and although extensively investigated will not be reiterated. The average daily excretion of both calcium and oxalate do not appear to be significantly enhanced in patients with IBD with or without an ileostomy. There are occasional series that note a rise in oxaluria following an ileostomy. Bambach and others have measured significant calcium oxalate and calcium phosphate supersaturations in patients with ileostomies. Volume appears to be the overwhelming risk factor according to these investigations. The exception to this observation is when larger segments of small bowel become involved and longer segments of bowel are removed. At this point the association with steatorrhea and enteric hyperoxaluria become critical. Figure 1 represents a case with this clinical scenario. After having undergone several abdominal explorations the patient is left with only 20 cm of small bowel and suffers from short gut syndrome. This is discussed in detail in the section on jejunoileal bypass.

Inhibitors might be the other significantly measurable abnormality promoting calcium-stone formation in these patients. Citrate is a major urinary inhibitor known to bind with calcium, decreasing urinary supersaturation *(25)*. In one large study of 66 patients with IBD, citrate urinary excretion in both ulcerative colitis and Crohn's disease were low before any bowel surgery was performed. Following any type of surgical resection, the urinary citrate levels were decreased further ($p < 0.0001$) *(26)*. Compared to citrate levels in healthy controls (654.0 ± 297 mg/24 h), ulcerative colitis patients before surgery have only 386.0 ± 207 mg citrate/d ($p < 0.01$). Following surgical resec-

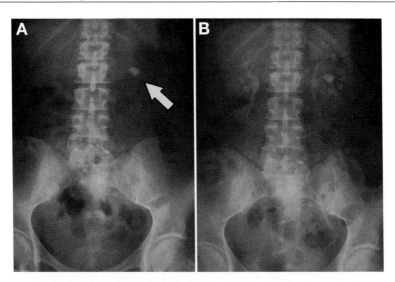

Fig. 1. A 45-yr-old white female presents with an incidentally found renal calculus at follow-up of her Crohn's disease. She has had numerous small bowel resections and currently has only 20 cm of small intestine remaining. **(A)** Scout film showing a 1.4 cm opaque midpole stone. **(B)** Intravenous urogram demonstrating no obstruction of the upper tracts.

tion this dropped further to 231.2 ± 161 mg citrate/d ($p < 0.0001$) *(26)*. In Crohn's disease patients before surgery the urinary citrate was 338.0 ± 233 mg/d ($p < 0.001$) and following surgery was noted to fall further to 215.0 ± 253 mg/d ($p < 0.001$). These authors further quantified stone forming risk in these patients by measuring crystalluria. In ulcerative colitis patients, crystalluria incidence was 30% with 93% being calcium oxalate dihydrate and 7% uric acid following surgical intervention. In Crohn's disease patients, crystalluria was significantly present before any surgical intervention (30%) and decreased marginally following surgery to 23.5% *(26)*.

Magnesium is another urinary inhibitor of calcium oxalate precipitation. Magnesium losses accrue secondary to loss in diarrheal stool. Systemic acidosis can lead to decreased urinary excretion and there may be some degree of gastrointestinal malabsorption of magnesium *(27)*. Using the data from Caudarella, urinary magnesium in healthy controls was 87.1 ± 35 mg/d compared to 82.6 ± 48 ($p < 0.005$) before surgery and 46.5 ± 17 ($p < 0.001$) following surgery in patients with ulcerative colitis. The Crohn's disease patient's urinary magnesium values were before surgery 54.4 ± 26 mg/d ($p < 0.005$) and 35.2 ± 25.4 ($p < 0.05$) following bowel resection *(26)*.

It has also been speculated that the increased risk of calcium oxalate stone formation of inflammatory bowel disease patients might be attributed to the high uric acid supersaturation. The model of heterogeneous nucleation would allow for the precipitation of calcium oxalate crystals on the readily available lattice of the uric acid crystals. No matter which mechanism is of greatest significance, these patients do represent a complex therapeutic dilemma.

Treatment

Having just outlined the primary pathophysiologic mechanisms of stone formation, a multifaceted method to medically treat these patients is now possible. As with prophylactic therapy in patients with "idiopathic" calcium stone disease, there exists very little data on the success of these therapies.

The most cost effective therapy is probably rehydration. These patients need to be encouraged to consume more fluids. The goal of getting urinary volumes to 2 or 2.5 L daily is critical. One effective method is encouraging these patients to consume small volumes more often. Patients should be encouraged to drink enough fluids so as to arise during sleep to urinate so that more fluid can be consumed during the sleep cycle when maximal urinary concentration is likely to occur. Although water is the classic fluid-of-choice, there are reports that lemonade and orange juice are excellent fluids for both uric acid and calcium stone formers (28,29). Citrus fruits are outstanding sources of dietary citrate and magnesium.

Chronic acidosis can likewise be treated. Sodium depletion can be corrected by the administration of oral sodium bicarbonate (30). Excess sodium loading can be detrimental to both uric acid and calcium stone prevention. Potassium-containing oral alkalizing agents have therefore assumed a greater role in the armamentarium for prophylaxis. Potassium citrate at doses from 30 to 80 meq/24 h increased urine pH from 5.3 to 6.19 and reduced new stone formation rate from 1.2 to 0.01 stones per year in patients with uric acid stone disease. Unfortunately, potassium citrate is associated with a large number of side effects, predominately gastrointestinal upset and the consequence to patients with IBD is not known. Compliance in the general stone population is known to be poor in long-term follow-up investigations. In one such study, Tiselius from Sweden noted that 62% of patients responding to a questionnaire reported compliance with citrate therapy (31). In an intermediate follow-up study, Lee reviewed 493 patients with a 34.2% stone recurrence rate and only 49.3% remained on medical prophylaxis longer than 12 mo (32). An additional study on patients with surgically active uric acid stones demonstrated that all patients were either partially or totally noncompliant with oral alkaline therapy for a variety of reasons including lack of physician-related information, concerns regarding possible side effects and medical neglect (33). Drop out rates might also be augmented by the inconvenience of multiple, timed, daily dosings necessary with potassium citrate (34).

Magnesium depletion remains the other identified parameter that can be treated in patients with inflammatory bowel disease. Magnesium, like citrate has gastrointestinal side effects ranging from 17 to 45% with exacerbation of diarrhea being foremost. Dietary methods of delivering magnesium were mentioned earlier by citrus fruit ingestion (28). Another study confirms the dietary efficacy demonstrating that navel oranges, Valencia oranges, and grapefruit all represent significant sources of magnesium and vitamin B6 (35). Confirmatory data exist for vitamin B6-magnesium supplements in recurrent stone formers both clinically and in experimental models (36,37). Vitamin B6 might augment the magnesium supplementation by acting in the liver to up-regulate enzymatic oxalate metabolism. The most recent possible therapeutic agent of interest in IBD is the combination of potassium-magnesium citrate (38). The ingestion of a meal with concurrent ingestion of citrate appears to decrease the gastrointestinal side effects without sacrifice of the physiologic or physicochemical actions (38). Potassium-magnesium citrate is capable of effectively correcting the magnesium, citrate, and potassium wasting effects of hydrochlorothiazide 50 mg/d in 242 investigational subjects (39). In follow-up studies, this same group studied the effect of varying the dose of potassium-magnesium citrate to correct hypokalemia and magnesium loss in thiazide-treated patients (40). Three dosages of potassium-magnesium citrate were randomized for 3 wk: four tablets (24 mEq K/12 mEq Mg/36 mEq citrate/d), 7 tablets (49 mEq K/ 24.5 mEq Mg/73.5 mEq citrate/d), and 10 tablets (70 mEq K/35 meq Mg/105 mEq citrate/d). All three doses resulted in increased potassium serum concentrations. Only the two higher doses resulted in significant elevations in serum magnesium. All three doses significantly increased urinary pH and citrate levels *(40)*. Another interesting drug used in the bowel preparation for radiologic evaluation is sodium picosulphate-magnesium citrate (Picolax). It has not been investigated as a supplement to reduce stone forming risks *(41)*.

Much clinical work remains to understand these complex patients with inflammatory bowel disease and stone formation. Both uric acid and calcium stone formation is possible at rates that exceed some of the "idiopathic" stone formers. One particular method of prophylaxis includes performing a total proctocolectomy in patients with ulcerative colitis, a mucosectomy of the anus with a continent ileal pull through and formation of a J-pouch reservoir. In one such nonrandomized comparative investigation, 13 patients with ulcerative colitis and an ileostomy were compared to 15 patients with J-pouches. The formation of the J-pouch requires more mobilization of the small bowel and as such, the patients were noted to have higher urinary concentrations of oxalate than those with ileostomy. Otherwise, the urinary physical chemistry appears to be quite similar to the ileostomy patients. The patients in both groups have lower urinary volumes, and subsequently higher concentrations of calcium, oxalate, and uric acid compared to control patients. Both groups likewise, had similarly lowered urinary pH *(42)*. There are thus few differences in the urinary physiology by modern methods of proctocolectomy and continent fecal diversion, and the long-term stone rates might still be similar to those of the ileostomy era *(43)*. The thought here is to minimize fluid loss by making a reservoir that will hold the ileal contents longer and eliminating the incontinent ileostomy. Studies on stone reduction have demonstrated that stone risk is reduced but still higher than in the nonoperated patients. Figure 2 is a case with a left-sided, asymptomatic calcium oxalate stone currently stable metabolically on magnesium and vitamin B6 plus potassium citrate therapy.

JEJUNOILEAL BYPASS SURGERY

Small bowel resection and bypass have long been associated with urolithiasis. The most common and best investigated groups are obese patients undergoing jejunoileal bypass (JIB) *(9–11)*. Other disease entities must also be considered as the pathophysiology is similar. Patients with Crohn's disease can have extensive involvement of not only the ileum, but other areas in the small bowel resulting in recurrent small-bowel resections. Infants can lose large sections of their small bowel secondary to vascular compromise and develop short gut syndromes *(44)*. Celiac sprue can compromise normal small-bowel function resulting in malabsorption syndromes, steathorrea, and chronic diarrhea *(45)*. Pancreatic and biliary obstruction or insufficiency can have profound effects on small-bowel function and result in steatorrhea and malabsorption syndromes. Other diseases can effect bowel function and lead to increased risk of urolithiasis including Hirsch sprung's disease. The mechanism from one review suggests that chronic constipation and enteric resections might be important to the 1.32% of stone patients seen in a group of 302 patients *(46)*. JIB surgery has been virtually reduced to a footnote in surgery, as other methods of bariatric surgery have come to the forefront of surgical practice, particularly laparoscopic techniques *(47–49)*. The

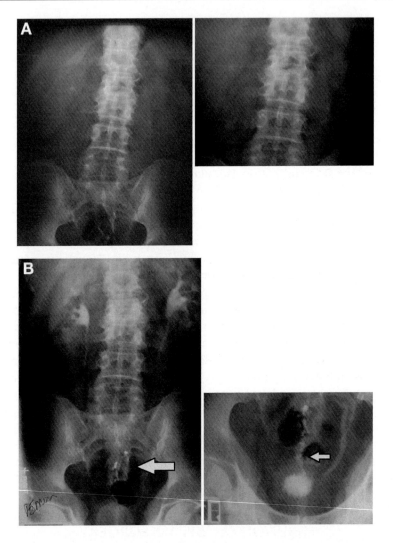

Fig. 2. This is a 64-yr-old white male with longstanding ulcerative colitis. He is status post total proctocolectomy with mucosectomy and a J-pouch. (**A**) Scout film showing small bilateral stones in clusters, left full KUB and right close tomographic view. (**B**) Intravenous urogram showing full details of unobstructed upper tracts (arrows pointing to the staple lines of his small bowel reconfiguration.

epilogue to JIB surgery remains of significant interest to students of stone disease because of the complex interactions between the bowel's absorptive and adaptive capacity and the relationship to diet, bone physiology, and stone formation *(50)*. These patients generally have normal gastrointestinal function before these procedures and the primary disruption and malabsorption that appears postoperatively has been extensively investigated.

JIB became a popular bariatric therapy for two decades, the 1970s and 1980s. There were two methods widely practiced, the Scott and the Payne anastomoses *(51)*. These

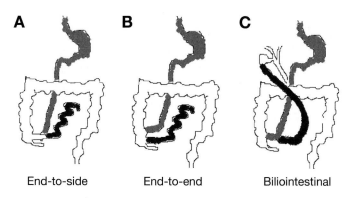

Fig. 3. Types of JIB and the amount of hyperoxaluria.

procedures included a 30–40-cm portion of the proximal jejunum that was attached to a 10–20-cm piece of distal ileum. A third operation was devised by Eriksson to minimize the metabolic consequences of JIB, the biliointestinal bypass thought to help by maintaining the enterohepatic circulation of bile and bile salts *(52)*. Individuals who underwent JIB have a high incidence of hyperoxaluria (60–88 %). The source of hyperoxaluria comes from intestinal oxalate absorption. Normally, humans absorb less than 20% of an administered dose of oxalate. If oxalate ingestion occurs with food, this absorption can be further reduced to <10%. In patients with small bowel resection (<50 cm) or JIB, absorption may range from 35% to <50%. Stone formation in JIB patients ranges from 8 to 40% *(53)*. The most common stone type is calcium oxalate, as expected (80–100%). Many patients begin to form stones quickly, within months after having the bypass procedure, but as many as 50% will not form their first stone until 3 yr postoperatively and there have been anecdotal reports of stones beginning 10 yr following JIB. The identification of the relationship of calcium oxalate stone formation led to a substantial number of investigations in these patients to better understand the complex interactions occurring in these individuals. In one investigation, all three types of JIB produced enteric hyperoxaluria; Paynes' end-to-side resulted in 863 ± 58 μmol oxalate/24 h, Scott's end-to-end produced 869 ± 65, and Eriksson's biliointestinal shunt was the worst with 1178 ± 68 (Fig. 3). The mean urinary oxalate excretion was 986 ± 49 μmol/24 h, all significantly greater than controls. There is no difference in oxalate excretion in stone formers with JIB vs nonstone formers *(54)*. Finally, numerous studies suggest that there is no decrease in hyperoxaluria over time.

In both animal experimental studies and radioisotope [$^{13}C_2$]oxalate ingestion studies, intestinal oxalate transport occurs in both the small and large bowel. There are both active and passive transport capacities involved. In addition, the distal small bowel is the site of absorption and reclamation of conjugated bile salts. In increasing quantity, these salts produce an osmotic secretion and net loss of intestinal water leading to increased diarrhea. After an ileal resection, it has been estimated that 13 mmol/L of bile acids can be found in fecal fluid of patients *(55)*. Finally, the stool normally contains little free fatty acids. Patients with JIB have malabsorption of these fatty acids with resultant steatorrhea. The effect of dietary fat consumption in individuals with fat malabsorption indicates that increasing dietary fat intake from 40 to 100 g/d increased fecal fat from 35 to 94 g/d. The fecal fat causes saponification with the calcium present from the diet. This complexation to the dietary calcium leaves the anion oxalate readily available for absorption. Therefore, fatty acids compete with oxalate for intestinal calcium complexation and this phenomenon is capable of being manipulated to decrease the adverse sequelae of hyperoxaluria. It is known that dietary calcium supplementation in patients with steatorrhea can reduce intestinal oxalate absorption. Finally, it has been noted that substituting medium-chain triglycerides for some of the dietary fat can produce a significant decrease in urinary oxalate excretion *(56)*.

One study suggests that the only measurable difference in stone forming patients with JIB was higher urinary magnesium excretion. At the University of Minnesota, a primary comparison between JIB (n=205) and gastric bypass (n=106) operations between 1975 and 1979 was undertaken. Weight loss was equivalent in each group but 7.1% of those in the JIB group developed urolithiasis whereas none from the gastric bypass group had a stone. In all, far fewer serious long-term complications were noted in the gastric bypass group *(57)*.

There are some final lessons important to mention before moving on to the bone diseases that increase the risk of stone formation. Patients having had a JIB also run the risk of chronic renal failure secondary to oxalate nephropathy *(58)*. Some have described this as a reversible phenomenon by conversion of the bypass back to small bowel continuity *(59)*. Renal failure can also occur secondary to renal amyloidosis, to which long-term JIB patients are prone *(60)*. It has been described in several investigations that stone disease occurring with the malabsorption of JIB can spontaneously disappear after reanastomosis *(61)*. One investigation quantified stone resolution in 86% of patients having reversal of JIB *(62)*.

IMMOBILIZATION SYNDROMES

Early in the clinical literature of urolithiasis it was documented that humans who are incapacitated and bed ridden are prone to kidney stones. In 1922, Paul from Toronto reported on 20 cases of nephrolithiasis occurring in men aged 22–37 (average 28.5) who developed renal calculi following war wounds. The average time from the wound to the first symptoms of stones was 17.7 mo. All patients had extensive injuries including osteomyelitis. Most of these patients were bedridden for prolonged times *(63)*. Pyrah followed by Pulvertaft both indicated that recumbency appeared to be the critical problem associated with calcium stone formation, not the degree of trauma *(64,65)*. The primary event increasing the risk of nephrolithiasis appears to be an acute mobilization of calcium from the skeletal reserves *(66)*. In some patients, hypercalciuria may be pronounced *(67)*. In these patients, indwelling Foley catheterization is also common and subsequent bladder infection makes upper tract seeding commonplace. Recurrent urinary tract infection therefore changes the primary stone risk in these patients with high urinary pH with the potential for ammonium production to form struvite stones *(68)*. In current practice with the emphasis on early mobilization and vigorous rehabilitation, no patients except perhaps those with global trauma (i.e., multiple organ injured individuals) run this risk. One current investigation on immobilization-related hypercalcemia studied five patients *(69)*. In this immobilized group, the hypercalcemia during 3 mo of observation could be reversed by administration of low-dose pamidronate (10 mg). In a review by Gordon and Reinstein, a discussion of common secondary problems associated with the management of complex trauma victims revealed that urolithiasis was a significant problem. In addition, the cost in managing this secondary problem was significant *(70)*. It would seem reasonable despite a paucity of published data, that immobilized patients are at higher risk and maintenance of adequate hydration would be a minimal recommendation. The use of bisphosphonates is more uncertain but indicated if hypercalcemia or urolithiasis develops. A final area of consideration is the effect of physical activity on calcium balance, calcium requirements, and bone mineral mass. Because of the aging population and the increasing risk of osteoporosis-induced risk of presbic fractures, a significant volume of research is becoming focused on these issues. In some studies, physical activity has been noted to have a more profound role in affecting enhanced bone mineral density before puberty *(71)*. The need for greater research and the potential for physical activity to have an effect on calcium balance are critical *(72)*.

Space Exploration

A corollary to the immobilization-related hypercalcemia and stone formation scenario is the possibility of placing humans in microgravity activity in outer space. With the advent of cooperative international endeavors such as the Space Station, plans for a manned mission to Mars, and the real probability that China might attempt a mission to the moon, these considerations have assumed more vigorous scientific scrutiny. The physiologic changes that occur to astronauts exposed to microgravity during space flight have been increasingly investigated. Body fluid volumes, electrolyte levels, and bone and muscle undergo significant changes as the body adapts to the weightless environment. There are both short-term space missions similar to those of Gemini, Apollo, and Space Shuttle flights and long-term missions such as Shuttle-Mir or Skylab *(73)*. In the former short-term space missions, negative calcium balance with bone mineral loss and associated hypercalciuria was noted during Gemini, Apollo, and Space Shuttle missions *(73)*. Additional alterations include elevated urinary phosphate, decreased fluid intake secondary to early flight space sickness (associated nausea and vomiting) with resulting decreased urinary volume and rising formation product *(74)*. Citrate has been shown to fall during space flight *(75)*. Whitson and coworkers have demonstrated that astronauts are at greater risk of forming calcium oxalate, calcium phosphate, and uric acid stones. In follow-up investigations, this same group studied more carefully six male astronauts with a mean age of 42.5 (range 36–49 yr old) flying Space Shuttle missions of 11–16 d *(75)*. Urine specimens were collected before, early in the mission (2–4 d), late in the mission (10–13 d), landing day, and 7–10 d after landing. Nutrition recommendations were rigorously controlled. Urine volume declined during the early flight but tended to equilibrate by post flight measurements. Urine output declined by 22–52% during spaceflight. Urine pH had a tendency toward increased acidity (lower pH), which also normalized by 7–10 d post flight. Urinary calcium levels increased for all members with individual variation being large (38–253 mg/d). Calcium excretion continued to increase during the flight. Urinary potassium was less during the early flight and urinary citrate was lower during the flight but neither was statistically different. The relative supersaturation of calcium oxalate, brushite, sodium urate, and uric acid all rose during early space flight. The calcium oxalate and brushite supersaturations remained statistically elevated throughout the entire space flight *(75)*.

Whitson and colleagues further speculate that dietary factors of the astronauts also play a role in risk for urolithiasis formation. Fluid restriction, protein, and calorie ingestion all increase urinary calcium and uric acid concentrations while decreasing urinary citrate. Dietary sodium can also promote renal calculus disease. Diets high in potassium and magnesium may have beneficial effects *(75)*. Zerwekh reviewed this metabolic data and generated specific nutritional recommendations for crew members on longer space missions. Pharmacologic intervention can raise urinary volumes, diminish bone losses, and prevent reductions in urine pH and citrate levels *(76)*.

There exists one published article suggesting that some cosmonauts have in fact formed stones during space missions *(77,78)*. Another report from NASA's Life Sciences Division suggests this to be a real probability *(79)*. In Pak's earlier investigations in stone formation by astronauts, he suggested that stone risk factors among applicants for spaceflight programs were environmental in origin *(80)*.

SARCOIDOSIS

Sarcoidosis is a systemic granulomatous disease of unknown etiology. Hypercalcemia varies from 2 to 63% of patients with sarcoidosis. This hypercalcemia has classically been ascribed to vitamin D formation when it was initially noted in 6 of 11 patients with this disease *(81)*. Henneman and colleagues noted that the calcium disorder of sarcoidosis was similar to vitamin D intoxication *(82)*. About 5 yr following this, the seasonal influence on serum calcium levels in patients with sarcoidosis led investigators to speculate on sunlight's influence and vitamin D consumption *(83)*. Adams, in 1983, suggested that alveolar macrophages synthesized $1,25$-$(OH)_2$-D_3 in patients with sarcoidosis showing that the hormone is produced outside of the kidney *(84)*.

In a large series from Italy, Rizzato and colleagues noted that in 618 cases of sarcoidosis, calculi were the presenting symptom in only 1% *(85)*. Stones have been noted to occur in about 10% of these individuals. Hypercalciuria represents a primary risk for stone formation *(86)*. Hypercalciuria is three times more common in sarcoid patients than is hypercalcemia. Current mechanisms proposed for this phenomenon include absorption secondary to $1,25$-$(OH)_2$-D_3 in the bowel, resorption with sarcoid involvement of the bones with resulting osteopenia, and finally osteoclast-activating factor perhaps produced by activated inflammatory cells (lymphocytes and monocytes) causing further bone resorption *(87)*.

Treatment of hypercalcemia in sarcoid patients is typically not necessary because their serum calcium levels are not critically elevated (often <14 mg/dL). More often therapy is indicated when hypercalciuria and urolithiasis ensue. Here the clinician should reduce oral vitamin D, calcium supplements, and dietary calcium consumption. Pushing oral fluids expands intravascular volume and promotes diuresis, lowering the formation product of calcium oxalate. To reduce endogenous production of $1,25$-$(OH)_2$-D_3, corticosteroids such as prednisone, 20–40 mg/d remains the treatment of choice. Steroid therapy will reduce serum calcium levels in patients with sarcoidosis in 3–5 d *(88)*. If this does not occur, the clinician should seek an additional diagnosis that is not secondary to systemic granulomatous disease. Once controlled, the prednisone dose is tapered over 4–6 wk while monitoring serum and urinary calcium levels. Chloroquine and hydrochloroquine have also been used in patients refractory or intolerant to corticosteroids *(89)*. Ketoconazole is an imidazole antimycotic drug that inhibits cytochrome P450-dependent enzymes and can reduce $1,25$-$(OH)_2$-D_1 *(90)*. Thiazide diuretics, phosphates, calcitonin, indomethacin, bisphosphonates, and plicamycin should not be considered in treating the hypercalcemia or hypercalciuria from sarcoidosis.

Before leaving this discussion mention must be made of granuloma-forming diseases that mimic sarcoidosis. These include tuberculosis, silicone-induced granulomatosis, berylliosis, disseminated candidiasis and leprosy. Berylliosis is an environmental chronic inflammatory disorder typically involving the lung from inhaled insoluble beryllium

(91). The clinical similarity of these diseases to sarcoidosis is striking but the therapy is different.

VITAMIN D INTOXICATION

Vitamin D was identified as a fat soluble "factor" found in the diet by Sir Edward Mellanby in 1919. Ricketts was a recognizable clinical problem at the outset of the 18th century. Ergosterol or vitamin D_2 was identified in the 1930s initially in plants, and Windaus discovered Vitamin D_3 in the skin of animals in 1936. It seems appropriate to discuss the clinical entity of vitamin D intoxication following sarcoidosis because the two clinical pictures are similar. Vitamin D intoxication and sarcoidosis have, in fact, been likened to the same clinical findings in patients with absorptive hypercalciuria, type I *(92)*. In health, serum 1,25- $(OH)_2$-D concentrations average about 85 pmol/L. Variations in dietary calcium across the usual normal range do not normally appear to alter 1,25- $(OH)_2$-D levels. Parathyroid hormone augments renal production as does dietary phosphate *(93)*. Sunlight exposure, particularly high-energy photons from the ultraviolet B (UVB) wavelengths between 295 and 305 nm are responsible for vitamin D synthesis in human skin. Most people rely on the cutaneous synthesis of vitamin D as the principle source of this hormone. Substantial amounts of vitamin D are present in fish and animal liver, egg yolks, and fish oils. The United States has had a longstanding policy of fortifying milk with vitamin D_2 and D_3 supplements. In other countries breads, cereals, and margarine might also contain vitamin D additives *(94)*. A particular concern with this process in the United States has been outbreaks of vitamin D intoxication, calling to question the methods used to evaluate the level of vitamin D in both infant formula and milk *(95)*. Thirteen brands of milk and five brands of infant formula purchased at random from local supermarkets in five Eastern states were investigated and high-performance liquid chromatography was used to measure vitamin D. Seven out of the 10 samples of infant formula contained 200% more of vitamin D than stated on the label. The highest concentration contained 419% more than the label *(96)*.

Vitamin D intoxication is a well known but increasingly rare clinical condition probably secondary to the use of histamine-2 blockers for the treatment of indigestion and gastric peptic disease. Patients exposed to excess vitamin D consumption have hypercalcemia and, occasionally, metastatic calcification secondary to mobilization of skeletal calcium. In addition, patients suffering from this malady also can have significant hypercalciuria, stone formation, nephrocalcinosis, and, occasionally, acute renal failure *(97)*. The incidence of this disease has been declining but the outbreaks have been reported with continued regularity. In one long-term crossover trial of the vitamins D in 6 patients with hypoparathyroidism the relative potencies were as follows (assigning vitamin D an arbitrary potency of 1): vitamin D_2, 1; dihydrotachysterol (DHT), 3; calcifediol, 10; alfacacidol, 750; and calcitriol, 1500 *(98)*. This study points out the two fold superiority of calcitriol over alfacacidol. In addition, an important subgroup of patients who are managed with vitamin D therapy is at risk for the development of vitamin D toxicity, namely those patients that have iatrogenic hypoparathyroidism. Several series of such patients indicate the significant potential risk of being over-treated with either alfacacidol or calcitriol and secondary development of toxicity. Several of these series have patients presenting with stone disease *(97,99,100)*. Figure 4 represents this type of case in which a surgically hypoparathyroid woman presented with numerous calcium phosphate renal calculi.

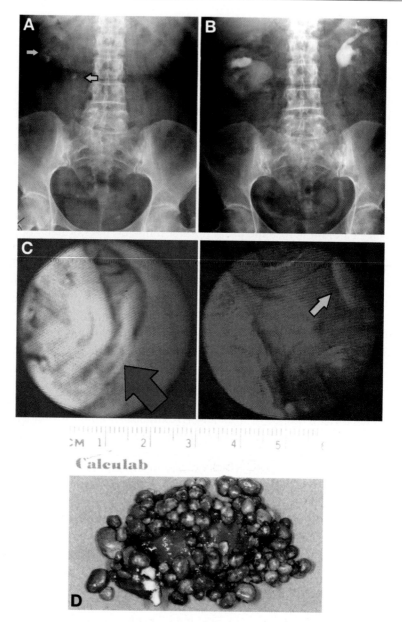

Fig. 4. This is a 68-yr-old female who is hypoparathyroid treated with Vitamin D (calcitriol) and calcium carbonate tablets for continued muscle cramps. She presents acutely after having passed predominately calcium phosphate stones with acute right renal colic. (**A**) Shown is a 9-mm stone wedged into her ureteropelvic junction. Behind this stone is literally a hundred smaller stones. (**B**) Her intravenous urogram showing hydronephrosis. (**C**) Percutaneous antegrade coagulum pyelolithotomy (blue arrow) and grasping lead stone (yellow arrow). (**D**) Stone analysis and photograph (80% apatite, 20% whewhellite).

Vitamin D intoxication should be treated aggressively. Hydration and restriction of dietary supplements is the first line therapy *(101)*. In some cases, the offending vehicle of vitamin D source is not found *(102)*. In cases of the milk-alkali syndrome the offending agents are readily identified during the history. In other cases, the offending agent can be quite exotic as in "enteque seco" an indigenous Argentinian disease from ingestion of the leaves of a toxic plant (*Solanum malacoxylon*) *(103)*. The use of steroids has classically been the next therapeutic intervention *(97,104)*. Prednisone has been reported to restore both mean serum calcium levels and mean calcium excretion within days in patients treated with vitamin D intoxication. Decrease in calcium mobilization from bone best accounts for the glucocorticoid-mediated amelioration of hypercalcemia in patients with toxicity *(104)*. The bisphosphonates have also been used to treat hypercalcemia in vitamin D toxicity. Pamidronate disodium, a bone resorption inhibitor through osteoclast mediation, has shown clinical effectiveness in lowering serum calcium levels within 24 h *(105)*. In a clinical investigation of six patients with hypervitaminosis D, two were treated with corticosteroids and three were treated with pamidronate. Pamidronate resulted in the most rapid decline in serum calcium levels with a more delayed response in the steroid treated group. These authors conclude that the bisphosphonates have a role in managing these patients *(106)*. But in refractory cases and chronic toxemia, at least one report suggests that the bisphosphonates can actually stimulate a rise in serum $1,25\text{-}(OH)_2$ D. These investigators speculate that possible factors predicting failure are body weight loss, hypoproteinemia, and phosphate depletion which can promote a bisphosphonte to stimulate PTH-independent production of $1,25\text{-}(OH)_2$ D *(100)*.

BONE DENSITY

The previous discussions should lead the reader to understand the complexity of categorizing patients with urolithiasis. In one paper, Pak and colleagues have identified 14 metabolic causes of calcium stone formation *(107)*. In other series, many if not most patients with calcium stones have more than one risk factor for stone formation. It should therefore be no great surprise that the coexistence of bone loss with the presence of calcium stone formation is controversial. The different causes of stone formation, particularly the hypercalciurias, not only vary widely from patient-to-patient, but significant variability of hypercalciuria can also be noted within the same patient from day-to-day. Fournier and colleagues point out that different densitometry methods employed in various published series do not always use standardized parameters and biochemical markers of bone remodeling.

Calcium is the most abundant mineral in the human body, accounting for 1.5–2% of an adult's body weight. Ninety nine percent of the body's calcium is found in bones and teeth complexed with phosphate as hydroxyapatite. The remaining calcium is used throughout the body for the biochemical processes necessary for life. Bone is therefore an important reservoir for calcium and constantly being turned over. Throughout the human life-cycle, there are three phases of bone growth and development. From birth to about age 20 the bones are in an active growth phase. Here bones are shaped and molded. This phase is overlapped by a phase of peak bone mass development from ages 12 to 40. Between the ages of 30 and 40, bone resorption begins resulting in a net loss of bone *(108)*. Bone mass itself is influenced in turn by many factors including physical activity, gonadal hormones and nutrition *(109)*. People of all ages and with a wide variety of co-morbid medical problems such as urolithiasis need dietary calcium to maintain positive calcium balance. The Committee on Dietary Allowances of the Food and Nutrition Board, National Academy of Sciences periodically evaluates research data and furnishes guidelines called Recommended Dietary Allowances (RDAs). Published RDAs for calcium are shown in evolution over time in Table 1. The 1994 Con-

Table 1
Evolving Estimates of Calcium Intake (milligrams)

Age	1984 RDA	1989 RDA	NIH 1994	1997 DRI
0–0.5 yr	360		400	
0.5–1 yr	540		600	
1–5 yr	800	800	800	500/800
6–10 yr	800	800	800–1200	800/1300
11–18 yr	1200	1200	1200–1500	1300/1000
19–24 yr	800	1200	1200–1500	1300/1000
25–65 yr	800	800	1000	1000/1200
>65 yr	800	800	1500	1200
Female over 50 not on estrogens			1500	
Pregnant/ lactating	1600	1200	1200–1500	1000

sensus Development Conference resolved that contemporary calcium requirement by both men and women are too low for optimal bone health (110).

Various bone densitometry methods have been employed to study bone loss in patients with calcium urolithiasis. Fournier and colleagues tabulated the world's literature to state that calcium stone formation adversely effects bone mineral density (111). The exceptions are those patients with absorptive hypercalciuria type I. Patients with dietary calcium-dependent hypercalciuria (type I) do not have more progressive bone mineral loss than age-matched controls. The patients with absorptive hypercalciuria and phosphate leak (type III) are the most likely to have bone mineral loss. The familial aggregation of this particular type of stone former has prompted numerous genetic investigations regarding the etiology of this disease. It appears that the heterozygous mutations of NPT 2a gene, a sodium-phosphate cotransporter, are the culprit (112).

As evidence mounts as to the potential for long-term sequelae of bone mineral loss in calcium stone formers and the potential for a protective effect by dietary calcium intake, prudent recommendations suggest not limiting calcium intake (113,114,). In addition to potential deleterious effects on the bone, dietary restriction of calcium can result in increased oxalate absorption (113). Loss of bone mineral density is a significant consideration because of the prevalence of osteoporosis, 25 million people in the United States, and the fact that it is the major underlying cause of bone fractures in postmenopausal women and the elderly. Surveys have revealed that 1.5 million fractures annually in the United States produce a $10 billion expenditure for our healthcare system (110). Compared to the 1986 fiscal impact of dealing with stone patients surgically, $2 billion, the impact in the United States alone is staggering (115).

CONCLUSIONS

It is always nice to bring the discussion full circle. In the introduction, the systemic nature of the diseases of the bowel and bone and their relationship to stone disease was stated. These are generally thought of as complex clinical scenarios even as far as stone disease goes. There is not a single best medical modality for every patient suffering from any of the disorders of the bowel or bone presented. As is often the case, each patient is unique and treatment should be individualized.

REFERENCES

1. Moran,ME. The founding fathers of calculous chemistry. Submitted to Urology.
2. Lindahl WW, Bargen,JA. Nephrolithiasis complicating chronic ulcerative colitis after ileostomy. J Urol 1941; 46: 183–192.
3. Worcester EM. Stones due to bowel disease. In: Kidney Stones: Medical and Surgical Management, (Coe FL, Favus MJ, Pak CYC, Park JH, Preminger GM, eds.). Lippincott-Raven, Philadelphia, PA, 1996; pp. 883–885.
4. Kreutzer N, Kruis W, Haupt G, Engelmann U. Kidney calculi in patients with Crohn's disease. J Urol 2002; 167: 270.
5. Deren JJ, Porush JG, Levitt MF, Khilani MT. Nephrolithiasis as a complication of ulcerative colitis and regional enteritis. Ann Intern Med 1962; 56: 8 43–53.
6. Grossman MS, Nugent FW. Urolithiasis as a complication of chronic diarhheal disease. Am J Digest Dis 1967; 12: 491–498.
7. Glezayd EA, Breuer RI, Kirsner JB. Nephrolithiasis in inflammatory bowel disease. Am J Digest Dis 1968; 13: 1027–1034.
8. Shield DE, Lytton B, Weiss RM, Schiff M Jr. Urologic complications of inflammatory bowel disease. J Urol 1976; 115: 701–706.
9. Smith LH, Hofmann AF, McCall JT, Thomas PJ. Secondary hyperoxaluria in patient with ileal resection and oxalate nephrolithiasis. Clin Res 1970; 18: 541.
10. Dowling RH, Rose GA, Sutor DJ. Hyperoxaluria and renal calculi in ileal disease. Lancet 1971; 1: 1103–1106.
11. Admirand WH, Ernest DL, Williams HE. Hyperoxaluria and bowel disease. Trans Assoc Am Physicians 1971; 84: 307–312.
12. McLeod RS, Churchill DN. Urolithiasis complicating inflammatory bowel disease. Am J Digest Dis 1968; 13: 1027–1034.
13. Dick WH, Lingeman JE, Preminger GM, Smith LH, Wilson DM, Shirrell WL. Laxative abuse as a cause for ammonium urate renal calculi. J Urol 1990; 143: 244–247.
14. Saito M, Takahashi C, Ishida G, Kadowaki H, Hirakawa S, Miyagana I. Acute renal failure associated with sulfur calculi. J Urol 2001; 165: 1985–1986.
15. Sillar DB, Kleining D. Sulphur calculi from ingestion of sulphasalazine. B J Urol 1993; 71: 750.
16. Allison MJ, Cook HM, Milne DB, Gallagher S, Clayman RV. Oxalate degradation by gastrointestinal bacteria from humans. Nutrition 1986; 116: 455–460.
17. Bargen JA, Jackman RJ, Kerr JG. Studies on the life histories of patients with chronic ulcerative colitis (thrombo-ulcerative colitis) with some suggestions for treatment. Ann Intern Med 1938; 12: 339–352.
18. Kennedy HJ, Al-Dujaili EAS, Edwards CRW, Truelove SC. Water and electrolyte balance in subjects with a permanent ileostomy. Gut 1983; 24: 702–705.
19. Kanaghinis T, Lubran M, Coghill NF. The composition of ileostomy fluid. Gut 1963; 4: 322–338.
20. Clarke AM, Chirnside A, Hill GL, Pope G, Stewart MK. Chronic dehydration and sodium depletion in patients with established ileostomies. Lancet 1967; 2: 740–743.
21. Turnberg LA, Morris AI, Hawler PC, Herman KJ, Shields RA, Horth CE. Intracellular electrolyte depletion in patients with ileostomies. Gut 1978; 19: 563–568.
22. Isaacs PET, Horth CE, Turnberg LA. The electrical potential difference across human ileostomy mucosa. Gastroenterol 1976; 70: 52–58.
23. Clarke AM, McKenzie RG. Ileostomy and the risk of uric acid stones. Lancet 1969; 2: 395–397.
24. Bambach CP, Robertson WG, Peacock M, Hill GL. Effect of intestinal surgery on the risk of urinary stone formation. Gut 1981; 22: 257–263.
25. Nicar MJ, Hill K, Pak CYC. Inhibition by citrate of spontaneous precipitation of calcium oxalate. J Bone Min Res 1987; 2: 215–220.
26. Caudarella R, Rizzoli E, Pironi N, et al. Renal stone formation in patients with inflammatory bowel disease. Scan Microsc 1993; 7: 371–380.
27. Galland L. Magnesium and inflammatory bowel disease. Magnesium 1988; 7: 78–83.
28. Seltzer MA, Low RK, McDonald M, Shami GS, Stoller ML. Dietary manipulation with lemonade to treat hypocitraturia. J Urol 1996; 156: 907–909.

29. Wabner CL, Pak CYC. Effect of orange juice consumption on urinary stone risk factors. J Urol 1993; 149: 1405–1408.

30. Pak CYC, Sakhaee K, Fuller C. Successful management of uric acid nephrolithiasis with potassium citrate. Kidney Int 1966; 30: 422–428.

31. Jendle-Bengton C, Tiselius HG. Long-term follow-up of stone formers trated with low dose of sodium potassium citrate. Scand J Urol Nephrol 2000; 34: 36–41.

32. Lee YH, Huang WC, Tsai JY, Huang JK. The efficiency of potassium citrate based medical prophylaxis for preventing upper urinary tract calculi: a midterm followup study. J Urol 1999; 161: 1453–1457.

33. Moran ME, Abrahams HM, Burday DE, Greene TD. Utility of oral dissolution therapy in the management of referred patients with secondarily treated uric acid stones. Urology 2002; 59: 206–210.

34. Cramer JA, Mattson RH, Prevey ML, Scheyer RD, Ouellete VL. How often is medication taken as prescribed? A novel assessment technique. JAMA 1989; 261: 3273.

35. Staroscik JA, Gregorio FU Jr, Reeder SK. Nutrients in fresh peeled oranges and grapefruit from California and Arizona. J Am Diet Assoc 1980; 77: 567–569.

36. Schneider HJ, Hesse A, Berg W, Kirsten J, Nickel H. Animal experimental studies on the effect of magnesium and vitamin B6 on calcium-oxalate nephrolithiasis. Zeit Urolog Nephrol 1977; 70: 419–427.

37. Gershoff SN, Prien EL. Effect of daily MgO and vitamin B6 administration to patients with recurring calcium oxalate kidney stones. Am J Clin Nutrit 1967; 20: 393–399.

38. Pak CYC. Citrate and renal calculi: an update. Mineral Electr Metab 1994; 20: 371–377.

39. Pak CYC. Correction of thiazide-induced hypomagnesemia by potassium-magnesium citrate from review of prior trials. Clin Nephrol 2000; 54: 271–275.

40. Ruml LA, Gonzalez G, Taylor R, Wuermser LA, Pak CY. Effect of varying doses of potassium-magnesium citrate on thiazide-induced hypokalemia and magnesium loss. Am J Therap 1999; 6: 45–50.

41. McDonagh AJ, Singh P, Pilbrow WJ, Youngs GR. Safety of Picolax (sodium picosulphate-magnesium citrate) in inflammatory bowel disease. Brit Med J 1989; 299: 776–777.

42. Christie PM, Knight GS, Hill GL. Comparison of relative risks of urinary stone formation after surgery for ulcerative colitis: conventional ileostomy vs. J-pouch. Dis Colon Rectum 1996; 39: 50–54.

43. Christie PM, Knight GS, Hill GL. Metabolism of body water and electrolytes after surgery for ulcerative colitis conventional versus J-pouch. Br J Surg 1990; 77: 149–151.

44. Ranganath L, Gould SR, Goddard PF. Renal calculi following superior mesenteric artery occlusion. Postgrad Med J 1998; 74: 303–305.

45. Gama R, Schweitzer FA. Renal calculus: a unique presentation of coeliac disease. Brit J Urol Int 1999; 84: 528–529.

46. Sarioglu A, Tanyel FC, Buyukpamukcu,N, Hicsonmez,A. Urolithiasis in patients with Hirschsprung's disease. Eur J Pediatr Surg 1997; 7: 149–151.

47. Nguyen NT, Wolfe BM. Laparoscopic bariatric surgery. Adv Surg 2002; 36: 39–63.

48. Fisher BL, Schauer P. Medical and surgical options in the treatment of severe obesity. Am J Surg 2002; 184: S9–S16.

49. Sugerman HL, Sugerman EL, DeMaria EJ, et al. Bariatric surgery for severely obese adolescents. J Gastointest Surg 2003; 7: 102–108.

50. Baddeley RM. An epilogue to jejunoileal bypass. World J Surg 1985; 9: 842–849.

51. Payne JM, DeWind LT. Surgical treatment of obesity. Am J Surg 1969; 118: 141–147.

52. Eriksson F. Biliointestinal bypass. Int J Obes 1981; 5: 437–447.

53. Annuk M, Backman U, Holmgren K, Vessby B. Urinary calculi and jejunoileal bypass operation. A long-term follow-up. Scand J Urol Nephrol 1998; 32: 177–180.

54. Nordenvall B, Backman L, Larsson L. The influence of gastrointestinal anatomy on oxalate excretion and kidney stone incidence in patients with enteric hyperoxaluria. Plenum Press

55. Hofmann AF, Poley JR. Role of bile acids malabsorption pathogenesis of diarrhea and steatorrhea in patients with ileal bowel resection. Gastroenterology 1972; 62: 918–934.

56. Earnest DL, Williams HE, Admirand WH. Treatment of enteric hyperoxaluria with calcium and medium chain triglycerides (MCT). Clin Res 1975; 23: 130A.

57. Rucker RD Jr, Horstmann J, Schneider BD, Varco RL, Buchwald H. Comparison between jejunoileal and gastric bypass operations for morbid obesity. Surgery 1982; 92: 241–249.

58. Hassan I, Jacobs LA, Milliner DS, Sarmiento JM, Sarr MG. Chronic renal failure secondary to oxalate nephropathy: a preventable complication after jejunoileal bypass. Mayo Clin Proc 2001; 76: 758–760.

59. Shah GM, Winer RL. Reversible acute renal failure after jejunoileal bypass for obesity. South Med J 1981; 74: 1535–1536.

60. Korzets Z, Smorjik Y, Zahavi T, Bernheim J. Renal AA amyloidosis- a long-term sequela of jejuno-ileal bypass. Nephrol Dial Transplant 1998; 13: 1843–1845.

61. Smith CL, Linner JH. Dissolution of calcium oxalate renal stones in patients with jejunoileal bypass after reanastomosis. Urology 1982; 19: 21–23.

62. Economou TP, Cullen W, Mason EE, Scott DH, Doherty C, Maher JW. Reversal of small intestinal bypass operations and concomitant vertical banded gastroplasty: long-term outcome. J Am Coll Surg 1995; 181: 160–164.

63. Paul HE. Bone suppuration the basic cause of renal calculus in twenty cases following war wounds. J Urol 1922; 9: 345–362.

64. Pyrah LN, Fowweather FS. Urinary calculi developing in recumbent patients. Brit J Surg 1938; 26: 98–112.

65. Pulvertaft RG. Nephrolithiasis occurring in recumbency. J Bone Joint Surg 1939; 21: 559–575.

66. Deitrick JE, Wheden GD, Shorr E. Effect of immobilization upon various metabolic and physiologic functions in normal men. Am J Med 1948; 4: 3–36.

67. Smith PH, Cook JB, Roberston WG. Stone formation in paraplegia. Paraplegia 1969; 7: 77–85.

68. Elliot JS, Todd HE. Calculus disease in patients with poliomyelitis. J Urol 1961; 86: 484–488.

69. Gallacher SJ, Ralston SH, Dryburgh FJ, et al. Immobilization-related hypercalceemia- a possible novel mechanism and response to pamidronate. Postgrad Med J 1990; 66: 918–922.

70. Gordon DL, Reinstein L. Rehabilitation of the trauma patient. Am Surg 1979; 45: 223–227.

71. Slemenda CW, Reister TK, Hui SL, Miller JZ, Christian JC, Johnston CC Jr. Influences on skeletal mineralization in children and adolescents: evidence for varying effects of sexual maturation and physical activity. J Pediatr 1994; 125: 201–207.

72. Weaver CM. Calcium requirements of physically active people. Am J Clin Nutr 2000; 72: 579S–584S.

73. Whitson PA, Pietrzyk RA, Pak CYC, Cintron NM. Alterations in renal stone risk factors after space flight. J Urol 1993; 150: 803.

74. Pietrzyk RA, Feiveson AH, Whitson PA. Mathematical model to estimate risk of calcium-containing renal stones. Mineral Electrol Metab 1999; 25: 199–203.

75. Whitson PA, Pietrzyk RA, Pak CYC. Renal stone risk assessment during Space Shuttle flights. J Urol 1997; 158: 2305–2310.

76. Zerwekh, JE. Nutrition and renal stone disease in space. Nutrition 2002; 18: 857–863.

77. Garilevich BA, Olefir IuV. Urolithiasis in flight personnel. Aviak Ekolog Medit 2002; 36: 49–53.

78. Arzamazov GS, Witson PA, Lavina ON, Pastushkova LKh, Pak CT. Assessment of the risk factors for urolithiasis in cosmonauts during long space flights. Aviak Ekolog Medit 1996; 30: 24–32.

79. Nicogossian AE, Rummel JD, Leveton L Teeter R. Development of countermeasures for medical problems encountered in space flight. Adv Space Res 1992; 12: 329–337.

80. Pak CY, Hill K, Cintron NM, Huntoon C. Assessing applicants to the NASA flight program for their renal stone-forming potential. Aviat Space Environ Med 1989; 60: 157–161.

81. Harrell GT, Fisher S. Blood chemical changes in Boeck's sarcoid with particular reference to protein, calcium and phophotase values. J Clin Inves 1939; 18: 678–693.

82. Henneman PH, Dempsey EF, Carol EJ et al. The causes of hypercalcemia in sarcoidosis and its treatment with cortisone and sodium phytate. J Clin Invest 1956; 35: 1229–1242.

83. Taylor RL, Lynch JJ Jr, Winsor WG. Seasonal influence of sunlight on the hypercalcemia in sarcoidosis. Clin Res 1963; 11: 220–225.

84. Adams J, Sharma OP, Gacad M, et al. Metabolism of 25-hydroxy vitamin D3 by cultured pulmonary alveolar macrophages in sarcoidosis. J Clin Inves 1983; 72: 1856–1860.

85. Rizzato G, Fraioli P, Montemurro L. Nephrolithiasis as a presenting feature of chronic sarcoidosis. Thorax 1995; 50: 555–559.

86. Muther R, McCarron D, Bennett W. Renal manifestation of sarcoidosis. Arch Intern Med 1981; 141: 643–645.

87. Sharma OP. Vitamin D, calcium, and sarcoidosis. Chest 1996; 109: 535–539.

88. Sharma OP. Pulmonary sarcoidosis and corticosteroids. Am Rev Respir Dis 1993; 147: 1598–1600.

89. Adams JS, Diz MM, Sharma OP. Effective reduction in the serum 1,25-dihydroxy vitamin D and calcium concentrations in sarcoidosis-associated hypercalcemia with short course chloroquine therapy. Ann Intern Med 1989; 111: 437, 438.

90. Glass AR, Eil C. Ketoconoazole-induced reduction in serum 1,25-dihydroxy vitamin D. J Clin Endocrin Metab 1986; 63: 766–768.

91. Saltini C, Amicosante M. Beryllium disease. Am J Med Scie 2001; 321: 89–98.

92. Zerwekh JE, Pak CYC, Kaplan RA, et al. Pathogenetic role of 1α,25-dihydroxyvitamin D in sarcoidosis and absorptive hypercalciuria: different response to prednisolone therapy. J Clin Endoc Metab 1980; 51: 381–386.

93. Maierhoger W, Gray RW, Lemann Jr, J. Phosphate deprivation increases serum 1,25 $(OH)_2$-vitamin D concentrations in healthy men. Kid Internat 1984; 25: 57.

94. Haddad JG. Vitamin D- solar rays, the milky way, or both? N Engl J Med 1992; 326: 1213–1215.

95. Jacobus CH, Holick MF, Shao Q, et al. Hypervitaminosis D associated with drinking milk. N Engl J Med 1992; 326: 1173–1177.

96. Holick MF, Shao Q, Liu WW, Chen TC. The vitamin D content in fortified milk and infant formula. N Engl J Med 1992; 326: 1178–1181.

97. Allen Sh, Shah JH. Calcinosis and metastatic calcification due to vitamin D intoxication. Horm Res 1992; 37: 68–77.

98. Stamp TC. Calcitriol dosage in osteomalacia, hypoparathyroidism and attempted treatment of myositis ossificans progressiva. Curr Med Res Opin 1981; 7: 316–336.

99. Ichioka K, Moroi S, Yamamoto S, et al. A case of urolithiasis due to vitamin D intoxication in a patient with idiopathic hypoparathyroidism. Acta Urolog Japon 2002; 48: 231–234.

100. Sato K, Emoto N, Toraya S, et al. Progressively increased serum 1,25-dihydroxyvitamin D2 concentration in a hypoparathyroid patient with protracted hypercalcemia due to vitamin D2 intoxication. Endoc J 1994; 41: 329–337.

101. Adams JS, Lee G. Gains in bone mineral density with resolution of vitamin D intoxication. Ann Intern Med 1997; 127: 203–206.

102. Koutkia P, Chen TC, Holick MF. Vitamin D intoxication associated with an over-the-counter supplement. N Engl J Med 2001; 345: 66, 67.

103. Boland RL. Solanum malacoxylon: a toxic plant which affects animal calcium metabolism. Biomed Environ Sci 1988; 1: 414–423.

104. Streck WF, Waterhouse C, Haddad JG. Glucocorticoid effects in vitamin D intoxication. Arch Intern Med 1979; 139: 974–977.

105. Lee DC, Lee GY. The use of pamidronate for hypercalcemia secondary to acute vitamin D intoxication. J Toxicol 1998; 36: 719–721.

106. Selby PL, Davies M, Marks JS, Mawer EB. Vitamin D intoxication causes hypercalcaemia by increased bone resorption which responds to pamidronate. Clin Endocrin 1995;43:;531–536.

107. Pak CYC, Britton F, Peterson R, et al. Ambulatory evaluation of nephrolithiasis. Classification, clinical presentation and diagnostic criteria. Am J Med 1980; 69: 19–30.

108. National Institutes of Health Consensus Development Conference Statement. Osteoporosis. Conference Statement 5(3), 1984.

109. Recker RR. Continuous treatment of osteoporosis: current status. Orthop Clin NA 1981; 12: 611–627.

110. NIH Consensus Development Panel on Optimal Calcium Intake. Optimal calcium intake. JAMA 1994; 272: 1942–1948.

111. Fournier A, Ghazali,A, Bataille P, et al. Bone involvement in idiopathic calcium-stone formers. In: Kidney Stones: Medical and Surgical Management, (Coe FL, Pavus MJ, Pak CYC, Park JH, Preminger GM, eds.). Lippincott-Raven, Philadelphia, PA, 1996; pp. 927.

112. Prie D, Huart V, Bakouh N, et al. Nephrolithiasis and osteoporosis associated with hypophosphatemia caused by mutations in the type 2a sodium-phosphate cotransporter. N Engl J Med 2002; 347: 983–991.

113. Bataille P, Chavasad G, Gregoire I, et al. Effect of calcium restriction on renal oxalate and the probability of stones in various pathophysiological groups with calcium stones. J Urol 1983; 130: 218–223.

114. Curhan GC, Willet WC, Rimm EB, Stampeer JM. A prospective study of dietary calcium and other nutrients and the risk of symptomatic kidney stones. J Engl J Med 1993; 328: 833–838.

115. Lingeman JE, Saywell RM Jr, Woods JR, Newman DM. Cost analysis of extracorporeal shock wave lithotripsy relative to other surgical and nonsurgical treatment alternatives for urolithiasis. Med Care 1986; 24: 1151–1160.

13

Medical Evaluation of Stone Disease

Clarita V. Odvina, MD *and Charles Y. C. Pak,* MD

Contents

Key Words: Nephrolithiasis; metabolic evaluation; etiology; urine collection.

INTRODUCTION

Medical management entails identification of causes of stone formation based largely on detection of abnormal urinary biochemistry (risk factors) *(1),* and application of dietary modification and pharmacological treatment designed to correct underlying disturbances *(2).* The importance of medical management is based on two important findings. Urolithiasis is characterized by a high recurrence rate *(3–6).* It is estimated that approx 60–80% of patients will form another stone within 10 yr of the first episode. Removal of existing stone does not prevent further stone formation *(7).*

It is now well recognized that a wide variety of biochemical derangements contribute to the formation of kidney stones. These abnormalities are "metabolic" (such as in cystinuria and primary hyperoxaluria) *(8,9)* or environmental (such as low urinary volume and high urinary sodium) *(10–13)* in origin, or combination of the two. The goals of clinical and laboratory evaluation of patients with history of nephrolithiasis should be directed toward obtaining sufficient information to guide the management and prevention of further stone formation. With proper evaluation and identification of risk factors, a treatment program can be developed that can alleviate further stone formation and avoid expensive urologic procedures *(2,13).*

In this chapter, we shall review diagnostic approaches to the medical evaluation of patients after the first stone episode ("single stone-formers"), as well as those with

From: Current Clinical Urology, *Urinary Stone Disease:*
A Practical Guide to Medical and Surgical Management
Edited by: M. L. Stoller and M. V. Meng © Humana Press Inc., Totowa, NJ

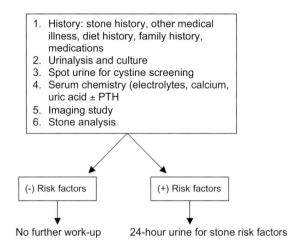

1. History: stone history, other medical
   illness, diet history, family history,
   medications
2. Urinalysis and culture
3. Spot urine for cystine screening
4. Serum chemistry (electrolytes, calcium,
   uric acid ± PTH
5. Imaging study
6. Stone analysis

(-) Risk factors   (+) Risk factors

No further work-up   24-hour urine for stone risk factors

Fig. 1. Simplified approach to evaluation of urolithiasis.

recurrent stone formation ("recurrent stone-formers"). Both simplified and detailed protocols will be described.

EVALUATION OF SINGLE STONE-FORMERS

The question of whether patients should be evaluated after a first stone episode has been a topic of considerable debate. Noting a relatively low morbidity associated with a first stone episode and somewhat high occurrence of side-effects with pharmacological therapy, some investigators have recommended that single stone-formers should not undergo elaborate or detailed evaluation *(14)*. However, patients with a single stone episode were shown to suffer from the same metabolic abnormalities as those with recurrent or multiple stones *(15)*. Single stone-formers are therefore at risk for recurrent stone formation, justifying a more detailed evaluation. In 1988, the National Institutes of Health (NIH) Consensus Conference recommended that all patients should at least have a serum chemistry panel checked for metabolic conditions (such as hyperparathyroidism) associated with nephrolithiasis *(16)*. Regardless, the decision to pursue a simple or comprehensive work-up should be made jointly by the patient and the physician, taking into consideration the estimated risk for new stone formation judged from medical history and laboratory tests.

Medical History

Complete medical history must be obtained for both single and recurrent stone-formers, whether a simple or detailed evaluation is contemplated (Fig. 1). A detailed medical history may provide clues to the underlying cause(s) of kidney stone. It should be focused on stone episodes, other medical illnesses, dietary habits, and information on current and previous medications (Table 1). Because some stone-forming conditions have a genetic predisposition, a careful family history of stones should also be obtained *(17)*.

The history should address other medical conditions associated with specific abnormalities, which could potentially cause or contribute to kidney stone formation. For instance, chronic diarrhea caused by inflammatory bowel disease or laxative abuse can

Table 1
Recommended Work-Up of First Time Stone-Former
at the First International Consultation on Stone Disease (Paris, France)

Medical history
- Stone history
- Other medical illness
- Family history
- Diet history
- Medications

Laboratory tests
- Imaging study (KUB or CT scan or ultrasound)
- Urinalysis ± culture
- Stone analysis
- Spot urine for cystine
- Serum chemistry (electrolytes, calcium, uric acid, ± PTH if indicated)
- 24-h urine for stone risk while on random (or usual diet)

lead to hypocitraturia from bicarbonate loss in the feces *(18)*. In addition, excessive fluid loss usually results in low urinary volume. Patients with malabsorption (secondary to pancreatic insufficiency, celiac sprue) are at risk of developing hyperoxaluria *(19)*. History of chronic or recurrent urinary tract infections may lead one to suspect infection lithiasis, which would warrant identification and eradication of the offending organism *(20)*. Prolonged bed rest or immobilization also increases the propensity for kidney stones, primarily through increased urinary calcium excretion *(21)*. History of peptic ulcer disease and skeletal involvement (nontraumatic appendicular fractures) may lead one to consider hyperparathyroidism *(22)*.

There is little doubt that diet plays a role in the development of kidney stones. Predisposing factors include high animal protein diet, which can produce hyperuricosuria, hypocitraturia, and hypercalciuria *(23)*. Two of the most common abnormalities found among stone-formers are low urine volume *(10,11)* and high urinary sodium *(12)*. Low urine volume results from inappropriately low fluid intake, excessive sweating, or intestinal fluid loss. High sodium intake can exaggerate stone disease by increasing urinary calcium, decreasing urinary citrate, and provoking sodium urate-induced calcium oxalate crystallization *(12)*. Diet high in oxalate and low in potassium-containing citrus fruit products *(24)* could also enhance the propensity to stone formation, by increasing urinary oxalate and lowering citrate.

A number of medications could either cause or increase the risk for stone formation. Carbonic anhydrase inhibitors such as acetazolamide can produce systemic acidosis, hypocitraturia and increased urinary pH *(25)*. A high dose of vitamin C increases urinary oxalate, without lowering urinary pH *(26)*. Other agents that can potentially promote stone formation include triamterene, vitamin D, calcium supplements, and protease inhibitors, particularly indinavir *(27,28)*.

Laboratory Tests

In addition to detailed medical history, patients presenting with kidney stones for the first time should have (1) urinalysis to rule out infection, (2) spot qualitative urine test

Table 2
Simplified Approach for Evaluating Patients With Recurrent Kidney Stones

First step
- Medical history
- Imaging study (KUB or CT scan or ultrasound)
- Spot urine sample for urinary sediments
- Serum chemistry (electrolytes, calcium, uric acid)
- 24-h Urine for stone risk while on random diet

Second step
- Short-term dietary modification based on the result of 24-h urine

Third step
- Repeat 24-h urine
- Identify metabolic risk factors and consider medical therapy

for cystine, (3) serum electrolytes, calcium and uric acid to identify metabolic causes of stone formation such as renal tubular acidosis, primary hyperparathyroidism, and gout, (4) appropriate imaging study [plain X-ray of kidneys, ureter, and bladder (KUB; CT scan or ultrasound)] to identify the presence of residual stone and detect anatomical abnormalities, and (5) stone analysis (if available), which may provide clues to the medical diagnosis (Fig.1).

Although the 1988 NIH Consensus Conference did not recommend it for single stone-formers except those at risk (Fig. 1) *(16)*, the First International Consultation on Stone Disease in 2001 suggested that a 24-h urine sample be analyzed for calcium, citrate, oxalate, uric acid, total volume, sodium and potassium in all single stone-formers *(29)* (Table 1). This recommendation was justified, because metabolic risk factors (such as hypercalciuria, hypocitraturia, hyperuricosuria, and low urinary pH) are frequently observed among single stone-formers *(15)*. In addition, the stone risk profile in a 24-h urine may help identify important dietary risk factors *(1,11)*.

EVALUATION OF RECURRENT STONE-FORMERS

Recurrence of stone formation suggests that underlying disturbances persist or are more severe than in single stone-formers. Thus, recurrent stone-formers merit a more thorough evaluation than single stone-formers. However, there is considerable disagreement as to what constitutes adequate work-up. In part, this controversy reflects considerable diversity in severity of recurrent stone disease, difficulty in conducting a comprehensive work-up in the setting of urologists in private practice, and cost-effectiveness of a detailed evaluation. For this reason, both simple and detailed approaches were recommended at the 2001 First International Consultation on Stone Disease *(29)*.

Simplified Approach

A simplified, step-by-step work-up for nephrolithiasis has been described previously *(30,31)*. This approach, applicable to routine uncomplicated cases of recurrent stone disease, is summarized in Table 2.

STEP 1

The initial evaluation should include detailed medical history as previously described, imaging study (KUB; CT scan or ultrasound), serum chemistry panel (electrolytes, calcium and uric acid), spot urine for urinary sediments and 24-h urine for calcium, oxalate, uric acid, citrate and pH to identify metabolic risk factors. Measurement of total volume, sodium, potassium, sulfate, phosphorous and magnesium will help define the environmental risk factors. A single 24-h urine sample on a random diet is felt to be adequate because abnormalities in stone risk factors had previously been shown to be remarkably reproducible *(32)*.

STEP 2

The second step involves placing the patient on a short-term dietary modification. For instance, if the urinary volume is less than 2 L/d, the patient should be instructed to increase fluid intake. If urinary sodium is greater than 200 meq/d, salt intake should be restricted. Usually, this modification can be achieved by advising patients to avoid using salt shakers during meals and limiting ingestion of salty and processed foods. If urinary oxalate is more than 45 mg/d, patients should be advised to avoid intake of high oxalate-containing food products such as tea, spinach, dark roughages, nuts, and chocolate. If urinary calcium is >250 mg/d, moderate calcium restriction should be advised especially if calcium intake is high. If urinary uric acid is >700 mg/d and sulfate is >30 mmol/d, intake of animal protein (beef, poultry, fish, and pork) should be limited to 6–8 oz/d. Lastly, if urinary pH, citrate and potassium are low, patients should be advised to increase intake of fruits, particularly with potassium-rich citrus products such as orange *(24)* and grapefruit.

STEP 3

In the third step, another 24-h urine sample is collected for stone risk profile, while subjects are maintained on a diet restricted in calcium, sodium, and oxalate for 1 wk. The results are compared with those obtained while on the usual (random) diet. Correction of abnormal risk factors on the restricted diet suggests that the abnormalities are environmental in origin. When environmental risk factors such as urine volume or urinary sodium remain abnormal after dietary intervention, the finding implies either poor compliance or inadequate dietary modification. Persistent abnormalities in metabolic factors (urinary calcium, citrate, pH, uric acid, and oxalate) despite dietary modification suggest the need for pharmacological intervention such as potassium citrate for persistently low pH and citrate, and thiazide for hypercalciuria. In even simpler version *(32)*, Step 3 is omitted.

Comprehensive Evaluation

A number of protocols are now available and are being used by different centers in the evaluation of kidney stone disease. These protocols may be applicable for use in centers specializing in the medical management of kidney stones and for evaluation of patients with severe or complicated stone disease.

THE UNIVERSITY OF CHICAGO PROTOCOL

In this protocol, three 24-h urine samples are collected while patients are on their usual diet, with corresponding blood samples *(5)*. Blood samples are drawn between 7 AM and

Table 3
Comprehensive Work-Up (UT Southwestern Protocol [33])

- Medical history
- Imaging study (KUB or CT scan or ultrasound)
- Urinalysis ± culture
- Three 24-h urine collections, 2 on random diet and one after dietary restriction of calcium, sodium & oxalate for 7 d
- Stone analysis
- Spot urine for cystine
- Serum chemistries corresponding to the urine collection, plus PTH in one sample
- "Fast and Ca load test"

---

9 AM after a 12-h fast. Urine samples are analyzed for calcium, magnesium, phosphorous, uric acid, oxalate, citrate, sulfate, ammonium, total volume, and pH. Concentrations of calcium, magnesium, phosphorous, uric acid and creatinine (plus sodium and potassium in one sample) are measured in the serum samples. Cystine screening is done on all patients using the nitroprusside reaction.

UNIVERSITY OF TEXAS SOUTHWESTERN PROTOCOL

The Stone Clinic at the Southwestern Medical Center uses an updated version of the 1978 ambulatory protocol (33). This protocol requires three outpatient visits (Table 3). Before the initial evaluation, patients are instructed to discontinue all medications that could affect the metabolism of calcium, uric acid and oxalate. Examples of such medications are thiazide, orthophosphate, allopurinol, vitamin C, acetazolamide, calcium, and vitamin D supplements.

On the first visit, a detailed history is obtained as described previously. Radiologic study (KUB; tomogram or intravenous pyelogram) is obtained to determine the presence of residual stone or any structural abnormality. Fresh spot urine is collected to rule out infection and for cystine screening. If not previously done and if the specimen is available, the stone is sent for analysis.

Three urine samples are collected. Two samples are obtained while the patient is on his or her customary diet and fluid intake. The third 24-h urine sample is collected after at least 7 d on a diet restricted in calcium (400 mg/d), sodium (100 meq/d), and oxalate (avoidance of chocolate, tea, nuts, and dark roughages). Urine samples are analyzed for calcium, magnesium, sodium, potassium, ammonium, uric acid, oxalate, citrate, phosphorus, sulfate, chloride, creatinine, pH, and total volume. Fasting venous blood sample is drawn during the random diet for chemistry panel (electrolytes, BUN, creatinine, calcium, phosphorous, magnesium, total protein, albumin, and uric acid).

Comparison of the results of urine analysis during random and restricted diets allows for the assessment of the role of certain environmental factors in the development of stones, as well as permit definition of certain abnormal risk factors. One week of the restricted diet also provides the necessary preparation for the "fast and load" test (34), which is performed to detect the presence of renal calcium leak and of intestinal hyperabsorption of calcium.

"Fast and load" testing involves collection of a fasting 2-h urine sample following an overnight fast, a fasting venous blood sample, and a 4-h urine sample after oral ingestion of 1-g calcium with a synthetic meal. Serum sample is analyzed for calcium, creatinine, and PTH; urine samples during fasting and following calcium load are measured for calcium and creatinine. The fasting urinary calcium, expressed as mg/dL glomerular filtrate, is a measure of renal calcium leak or skeletal calcium mobilization. The increment in 4-h urinary calcium over the fasting value, expressed as mg calcium/dL glomerular filtrate, provides an indirect assessment of intestinal calcium absorption.

When hypercalciuria is present, bone density is measured in the spine, hip and radius. This procedure recognizes the association of low bone density with hypercalciuric nephrolithiasis (35).

MISCELLANEOUS CONSIDERATIONS

Centralized vs Institutional Laboratories

For physicians practicing in the community, it may be convenient to use the commercially available tests of urine for stone risks factors. Several specialized laboratories can now provide kits that allow standardized biochemical assays and physicochemical measurements to identify the risk factors for stone formation.

THE MISSION PHARMACAL COMPANY (SAN ANTONIO, TX)

This kit contains a volume marker and appropriate preservatives (1). The patient is instructed to collect a 24-h urine sample after which two small (30 mL) aliquots are sent to a central laboratory. The laboratory calculates the total volume from the dilution of the volume marker and analyzes urinary metabolic risk factors (calcium, oxalate, uric acid, citrate, and pH) and environmental risk factors (total volume, sodium, sulfate, phosphorous, and magnesium). From the analyzed values, physicochemical risk factors are calculated. The laboratory provides a visual display of all available data in a single report. Each risk factor is assigned a vertical line on a linear scale, and the risk factors are grouped into metabolic, environmental, and physicochemical risks. A horizontal line intersecting each vertical scale at an approximate midpoint represents upper or lower normal limit. Values below the horizontal line represent normal values (or reduced risk) and values above the line represent increased risk. For the physicochemical risks, values above the horizontal dashed line represent supersaturation beyond the mean values in normal subjects with respect to four stone-forming salts (calcium oxalate, brushite, or calcium phosphate, monosodium urate, and uric acid). Although the profile provided by the laboratory has diagnostic utility, additional information such as medical history, serum chemistry, and appropriate X-rays are still necessary to come up with a more definite diagnosis.

THE LITHOLINK (CHICAGO, ILLINOIS)

This kit contains a urine collection container, a green topped tube for urine aliquot and a collection data sheet. Patients are instructed to record the start and stop times and the urinary volume on the data collection sheet. At the completion of the urine collection, urine aliquot is collected and is sent with the data sheet to the laboratory. The laboratory also provides a full evaluation of stone risk factors (metabolic, environmental and physicochemical). However, unlike the visual display provided by Mission, Litholink sends the ordering physician a tabulated report. Bigger and bolder fonts indicate that a given measurement is closer to that of a stone-forming population (therefore, increased risk). Litholink also provides time sequential data that allows the physician to evaluate the progress of the patient during treatment.

Adequancy of Urine Collection

Accurate interpretation of the results of urinary biochemistry depends on completeness of urinary collection. Correction of urinary creatinine by bodyweight can help assess the adequacy of urine collection. The average urinary creatinine is 13–21 mg/kg for women and 17–27 mg/kg for men. A value that is below the lower end would suggest undercollection. On the other hand, a value that is at the upper end would be consistent with overcollection.

Clues to Detecting Dietary Influences From Urinary Stone Risks

The effects of environmental risk factors can be assessed by comparing the urinary chemistries while on usual (random diet) vs those obtained during the restricted diet. Diet-induced hypercalciuria should be suspected if the urinary calcium is normalized by dietary modification. This finding may indicate excessive calcium intake or high intake of sodium or animal proteins.

Hyperuricosuria in a patient with normal serum uric acid concentration suggests increased intake of purine-rich foods (meat products). Urinary oxalate >45 mg/d in a patient without history of malabsorption indicates either high oxalate consumption or intake of large doses of vitamin C. Normalization of urinary oxalate during dietary restriction would confirm this impression. Low urinary volume usually indicates inadequate fluid intake or excessive fluid loss either from diarrhea or excessive sweating.

Interpretation of Response to "Fast and Load" Test

For accurate interpretation of the fasting urinary calcium, it is important to place the patients on a diet limited in calcium and sodium before the test is preformed. Patients with intestinal hyperabsorption of calcium (absorptive hypercalciuria) may have high fasting urinary calcium if this precaution is not followed. Without this preparation, fasting hypercalciuria may be present from the delayed clearance of absorbed calcium and persistent PTH suppression (which reduces renal tubular reabsorption of calcium). Fasting urinary calcium is expressed as mg/dl glomerular filtrate to reflect renal function rather than muscle mass. This derivation is obtained by multiplying urinary calcium in mg/mg creatinine by the corresponding serum creatinine in mg/dl. Normal value for fasting urinary calcium is <0.11 mg/dL glomerular filtrate. Fasting hypercalciuria in the setting of normal serum calcium and PTH is indicative of renal hypercalciuria.

The increase in urinary calcium excretion after 1 gram calcium load provides an indirect assessment of intestinal calcium absorption. A "post-load" urinary calcium of >0.2 mg/dL glomerular filtrate or mg/mg creatinine in a patient with normal values for serum PTH and fasting urinary calcium indicates absorptive hypercalciuria *(34)*.

CONCLUSION

This chapter describes the different protocols that one may use in evaluating patients with nephrolithiasis. The extent of the work-up should be based on whether (a) the patient is presenting with an acute stone episode for the first time or (b) the patient has recurrent or complicated kidney stone disease. In the majority of patients, the simplified step-by-step approach may be sufficient. However, in certain instances, particularly for those presenting with complicated or severe stone disease, a more comprehensive work-up maybe warranted to identify the pathophysiological mechanism for stone formation.

REFERENCES

1. Pak CYC, Skurla C, Harvey J. Graphic display of urinary risk factors for renal stone formation. J Urol 1985; 134: 867.
2. Pak CYC. Medical management of nephrolithiasis. J Urol 1982; 128: 1157.
3. Marshall N, White RH, De Saintonge MC, et al. The natural history of renal and ureteric calculi. Br J Urol 1975; 47: 117.
4. Johnson CM, Wilson DM, O'Fallon WM, et al. Renal stone epidemiology: a 25-year study in Rochester, Minnesota. Kid Int 1979; 16: 624.
5. Sutherland JW, Parks JH, Coe FL. Recurrence after a single renal stone in a community practice. Miner Electrolyte Metab 1985; 11: 267.
6. Coe FL, Keck J, Norton ER. The natural history of calcium urolithiasis. J Am Med Assoc 1977; 238: 519.
7. Fine JK, Pak CYC, Preminger GM. Effect of medical management and residual fragments on recurrent stone formation following shock wave lithotripsy. J Urol 1995; 153: 27.
8. Crawhall JC, Purkiss P, Watts RWE, Young EP. The excretion of amino acids by cystinuric patients and their relatives. Ann Human Genet 1969; 33:149.
9. Danpure CJ, Smith LH. The primary hyperoxalurias. In: Kidney Stones: Medical and Surgical Management, (Coe FL, Favus MJ, Pak CYC, Parks JH, Preminger GM, eds.). Lippincott Raven, Philadelphia, PA, 1996; p. 859.
10. Pak CYC, Sakhaee K, Crowther C, Brinkley L. Evidence justifying high fluid intake in the treatment of nephrolithiasis. Ann Inter Med 1980; 93: 36.
11. Borghi L, Meschi T, Amato F, et al. Urinary volume, water and recurrences in idiopathic calcium nephrolithiasis: a 5-year randomized prospective study. J Urol 1996; 155: 839.
12. Sakhaee K, Harvey JA, Padalino PK, et al. Potential role of salt abuse on the risk of kidney stone formation. J Urol 1991; 150: 310.
13. Robertson WG, Peacock M, Heyburn PJ. Risk factors in calcium stone disease of the urinary tract. Br J Urol 1978; 50: 449.
14. Uribarri J, Oh MS, Carroll HJ. The first kidney stone. Ann Intern Med, 1989; 111: 1006.
15. Pak CYC. Should patients with single renal stone formation undergo diagnostic evaluation? J Urol 1982; 127: 854.
16. Consensus Conference: prevention and treatment of kidney stones. J Am Med Assoc 1988; 260: 977.
17. Curhan GC, Willett WC, Rimm EB, Stampfer MJ. Family history and risk of kidney stone. J Am Soc Nephrol 1997; 8:1568.
18. Rudman D, Dedonis JL, Fountain MT, et al. Hypocitraturia in patients with gastrointestinal malabsorption. N Eng J Med 1980; 303: 657.
19. Smith LH, Fromm H, Hofmann AF. Acquired hyperoxaluria, nephrolithiasis and intestinal disease: description of a syndrome. N Eng J Med 1972; 286:1371.
20. Griffith DP, Musher DM. Prevention of infected urinary stone by urase inhibition. Invest Urol 1973; 11: 228.
21. Hwang TIS, Hill K, Schneider V, Pak CYC. Effect of prolonged bedrest on propensity for renal stone formation. J Clin Endo Metab 1988, 66: 109.
22. Klugman V, Pak CYC, Favus MJ. Nephrolithiasis in primary hyperparathyroidism. In: The Parathyroids: Basic and Clinical Concepts, 2nd Ed., (Bilezikian JP, Marcus R, Levine MA, eds.). Academic Press, San Diego, CA, 2001; pp. 437–450.
23. Reddy, S.T., Wang, C.Y., Sakhaee, K. et al.: Effect of low-carbohydrate high-protein diets on acid-base balance, stone-forming propensity, and calcium metabolism. Am J Kid Dis, 2002; 40: 265.
24. Wabner CL, Pak CYC. Effect of orange juice consumption on urinary stone risk factors. J Urol 1993; 149: 1405.

25. Higashihara E, Nutahara K, Takeuchi T, et al. Calcium metabolism in acidotic patients induced by carbonic anhydrase inhibitors: responses to citrate. J Urol 1991; 145: 942.
26. Auer BL. Auer D, Rodger AL. Relative hyperoxaluria, crystalluria and haematuria after megadose ingestion of vitamin C. Eur J Clin Invest 1998; 28: 695.
27. Ettinger B, Oldroyd NO, Sorgel F. Triamterene nephrolitiasis. J Am Med Assoc 1980; 244: 2443.
28. Berns JS, Cohen RM, Silverman M, Turner J. Acute renal failure due to indinavir crystalluria and nephrolithiasis: report of 2 cases. Am J Kidney Dis 1997; 30: 558.
29. Pak CYC, Asplin JR, Ogawa Y, et al. Evaluation of stone-forming patients. Paris Consultation on Stone Disease. Paris, France. July 4–5, 2001.
30. Pak CYC. Medical management of nephrolithiasis: a new, simplified approach for general practice. Am J Med Sci 1997; 313: 215.
31. Pak CYC, Resnick MI. Medical therapy and new approaches to management of urolithiasis. Urol Clin North Am 2000; 27: 243.
32. Pak CYC, Peterson R, Pondexter JR. Adequacy of a single stone risk analysis in the medical evaluation of urolithiasis. J Urol 2001; 165: 378.
33. Levy FL, Adams-Huet B, Pak CYC. Ambulatory evaluation of nephrolithiasis: an update of a 1980 protocol. Am J Med 1995; 98: 509.
34. Pak CYC, Kaplan RA, Bone II, et al. A simple test for the diagnosis of absorptive, resorptive and renal hypercalciurias. N Engl J Med 1975; 292:497.
35. Pietchmann F, Breslau NA, Pak CYC. Reduced vertebral bone density in hypercalciuric nephrolithiasis. J Bone Min Res 1992; 7:1383.

14 Pharmacologic Prophylaxis of Calcium Stones

Yeh Hong Tan, MD and Glenn M. Preminger, MD

Key Words: Nephrolithiasis; medical management; prophylaxis; calcium; diuretic.

INTRODUCTION

The management of nephrolithiasis forms an important part of urologic practice. The recurrence rate after forming an initial stone is reported to be as high as 50% at 5 yr and 80–90% at 10 yr, highlighting the importance of medical prophylactic therapy. A better understanding of pathophysiology and formulation of diagnostic criteria for different

From: Current Clinical Urology, *Urinary Stone Disease:*
A Practical Guide to Medical and Surgical Management
Edited by: M. L. Stoller and M. V. Meng © Humana Press Inc., Totowa, NJ

etiologies of nephrolithiasis have made feasible the adoption of selective treatment programs. The objectives of medical stone management should be:

1. Correct the underlying physicochemical and physiologic derangements
2. Prevent new stone formation
3. Avoid nonrenal complications of the disease process
4. Be free of serious side-effects

The background for the selection of certain medical treatment programs is the assumption that specific physicochemical and physiological abnormalities identified with a given disorder are etiologically important in the formation of renal stones, and that the correction of these disturbances would prevent stone formation. Moreover, it is assumed that such a selective treatment program would be more effective and safe than a "random" treatment approach.

These hypotheses appear reasonable and logical. For many pharmacologic treatment programs recommended for the prevention of recurrent nephrolithiasis, sufficient information is now available to characterize their physicochemical and physiological actions.

PATHOPHYSIOLOGY OF HYPERCALCIURIA

Hypercalciuria is defined as the excretion of urinary calcium exceeding 200 mg/24 h (or an excess of 4 mg of calcium/kg/24 h). The association of hypercalciuria with recurrent calcium nephrolithiasis has long been recognized, although the exact nature of this relationship continues to be investigated. Nephrolithiasis resulting from hypercalciuria is heterogeneous in origin, and comprises several entities.

Absorptive Hypercalciuria

The primary abnormality in absorptive hypercalciuria is increased intestinal absorption of calcium *(1)*. The exact cause for the hyperabsorption of calcium is not fully understood. A subsequent increase in serum calcium concentration enhances the renal filtered load and suppresses parathyroid function (Fig. 1). The combination of an increase in the filtered load and a decrease in renal tubular reabsorption of calcium, caused by parathyroid suppression, results in development of hypercalciuria and potential stone formation. The excessive renal loss of calcium compensates for the intestinal hyperabsorption, thereby maintaining serum calcium in the normal range.

Absorptive hypercalciuria type I (AH-I) is the most severe form of absorptive hypercalciuria, characterized by a urine calcium level >200mg/d, with high or low dietary calcium intake. In AH-I, patients have normal serum levels of calcium and phosphorus and a normal or low serum PTH level. Fasting urinary calcium is normal, whereas an oral calcium load results in exacerbated hypercalciuria. Absorptive hypercalciuria Type II (AH-II) is a mild to moderate form of this disorder in which hypercalciuria only occurs with high calcium intake. These patients have normal urinary calcium excretion either while fasting or on a restricted calcium diet.

Renal Hypercalciuria

The underlying abnormality in renal hypercalciuria (or "renal leak" hypercalciuria) is thought to be impairment of renal tubular reabsorption of calcium *(1)*. The consequent reduction in serum calcium concentration stimulates parathyroid function (Fig. 2). Parathyroid hormone (PTH) excess results in mobilization of calcium from bone and enhanced intestinal absorption of calcium, with ensuing stimulation of renal synthesis

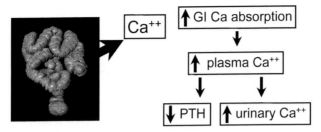

Fig. 1. Absoptive hypercalciuria.

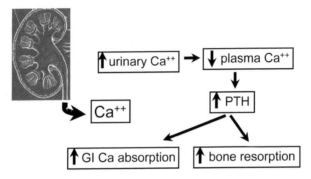

Fig. 2. Renal hypercalciuria.

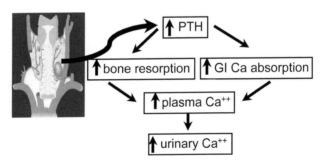

Fig. 3. Resorptive hypercalciuria.

of 1,25-$(OH)_2D$. These events lead to an increase in the circulating concentration and renal filtered load of calcium, often causing significant hypercalciuria, even during the fasting state. Unlike primary hyperparathyroidism, patients with renal hypercalciuria have normal serum calcium level. As the elevated PTH (secondary hyperparathyroidism) is a response to the renal calcium leak, an oral calcium load may suppress the hyperparathyroidism in these individuals.

Resoprtive Hypercalciuria

Primary hyperparathyroidism is the cause of resorptive hypercalciuria. The initial event in this condition is hypersecretion of PTH, resulting in excessive bone resorption and an increase in serum calcium levels (Fig. 3). Intestinal absorption of calcium is often secondarily elevated owing to PTH-dependent stimulation of renal synthesis of 1,25-$(OH)_2D$. These effects cause significant hypercalciuria through an increase in the circu-

Table 1
Differential Diagnosis of Hypercalciuria

	Absorptive	Renal	Resorptive
• Serum calcium	Normal	Normal	Elevated
• Parathyroid function	Suppressed (secondarily)	Stimulated (primarily)	Stimulated
• Fasting urinary calcium	Normal	Elevated	Elevated
• Intestinal calcium absorption	Elevated (primarily)	Elevated (secondarily)	Elevated (secondarily)

lating concentration and renal filtered load of calcium. Elevated PTH also enhances renal reabsorption of calcium and the excretion of phosphate. Fasting urinary calcium levels remain elevated as in patients with renal hypercalciuria.

Differential Diagnosis of Hypercalciuria

Different forms of hypercalciuria can be differentiated from their biochemical and physiological pictures (Table 1). Although the serum calcium is normal in absorptive hypercalciuria and renal hypercalciuria, patients with resorptive hypercalciuria have elevated circulating calcium levels. Serum PTH concentration is primarily elevated in resorptive hypercalciuria and secondarily elevated in renal hypercalciuria, whereas parathyroid activity is normal or suppressed in absorptive hypercalciuria. Fasting urinary calcium is normal in patients with absorptive hypercalciuria but is elevated in renal hypercalciuria and resorptive hypercalciuria. Finally, all three forms of hypercalciuria are accompanied by an intestinal hyperabsorption of calcium. However, this disturbance is a primary defect in patients with absorptive hypercalciuria and a secondary defect in renal hypercalciuria and resorptive hypercalciuria.

Some patients may present with fasting hypercalciuria and normal serum PTH (unclassified hypercalciuria) (2). This disorder exhibits features of both absorptive and renal hypercalciuria. However it lacks the characteristics required for clear differentiation. Fasting hypercalciuria suggests a renal calcium leak, although hyperparathyroidism is not evident. A lack of PTH elevation resembles absorptive hypercalciuria, but the fasting urinary calcium is elevated. The picture of unclassified hypercalciuria is most commonly caused by inadequate dietary preparation.

MANAGEMENT OF HYPERCALCIURIA

Sodium Cellulose Phosphate

Sodium cellulose phosphate can be used in selected patients with absorptive hypercalciuria (3,4). However, sodium cellulose phosphate is not routinely used for prevention of stone recurrence (5). This medication is more commonly used as a diagnostic tool in patients with absorptive hypercalciuria.

Sodium cellulose phosphate may decrease urinary magnesium, increase urinary oxalate, and have a limited hypocalciuric action or cause negative calcium balance in the absence of increased calcium absorption or in the presence of renal calcium leak (4).

When sodium cellulose phosphate is administered, this nonabsorbable resin binds calcium and inhibits intestinal calcium absorption. However, this inhibition is caused by limiting the amount of intraluminal calcium available for absorption, not by correcting the basic disturbance in calcium transport.

The common side effects of cellulose phosphate are hyperoxaluria, hypomagnesiuria and diarrhea *(6)*. The potential complications of sodium cellulose phosphate therapy can be explained by its mechanism of action. First, this medication may cause a negative calcium balance and parathyroid stimulation when used in patients with normal intestinal calcium absorption or with renal or resorptive hypercalciuria. Second, the treatment may cause magnesium depletion by binding magnesium in the gut. Finally, sodium cellulose phosphate may produce secondary hyperoxaluria by binding divalent cations in the intestinal tract, reducing divalent cation-oxalate complexation, and making more oxalate available for absorption. These complications may be overcome by using the drug only in documented cases of absorptive hypercalciuria Type I, providing oral magnesium supplementation (given independent from sodium cellulose phosphate), and imposing a moderate dietary restriction of oxalate *(4)*.

When these precautions are followed, sodium cellulose phosphate at a dosage of 10–15 g/d (given with meals) has been shown to reduce urinary calcium and the saturation of calcium salts (calcium phosphate as well as calcium oxalate), maintain stable bone density and to be clinically effective.

Thiazides

Thiazide diuretics are ideally indicated for the treatment of renal hypercalciuria. Several studies have demonstrated the beneficial effects of thiazide in preventing stone recurrence. Thiazides have been demonstrated to correct the renal leak of calcium by augmenting calcium reabsorption in the distal tubule and by causing extracellular volume depletion and stimulating proximal tubule reabsorption of calcium *(7–9)*. The subsequent correction of secondary hyperparathyroidism restores normal serum 1,25-$(OH)_2D$ and intestinal calcium absorption. Thiazides provide a sustained correction of hypercalciuria commensurate with a restoration of normal serum 1,25-$(OH)_2D$ and intestinal calcium absorption for up to 10 yr of therapy. Physicochemically, the urinary environment becomes less saturated with respect to calcium oxalate and brushite during thiazide treatment, largely because of the reduced calcium excretion. In addition, urinary inhibitor activity, as reflected in the limit of metastability, is increased. The above effects are shared by hydrochlorothiazide (50 mg twice per day), chlorothalidone (50 mg/d) or indapamide (1.5 mg/d). Potassium supplementation (approx 40 meq/d) is required to prevent hypokalemia and attendant hypocitraturia with all of these agents. Potassium citrate has been shown to be effective in averting hypokalemia and in increasing urinary citrate when administered to patients with calcium nephrolithiasis who are taking thiazides *(10,11)*. Concurrent use of triamterene, a potassium-sparing agent, should be undertaken with caution because of recent reports of triamterene stone formation *(12,13)*. Thiazide is contraindicated in primary hyperparathyroidism because of potential aggravation of hypercalcemia.

Thiazide is not considered a selective therapy for absorptive hypercalciuria, because it does not decrease intestinal calcium absorption in this condition. However, this drug has been used widely to treat absorptive hypercalciuria because of its hypocalciuric action and the high cost and inconvenience of alternative therapy (sodium cellulose phosphate).

Current studies indicate that thiazide may have a limited long-term effectiveness in AH-I *(14)*. Despite an initial reduction in urinary calcium excretion, the intestinal calcium absorption remains persistently elevated. These studies suggest that the retained calcium may be accreted in bone at least during the first few years of therapy. Bone density may increase during thiazide treatment in AH *(15)*. With continued treatment, however, the rise in bone density stabilizes and the hypocalciuric effect of thiazide becomes attenuated. These results suggest that thiazide treatment has caused a low turnover state of bone that interferes with a continued calcium accretion in the skeleton. The "rejected" calcium would then be excreted in urine. In contrast, bone density is not significantly altered in renal hypercalciuria, where thiazide causes a decline in intestinal calcium absorption commensurate with a reduction in urinary calcium.

Besides hypokalemia, the side effects of thiazide include erectile dysfunction, gout raised serum cholesterol and glucose intolerance.

Guidelines for the Use of Sodium Cellulose Phosphate or Thiazides in Absorptive Hypercalciuria Type I

There is currently no treatment program capable of correcting the basic abnormality of AH-I. Neither sodium cellulose phosphate nor thiazides corrects the basic, underlying physiologic defect in AH. Some guidelines are offered until more selective therapy can be developed.

Sodium cellulose phosphate might be used in patients with severe AH-I (urinary calcium greater than 350 mg/d) or in those resistant to or intolerant of thiazide therapy. In patients with AH-I who may be at risk for bone disease (growing children, postmenopausal women) or who already have bone loss, thiazides may be the first choice. If thiazides lose their hypocalciuric action (after long-term treatment), sodium cellulose phosphate may be temporarily substituted for approx 6 mo; thiazide treatment may then be resumed. Continued monitoring of urinary calcium excretions is essential to assure that the hypocalciuric action of thiazides persist.

Orthophosphate (Including Slow-Releasing Potassium Phosphate)

The most common form of absorptive hypercalciuria is secondary to increased intestinal calcium absorption. Various theories exist regarding the exact pathophysiology of absorptive hypercalciuria including both vitamin D dependent as well as vitamin D independent absorptive hypercalciuria. It is believed that in a significant subset of patients, increased 1-25 $(OH)_2$ D (vitamin D) levels may be responsible for enhanced intestinal calcium absorption in patients with absorptive hypercalciuria.

There are two types of orthophosphate (acidic and neutral) that have been used clinically in patients with nephrolithiasis. Previous studies have demonstrated that neutral phosphates may indeed be a useful preparation to reduce serum vitamin D levels as well as to inhibit urinary calcium excretion in patients with AH *(16)*. However, there are a number of problems available with current forms of orthophosphate therapy. These preparations provide rapid-release of neutral phosphate that may cause gastrointestinal upset and diarrhea from an increased osmotic load. The side effects include diarrhea, nausea, vomiting and abdominal colic. In addition, many orthophosphate preparations provide an inadequate hypocalciuric response as compared to thiazides or sodium cellulose phosphate preparations owing to the renal effect of sodium contained in most currently available orthophosphate preparations (see section on dietary sodium intake). Finally, previous studies have also demonstrated that orthophosphate preparations may increase the urinary saturation of calcium phosphate (brushite) owing to a substantial rise in urinary pH, caused by the increased alkalinity of most available orthophosphate preparations.

A new formulation of slow-release, neutral potassium phosphate has been developed to obviate the problems with currently available orthophosphate preparations (17,18). This potassium phosphate preparation (UroPhos-K) is prepared in a wax matrix to provide slow release of the orthophosphate. This restricted release limits the amount of GI upset found with most current orthophosphate preparations. In addition, UroPhos-K contains phosphate salts of potassium and no sodium. Therefore, this preparation does not provide a sodium load that could offset the hypocalciuric action of the orthophosphate. Finally, this medication is designed to yield a pH of 7.0 as compared to 7.3 for some available orthophosphate preparations. Therefore, it is less likely that the crystallization of calcium phosphate may occur in the urine.

Randomized prospective double-blind trials were performed to assess the impact of this new medication on patients with documented stone formation and AH-I (18,19). Patients received either UroPhos-K or placebo in a double-blinded fashion. No significant gastrointestinal side effects were noted with the slow-release potassium phosphate preparation nor was there a significant increase in fasting serum potassium or phosphorus. However, the UroPhos-K treatment did significantly reduce urinary calcium without altering oxalate excretion. Moreover, the urinary saturation of calcium oxalate was significantly reduced without altering brushite saturation. Also noted was a significant increase of inhibitor activity secondary to increased urinary citrate and pyrophosphate, thereby inhibiting the potential crystallization of calcium oxalate in the urine.

PATHOPHYSIOLOGY OF HYPERURICOSURIC CALCIUM OXALATE NEPHROLITHIASIS

Hyperuricosuria is found in about 10% of patients with calcium oxalate nephrolithiasis. The features of hyperuricosuric calcium oxalate nephrolithiasis include elevated urinary uric acid >600mg/d, a normal serum calcium level, normal urinary calcium and oxalate levels, normal fasting and calcium load response, and urinary pH typically >5.5 (20,21).

Although excessive uric acid excretion can be found in primary gout, it may also be seen in secondary conditions of purine overproduction (e.g., myeloproliferative disease, glycogen storage disease and malignancy). Excessive dietary intake of purine-rich foods is another potential cause for this condition. It is believed that monosodium urate is formed in a supersaturated environment in hyperuricosuric patients. Monosodium urate (colloidal or crystalline) may then initiate calcium stone formation through direct induction of heterogeneous nucleation of calcium oxalate or by adsorption of certain macromolecular inhibitors of stone formation (22).

MANAGEMENT OF HYPERURICOSURIC CALCIUM OXALATE NEPHROLITHIASIS
Allopurinol

Allopurinol (300 mg/d), a xanthine oxidase inhibitor, is the drug of choice in hyperuricosuric calcium oxalate nephrolithiasis resulting from uric acid overproduction because of its ability to reduce uric acid synthesis and lower urinary uric acid *(23)*. Besides reducing urate production and the serum urate concentration, allopurinol also decreases urate excretion in urine. Its use in hyperuricosuria associated with excessive dietary purine intake may be necessary if dietary purine restriction cannot be achieved. Changes ensuing from restoration of normal urinary uric acid include an increase in the urinary limit of metastability of calcium oxalate. Thus, the spontaneous nucleation of calcium oxalate is retarded by treatment, probably via inhibition of monosodium urate-induced calcium oxalate crystallization. Because sodium could exaggerate monosodium urate-induced calcium oxalate crystallization, a moderate sodium restriction (100 meq/d) is also advisable. The side effects from allopurinol are not common and these include hypersensitivity reaction, skin rash, drowsiness, nausea and diarrhea.

Potassium Citrate

Potassium citrate represents an effective alternative to allopurinol in the treatment of hyperuricosuria *(24,25)*. Administration of potassium citrate (at a dose of 40-60 meq/d in divided doses) to patients with hyperuricosuric calcium oxalate nephrolithiasis may reduce the urinary saturation of calcium oxalate (by complexing calcium), and inhibit urate-induced crystallization of calcium oxalate. Potassium citrate may be particularly useful in patients with mild-to-moderate hyperuricosuria (<800 mg/d) in whom hypocitraturia is also present. However, allopurinol is probably preferred in patients with more marked hyperuricosuria, especially if hyperuricemia coexists.

PATHOPHYSIOLOGY OF HYPEROXALURIA

Hyperoxaluria is defined by urinary oxalate excretion in excess of 45 mg/d. A mild-to-moderate elevation (45–80 mg/d) may be caused by dietary hyperoxaluria. At levels >80 mg/d, the diagnosis of nephrolithiasis is likely caused by either enteric or primary hyperoxaluria.

Dietary Hyperoxaluria

The majority (80–90%) of urinary oxalate is synthesized in the liver, whereas the rest is derived from dietary oxalate or ascorbic acid (vitamin C). Therefore, dietary intake in oxalate-rich foods or excessive ascorbic acid ingestion can contribute to hyperoxaluria through intestinal absorption of oxalate. However, controversy persists regarding the importance of dietary ascorbic acid. Recent studies have demonstrated that high doses of vitamin C do not increase the risk of calcium oxalate stone disease. Ascorbate excretion increases when vitamin C ingestion is initiated, but will level out after 24 h, suggesting that once the metabolic pool is saturated, ingested ascorbic acid is excreted unmetabolized in the urine *(26,27)*. In addition, no association between serum ascorbic acid levels and the prevalence of kidney stones has been found in women or men *(28)*. Moreover, a prospective study of 85,557 women with 14-yr follow up demonstrated that vitamin C intake was not associated with risk of stone formation. Routine restriction of vitamin C to prevent stone formation appears unwarranted *(29)*. Studies suggest that a daily intake of up to 4 gm of vitamin C can be allowed with no significant risk of stone formation *(30)*. However, recurrent stone formers and patients with renal failure who have a defect in ascorbic acid or oxalate metabolism should probably restrict daily vitamin C intakes to approx 100 mg

Enteric Hyperoxaluria

The cause of calcium stone formation in the majority of hyperoxaluric patients is enteric hyperoxaluria *(31,32)*. Ileal disease is responsible for increased intestinal absorption of oxalate that leads to hyperoxaluria. This disorder may be encountered in patients with inflammatory bowel disease, gastric or small bowel resection, or jejunoileal bypass *(33)*.

Two processes are likely responsible for the intestinal hyperabsorption of oxalate. Bile salts and fatty acids increase the permeability of the intestinal mucosa that results in a primary increase in the intestinal transport of oxalate. Fat malabsorption, characteristic of ileal disease, leads to calcium soap formation. This factor limits the amount of free calcium that can complex with oxalate, thereby raising the oxalate pool available for absorption and promoting the development of stones.

In enteric hyperoxaluria, stone formation may also be the result of additional factors such as low urinary output from intestinal fluid loss, low urinary citrate caused by hypokalemia and metabolic acidosis, and low urinary magnesium caused by impaired intestinal magnesium absorption.

Primary Hyperoxaluria

Primary hyperoxaluria type I is an autosomal recessive disorder due in a defect of the hepatic enzyme alanine-glyoxylate aminotransferase (AGT). In the normal liver, AGT functions in catalyzing the transamination of glyoxylate to glycine in hepatic peroxisomes. The deficiency, or altered migration of this enzyme, in primary hyperoxaluria type I results in the conversion of glyoxylate to oxalate, leading to increased urinary excretion of oxalic, glycolic, and glyoxylic acids *(34,35)*.

This condition is characterized by nephrocalcinosis, oxalate deposition in tissues (oxalosis), and renal failure resulting in death before the age of 20 when untreated *(36)*. The diagnosis can definitively be made by assaying the amount and distribution of AGT in liver specimens obtained by percutaneous biopsy.

Primary hyperoxaluria type II is very rare and results in deficiencies in the hepatic enzymes D-glycerate dehydrogenase and glyoxylate reductase, leading to increased urinary oxalate and glycerate excretion *(37)*. Both types of primary hyperoxaluria cause stone formation beginning in childhood, with subsequent development of nephrocalcinosis, tubulointerstitial nephropathy, and chronic renal failure. In addition to high levels of urinary oxalate, serum oxalate levels are also elevated.

MANAGEMENT OF HYPEROXALURIA

Dietary Hyperoxaluria

Less than 10–15% of urinary oxalate is usually derived from dietary sources. Foodstuffs that are rich in oxalate include spinach, chocolate, nuts, and tea. Although general advice on a restricted oxalate intake might be given to patients with recurrent nephrolithiasis, a low oxalate diet would be most useful in patients with enteric hyperoxaluria or those with underlying bowel abnormalities.

Enteric Hyperoxaluria

Oral administration of large amounts of calcium (0.25–1.0 g four times per day) or magnesium has been recommended for the control of calcium nephrolithiasis of ileal disease. Although urinary oxalate may decrease (probably from binding of oxalate by divalent cations), the concurrent rise in urinary calcium may obviate the beneficial effect of this therapy, at least in some patients. Cholestyramine does not cause a sustained reduction in urinary oxalate. The replacement of dietary fat with medium chain triglycerides may be helpful in those patients who also have malabsorption.

Patients may exhibit hypomagnesiuria caused by impaired intestinal absorption of magnesium. Because magnesium has been shown to complex oxalate, hypomagnesiuria may increase the urinary saturation of calcium oxalate. Although oral magnesium supplements may correct hypomagnesiuria, they may also provoke further diarrhea. Treatment with potassium citrate (60–120 meq/d) may correct the hypokalemia and metabolic acidosis and in some patients, increase urinary citrate toward normal. A liquid form of potassium citrate is preferable owing to the rapid gastrointestinal transit time in many individuals with enteric hyperoxaluria.

A high fluid intake is recommended to assure adequate urine volume in patients with enteric hyperoxaluria. Because excessive fluid loss may be present, an antidiarrheal agent may be necessary before sufficient urine output can be achieved. Calcium citrate may theoretically have a role in management of enteric hyperoxaluria. This treatment may lower urinary oxalate by binding oxalate in the intestinal tract. Calcium citrate may also raise the urinary citrate and pH by providing an alkali load. Finally, calcium citrate may correct the malabsorption of calcium and adverse effects on skeleton by providing an efficiently absorbed calcium supplement.

Primary Hyperoxaluria

Overall, the prognosis of patients with primary hyperoxaluria has been unfavorable. These patients usually develop renal failure and early death. Routine renal transplantation fails because of progressive systemic oxalosis (38). An alternate option of combined liver and kidney transplantation, aims to replace the deficient enzyme, peroxisomal AGT, and to re-establish normal kidney function. However, this treatment carries significant operative morbidity and mortality (39). Bilateral nephrectomies of native kidneys, which are a major source of oxalate, have to be considered because of persistent systemic oxalosis (40).

Currently, pharmacologic therapy plays little part in treatment of primary hyperoxaluria. Pyridoxine is useful only in a minority of patients. Long-term administration of orthophosphate and pyridoxine might decrease urinary oxalate crystallization and might preserve renal function in selected patients. In addition, long-term administration of alkali citrate might be beneficial in some patients (41,42). The key to successful management of primary hyperoxaluria is early diagnosis, testing for pyridoxine response and early planning for definitive therapy when renal function deteriorates.

PATHOPHYSIOLOGY OF HYPOCITRATURIC CALCIUM OXALATE NEPHROLITHIASIS

Hypocitraturic calcium nephrolithiasis may exist as an isolated abnormality (10%) or in combination with other metabolic disorders (50%). Acid–base disorder, especially acidosis, is the most important factor that affects the renal handling of citrate, with increased acid levels resulting in diminished endogenous citrate production (43,44). Citrate lowers urinary saturation of calcium salts by forming soluble complexes with calcium, as well as directly inhibiting the crystallization of calcium salts (45,46). In the setting of hypocitraturia, the urinary environment is more supersaturated with respect to calcium salts, thus promoting nucleation, growth, and aggregation, resulting in stone formation. Mean normal urinary citrate excretion is 640 mg/d, whereas the lower limit of normal is 320 mg/d.

In patients with hypocitraturic calcium oxalate nephrolithiasis, potassium citrate treatment is capable of restoring normal urinary citrate, lowering the urinary saturation and inhibiting crystallization of calcium salts (10,47,48). Moreover, a recent study demonstrates that potassium citrate therapy might have beneficial effect in preventing age dependent bone loss (49). Because hypocitraturia is found in a number of different conditions, each will be addressed individually.

Distal Renal Tubular Acidosis

One of the more common causes of hypocitraturia is distal renal tubular acidosis (RTA). Acidosis impairs urinary citrate excretion by enhancing renal tubular reabsorption of citrate as well as by reducing its synthesis (50). Distal RTA may occur in a complete or incomplete form. The complete form is characterized by hyperchloremic metabolic acidosis, hypokalemia, and elevated urinary pH, whereas the incomplete form is characterized by normal serum electrolyte levels and an inability to acidify urine following an ammonium chloride load. Hypercalciuria and profound hypocitraturia may be associated with either complete or incomplete RTA. In combination with alkaline urine, the patient is at risk for developing calcium oxalate or calcium phosphate stones (51).

Potassium citrate therapy may correct the metabolic acidosis and hypokalemia found in patients with distal renal tubular acidosis. In addition, it is capable of restoring normal urinary citrate, although large doses (up to 120 meq/d) may be required in severe acidotic states (51). With correction of the acidosis, urinary calcium should decline into the normal range. Because urinary pH is generally high to begin with in patients with renal tubular acidosis, the overall rise in urinary pH is usually small.

Potassium citrate therapy may produce a sustained decline in the urinary saturation of calcium oxalate (from reduction in urinary calcium and from citrate complexation of calcium). The urinary saturation of calcium phosphate does not increase because the rise in phosphate dissociation is relatively small and is adequately compensated by a decline in ionic calcium concentration. In addition, the inhibitory activity against the crystallization of calcium oxalate and calcium phosphate is augmented owing to the direct action of citrate.

Chronic Diarrheal Syndromes

Patients with these conditions lose alkali in the form of bicarbonate via their gastrointestinal tract. This bicarbonate loss results in metabolic acidosis with a subsequent impairment in citrate synthesis (52). Decreased citrate production is responsible for the lower urinary concentration of citrate. Besides hypocitraturia, patients with chronic diarrheal syndrome may have additional risk factors for stone formation such as low urine volumes and hyperoxaluria.

Potassium citrate therapy in patients with hypocitraturia secondary to chronic diarrheal states has been shown to significantly reduce the stone formation rate and produce remission in 70% of patients (45,53). The dose of potassium citrate will be dependent on the severity of hypocitraturia in these patients. Dosages of potassium citrate range from 60 meq in three to four divided doses to 120 meq/d.

It is recommended that a liquid preparation of potassium citrate be used rather than the slow-release tablet preparation because the slow-release medication may be poorly absorbed owing to rapid intestinal transit time. In addition, frequent dose schedules (three to four times per day) for the liquid preparation are necessary because this form of the medication has a relatively short duration of biological action. A less frequent dose schedule (two to three times per day) is acceptable if the solid preparation is used because of its slow-release characteristic.

Thiazide-Induced Hypocitraturia

Thiazide diuretics can produce hypokalemia that leads to intracellular acidosis. The acidotic state inhibits the synthesis of citrate, resulting in hypocitraturia. The essential mechanism is the inhibition of citrate production that is a consequence of chronic acidosis *(10,11)*. Therefore, potassium supplementation, preferably in the form of potassium citrate, should be administered to patients receiving thiazides during treatment of hypercalciuria. Potassium citrate is equally effective as potassium chloride in correcting thiazide-induced hypokalemia, except in severe chloride deficiency. Moreover, potassium citrate will enhance citrate excretion.

Idiopathic Hypocitraturia

This entity includes hypocitraturia occurring alone, as well as in conjunction with other abnormalities (i.e., hypercalciuria or hyperuricosuria). Mechanisms that account for hypocitraturia in this condition include a high animal protein diet (with an elevated acid-ash content), strenuous physical exercise (causing lactic acidosis), high sodium intake, and intestinal malabsorption of citrate.

Stones formed in this condition are predominantly composed of calcium oxalate. Potassium citrate therapy has been shown to produce a sustained increase in urinary citrate excretion from initially low values to within normal limits *(54)*.

Thus, potassium citrate can be used in a variety of conditions. A liquid preparation of potassium citrate with a frequent dose schedule (three to four times per day) is recommended in chronic diarrheal states. In other conditions, a solid preparation given on a twice-daily schedule is generally preferred.

PATHOPHYSIOLOGY OF HYPOMAGNESURIA

Hypomagnesuric calcium oxalate nephrolithiasis occurs in less than 5% of patients with recurrent calcium stones. Hypomagnesuria is defined as urinary magnesium excretion <50 mg/d. This condition may co-exist with hypocitraturia in approx 65% of patients, and low urine volume (<1 L/d) in approx 40% of patients *(55)*. Many patients with nephrolithiasis will report a limited intake of magnesium-rich foods such as nuts and chocolate, suggesting the dietary basis of this condition.

Magnesium is known to be an inhibitor of calcium nephrolithiasis by apparently increasing the solubility product of calcium oxalate and calcium phosphate. Magnesium forms complexes with oxalate, thereby reducing the supersaturation with calcium oxalate. Magnesium has some direct inhibitory effect on crystal growth of calcium phosphate and oxalate. Besides, the urinary excretion of magnesium and citrate is increased, whereas the pH is elevated.

Magnesium hydroxide and oxide have been used clinically to treat stone recurrence. However, both preparations are poorly absorbed and produce slight increase in urinary magnesium. Besides, the administration of magnesium produces an increase in urinary calcium *(56)*. In a randomized trial, the use of magnesium hydroxide did not significantly reduce the recurrence rate of calcium nephrolithiasis *(9)*. However, in a recent prospective study, potassium-magnesium citrate reduced the 3-yr recurrence rate of calcium oxalate formation *(57)*. Magnesium therapy may results in side effects in gastrointestinal (diarrhea) and central nervous systems (paresis and sleepiness). At the present moment, their clinical application as a monotherapy is rather limited other than in patients with hypomagnesuric calcium oxalate nephrolithiasis. Moreover, some suggest that the protective effect of magnesium administration may be due primarily to magnesium's effect on urinary citrate excretion *(58)*.

DRUG-INDUCED CALCIUM NEPHROLITHIASIS

Certain medications (e.g., acetazolamide and lithium) used to treat other medical conditions are known to be associated with calcium stone formation. If possible, these medications should be discontinued or alternative therapy should be employed.

Acetazolamide

Acetazolamide is used to manage elevated intraocular pressure in glaucoma, and is also used to prevent acute mountain sickness (altitude sickness). This medication can also be a component of treatment plans for congestive heart failure and seizure disorders. Long-term use of acetazolamide is known to cause nephrolithiasis and nephrocalcinosis *(59,60)*. Acetazolamide, a carbonic anhydrase inhibitor, may raise the urinary pH initially because of renal bicarbonate loss. However, the resultant metabolic acidosis often results in lowering urinary pH with hypocitraturia, eventually causing the formation of renal calculi. Long-term treatment with acetazolamide markedly decreases urinary citrate, which will result in an increased ion-activity product of calcium phosphate and decreased inhibition of calcium phosphate crystallization. Treatment with acetazolamide has also been shown to increase urinary oxalate, which together with hypocitraturia, might further increase the risk of calcium oxalate crystallization *(61)*.

The use of alkali to buffer acidosis and prevent the urinary abnormalities associated with these medications is often inadequate. The concurrent use of sodium bicarbonate further potentiates the risk of stone formation.

Lithium

Lithium carbonate has proved to be a highly effective medication to manage bipolar mood disorders and an increasing number of patients are receiving long-term lithium therapy. However, the long-term use of lithium has been associated with hyperparathyroidism and hypercalcemia. Because of the first report of lithium-induced hyperparathyroidism in 1973, more than 40 cases have been uncovered *(62–65)*. However, nephrolithiasis has rarely been reported. Renal calculi and hypercalciuria are common with primary hyperparathyroidism, whereas calculi and renal calcium excretion is variable in the lithium-induced state *(66)*. The exact mechanism is not well studied. By interfering with adenylate cyclase, lithium affects thyroid and parathyroid function, causing hyperparathyroidism, hypercalcemia, and hypothyroidism. Although primary hyperparathyroidism is usually associated with hypercalciuria, there is decreased urinary calcium excretion in patients taking lithium. Lithium may act independently of parathyroid hormone on the renal tubule to increase calcium absorption. The hypocalciuric effect probably results in the low risk of nephrolithiasis of lithium-induced hyperparathyroidism *(67)*.

CONCLUSIONS

Significant progress has been made over last decades in the metabolic evaluation and management of nephrolithiasis. In addition to conservative measures like dietary and fluid regimens, selective medical therapy is effective in preventing new stone formation. Remission rate of greater than 80% and overall reduction in individual stone formation rate of greater than 90% can be achieved in patients with recurrent nephrolithiasis. Despite initial higher cost of diagnostic protocols and medical therapy, an effective pharmacologic prophylactic program could significantly reduce the need for stone removal, thereby potentially reducing the long-term costs associated with recurrent nephrolithiasis.

REFERENCES

1. Pak CY. Physiological basis for absorptive and renal hypercalciurias. Am J Physiol 1979; 237: F415–F423.
2. Preminger GM, Peterson R, Pak CYC. Differentiation of unclassified hypercalciuria utilizing a sodium cellulose phosphate trial. In: Nephrolithiasis, (Walker VR, Sutton AL, Pak CYC, Robertson WG, eds.). Plenum Press, New York, NY, 1989; pp. 325–340.
3. Pak CY. Clinical pharmacology of sodium cellulose phosphate. J Clin Pharmacol 1979; 19: 451–457.
4. Pak CY. A cautious use of sodium cellulose phosphate in the management of calcium nephrolithiasis. Investig Urol 1981; 19: 87–190.
5. Backman U, Danielson BG, Johansson G, Ljunghall S, Wikstrom B. Treatment of recurrent calcium stone formation with cellulose phosphate. J Urol 1980; 123: 9–13.
6. Hautmann R, Hering FJ, Lutzeyer W. Calcium oxalate stone disease: effects and side effects of cellulose phosphate and succinate in long-term treatment of absorptive hypercalciuria or hyperoxaluria. J Urol 1978; 120: 712–715.
7. Mortensen JT, Schultz A, Ostergaard AH. Thiazides in the prophylactic treatment of recurrent idiopathic kidney stones. Int Urol Nephrol 1986; 18: 265–269.
8. Ohkawa M, Tokunaga S, Nakashima T, Orito M, Hisazumi H. Thiazide treatment for calcium urolithiasis in patients with idiopathic hypercalciuria. Br J Urol 1992; 69: 571–576.
9. Ettinger B, Citron JT, Livermore B, Dolman LI. Chlorthalidone reduces calcium oxalate calculous recurrence but magnesium hydroxide does not. J Urol 1988; 139: 679–684.
10. Pak CY, Peterson R, Sakhaee K, Fuller C, Preminger GM, Reisch J. Correction of hypocitraturia and prevention of stone formation by combined thiazide and potassium citrate therapy in thiazide-unresponsive hypercalciuric nephrolithiasis. Am J Med 1985; 79: 284–288.
11. Nicar MJ, Peterson R, Pak CY. Use of potassium citrate as potassium supplement during thiazide therapy of calcium nephrolithiasis. J Urol 1984; 131: 430–433.
12. Carr MC, Prien EL, Jr, Babayan RK. Triamterene nephrolithiasis: renewed attention is warranted. J Urol 1990; 144: 1339, 1340.
13. Ettinger B, Weil E, Mandel NS, Darling S. Triamterene-induced nephrolithiasis. Ann Int Med 1979; 91: 745, 746.
14. Preminger GM, Pak CY. Eventual attenuation of hypocalciuric response to hydrochlorothiazide in absorptive hypercalciuria. J Urol 1987; 137: 1104–1109.
15. Adams JS, Song CF, Kantorovich V. Rapid recovery of bone mass in hypercalciuric, osteoporotic men treated with hydrochlorothiazide. Ann Int Med 1999; 130: 658–660.
16. Ettinger B. Recurrent nephrolithiasis: natural history and effect of phosphate therapy. A double-blind controlled study. Am J Med 1976; 61: 200–206.
17. Heller HJ, Reza-Albarran AA, Breslau NA, Pak CY. Sustained reduction in urinary calcium during long-term treatment with slow release neutral potassium phosphate in absorptive hypercalciuria. J Urol 1998; 159: 1451–1456.

18. Breslau NA, Heller HJ, Reza-Albarran AA, Pak CY. Physiological effects of slow release potassium phosphate for absorptive hypercalciuria: a randomized double-blind trial. J Urol 1998; 160: 664–668.

19. Breslau NA, Padalino P, Kok DJ, Kim YG, Pak CY. Physicochemical effects of a new slow-release potassium phosphate preparation (UroPhos-K) in absorptive hypercalciuria. J Bone Mineral Res 1995; 10: 394–400.

20. Coe FL, Kavalach AG. Hypercalciuria and hyperuricosuria in patients with calcium nephrolithiasis. [Review]. N Engl J Med 1974; 291: 1344–1350.

21. Coe FL. Uric acid and calcium oxalate nephrolithiasis. Kid Int 1983; 24: 392–403.

22. Zerwekh JE, Holt K, Pak CY. Natural urinary macromolecular inhibitors: attenuation of inhibitory activity by urate salts. Kid Int 1983; 23: 838–841.

23. Ettinger B, Tang A, Citron JT, Livermore B, Williams T. Randomized trial of allopurinol in the prevention of calcium oxalate calculi. N Engl J Med 1986; 315: 1386–1389.

24. Lee YH, Huang WC, Tsai JY, Huang JK. The efficacy of potassium citrate based medical prophylaxis for preventing upper urinary tract calculi: a midterm followup study. J Urol 1999; 161: 1453–1457.

25. Pak CY, Peterson R. Successful treatment of hyperuricosuric calcium oxalate nephrolithiasis with potassium citrate. Arch Int Med 1986; 146: 863–867.

26. Gerster H. No contribution of ascorbic acid to renal calcium oxalate stones. Ann Nutr Metab 1997; 41: 269–282.

27. Auer BL, Auer D, Rodgers AL. The effect of ascorbic acid ingestion on the biochemical and physicochemical risk factors associated with calcium oxalate kidney stone formation. Clin Chem Lab Med 1998; 36: 143–147.

28. Simon JA, Hudes ES. Relation of serum ascorbic acid to serum vitamin B12, serum ferritin, and kidney stones in US adults. Arch Int Med 1999; 159: 619–624.

29. Curhan GC, Willett WC, Speizer FE, Stampfer MJ. Intake of vitamins B6 and C and the risk of kidney stones in women. J Am Soc Nephrol 1999; 10: 840–845.

30. Auer BL, Auer D, Rodgers AL. Relative hyperoxaluria, crystalluria and haematuria after megadose ingestion of vitamin C. Eur J Clin Investig 1998; 28: 695–700.

31. Smith LH, Fromm H, Hofmann AF. Acquired hyperoxaluria, nephrolithiasis, and intestinal disease. Description of a syndrome. N Engl J Med 1972; 286: 1371–1375.

32. Barilla DE, Notz C, Kennedy D, Pak CY. Renal oxalate excretion following oral oxalate loads in patients with ileal disease and with renal and absorptive hypercalciurias. Effect of calcium and magnesium. Am J Med 1978; 64: 579–585.

33. Clayman RV, Buchwald H, Varco RL, DeWolf WC, Williams RD. Urolithiasis in patients with a jejunoileal bypass. Surg Gynecol Obstet 1978; 147: 225–230.

34. Menon M, Mahle CJ. Oxalate metabolism and renal calculi. J Urol 1982; 127: 148–151.

35. Danpure CJ. Molecular and cell biology of primary hyperoxaluria type I. Clin Investig Med - Medecine Clinique Et Experimentale 1994; 72: 725–727.

36. Williams HE, Smith LHJ. L-glyceric aciduria: A new genetic variant of primary hyperoxaluria. N Engl J Med 1978; 278: 233–238.

37. Chlebeck PT, Milliner DS, Smith LH. Long-term prognosis in primary hyperoxaluria type II (L-glyceric aciduria). Am J Kid Dis 1994; 23: 255–259.

38. Scheinman JI. Primary hyperoxaluria. Min Electrol Metabol 1994; 20: 340–351.

39. Toussaint C, Vienne A, De Pauw L, et al. Combined liver-kidney transplantation in primary hyperoxaluria type 1. Bone histopathology and oxalate body content. Transplantation 1995; 59: 1700–1704.

40. Mizusawa Y, Parnham AP, Falk MC, et al. Potential for bilateral nephrectomy to reduce oxalate release after combined liver and kidney transplantation for primary hyperoxaluria type 1. Clin Transplant 1997; 11: 361–365.

41. Holmes RP. Pharmacological approaches in the treatment of primary hyperoxaluria. J Nephrol 11 Suppl 1998; 1: 32–35.

42. Leumann E, Hoppe B, Neuhaus T. Management of primary hyperoxaluria: efficacy of oral citrate administration. Pediatr Nephrol 1993; 7: 207–211.

43. Danielson BG, Pak CY, Smith LH, Vahlensieck W, Robertson WG. Treatment of Idiopathic calcium stone disease. Calcified Tissue Int 1983; 35: 715–719.

44. Nicar MJ, Skurla C, Sakhaee K, Pak CY. Low urinary citrate excretion in nephrolithiasis. Urology 1983; 21: 8–14.

45. Pak CY, Skurla C, Brinkley L, Sakhaee K. Augmentation of renal citrate excretion by oral potassium citrate administration: time course, dose frequency schedule, and dose-response relationship. J Clin Pharmacol 1984; 24: 19–26.

46. Kok DJ, Papapoulos SE, Bijvoet OL. Excessive crystal agglomeration with low citrate excretion in recurrent stone-formers. Lancet 1986; 1: 1056–1058.

47. Pak CY, Fuller C, Sakhaee K, Preminger GM, Britton F. Long-term treatment of calcium nephrolithiasis with potassium citrate. J Urol 1985; 134: 11–19.

48. Preminger GM, Harvey JA, Pak CY. Comparative efficacy of specific potassium citrate therapy versus conservative management in nephrolithiasis of mild to moderate severity. J Urol 1985; 134: 658–661.

49. Pak CY, Peterson RD, Poindexter J. Prevention of spinal bone loss by potassium citrate in cases of calcium urolithiasis. J Urol 2002; 168: 31–34.

50. Pak CY, Nicar M, Northcutt C. The definition of the mechanism of hypercalciuria is necessary for the treatment of recurrent stone formers. [Review]. Contributions Nephrol 1982; 33: 136–151.

51. Preminger GM, Sakhaee K, Skurla C, Pak CY. Prevention of recurrent calcium stone formation with potassium citrate therapy in patients with distal renal tubular acidosis. J Urol 1985; 134: 20–23.

52. Rudman D, Dedonis JL, Fountain MT, et al. Hypocitraturia in patients with gastrointestinal malabsorption. N Engl J Med 1980; 303: 657–661.

53. Pak CY. Citrate and renal calculi: new insights and future directions. Am J Kid Dis 1991; 17: 420–425.

54. Barcelo P, Wuhl O, Servitge E, Rousaud A, Pak CY Randomized double-blind study of potassium citrate in idiopathic hypocitraturic calcium nephrolithiasis. J Urol 1993; 150: 1761–1764.

55. Preminger GM, Baker S, Peterson R, Poindexter J, Pak CYC Hypomagnesiuric hypocitraturia: An apparent new entity for calcium nephrolithiasis. J Lithotripsy Stone Dis 1989; 1: 22–25.

56. Tiselius HG, Ahlstrand C, Larsson L. Urine composition in patients with urolithiasis during treatment with magnesium oxide. Urolog Res 1980; 8: 197–206.

57. Ettinger B, Pak CY, Citron JT, Thomas C, Adams-Huet B, Vangessel A. Potassium-magnesium citrate is an effective prophylaxis against recurrent calcium oxalate nephrolithiasis. J Urol 1997; 158: 2069–2073.

58. Schwartz BF, Bruce J, Leslie S, Stoller ML. Rethinking the role of urinary magnesium in calcium urolithiasis. J Endourol 2001; 15: 233–235.

59. Sutton RA, Walker VR. Responses to hydrochlorothiazide and acetazolamide in patients with calcium stones. Evidence suggesting a defect in renal tubular function. N Engl J Med 1980; 302: 709–713.

60. Tawil R, Moxley RT, Griggs RC. Acetazolamide-induced nephrolithiasis: implications for treatment of neuromuscular disorders. Neurology 1993; 43: 1105, 1106.

61. Parfitt AM. Acetazolamide and renal stone formation. Lancet 1970; 2: 153.

62. Stancer HC, Forbath N; Hyperparathyroidism, hypothyroidism, and impaired renal function after 10 to 20 years of lithium treatment. Arch Int Med 1989; 149: 1042–1045.

63. Garfinkel PE, Ezrin C, Stancer HC. Hypothyroidism and hyperparathyroidism associated with lithium. Lancet 1973; 2: 331, 332.

64. Pieri-Balandraud N, Hugueny P, Henry JF, Tournebise H, Dupont C. Hyperparathyroidism induced by lithium. A new case. Revue de Medecine Interne 2001; 22: 460–464.

65. Brochier T, Adnet-Kessous J, Barillot M, Pascalis JG. Hyperparathyroidism with lithium. Encephale 1994; 20: 339–349.

66. Nordenstrom J, Elvius M, Bagedahl-Strindlund M, Zhao B, Torring O. Biochemical hyperparathyroidism and bone mineral status in patients treated long-term with lithium. Metabol Clin Exp 1994; 43(12): 1563–1567.

67. McHenry CR, Rosen IB, Rotstein LE., Forbath N, Walfish PG. Lithiumogenic disorders of the thyroid and parathyroid glands as surgical disease. Surgery 1990; 108(6): 1001–1005.

15 Diet and Urolithiasis

William K. Johnston, III, MD and Roger K. Low, MD

CONTENTS

Key Words: Nephrolithiasis; diet; fluid; calcium; protein; sodium.

INTRODUCTION

Nephrolithiasis is a common disorder affecting approx 8–13% of the US population *(1,2)*. After experiencing renal colic and/or treatment for urinary stones, nearly every patient expresses interest in diet and specific dietary changes useful in lowering the risk for future stones.

The pathophysiology of nephrolithiasis is complex and involves multiple factors. Diet plays a major role in the concentration of a number of urinary solutes and inhibitors involved in crystallization and stone growth. Determining the impact of one's diet on future stone risk begins with a dietary history and subsequent metabolic testing. Metabolic testing usually reveals that an individual's risk is caused by a combination of metabolic and environmental factors, many of which can be improved with dietary modification. In this chapter, we will outline how diet impacts urinary stone formation and offer dietary recommendations for individuals with specific types of urinary stone.

From: Current Clinical Urology, *Urinary Stone Disease:*
A Practical Guide to Medical and Surgical Management
Edited by: M. L. Stoller and M. V. Meng © Humana Press Inc., Totowa, NJ

FLUIDS

Patient inquiries on the influence of fluid intake on stone formation are perhaps the most common during discussion of stone prevention. Many patients come with a preconceived notion that forcing oral fluids not only decreases stone risk but also influences spontaneous stone passage. Little evidence supports this practice during the acute phase of stone passage; however, the importance of fluid intake on the prevention of future stones recurrences cannot be overemphasized.

Current theories on stone formation are based on crystal formation caused by supersaturation of urinary salts. Saturation, determined by the concentration of urinary salts, is proportional to excreted substrate and inversely proportional to urinary volume. In theory, increasing urinary volume should decrease the supersaturation capabilities of urine and increasing oral fluid intake should be beneficial to patients with all types of stones. Evidence supporting this practice is less convincing. Although some studies do demonstrate a lower oral fluid intake *(3,4)* in stone formers vs controls, others do not *(5–7)*. There is also a concern that hydration may actually be detrimental by diluting inhibitors present within the urine.

Despite less than convincing evidence, there is a consensus that fluid intake to achieve a daily urine output in excess of 2 L should be recommended to all patients with a history of urolithiasis *(8)*. For most patients, this requires a daily fluid intake of more than 3 L/d. This daily intake of fluid typically requires 12 oz of fluid to be ingested with meals, in between meals, at bedtime, and again during the night. It is useful to explain to patients the utility of using the appearance of their urine as a gauge as to the adequacy of hydration. Fluid consumption to produce urine nearly free of coloration is encouraged. Although hydration is encouraged to all patients, successful incorporation of this dietary change is often challenging because of patients' social and occupational lifestyles.

Most would agree that water is the preferred fluid for stone formers to consume. Does water "hardness" influence the risk of forming stones? Water "hardness" relates to the amount of dissolved calcium and magnesium. Numerous population studies have attempted to attribute regional differences in urolithiasis incidence to differences in water hardness. The small concentration differences of calcium and magnesium between "hard" and "soft" water relative to those found in the urine make this factor probably unimportant *(9)*.

Although much is made about the risk of specific types of beverages on stone risk, most studies indicate a benefit to consumption of nearly any fluid. Beverages such as coffee, tea, and alcohol have been found to reduce stone formation *(4,10)*. Although alcoholic beverage consumption promotes urinary calcium and uric acid excretion, studies suggest a negative correlation between consumption and stone risk. Krieger et al. found the consumption of as little as 8 oz of beer per week reduces the risk of having a stone event *(11)*. The beneficial effects of caffeinated coffee and alcohol may be attributable to induction of diuresis from either blunting of the effects of antidiuretic hormone or limiting its secretion *(12)*.

With the exception of grapefruit and apple juice, consumption of fruit juices produce no increased stone risk *(10)*. This increased risk may be caused by their high oxalate content. In general, citrus juices tend to be beneficial to stone formers by alkalinizing the urine and promoting an increase in urinary citrate, a known inhibitor of calcium stone formation. In a study of 12 patients with a history of refractory hypocitraturia, Seltzer et al. found lemonade consumption of 2 L/d increased urinary citrate an average of 204

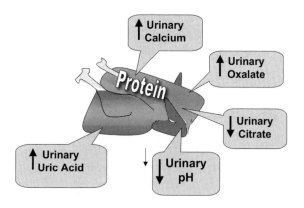

Fig. 1. Effects of dietary protein.

mg/d *(13)*. The antibacterial effects of cranberry juice ingestion has been debated *(14)*; however, dietary cranberry juice lowers urinary pH, increases urinary oxalate, and increases the urinary saturation of uric acid *(15)*. In contrast, ingestion of blackcurrant juice increases urinary pH, increases urinary citrate, and could be useful in metaphylaxis of uric acid stones *(15)*.

The consumption of soft drinks and oxalate-containing sodas has long been associated with stone formation. Nevertheless, controlled studies have been unable to show a significant increased risk with cola consumption *(10)*. Many sodas contain caffeine and induce diuresis from both fluid ingestion and an antidiuretic effect. Skim and whole milk both have been shown to reduce stone formation risk likely secondary to the binding of intestinal oxalate.

In summary, the intake of nearly all beverages is useful in reducing the risk of recurrent kidney stones. Fluid consumption should be encouraged in all patients with urolithiasis. Any type of beverage is acceptable in moderation, however water is probably the preferred fluid given its availability and lack of stone enhancing solutes.

PROTEIN

A diet high in protein is associated with an increased risk of urinary stone formation. Epidemiological studies relate a high socioeconomic status with stone formation attributable to diets high in protein *(16)*. Curhan et al., in a prospective study of male healthcare workers, reported a 1.33 relative risk of stone formation for the group with the highest animal protein consumption vs individuals on an animal protein free diet *(17)*. Multiple metabolic changes are induced by dietary protein consumption including hypercalciuria, hyperuricosuria, hypocitraturia and possibly hyperoxaluria (Fig. 1). These changes in urinary milieu predispose individuals to the formation of both calcium and uric acid stones.

The mechanism by which dietary protein increases the risk of calcium stones is complex and involves changes in calcium metabolism and other ions influencing calcium stone formation. Dietary proteins possess sulfur-containing amino acids that, on oxidation, yield sulfate. Sulfate represents an acid load and promotes a state of metabolic acidosis. The presence of sulfate and metabolic acidosis promotes hypercalciuria by increasing calcium resorption from bone and decreasing tubular calcium resorption caused by binding of urinary calcium with sulfate. This increase in filtered calcium, coupled with decrease in tubular resorption, account for the increase in urinary calcium. In normal subjects, the addition of 75 g of protein raises urinary calcium excretion approx 100 mg/d *(18)*. The metabolic acidosis caused by protein consumption also decreases urinary citrate. Lastly, hepatic metabolism of sulfur-containing amino acids produces uric acid. The resultant increase in urinary uric acid excretion can also increase the risk of calcium oxalate stone formation through heterogeneous nucleation. An increase in urinary oxalate following high dietary protein ingestion has been demonstrated in adult females but not in adult males *(19)*. The explanation for an increase in urinary oxalate may be owing to an increase in production of glycolate, a precursor to oxalate. In summary, dietary protein adversely influences multiple urinary solutes important to calcium oxalate stone formation. Consumption of large amounts of dietary protein should be avoided in all patients with a history of calcium nephrolithiasis.

Dietary protein ingestion not only increases the risk of calcium stones but also uric acid stones. Protein consumption is associated with both hyperuricosuria and urinary acidification, factors known to promote uric acid stone formation. Dietary protein is a source of amino acids, which on hepatic metabolism, increase endogenous production of uric acid. In addition, the previously described metabolic acidosis resulting from protein ingestion promotes urinary acidification. Hyperuricosuria and an acidic urinary environment are two important factors adversely influencing the risk of uric acid stone formation. Protein restriction is beneficial in those with a history of uric acid stones and hyperuricosuric calcium nephrolithiasis, often attributable to dietary indulgence of animal protein.

The type of dietary protein may influence stone risk. The highest risk is associated with a diet high in animal protein, represented primarily by meats. Breslau et al. examined the urinary effects of three different types of dietary protein *(20)*. Subjects were evaluated after the ingestion of diets containing animal protein, soy protein, and a combination of soy and egg protein. Calcium and uric acid excretion were highest and urinary citrate lowest after the ingestion of the animal protein diet. This increased risk associated with animal protein has been attributed to meats containing the highest amounts of the sulfur rich amino acids: cystine and methionine.

CARBOHYDRATES

There is little evidence suggesting dietary carbohydrates significantly affect one's risk for urolithiasis. Carbohydrate consumption is similar in stone formers compared to controls *(21,22)*. In addition, patients on a prolonged high carbohydrate diet have not been found to have an increased incidence of urolithiasis *(23)*. Ingestion of carbohydrates has been associated with increased urinary calcium and oxalate. Dietary carbohydrates increase intestinal absorption and decrease renal tubular resorption of calcium *(24–27)*. An increase in urinary oxalate has been demonstrated in control subjects following a glucose load, probably caused by an increase in endogenous hepatic metabolism *(26,28)*. The available literature suggests that although dietary carbohydrates influence key urinary substrates, they do not definitively increase one's risk of urolithiasis.

FAT

The effect of dietary fat intake on the risk for urolithiasis is unclear. Most studies demonstrate a similar dietary fat intake between stone formers and controls *(17,21,29)*.

The focus on dietary fat and stone risk has centered on eicosapentanoic acid, an inhibitor of arachidonic acid metabolism. Fish oil is high in eicosapentaenoic acid and a dietary staple of Greenland Eskimos, who have a very low incidence of urinary stones *(30)*. Studies of stone formers who supplement their diet with fish oil have demonstrated a reduction in both urinary calcium and oxalate *(31,32)*. Additional clinical studies are needed to verify the apparent benefit of fish oil in reducing the risk of urolithiasis.

CALCIUM

It is important to recognize that many urinary substrates influence calcium stone formation including calcium, oxalate, citrate, sodium, and uric acid. The most common identifiable abnormality in those with calcium stones is hypercalciuria related to dietary hyperabsorption *(33,34)*. It would seem logical that all patients with calcium stones would benefit from limiting their dietary calcium intake. There is a linear relationship between dietary calcium intake and urinary calcium *(35,36)*. However, dietary calcium restriction may result in higher levels of urinary oxalate, believed to be caused by a decreased oxalate binding with calcium in the intestine *(37)*. In addition, two cohort studies by Curhan et al. suggest a protective rather than detrimental effect of a high calcium intake on stone formation risk *(17,29)*. These studies also found that supplemental calcium decreased, rather than increased, the risk of stone formation; this difference was only statistically significant in women.

Recently, Borghi et al. published the only long-term study evaluating stone formation risk associated with dietary calcium intake *(38)*. They evaluated 120 men with unclassified hypercalciuria and a history of calcium oxalate nephrolithiasis. Subjects were assigned a specific diet for a period of at least 5 yrs. Patients were randomized to either a low calcium diet (400 mg/d) or a normal calcium diet (1200 mg/d) with restricted sodium (2900 mg/d) and animal protein (52 g/d). Both groups were instructed to limit their oxalate intake and encouraged to drink fluids. A diet restricted in animal protein and salt was chosen because both of these substances are associated with increased urinary calcium; combining this diet with normal dietary calcium intake may minimize the risk of hyperoxaluria. Patients were followed radiographically for development of stone recurrences and metabolically with annual quantitative urinary chemistries.

At 5 yrs, the relative risk of forming recurrent stones was higher in the low dietary calcium group vs the group on a normal calcium, restricted protein and sodium diet. Twenty-three of 60 men on the low calcium diet vs only 12 of the 60 men on the normal calcium diet developed stone recurrences. The relative risk of stone formation for those patients on the normal calcium, low protein and sodium diet was 0.49 compared to the men on the low calcium diet. Urinary chemistries documented lower urinary calcium levels in both groups; however, a lower calcium oxalate product and saturation were found in those patients on the normal calcium, low sodium and protein diet. This was caused by urinary oxalate levels, which rose in the low calcium diet and fell in the normal calcium, protein and sodium restricted diet. These results suggest that patients with hypercalciuria and calcium oxalate stones benefit from a diet that allows a moderate intake of dietary calcium but limits dietary protein and sodium. This study was performed with men only and it would be beneficial if similarly validated with women. In addition, some forms of hypercalciuria, such as resorptive and renal hypercalciuria, require surgical or pharmacologic intervention to prevent stone recurrences; it is unclear how many of these patients were classified in this way.

OXALATE

Calcium oxalate stones are the most common urinary calculi. Many patients with calcium oxalate stones assume that lowering dietary oxalate consumption will curb future stone formation. Literature supporting this practice is lacking. The dietary oxalate intake of stone formers vs controls has been found to be similar (22). Urinary oxalate originates from two sources, endogenous production from hepatic metabolism and dietary oxalate resulting from intestinal absorption. Until recently, the endogenous oxalate production from hepatic metabolism was thought to account for the majority of urinary oxalate with dietary oxalate contributing only 10–15% (39,40).

Recent work by Holmes and Assimos suggests a much higher contribution of dietary oxalate to urinary oxalate (41). They found a nonlinear relationship between dietary oxalate intake and absorption with a 45% mean contribution of diet to urinary oxalate. In addition, marked individual variance in absorption was observed ranging from 10–72% (42). Much of the difficulty in determining the influence of dietary oxalate on urinary oxalate relates to lack of information on oxalate content of dietary foodstuffs and inaccurate methods of oxalate quantification. Previous methods used to quantify oxalate content relied on indirect enzymatic and calorimetric assays, which underestimate oxalate content. Evidence also suggests there may be a genetic component, which may explain the variability among individuals (43).

The main dietary sources of oxalate are green leafy vegetables, chocolate, and tea. In general spinach and rhubarb have abundant oxalate, however the actual content may vary with source, location, brand, or even growth conditions (42). The oxalate contained within tea can vary with type and producer (44,45). In addition to these variables, food processing and preparation influence oxalate bioavailability (42). Intestinal oxalate absorption is passive and affected by binding with intestinal cations, such as calcium and magnesium. Intestinal oxalate complexes with calcium and magnesium and limits the amount available for absorption. Patients with fat malabsorption syndromes are at highest risk for developing hyperoxaluria. Intestinal transit time and the presence of oxalate-degrading bacteria may also influence oxalate availability. *Oxalobacter formigenes* is a common colonic bacterium capable of degrading intestinal oxalate. Typically, 70% of adults are colonized with the bacterium (46). Absence of intestinal *O. formigenes* has been linked with hyperoxaluria and an increase in severity of stone disease (47,48).

Although the influence of dietary oxalate on urinary oxalate remains controversial, the risk of hyperoxaluria on calcium oxalate urinary stone formation is well documented. Most would agree that avoidance of foods that are high in oxalate is beneficial in those with a history of calcium oxalate stone disease.

SODIUM

Sodium is an important dietary element influencing urolithiasis risk. An increase in dietary sodium intake has been associated with hypercalciuria, hypocitraturia, and cystinuria (Fig. 2). As a result, dietary sodium should be restricted in those patients at risk for calcium and cystine stones.

Because of similar renal tubular handling of sodium and calcium, dietary sodium and natriuresis are associated with calciuria (49). A 100 mmol increase in dietary sodium intake increases urinary calcium an average of 25 mg/d (50). In addition, hypercalciuric patients may have an increased sensitivity to the calciuric effects of dietary sodium (51). Although the sodium intake of stone formers has been found to be similar compared with

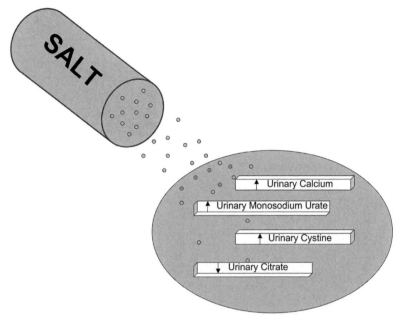

Fig. 2. Effects of salt on urinary constituents.

controls *(21,17)*, dietary sodium restriction in hypercalciuric stone formers has been shown to reduce urinary calcium *(52,53)*. For these reasons, dietary sodium restriction should be recommended to all hypercalciuric patients.

In addition to promoting hypercalciuria, dietary sodium intake influences calcium stone formation through promotion of epitaxial calcium oxalate crystal growth and reduction of urinary stone inhibitors. Natriuresis increases urinary supersaturation of monosodium urate and heterogeneous nucleation of calcium oxalate *(54)*. Dietary intake of sodium also lowers urinary citrate levels *(55)*. For all the above reasons, dietary intake of sodium should be restricted in patients with a history of calcium stone disease. Patients should be instructed to limit their intake of sodium to less than 200 mEq/d (11 g/d) *(56)*.

Dietary sodium restriction is beneficial in those with calcium stones, and in cystinuric patients. Dietary sodium intake increases dibasic amino acid excretion including urinary cystine. Jaeger et al. demonstrated that a reduction of 150 mEq (8.8 g) in dietary sodium chloride reduced urinary cystine by 156 mg/d *(57)*. The cystinuric effect of sodium also explains why potassium citrate preparations are preferred over sodium bicarbonate as an alkalinizing agent for the treatment of cystinuria. Potassium citrate preparations lack the sodium load and thereby minimize urinary cystine while still providing urinary alkalinization.

VITAMINS AND SUPPLEMENTS

Nutritional supplementation is promoted by our health conscious society and aging population concerned about senescence. Physicians must be aware of the potential risks of vitamin and nutritional supplementation on stone formation risk. Much of the difficulty in determining the risks of nutritional and herbal supplements is related to our lack of formal education and federal regulation of commercially available products.

Table 1
Recommended Diets

Stone type	Recommendations
Calcium	• Decrease meat consumption • Minimize salt intake • Moderate calcium intake (1200 mg/d)
Uric acid	• Decrease meat consumption • Encourage citrus juices
Cystine	• Minimize salt intake • Limit meat and milk intake
Struvite	• Encourage fluid intake

Note: Meat = beef, poultry, or fish.

Much has been written about the potential risk of vitamin C intake. Dietary ascorbic acid is metabolized in the liver to form oxalate, which is then excreted in the urine. The recommended daily dose of vitamin C is 60 mg/d. Linus Pauling is responsible for promoting the ingestion of supraphysiologic quantities of vitamin C to maintain health. An increase in urinary oxalate has been shown in both stone formers and normal controls after the ingestion of 1 g of ascorbic acid per day *(58)*. Other studies have found either a similar or decreased risk of stones in patients who take supplemental vitamin C *(59,60)*. In summary, vitamin C ingestion is associated with increasing urinary oxalate, however if taken in moderate quantities (500 mg/d), its use probably does not significantly influence one's risk for stone formation.

Nutritional supplementation to enhance muscle mass is in vogue predominantly in athletes and young men. Unfortunately, many of these supplements contain large amounts of protein. As discussed, dietary supplementation with many of these compounds can be associated with a significant increased risk of stone formation. Protein supplementation can be associated with hypercalciuria, hyperuricosuria, hypocitraturia, and possibly hyperoxaluria. These associated urinary changes increase the risk for both calcium and uric acid stones. Patients taking such supplements should be warned about the associated risks of their usage and importance of fluid intake during exertional exercise.

The beneficial effect of cranberry juice in preventing urinary tract infections has been popularized. Many health food stores offer cranberry extract tablets promoting its use as being "healthy for the urinary tract". Cranberries contain oxalate, and unfortunately these supplements have been associated with the development of calcium oxalate stones *(61)*. Terris et al. found that use of cranberry extract tablets in five nonstone forming adults increased their mean urinary oxalate level an average of 43% *(61)*. Cranberry extract tablets not only contain oxalate but also supplemental vitamin C.

RECOMMENDATIONS FOR SPECIFIC STONE TYPES (TABLE 1)

Calcium Stones

Known risk factors for calcium oxalate stones include: hypercalciuria, hyperoxaluria, hypocitraturia, hyperuricosuria and unduly concentrated urine. In general, any abnormality identified benefits from dietary restriction or dietary augmentation in the case of hypocitraturia and dehydration.

The most common identifiable abnormality in patients with calcium stones is hypercalciuria related to intestinal absorption. Traditionally, extensive metabolic testing has been recommended to classify patients and selectively treat patients accordingly. General dietary measures are recommended to all patients. These measures include dietary fluid intake to maintain a urine output of at least 2 L/d, avoidance of dietary overindulgence of sodium and animal protein, and regulated amounts of calcium. Patients with milder forms of absorptive hypercalciuria can be selectively managed with a calcium restricted diet (400–600 mg/d). Borghi et al. demonstrated the importance of dietary protein and sodium on influencing urinary calcium excretion. Their findings suggest that dietary restriction of sodium and protein coupled with a normal amount dietary calcium intake provides greater protection from recurrent calcium stones than a low-calcium diet *(38)*. Dietary calcium restriction may be detrimental in some patients with hypercalciuria. Dietary calcium restriction in patients with renal hypercalciuria can exacerbate the secondary hyperparathyroidism associated with a renal calcium leak. In addition, growing children and postmenopausal women may be at risk for bony loss from limiting their dietary calcium intake.

In summary, a high fluid intake along with dietary sodium and protein restriction is beneficial in reducing the risk for recurrent calcium stones. These dietary modifications in combination with a normal calcium intake have been shown to lower stone recurrence rates in men with a history of hypercalciuria and calcium stones. Dietary calcium restriction is capable of lowering urinary calcium in all forms of hypercalciuria, excluding renal hypercalciuria, but must be practiced in conjunction with dietary oxalate restriction to prevent hyperoxaluria. Specific groups at risk for negative calcium balance such as growing children, post-menopausal women, or adults with documented bony loss are best served by adhering to a diet with a normal amount of daily calcium but restricted amounts of dietary sodium and animal protein. In addition, differentiation between the various forms of hypercalciuria remains useful in identifying patients who would benefit from additional pharmacologic intervention.

Uric Acid Stones

Urinary uric acid solubility relates to uric acid concentration and pH. Of these, urinary pH is most important. Uric acid stones form in patients with unduly acidic urine (pH <5.5). These include patients with gout, chronic diarrhea states, and those who participate in frequent exercise. As with all stone patients, patients with a history of uric acid stones benefit from maintaining a high dietary fluid intake to maintain dilute urine. Fruit juices, a source of alkali, may be particularly useful owing to their urinary alkalinizing effects.

Uric acid is the end product of purine metabolism and is derived from three sources: diet, de novo synthesis, and tissue catabolism. Diet normally contributes approximately one-half (400 mg) of the uric acid produced by the body each day. The main dietary source of purines comes from meat, poultry, and fish. Both serum and urinary levels of uric acid reflect changes in dietary purine intake. Individuals placed on a low-purine diet exhibit urinary uric acid levels of 300 mg/d as opposed to the normal 600 mg/d *(62)*. As a result, it is recommended that patients with uric acid stones limit their intake of animal meat. Complete abstinence of meat is impractical, however reduction of the frequency and size of meat portions is beneficial. It has been recommended that individuals limit their dietary protein intake to 1 gm/Kg ideal body weight/d *(63)*.

The most effective method of preventing uric acid stones is urinary alkalinization. First time stone formers are encouraged to make necessary dietary changes and to be monitored closely. Urinary alkalinizing agents should be implemented in those who fail dietary therapy.

Cystine Stones

The goal in prophylaxis against recurrent urinary cystine stones is to maintain urinary cystine levels below its solubility limit of 200 mg/L. To this end, hydration to maintain urinary volumes in excess of 2 L/d is a mainstay of therapy. Hydration alone has been reported to be successful in preventing stone recurrences in up to two-thirds of cystinuric patients (64). Continued hydration even throughout the night is recommended to maintain urinary cystine concentrations below its solubility limit. Hydration with any type of beverage is probably useful; however, avoidance of milk due its methionine content and sodium rich beverages are encouraged. Alkali-containing fruit juices are preferred given their ability to augment urinary citrate and urinary alkalinizing effects.

Aside from hydration, avoidance of sodium is perhaps the most important dietary principle for cystinuric patients. Dietary sodium increases urinary cystine excretion by a poorly understood mechanism. Jaeger et al. demonstrated a reduction of dietary sodium of 150 mEq/d could reduce urinary cystine by 156 mg/d (57). The main dietary source of urinary cystine comes from methionine incorporated in protein. Common sources of dietary methionine are animal meats, milk, eggs, wheat, and peanuts. It is impractical to require dietary restriction of methionine containing foodstuffs because of poor palatability; however, overindulgence of these foodstuffs should be avoided.

Struvite Stones

Dietary manipulation has a limited role in the prevention of stone recurrences in patients with infection related stone disease. Rendering a patient stone and infection free is the mainstay of therapy for those with either struvite or carbonate apatite stones. As in patients with other stone types, hydration is encouraged to maximize ion solubility and minimize bacterial colonization.

A low phosphorus diet in combination with aluminum hydroxide was popularized by Shorr and colleagues. Aluminum hydroxide binds intestinal phosphate and, when coupled with a low phosphorus diet, is capable of lowering urinary phosphorus (65). Clinical trials in patients treated with this regimen demonstrate not only a reduction of stone growth but enhanced stone dissolution in some patients (65,66). Unfortunately, the Shorr regimen is poorly tolerated and dietary compliance difficult. Takeuchi et al. studied the effects of dietary magnesium and calcium in rats. They demonstrated that a low magnesium diet resulted in decreased urinary magnesium excretion and decreased stone growth. Similarly, a high calcium diet led to lower urinary phosphate and magnesium levels thought to be related to intestinal calcium binding (67).

In theory, urinary acidification would be beneficial in those patients with infection related stones. Urinary acidification would not only increase urinary solubility of magnesium ammonium phosphate and carbonate apatite but also may increase the antimicrobial effects of some penicillins (68,69). Unfortunately, no dietary changes have been found to be capable of providing sustained urinary acidification. Murphy et al. demonstrated urinary acidification from ingestion of ascorbic acid when given in combination with antimicrobials (70). Pharmacologic doses of ammonium sulfate and ammonium

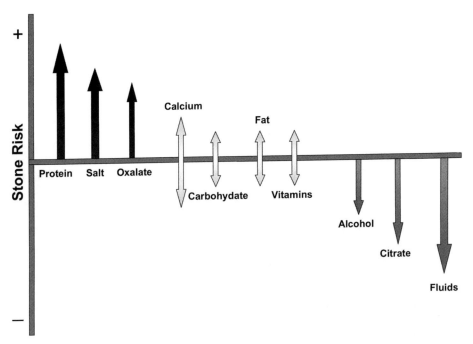

Fig. 3. Dietary stone risk.

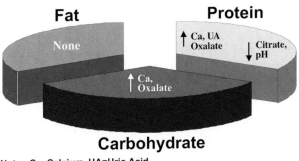

Note: Ca=Calcium, UA=Uric Acid

Fig. 4. Impact of major food groups.

nitrite are also capable of urinary acidification but are poorly tolerated and available only in Europe.

CONCLUSION

Diet plays a major role in the majority of patients with urolithiasis. Excluding patients with infection related stones, all patients benefit from a detailed dietary history, metabolic evaluation, and dietary counseling on stone prevention. Dietary modification can reduce and often prevent stone recurrences and is adjunctive in patients requiring pharmacologic therapy. Physician's awareness of the importance of diet and urolithiasis will benefit patients who suffer from urinary stone disease (Figs. 3 and 4).

REFERENCES

1. Ramello A, Vitale C, Marangella M. Epidemiology of nephrolithiasis. J Nephrol 2000; 13 Suppl 3: S45–50.

2. Johnson CM, Wilson DM, O'Fallon WM, et al. Renal stone epidemiology: a 25-year study in Rochester, Minnesota. Kid Int 1979; 16: 624–631.

3. Borghi L, Meschi T, Amato F, Briganti A, Novarini A, Giannini A. Urinary volume, water and recurrences in idiopathic calcium nephrolithiasis: a 5-year randomized prospective study. J Urol 1996; 155(3): 839–843.

4. Curhan GC, Willett WC, Speizer FE, Stampfer MJ. Beverage use and risk for kidney stones in women. Ann Intern Med 1998; 128(7): 534–540.

5. Ryall RL, Marshall VR. The value of the 24-hour urine analysis in the assessment of stone-formers attending a general hospital outpatient clinic. Br J Urol 1983; 55(1): 1–5.

6. Power C, Barker DJ, Nelson M, Winter PD. Diet and renal stones: a case-control study. Brit J Urol 1984; 56: 456.

7. Ljunghall S, Waern AU. Urinary electrolytes in renal stone formers and healthy subjects. A population study of 60-year-old men. Scand J Urol Nephrol. 1977; 41(11 Suppl): 55 abstract.

8. Consensus conference. Prevention and treatment of kidney stones. JAMA 1988; 260: 977.

9. Shuster J, Finlayson B, Scheaffer R, Sierakowski R, Zoltek J, Dzegede S. Water hardness and urinary stone disease. J Urol 1982; 128(2): 422–425.

10. Curhan GC, Willett WC, Rimm EB, Spiegelman D, Stampfer MJ. Prospective study of beverage use and the risk of kidney stones. Am J Epidemiol 1996; 143(3): 240–247.

11. Krieger JN, Kronmal RA, Coxon V, Wortley P, Thompson L, Sherrard DJ. Dietary and behavioral risk factors for urolithiasis: potential implications for prevention. Am J Kidney Dis 1996; 28(2): 195–201.

12. Kovacs L, Robertson GL. Syndrome of inappropriate antidiuresis. Endocrinol Metab Clin North Am 1992; 21(4): 859–875.

13. Seltzer MA, Low RK, McDonald M, Shami GS, Stoller ML. Dietary manipulation with lemonade to treat hypocitraturic calcium nephrolithiasis. J Urol 1996; 156(3): 907–909.

14. Lee YL, Owens J, Thrupp L, Cesario TC. Does cranberry juice have antibacterial activity? JAMA 2000; 283(13): 1691.

15. Kessler T, Jansen B, Hesse A. Effect of blackcurrant-, cranberry- and plum juice consumption on risk factors associated with kidney stone formation. Eur J Clin Nutr 2002; 56(10): 1020–1023.

16. Anderson DA. Environmental factors in the etiology of urolithiasis. In: Urinary Calculi, (Cifuentes-Delatte A, Rapado A, Hodgkinson A, eds.). Basel, Karger, 1973; p.130.

17. Curhan GC, Willett WC, Rimm EB, Stampfer MJ. A prospective study of dietary calcium and other nutrients and the risk of symptomatic kidney stones. N Engl J Med 1993; 328(12): 833–838.

18. Licata AA, Bou E, Bartter FC, Cox J. Effects of dietary protein on urinary calcium in normal subjects and in patients with nephrolithiasis. Metabolism 1979; 28(9): 895–900.

19. Holmes RP, Goodman HO, Hart LJ, Assimos DG. Relationship of protein intake to urinary oxalate and glycolate excretion. Kidney Int 1993; 44(2): 366–372.

20. Breslau NA, Brinkley L, Hill KD, Pak CY. Relationship of animal protein-rich diet to kidney stone formation and calcium metabolism. J Clin Endocrinol Metab 1988; 66(1): 140–146.

21. Fellstrom B, Danielson BG, Karlstrom B, Lithell H, Ljunghall S, Vessby B. Dietary habits in renal stone patients compared with healthy subjects. Br J Urol 1989; 63(6): 575–580.

22. Trinchieri A, Mandressi A, Luongo P, Longo G, Pisani E. The influence of diet on urinary risk factors for stones in healthy subjects and idiopathic renal calcium stone formers. Br J Urol 1991; 67(3): 230–236.

23. Garg A, Bonanome A, Grundy SM, Unger RH, Breslau NA, Pak CY. Effects of dietary carbohydrates on metabolism of calcium and other minerals in normal subjects and patients with noninsulin-dependent diabetes mellitus. J Clin Endocrinol Metab 1990; 70(4): 1007–1013.

24. Barilla DE, Townsend J, Pak CY. An exaggerated augmentation of renal calcium excretion after oral glucose ingestion in patients with renal hypercalciuria. Invest Urol 1978; 15(6):486–488.

25. Nguyen NU, Dumoulin G, Henriet MT, Regnard J. Effects of i.v. insulin bolus on urinary calcium and oxalate excretion in healthy subjects. Horm Metab Res 1998; 30(4): 222–226.

26. Nguyen NU, Dumoulin G, Wolf JP, Bourderont D, Berthelay S. Urinary oxalate and calcium excretion in response to oral glucose load in man. Horm Metab Res 1986; 18(12): 869, 870.

27. Wood RJ, Gerhardt A, Rosenberg IH. Effects of glucose and glucose polymers on calcium absorption in healthy subjects. Am J Clin Nutr 1987; 46(4): 699–701.

28. Nguyen NU, Henriet MT, Dumoulin G, Widmer A, Regnard J. Increase in calciuria and oxaluria after a single chocolate bar load. Horm Metab Res 1994; 26(8): 383–386.

29. Curhan GC, Willett WC, Speizer FE, Spiegelman D, Stampfer MJ. Comparison of dietary calcium with supplemental calcium and other nutrients as factors affecting the risk for kidney stones in women. Ann Intern Med 1997; 126(7): 497–504.

30. Modlin M. Urinary sodium and renal stone. In: Hodgkinson A, Nordin BEC (eds). Renal Stone Research Symposium. London J and Churchill A, pp. 209–220, 1969.

31. Buck AC, Davies RL, Harrison T. The protective role of eicosapentaenoic acid [EPA] in the pathogenesis of nephrolithiasis. J Urol 1991; 146(1): 188–194.

32. Rothwell PJ, Green R, Blacklock NJ, Kavanagh JP. Does fish oil benefit stone formers? J Urol 1993; 150(5 Pt 1): 1391–1394.

33. Broadus AE, Erickson SB, Gertner JM, Cooper K, Dobbins JW. An experimental human model of 1,25-dihydroxyvitamin D-mediated hypercalciuria. J Clin Endocrinol Metab 1984; 59(2): 202–206.

34. Asplin JR, Favus ME, Coe FL. Nephrolithiasis. In: Brenner & Rector's the Kidney, 6th Ed, Vol. 2., (Brenner BM, ed.). W.B. Saunders, Philadelphia, PA, 2000; pp. 1774–1819.

35. Bleich HL, Moore MJ, Lemann J Jr, Adams ND, Gray RW. Urinary calcium excretion in human beings. N Engl J Med 1979; 301(10): 535–541.

36. Robertson WG. Diet and calcium stones. Miner Electrolyte Metab 1987; 13(4): 228–234.

37. Bataille P, Achard JM, Fournier A, et al. Diet, vitamin D and vertebral mineral density in hypercalciuric calcium stone formers. Kidney Int 1991; 39(6): 1193–1205.

38. Borghi L, Schianchi T, Meschi T, et al. Comparison of two diets for the prevention of recurrent stones in idiopathic hypercalciuria. N Engl J Med 2002; 346(2): 77–84.

39. Hagler L, Herman RH. Oxalate metabolism. IV. Am J Clin Nutr 1973; 26(10): 1073–1079.

40. Menon M, Mahle CJ. Oxalate metabolism and renal calculi. J Urol 1982; 127(1): 148–151.

41. Holmes RP, Goodman HO, Assimos DG. Contribution of dietary oxalate to urinary oxalate excretion. Kidney Int 2001; 59(1): 270–206.

42. Holmes RP, Kennedy M. Estimation of the oxalate content of foods and daily oxalate intake. Kidney Int 2000; 57(4): 1662–1667.

43. Holmes RP, Assimos DG, Goodman HO. Genetic and dietary influences on urinary oxalate excretion. Urol Res 1998; 26(3): 195–200.

44. Kasidas GP, Rose GA. Oxalate content of some common foods: determination by an enzymatic method. J Hum Nutr 1980; 34(4): 255–266.

45. McKay DW, Seviour JP, Comerford A, Vasdev S, Massey LK. Herbal tea: an alternative to regular tea for those who form calcium oxalate stones. J Am Diet Assoc 1995; 95(3): 360–361.

46. Kwak C, Jeong BC, Lee JH, Kim HK, Kim EC, Kim HH. Molecular identification of Oxalobacter formigenes with the polymerase chain reaction in fresh or frozen fecal samples. BJU Int 2001; 88(6): 627–632.

47. Kumar R, Mukherjee M, Bhandari M, Kumar A, Sidhu H, Mittal RD. Role of Oxalobacter formigenes in calcium oxalate stone disease: a study from north India. Eur Urol 2002; 41(3): 318–322.

48. Troxel SA, Low RK, Sidhu H. Intestinal Oxalobacter Forminges colonization in calcium oxalate stone formers. Abstract 1011, AUA meeting, Orlando, Fl, 2002.

49. Agus ZS, Goldfarb S, Wasserstein A. Calcium transport in the kidney. Rev Physiol Biochem Pharmacol 1981; 90: 155–169.

50. McCarron DA, Rankin LI, Bennett WM, Krutzik S, McClung MR, Luft FC Urinary calcium excretion at extremes of sodium intake in normal man. Am J Nephrol 1981; 1(2): 84–90.

51. Wasserstein AG, Stolley PD, Soper KA, Goldfarb S, Maislin G, Agus Z. Case-control study of risk factors for idiopathic calcium nephrolithiasis. Miner Electrolyte Metab 1987; 13(2): 85–95.

52. Silver J, Rubinger D, Friedlaender MM, Popovtzer MM. Sodium-dependent idiopathic hypercalciuria in renal-stone formers. Lancet 1983; 27; 2(8348): 484–486.

53. Muldowney FP, Freaney R, Moloney MF. Importance of dietary sodium in the hypercalciuria syndrome. Kidney Int 1982; 22(3): 292–296.
54. Sarig S. The hyperuricosuric calcium oxalate stone former. Miner Electrolyte Metab 1987; 13(4): 251–256.
55. Simpson DP. Citrate excretion: a window on renal metabolism. Am J Physiol 1983; 244(3): F223–F234.
56. Pak C. General guidelines in management. In: Urolithiasis. W.B. Saunders, Philadelphia, PA, 1990; p. 176.
57. Jaegar P, Portmann L, Saunders A, et al: Anticystinuric effects of glutamine and of dietary sodium restriction. N Eng J Med 1986; 315: 1120.
58. Traxer O, Huet B, Pak CYC, Pearle MS. Stone forming risk of ascorbic acid. J. Endourol 2000; 14 (Supp 1): A9.
59. Simon JA, Hudes ES. Relation of serum ascorbic acid to serum vitamin B12, serum ferritin, and kidney stones in US adults. Arch Intern Med 1999; 159(6): 619–624.
60. Curhan GC, Willett WC, Speizer FE, Stampfer MJ. Intake of vitamins B6 and C and the risk of kidney stones in women. J Am Soc Nephrol 1999; 10(4): 840.
61. Terris MK, Issa MM, Tacker JR. Dietary supplementation with cranberry concentrate tablets may increase the risk of nephrolithiasis. Urology 2001; 57(1): 26–29.
62. Pak CY, Barilla DE, Holt K, Brinkley L, Tolentino R, Zerwekh JE. Effect of oral purine load and allopurinol on the crystallization of calcium salts in urine of patients with hyperuricosuric calcium urolithiasis. Am J Med 1978; 65(4): 593–599.
63. Rodman JS, Sosa RE, Lopez MA. Diagnosis and Treatment of Uric Acid Calculi. In: Kidney Stone. Lippincott-Raven, Philadelphia, PA, 1996; p. 980.
64. Dent CE, Friedman M, Green H, et al. Treatment of Cystinuria. Br J Urol 1955; 27: 317.
65. Shorr E, Carter AC. Aluminum gels in the management of renal phosphate calculi. JAMA 1950, 144: 1549–1556.
66. Lavengood RW Jr, Marshall VF. The prevention of renal phosphatic calculi in the presence of infection by the Shorr regimen. J Urol 1972; 108(3): 368–371.
67. Takeuchi H, Ueda M, Satoh M, Yoshida O. Effects of dietary calcium, magnesium and phosphorus on the formation of struvite stones in the urinary tract of rats. Urol Res 1991; 19(5): 305–308.
68. Andersen JA. Benurestat, a urease inhibitor for the therapy of infected ureolysis. Invest Urol 1975; 12(5): 381–386.
69. Williams JJ, Rodman JS, Peterson CM. A randomized double-blind study of acetohydroxamic acid in struvite nephrolithiasis. N Engl J Med 1984; 311(12): 760–764.
70. Murphy FJ, Zehman S, Mau W. Ascorbic acid as a urinary acidifying agent. Its role in chronic urinary tract infection. J. Urol 1965; 94: 300–303.

16 Uric Acid Urolithiasis

Bodo E. Knudsen, MD, Darren T. Beiko, MD, and John D. Denstedt, MD

CONTENTS

Key Words: Nephrolithiasis; uric acid; pH; dissolution.

INTRODUCTION

Uric acid calculi are responsible for 5–10% of calculi in the North American population. These radiolucent stones are of particular interest because of their ability to be successfully managed with both medical therapy and surgical intervention. The pathophysiology is unique and important to understand when treatment is being planned.

EPIDEMIOLOGY

The worldwide prevalence of uric acid stones ranges from 5 to 40%. The prevalence varies geographically with a rate of 5–10% in North America but as high as 40% in Israel *(1–6)*.

URIC ACID: PATHOPHYSIOLOGY

The final product of purine metabolism is uric acid (2,6,8-trioxypurine). It performs no known physiologic function in humans. In most mammals uric acid is further converted

From: Current Clinical Urology, *Urinary Stone Disease:*
A Practical Guide to Medical and Surgical Management
Edited by: M. L. Stoller and M. V. Meng © Humana Press Inc., Totowa, NJ

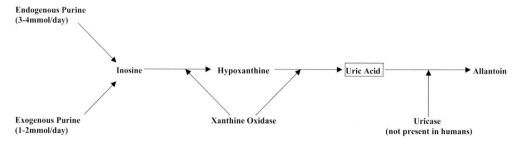

Fig. 1. Purine metabolism.

to allantoin by uricase. However humans lack this enzyme and therefore are unable to produce the 10–100 times more soluble allantoin.

The volume of urine and the amount of uric acid excreted determine urinary concentration. Nevertheless urine pH remains the single most important determinant of uric acid solubility. Uric acid has two dissociation constants (pKa): each governs the loss of a single proton from uric acid, at pH of 5.5 and 10.3 respectively. At the first pKa of 5.5, the conversion of uric acid to the more soluble anionic urate is controlled. The second pKa of 10.3 is not clinically significant because mean human urine pH is 5.9 and normally ranges from 4.8 to 7.4 (7,8). At a urinary pH <5.5 nearly 100% of uric acid is undissociated and urine becomes supersaturated with uric acid. Conversely, at a pH of >6.5 the majority of the uric acid exists as anionic urate.

There are both endogenous and exogenous sources of uric acid. Endogenous sources include *de novo* synthesis and tissue catabolism. Approximately 300–400 mg/d is produced under normal circumstances. Certain disease processes are associated with overproduction of uric acid. These include gout, myeloproliferative disorders, and certain congenital metabolic defects. Patients receiving chemotherapy may also have elevated uric acid levels secondary to rapid cell turnover.

Exogenous sources of purine are obtained from the diet and can vary greatly from individual to individual. Purine is broken down in the intestinal tract into free nucleic acids and then to inosinic acid. The next step is the conversion to hypoxanthine, which is subsequently converted to xanthine and finally uric acid by xanthine oxidase (Fig. 1). Foods highest in purine include fish, meats (especially liver, kidney, and heart), sweetbreads, and yeast (Table 1).

Two-thirds of uric acid elimination is handled by the kidney. The remaining third is cleared by extra-renal routes, including the skin, nails, hair, saliva, and the gastrointestinal tract (9,10). Bacteria in the bowel convert a portion of the uric acid to carbon dioxide and ammonia. Carbon dioxide is expelled as gas. The ammonia may be used by bacteria as an energy source or absorbed and consequently excreted in the urine (11).

Ninety-five percent of serum uric acid exists as monosodium urate, which is freely filtered at the glomerulus, whereas the remaining 5% is protein bound. A series of steps involving reabosrption, secretion, and further reabsorption occurs. Ninety-nine percent of the filtered urate is reabsorbed in the proximal convoluted tubule (PCT). However 50% is then secreted back into the PCT. Postsecretory absorption of 80% of this urate occurs distally but still within the PCT. Ultimately about 10% of the filtered urate is excreted in the urine. The fractional excretion of urate does vary with age ranging from 60% in a premature neonate to 12% in a 3 yr old and 7% in the adult (12) population.

Table 1
Foods High in Purine

• *Meats*	• *Fish*	• *Vegetables*	• *Mushrooms*
○ Organ meats	○ Anchovies	○ Peas	
liver	○ Herring	○ Legumes	• *Yeast*
kidneys	○ Sardines	○ Spinach	
heart	○ Mackerel	○ Lentils	• *Nuts*
○ Red meat	○ Fish roe	○ Beans	
○ Poultry	○ Shellfish	○ Asparagus	• *Alcohol*
wild game	○ Mussels	○ Cauliflower	○ Beer
	○ Shrimp		○ Wine
	○ Scallops		

Factors that can affect the renal handling of uric acid include the patient's volume status and urine output, serum urate concentration, as well as numerous medications. Extra-cellular volume expansion is inversely related to serum urate concentration. Medications such as salicyclates, sulfinpyrazone, and probenecid are uricosuric by way of impairing urate absorption in the PCT. Thiazides may cause hyperuricosuria by producing extra-cellular volume contraction, leading to increased urate secretion in the PCT *(13,14)*. Pregnancy is associated with hyperuricosuria. This is thought to be the result of a combination of the increased intravascular volume of pregnancy and fetal urate production *(11,15)*.

ASSOCIATED CONDITIONS

Three factors are primarily responsible for uric acid stone formation. These include (1) low urine pH, (2) low urine output, and (3) high urinary uric acid concentration. The most important of these factors is low urine pH, but all three interact and influence subsequent stone formation.

Gastrointestinal Conditions Associated With Uric Acid Lithiasis

Patients with inflammatory bowel disease, ileostomy, or multiple bowel resections, especially involving the terminal ileum, are at an increased risk of uric acid nephrolithiasis. Patients with ulcerative colitis have a 0.5–3.2% incidence of urolithiasis *(16–18)*. Ileostomy patients have a reported incidence of 50–70% and Crohn's disease patients with terminal ileal involvement as high as 80% *(19)*. These patients have a persistently low urinary pH but otherwise have normal serum and urine uric acid levels. They become dehydrated as a result of the ongoing water loss from the gastrointestinal tract. This also results in excessive bicarbonate losses with a resultant metabolic acidosis, hypocitraturia and low urinary pH. Such patients are at risk for both uric acid and calcium oxalate lithiasis. Patients with an ileostomy encounter similar difficulties.

Other situations that predispose to chronic dehydration such as working in a hot environment, heavy physical activity without fluid replacement, or living in an arid climate can result in increased uric acid stone formation. This may account for the increased incidence of uric acid stones in the Middle East *(20)*.

Gout and Stones

Primary gout is an inherited disorder characterized by hyperuricemia, persistently acidic urine and in some patients hyperuricosuria. A recurrent acute or chronic arthritis of peripheral joints develops that is the result of deposition of monosodium urate crystals in and about the joints and tendons *(21)*. Sustained hyperuricemia is a function of decreased renal clearance of urate. This may be caused by a tubular defect that results in decreased secretion of urate *(21)*. Patients on chronic diuretics or those with a decreased glomerular filtration rate (GFR) secondary to primary renal disease are particularly at risk. Longer duration and higher levels of hyperuricemia are associated with an increased incidence of gouty arthritis. In 10% of cases increased purine synthesis is responsible for the development of gout *(11,21)*.

The incidence of uric acid stones in individuals with primary gout is 10–20% *(21–24)*. In 40% of these patients stones develop before the onset of articular symptoms *(24)*. The majority of stone formers are men in the third to fifth decades of life. The patients universally have acidic urine that promotes the formation of uric acid calculi *(25–27)*. Hyperuricosuria only occurs in the 10% of patients who have an increase in *de novo* synthesis of purines. In fact, patients with gout have a lower rate of hyperuricosuria compared to normal controls *(28)*.

In normal individuals a postprandial increase in urinary pH occurs, referred to as an alkali tide *(29)*. This results from the secretion of bicarbonate into the serum by parietal cells of the stomach in response to gastric acid secretion. This produces an increased urinary pH, which promotes dissolution of uric acid and reduces precipitation and subsequent calculi formation. Patients with gout, and also some idiopathic uric acid stone formers, may lack this postprandial increase in urinary pH *(30,31)*. The exact mechanism for this phenomenon remains unclear. One theory is that there is impaired renal ammonium excretion and that this defect may worsen with aging *(24,32–35)*. However this theory has not universally been accepted *(36–38)* and in fact the etiology may be multifactorial.

Increased Catabolism

As many as 40% of patients with myelo- or lympho-proliferative disorders develop uric acid calculi *(24)*. With these disorders there is an increase in the production and turnover of nucleic acids. In patients receiving chemotherapy an enormous increase in the endogenous purine pool may occur as a result of tissue necrosis. This can lead to acute urinary obstruction because of severe crystalluria.

Other benign disorders that are associated with uric acid lithiasis include thalassemia, hemolytic anemia, polycythemia, and sickle cell disease *(39)*.

Enzymatic Defects Associated With Uric Acid Lithiasis

Hypoxanthine guanine phosphoribosyl transferase (HGPRT) is an enzyme whose function is to convert hypoxanthine to inosinic acid and guanine to guanylic acid. A partial or complete HGPRT deficiency may occur as an inborn error of metabolism. The complete form, known as Lesch–Nyhan syndrome, is X-linked and therefore seen only in males. It is characterized by self-mutilating behaviors, mental retardation, gout, and uric acid lithiasis. Infants may present with orange crystal-like deposits in their diapers, which are a result of uricosuria *(40)*.

Patients with type 1 glycogen storage diseases (GSDs) have either a primary defect in or impaired function of glucose-6-phosphatase. It is associated with an increased incidence of uric acid lithiasis. Patients develop hyperuricemia, hyperuricosuria, metabolic acidosis, hypoglycemia, hepatic adenomas, and chronic renal disease *(21)*.

Phosphoribosyl pyrophosphate (PRPP) synthetase overactivity is another X-linked disorder associated with uric acid lithiasis. PRPP synthetase is responsible for the formation of PRPP from ribose-5-phosphate and adenosine triphosphate. Increased PRPP synthetase activity results in hyperuricemia and hyperuricosuria *(41)*.

Diet

A diet high in animal protein may result in aciduria and hyperuricosuria with a resultant increase in uric acid lithiasis *(31)*. Patients generally have normal serum uric acid levels.

Familial

An autosomal dominant inherited form of uric acid lithiasis has been reported in a group of Israeli Jews. It appears to affect men and women equally, unlike primary gout. A persistent low urinary pH is manifested and stones may occur at an early age *(42)*.

Idiopathic

Some patients have neither a family history nor any predisposing conditions that can contribute to uric acid calculi. In one study, a noninherited idiopathic form of uric acid lithiasis was described in 15% of the population in central Europe. This group of patients had normouricemia and normouricosuria but did have a persistently low urinary pH *(30)*.

DIAGNOSIS

A detailed history is a key element in the work up of any patient with suspected uric acid urolithiasis. Items that must be covered include whether the patient has a past history of uric acid lithiasis, history of bowel disease or previous bowel surgery, risk factors for dehydration, family history of stones, history of gout, diet specifics, and any other major medical problems. It is also important to review any medications the patient is taking as well inquire about the patient's occupation.

Serum electrolytes, creatinine and urinalysis should be performed in all patients presenting with renal colic. Urinary pH should be recorded. A pH of <5.5 should alert the physician to the possibility of uric acid lithiasis in a patient with renal colic. If uric acid stones are suspected, then a serum uric acid and a complete blood count to screen for myeloproliferative disorders are recommended.

Initial imaging will vary based on what is available at the presenting institution. A plain kidney, ureters, and bladder (KUB) radiograph will fail to demonstrate pure uric acid stones because of their radiolucent nature (Fig. 2A). Stones that are composed of a combination of uric acid and calcium oxalate may however be visible. An intravenous pyelogram (IVP) can be performed as a first-line investigation. A radiolucent filling defect is suggestive of a uric acid stone (Fig. 2B). An IVP may also provide information regarding the degree of obstruction that a stone is causing. Information regarding stone size and location can also be obtained.

Many institutions are now performing noncontrast enhanced computerized tomography (CT) as a first line radiographic investigation for renal colic. Uric acid calculi are readily apparent on CT images (Fig. 2C). Hounsfield units (HU) between 300 and 600

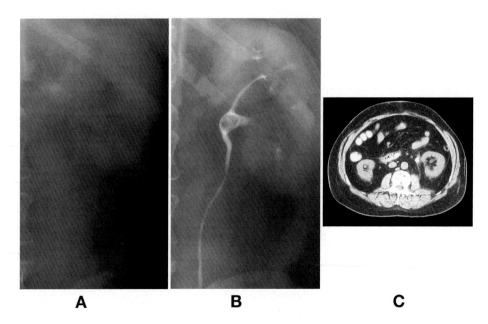

Fig. 2. Radiographic imaging of uric acid stone. **(A)** KUB demonstrating lack of radiopaque stone. **(B)** IVP showing filling defect in left renal pelvis. **(C)** CT scan with corresponding stone demonstrated.

are typical of pure uric acid calculi. HUs are generally somewhat lower for uric acid compared to calcium oxalate calculi *(43–45)*. A radiolucent filling defect on IVP has a broad differential diagnosis including blood clot, fungal ball, papillary necrosis, and transitional cell carcinoma. A CT scan can aid in differentiating these possibilities based both on the appearance of the lesions and their HU, which are between 20 and 55 HU for soft tissues *(46)*.

Renal ultrasound is a reasonable imaging option especially when used to follow patients with a history of uric acid lithiasis or in pregnancy. It offers the advantage of no radiation exposure but is less sensitive when compared to CT or IVP for detecting ureteric calculi and misses 20–30% of acute obstructions caused by a ureteric stone *(47)*.

With respect to metabolic evaluation, hyperuricosuria is a known risk factor for uric acid lithiasis. Pak defines hyperuricosuria as a mean 24-h urinary excretion of greater than 600 mg/d on two of three collected samples *(48)*.

TREATMENT

General Measures

Therapeutic goals include first achieving a stone free state and secondarily preventing new stone formation. In order to achieve these goals uric acid concentration must be reduced below the supersaturation point in the urine. Treatments are aimed at increasing the daily urinary volume, increasing the urinary pH, and reducing the amount of uric acid excreted.

General measures include encouraging patients to maintain a daily urine output of greater than 2 L and dietary counseling to reduce intake of purine rich food.

Chemolysis of Uric Acid Lithiasis

Uric acid stones are one of the few stone types that are amenable to dissolution therapy either in the form of oral or intravenous (IV) therapy, or via direct instillation of irrigating agents. Dissolution is an attractive treatment option especially for patients who have little or no symptoms, no associated infection, and do not have high-grade obstruction. Surgical drainage of the kidney is required first in the form of a stent or nephrostomy if one or more of the above are present. Dissolution therapy however remains an option after the kidney is appropriately drained and any infection treated.

As previously stated, uric acid has two dissociation constants, one at a pKa of 5.5 where the conversion of uric acid to the more soluble anionic urate is controlled and a second, clinically insignificant one at a pKa of 10.3. The goal is therefore to raise the urinary pH to a level where the stones can be dissolved. At a pH of 5.0, the solubility of uric acid is 6–8 mg/100 mL. At a pH of 7.0 this increases to 158 mg/100 mL. Therefore the goal is to increase the pH to approx 6.5 (49). Raising the pH higher than this, especially with oral therapy, increases the risk of calcium phosphate stone formation (50).

Oral Dissolution

In a patient with good renal function in the affected kidney and a stone size of 1 cm or less, oral dissolution therapy is an excellent option with success rates in excess of 80%. It may however take several months for the stones to dissolve (51,52).

Oral alkalinization of urine can be achieved with either sodium bicarbonate or potassium citrate. The dose of sodium bicarbonate is 650–1000 mg three to four times per day. The sodium load may prove problematic in patients with congestive heart failure or in the elderly. Potassium citrate is a better option and is administered at a dose of 15–30 meq three to four times per day. Caution is advised in patients with renal insufficiency because of the potassium load. Patients should be given either nitrazine paper or pH strips in order to optimize therapy to a urinary pH of 6.5. Care should be taken not to over correct the pH as calcium phosphate stone formation can occur at a pH greater than 7.0 (49). Potassium citrate administration may also act as a stone inhibitor and prevent new stones from developing (25). Stone dissolution rates can be expected to be approx 1 cm of stone radius per month. Patients should be imaged regularly during treatment to ensure active dissolution.

In addition to alkalinizing the urine with sodium bicarbonate or potassium citrate, allopurinol may be added to the treatment protocol. Some favor adding allopurinol only in patients with hyperuricosuria and hyperuricosemia (49). It is not unreasonable however to add it in all patients with uric acid stones undergoing dissolution therapy provided that there is no contraindication. Allopurinol is an inhibitor of the enzymes xanthine oxidase and hypoxanthine oxidase, which convert hypoxanthine to xanthine and xanthine to uric acid, respectively. Hypoxanthine and xanthine are both much more soluble than uric acid and are excreted by the kidney. De novo purine synthesis is also decreased with the administration of allopurinol. The recommended dose is 300 mg once per day. The dose should be adjusted in patients with renal insufficiency. The medication is well tolerated but approx 20% of patients may develop a fever, rash, or gastrointestinal upset. Liver enzymes should be periodically monitored as they may become elevated and hepatitis can develop. The most severe complication is Stevens–Johnson syndrome, which may lead to a fatal vasculitis. Pruritus usually is the initial complaint and precedes the hemorrhagic skin lesions and vasculitis. The onset of pru-

ritus in a patient taking allopurinol should prompt the physician to immediately stop it
(11,49,53,54).

Intravenous Dissolution

Intravenous alkalinization can be performed but is usually reserved for hospitalized
patients with acute urinary obstruction. Intravenous therapy raises urinary pH faster and
to a greater degree than oral dissolution therapy. One-sixth molar lactate solution, which
is metabolized to bicarbonate, has been used to dissolve uric acid calculi *(49,55)*.

Direct Dissolution

Direct dissolution of uric acid calculi, via an antegrade nephrostomy or retrograde
catheters, can be performed. Its primary use it to treat residual stones following a surgical
procedure or after shockwave lithotripsy. Tromethamine (THAM, pH 8.6), 0.3 *M*
tromethamine E (THAM-E pH 10.5), and sodium bicarbonate (pH 7.0–9.0) may all be
used. Patients however must be hospitalized to receive the treatment, which contributes
significantly to costs. Furthermore, recent advances in endourology have increased
surgical stone-free rates and therefore direct dissolution is becoming a historical option
(11,49,56).

Surgical Treatment of Uric Acid Calculi

Uric acid calculi are amenable to extracorporeal shockwave lithotripsy. However
targeting these radiolucent stones with fluoroscopy may not be possible unless they are
mixed stones with a significant calcium component. Retrograde instillation or intravenous infusion of contrast via a ureteric catheter can facilitate visualization. Alternatively, ultrasound can be used to target uric acid calculi *(57)*.

Ureteroscopy with intracorporeal lithotripsy and percutaneous nephrolithotripsy are
both effective modalities for treating uric acid calculi. Electrohydraulic, ultrasonic,
pneumatic, or Holmium:YAG laser lithotripsy are all effective fragmentation devices.
Holmium:YAG laser lithotripsy results in the production of cyanide. No clinical toxicity
or side effects have been demonstrated by its production *(58)*.

CONCLUSION

Uric acid calculi are a relatively common problem but may be amenable to appropriate
medical dissolution therapy. Effective medical treatment options include dissolution
therapy using oral sodium bicarbonate or potassium citrate, intravenous one-sixth molar
lactate solution or direct instillation of THAM, THAM-E, or sodium bicarbonate. When
medical therapy fails or an indication for surgical intervention is present, uric acid calculi
may be successfully treated by any of the available endourologic treatment options,
including extracorporeal shockwave lithotripsy, ureteroscopic lithotripsy, or percutaneous nephrolithotripsy. Knowledge of the size and location of the stone, along with an
understanding of the pathophysiology of uric acid urolithiasis and the associated conditions is paramount in determining the best treatment option.

REFERENCES

1. Gutman AB, Yu TF. Uric acid nephrolithiasis. Am J Med 1968; 45: 756.
2. Hesse A, Schneider HJ, Berg W, Hienzsch E. Uric acid dihydrate as urinary calculus component.
   Invest Urol 1975; 12: 405.

3. Scholz D, Schwille PO, Ulbrich D, Bausch WM, Sigel A. Composition of renal stones and their frequency in a stone clinic: relationship to parameters of mineral metabolism in serum and urine. Urol Res 1979; 7: 161.

4. Grenabo L, Hedelin H, Pettersson S. The severity of infection stones compared to other stones in the upper urinary tract. Scand J Urol Nephrol 1985; 19: 285.

5. Atsmon A, de Vries A, Frank M. Uric Acid Lithisasis. Elsevier, New York, NY, 1963.

6. Pak CYC, Resnick MI. Introduction. In: Urolithiasis: A medical and Surgical Reference, (Resnick MI, Pak CYC, eds.). WB Saunders, Philadelphia, PA, 1990; p. 1.

7. Elliot JS, Sharp RF, Lewis L. Urinary pH. J Urol 1959; 81: 339.

8. Finlayson B, Smith A. Stability of first dissociable proton of uric acid. Chem Eng 1974; 19: 94.

9. Bolliger A, Gross R. Ammonia, urea and uric acid content of toenails in renal insufficiency and gout. Aust J Biol Med Sci 1953; 31: 385.

10. Breslau NA, Brinkley L, Hill KD, et al. Relationship of animal protein-rich diet to kidney stone formation and calcium metabolism. J Clin Endocrinol Metab 1988; 66: 140.

11. Shekarriz B Stoller ML. Uric acid nephrolithiasis: current concepts and controversies. J Urol 2002; 168: 1307.

12. Camron JS, Moro F. Gout, uric acid, and purine metabolism in pediatric nephrology. Pediatric Nephrol 1993; 7: 105–118.

13. Pak CYC. Hyperuricosuric calcium nephrolithiasis. In: Urolithiasis. A Medical and Surgical Reference, (Resnick MI, Pak CYC, eds.). WB Saunders, Philadelphia PA, 1990; p. 79.

14. Pak CYC, Tolentino R, Stewart A, et al. Enhancement of renal excretion of uric acid during long-term thiazide therapy. Invest Urol 1978; 3: 191.

15. Semple PF, Carswell W, Boyle JA. Serial studies of the renal clearance of urate and inulin during pregnancy and after the puerperium in normal women. Clin Mol Med 1974; 47: 559.

16. Bargen JA, Jackman RJ, Kerr J. Studies of the life histories of patients with ulcerative colitis (thromboulcerative colitis), with some suggestions for treatment. Ann Intern Med 1938; 12: 339.

17. Grossman MS Nugent FW. urolithiasis as a complication of chronic diarrheal disease. Am J Dig Dis 1967; 12: 491.

18. Maratka Z, Nedbal J. Urolithiasis as a complication of the surgical treatment of ulcerative colitis. Gut 1964; 5: 214.

19. Gelzayd EA, Breuer RI Kirsner JB. Nephrolithiasis in inflammatory bowel disease. Am J Digest Dis 1968; 13: 1027.

20. Sakhaee K, Nigam S, Snell P, et al. Assessment of the pathogenic role of physical exercise in renal stone formation. J Clin Endocrinol Metab 1987; 65: 974.

21. McCarty DJ. Crystal-induced conditions. In: The Merck Manual, (Beers MH, Berkow R,eds.). Merck Research Laboratories, Whitehouse Station, NJ, 1999; pp. 460–465.

22. Gutman AB, Yu TF. Uric acid nephrolithiasis. Am J Med 1968; 45: 756.

23. Stoller ML. Gout and stones or stones and gout? J Urol 1995; 154: 1670.

24. Yu TF, Gutman AB. Uric acid nephrolithiasis in gout. Predisposing factors. Ann Intern Med 1967; 67: 1133.

25. Pak CYC, Sakhaee K, Fuller C. Successful management of uric acid nephrolithiasis with potassium citrate. Kidney Int 1986; 30: 422.

26. Pak CYC, Poy RK. Urinary pH in gout. Aust Ann Med 1965; 14: 35.

27. Serane J, Bonniot R. Etude clinique de 136 cas de goutte masculine. Presse Med 1954; 62: 507.

28. Khatchadourian J, Preminger GM, Whitson PA, Adams-Huet, B, Pak CYC. Clinical and biochemical presentation of gouty diathesis: comparison of uric acid versus pure calcium stone formation. J Urol 1995; 154: 1665.

29. Moore EW. The alkaline tide. Gastroenterology 1967; 52: 1052.

30. Zechner O, Pflüger H, Scheiber V. Idiopathic uric acid lithiasis: epidemiologic and metabolic aspects. J Urol 1982; 128: 1219.

31. Breslau NA, Brinkley L, Hill KD, Pak CYC. Relationship of animal protein-rich diet to kidney stone formation and calcium metabolism. J Clin Endocrinol Metab 1988; 66: 140.

32. Gutman AB, Yu TF. On the nature of the inborn metabolic error(s) of primary gout. Trans Assoc Am Physicians 1963; 76: 141.

33. Gutman AB, Yu TF. Urinary ammonium excretion in primary gout. J Clin Invest 1965; 44: 1474.

34. Henneman PA, Wallach S, Dempsey EF. The metabolic defect responsible for uric acid stone formation. J Clin Invest 1962; 41: 537.

35. Barzel US, Sperling O, Frank M, et al. Renal ammonium excretion and urinary pH in idiopathic uric acid lithiasis. J Urol 1964; 92: 1.

36. Metcalfe-Gibson A, McCallum FM, Morrison RBI, Wrong O. Urinary excretion of hydrogen ion in patients with uric acid calculi. Clin Sci 1965; 28: 325.

37. Plante GE, Durivage J, Lemieux G. Renal excretion of hydrogen in primary gout. Metabolism 1968; 17: 377.

38. Falls WF, Jr. Comparison of urinary acidification and ammonium excretion in normal and gouty subjects. Metabolism 1972; 21: 433.

39. Low RK, Stoller ML. Uric acid-related nephrolithiasis. Urol Clin North Am 1997; 24: 135.

40. Lesch M, Nyan WL. A familial disorder of uric acid metabolism and central nervous system function. Am J Med 1964; 36: 561.

41. Becker MA, Meyer LJ, Seegmiller JE. Gout with purine overproduction due to increased phosphoribosyltransferase deficiency. Am J Med 1973; 55: 232.

42. de Vries A. Frank M, Atsmon A. Inherited uric acid lithiasis. Am J Med 1962; 33: 880.

43. Resnick MI, Kursh ED, Cohen AM. Use of computerized tomography in the delineation of uric acid calculi. J Urol 1984; 131: 9.

44. Nakada SY, Hoff DG, Attai S, Heisey D, Blankenbaker D, Pozniak M. Determination of stone composition by noncontrast spiral computed tomography in the clinical setting. Urology 2000; 55: 816.

45. Spencer BA, Wood BJ, Dretler SP. Helical CT and ureteral colic. Urol Clin North Am 2000; 27: 231.

46. Clayman RV, Kavoussi L. Endosurgical techniques for the diagnosis and treatment of noncalculus disease of the ureter and kidney. In: Campbells Urology, (Walsh PC, Retik AB, Stamey TA, Vaughn ED, Jr, eds.). WB Saunders, Philadelphia, PA, 1992.

47. Platt JF, Rubin JM, Ellis JH. Acute renal obstruction: evaluation with intra-renal duplex Doppler and conventional US. Radiology 1993; 186: 685.

48. Pak CYC, Holt K, Peterson R, et al. Ambulatory evaluation of nephrolithiasis: Classification, clinical presentation and diagnostic criteria. AM J Med 1980; 69: 19.

49. Bernardo NO, Smith AD. Chemolysis of urinary calculi. Urol Clin North Am 2000; 27: 355.

50. Parks JH, Coward M, Coe FL. Correspondence between stone composition and urine supersaturation in nephrolithiasis. Kidney Int 1997; 51: 894.

51. Moran ME, Abrahams HM, Burday BE, Greene TD. Utility of oral dissolution therapy in the management of referred patients with secondarily treated uric acid stones. Urology 2002; 59: 206.

52. Uhlir K. The peroral dissolution of renal calculi. J Urol 1970; 104: 239.

53. Greene ML, Fujimoto WY, Seegmiller JE. Urinary xanthine stones – a rare complication of allopurinol therapy. N Engl J Med 1969; 280: 426.

54. Potter JL, Silvidi AA. Xanthine lithiasis, nephrocalcinosis, and renal failure in a leukemia patient treated with allopurinol. Clin Chem 1987; 33: 2314.

55. Lewis R, Roth J, Polanka E, et al. Molar lactate in the management of uric acid renal obstruction. J Urol 1981; 125: 87.

56. Gordon M, Carrion J, Politano V. Dissolution of uric acid calculi with THAM irrigation. Urology 1978; 12: 393.

57. Royce PL, Fuchs GJ, Lupu An N, Chaussy CG. The treatment of uric acid calculi with extracorporeal shock wave lithotripsy. Br J Urol 1987; 60: 6.

58. Teichman JMH, Champion PC, Wollin TA, Denstedt JD. Holmium:YAG lithotripsy of uric acid calculi. J Urol 1998; 160: 2130.

17 Struvite Stones

D. Brooke Johnson, MD and Margaret S. Pearle, MD, PhD

Key Words: Struvite stone; urinary infection; urease; staghorn.

INTRODUCTION

The occurrence of urinary infection in patients with nephrolithiasis is not uncommon. Although stones of any composition may occur in patients who experience urinary tract infections owing to a variety of urinary pathogens, the term "infection stone" is reserved for calculi that form as a direct consequence of infection with urease-producing bacteria and the urinary environment they promote. This chapter will focus on current concepts regarding infection stones, including their pathogenesis, clinical diagnosis and treatment.

COMPOSITION

Infection calculi are composed primarily of magnesium ammonium phosphate hexahydrate ($MgNH_4PO_4 \times 6H_2O$) but may, in addition, contain calcium phosphate in the form of carbonate apatite ($Ca_{10}[PO_4]_6 \times CO_3$) *(1,2)*. Because infection calculi are

From: Current Clinical Urology, *Urinary Stone Disease:*
A Practical Guide to Medical and Surgical Management
Edited by: M. L. Stoller and M. V. Meng © Humana Press Inc., Totowa, NJ

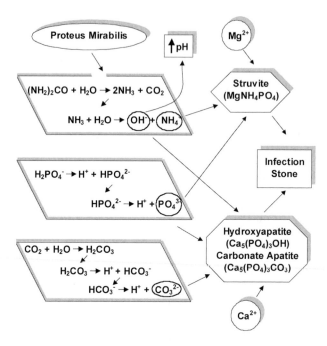

Fig. 1. Schematic depicting concurrent events leading to struvite stone formation.

composed of three different cations (Ca^{2+}, Mg^{2+}, and NH_4^+) in combination with one anion (PO_4^{3-}) the term "triple-phosphate stones" has been applied as well *(1,2)*. Magnesium ammonium phosphate hexahydrate is also known as "struvite," a moniker denoted by the German chemist George Ludwig Ulex who first identified the mineral and was a student of the Russian diplomat and naturalist Heinrich Christian Gottfried von Struve *(3)*. Hence the term "struvite stone" is often used interchangeably with "infection stone." Likewise, the term "urease stone" is also used to describe these calculi, because the presence of urease-producing bacteria is requisite to their formation.

PATHOGENESIS

Calcium, magnesium, phosphate, and urea are normal constituents of urine at concentrations sufficient for stone formation. On the other hand, ammonia, bicarbonate, and carbonate achieve concentrations sufficient for stone formation only during the process of ureolysis *(see* below) *(4)*. In order for crystallization to occur, not only must the constituent ions and ammonia be present in adequate concentration, but urinary pH must be 7.2 or greater also *(5)*.

The process of ureolysis provides the alkaline urinary environment and necessary carbonate and ammonia concentrations to induce infection stone formation. Because urease is not present in sterile human urine, infection with urease-producing bacteria is a prerequisite for the formation of infection stones *(6)*. A cascade of chemical reactions generates the conditions conducive to the formation of infection stones (Fig. 1). First, urease catalyzes the enzymatic breakdown of urea to ammonia and carbon dioxide:

$$(NH_2)_2CO + H_2O \quad 2NH_3 + CO_2$$

Ammonia then accepts a hydrogen ion from water to form ammonium:

$$NH_3 + H_2O \quad NH_4^+ + OH^- \quad pK = 9.0$$

Under physiologic conditions, alkaline urine contains low levels of ammonia. However, the presence of urease enables the generation of additional ammonia despite an alkaline urine, thereby further increasing urinary pH. In an alkaline environment, carbon dioxide is hydrated to carbonic acid that then dissociates into bicarbonate and hydrogen ion. Bicarbonate further dissociates into carbonate and two hydrogen ions:

$$CO_2 + H_2O \quad H_2CO_3 \qquad pK = 4.5$$

$$H_2CO_3 \quad H^+ + HCO_3^- \qquad pK = 6.3$$

$$HCO_3^- \quad H^+ + CO_3^{2-} \qquad pK = 10.2$$

At the same time, the alkaline urinary conditions promote the dissociation of phosphate:

$$H_2PO_4^- \quad H^+ + HPO_4^{2-} \qquad pK = 7.2$$

$$HPO_4^{2-} \quad H^+ + PO_4^{3-} \qquad pK = 12.4$$

This chemical cascade occurring within physiologic urine leads to sufficient concentrations of magnesium, ammonium, and phosphate for precipitation of struvite, and ultimately the formation of struvite stones. In addition, the concentrations of calcium, phosphate and carbonate allow precipitation of carbonate apatite and hydroxyapatite, thus accounting for the triad of mineral constituents of human infection stones.

BACTERIOLOGY

Infection of the urinary tract with urease-producing organisms is required for the formation of infection stones in humans. Although the species Enterobacteriaceae comprises the majority of urease-producing pathogens, a variety of gram-positive and gram-negative bacteria and some yeasts and mycoplasma species have the capacity to synthesize urease (Table 1) (3). In all, over 200 species of bacteria have been shown to have urease activity (4) which they use to provide a nitrogen source by incorporating the NH_3 produced from urea into glutamate and glutamine (7). The largest population of urease-producing bacteria resides within the gastrointestinal tract, and in this setting, the organisms are symbiotic. However, a pathologic urinary tract infection may be derived from the gastrointestinal urease-producing flora (4). The most common organism associated with infection stones is *Proteus mirablis (8)*.

EPIDEMIOLOGY

Historically infection stones have been thought to account for 7–31% of urinary calculi in the Western world (9). However, a search of the database of a large stone analysis laboratory revealed only a 2.1% (795 of 37,400) incidence of struvite-containing stones among the specimens (10). In contrast, struvite/carbonate apatite was found to comprise the most common composition of stones in a study of urinary lithiasis in African American patients in Ohio, accounting for a third of stones in males and nearly 50% in females in this population (11). Infection stones are most likely to occur in patients who are pre-disposed to frequent or persistent urinary tract infections. Struvite stones occur more often in women than men by a ratio of 2:1, most likely because of the higher incidence of urinary tract infections in women compared with men (12). New-

Table 1
Organisms Commonly Associated
With Urease Production

Category	Organism
• Gram Negative	*Proteus mirabilis*
	Proteus morganii
	Proteus rettgeri
	Proteus vulgaris
	Providencia stuartii
	Haemophilus influenzae
	Bordetella pertussis
	Bacteroides corrodens
	Yersinia enterocolitica
	Brucella spp.
	Flavobacterium spp.
• Gram Positive	*Corynebacterium hofmanii*
	Corynebacterium ovis
	Corynebacterium renale
	Corynebacterium ulcerans
	Micrococcus varions
	Staphylococcus aureus
• Mycoplasma	T-strain *Mycoplasma*
	Ureaplasma urealyticum
• Yeast	*Cryptococcus humicola*
	Cryptococcus
	Sporobolmyces
	Rhodotorula
	Trichosporon cutaneum

Adapted from Gleeson, Kobiashi, et al. *(3)*.

borns, especially those born prematurely or with congenital urinary tract malformations, are also at increased risk for infection stones *(7)*. Both elderly men and women are prone to developing infection stones because susceptibility to urinary tract infections increases with age *(13)*.

Urinary stasis associated with urinary tract obstruction, urinary diversion or neurologic disorders also pre-disposes to urinary tract infection and infection stones. Spinal cord injury patients are at increased risk for both infection and metabolic stones due to neurogenic urinary tract dysfunction and hypercalciuria related to immobility. Patients with a functionally complete cord transection are at highest risk of developing a staghorn calculus *(14)*. Patients with diabetes mellitus or those consuming excessive amounts of laxatives or analgesics are at increased risk for struvite stone formation as well *(15)*. Lastly conclusion, a foreign body or a calcium stone nidus may become colonized with bacteria leading to the formation of struvite stones in conjunction with existing calcium stone disease *(10)*.

CLINICAL PRESENTATION

Signs and Symptoms

A variety of clinical signs and symptoms have been associated with infection stones, although up to 25% of patients may be asymptomatic *(16,17)*. In many patients, symptoms are not due to the stone itself, but rather are attributable to the underlying conditions predisposing to stones, such as recurrent urinary tract infections or neurogenic bladder. When symptoms due to the stone are present they are typical of urinary tract infection and/or renal calculi, such as flank pain, fever, dysuria, urgency, frequency, and hematuria. A palpable mass, hydronephrosis, acute pyelonephritis and sepsis may develop in severe cases and may progress to acute pyonephrosis or intrarenal or perirenal abscess. In some patients, particularly those with diabetes mellitus, xanthogranulomatous pyelonephritis may occur in which renal parenchyma is replaced with lipid-laden macrophages. Progression to pyonephrosis, end-stage hydronephrosis, and xanthogranulomatous pyelonephritis is usually associated with complete obstruction *(17)*.

Laboratory Testing

Because it is nearly impossible to eradicate bacteria from infection stones, patients commonly present with bacteriuria and/or pyuria. An abnormal urinalysis may provide the first evidence suggesting struvite stones. Infection with a urease-positive organism will be associated with an alkaline urine, and on microscopic examination bacteria, leukocytes and "coffin lid-shaped" crystals may be evident *(18)*. A urine culture is essential for identification of the urease-producing organism and for obtaining antibiotic sensitivities to guide treatment prior to surgery. In cases where the urine culture is negative but the suspicion of a struvite stone is high, infection with atypical organisms such as *Ureaplasma urealyticum (19)*, *Corynebacterium urealyticum* or fungal species should be considered *(20)*. If cultures are positive only for a non-urease-producing organism (e.g., *Escherichia coli*) and a staghorn stone is present, the stone is likely composed of a material other than struvite *(21)*.

An elevated serum creatinine may suggest loss of renal function as a result of obstruction or parenchymal scarring due to recurrent urinary tract infections and pyelonephrits. The urinary conditions predisposing to struvite stones place both kidneys at risk, although involvement of only one kidney is common. Determination of differential renal function may be necessary to establish the utility of kidney salvage versus nephrectomy.

Although the urine of patients with struvite stones is usually chronically infected, symptoms of systemic disease may be intermittent. A complete blood count can indicate ongoing pyelonephritis or early sepsis. In some elderly or debilitated patients typical signs of infection, such as fever, may be absent.

Radiographic Studies

Because of their characteristic appearance, struvite calculi may be suspected based on radiographic imaging studies. Struvite stones typically grow rapidly and may fill the entire collecting system, giving the appearance of a "staghorn", before causing symptoms. The majority of staghorn stones are composed of struvite despite the relative infrequency of struvite stones compared to calcium calculi *(21)*. Approximately 75% of staghorn stones are composed of a mixture of struvite, carbonate apatite and matrix *(3)*.

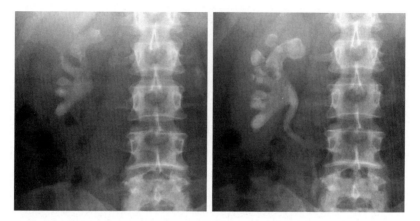

Fig. 2. Plain abdominal radiograph and intravenous urogram depicting a complete right staghorn calculus associated with minimal obstruction.

Although most infection stones are radiopaque, they appear less dense than calcium stones on plain radiographs due to their lower mineral content *(3)*.

Although a plain abdominal radiograph will identify most staghorn calculi, an intravenous urogram is advisable to determine the degree of obstruction and to clarify renal anatomy in anticipation of surgery (Fig. 2). Surprisingly, many staghorn calculi are associated with minimal obstruction despite their large size.

Determination of renal function is prudent if the possibility of surgical intervention is entertained. Although global renal function can be determined by serum creatinine or creatinine clearance, differential renal function should be assessed by nuclear reno graphy if contrast imaging studies such as intravenous urogram or contrast computerized tomography (CT) suggest equivocal unilateral renal function *(21)*.

Helical CT, with its multiple overlapping images, can provide precise 3-dimensional reconstruction of the stone and collecting system that can be used to assist in surgical planning. However, CT imaging has not been shown to be superior to plain films and intravenous urograms solely for this purpose, and consequently CT is not currently recommended for routine pre-operative use *(22)*. In vitro studies have suggested that thin-cut CT may be capable of differentiating struvite from other stone compositions which could help treatment planning *(23)*; unfortunately, the overlapping ranges of Hounsfield units for stones of different compositions currently precludes use of this technology in vivo for the definitive preoperative diagnosis of struvite stones.

NONSURGICAL TREATMENT

The treatment of struvite stones involves removal of the urinary calculus and eradication of infection with urease-producing bacteria. Only by accomplishing both these goals is the risk to renal function eliminated and the prevention of recurrent struvite stones assured. Without removing the stone, eradication of infections associated with struvite stones is virtually impossible, as the stones harboring bacteria cannot be penetrated by systemic antibiotics. Once a patient is rendered stone free, prevention of further infection is critical to prevent future stone formation. Consequently, treatment of struvite calculi requires a multi-modal approach, utilizing both medical and surgical therapy to achieve the optimal results.

Diet

Early investigators attempted to treat struvite and other phosphate-containing stones with dietary modification based on a low calcium, low phosphorus, high fluid (3 L/d) diet, along with aluminum gel supplementation *(24,25)*. The aluminum gel served to bind phosphate in the intestinal lumen, thereby reducing intestinal phosphate absorption and subsequent urinary phosphate excretion. Retrospective evaluation of stone formers maintained on this regimen demonstrated a reduced stone recurrence rate, particularly when the dietary regimen was combined with antimicrobial sterilization of the urine *(26)*. However, compliance with this diet was difficult as it was cumbersome, constiptating and somewhat unpalatable *(26)*.

In the 1930s, dietary deficiency of vitamin A was thought to contribute to the formation of struvite calculi *(27,28)*. However, vitamin A dietary supplementation is now thought to provide little benefit in stone prevention *(3)*.

Antimicrobial Agents

Antimicrobial treatment is directed at eradicating the causative organism, thereby eliminating urease-production and alkaline urine. Earlier in vitro studies showed dissolution of struvite crystals when they were perfused with sterile, undersaturated urine *(29)*, and in vivo studies demonstrated at least partial dissolution of infection calculi in urine that had been rendered sterile *(30,31)*. However, sterilization of the urine is impeded by the protection from antibiotics afforded bacteria that dwell within the interstices of the stone *(32)*. Even if sterile urine can be maintained for a time, cessation of antibiotic therapy usually results in re-infection of the urine by the organisms residing within the stone, re-establishing the conditions conducive for struvite stone formation. Moreover, long-term suppressive antibiotic therapy may lead to colonization with more virulent, resistant organisms *(33)*. Consequently, antibiotic therapy alone does not provide definitive treatment for struvite calculi.

Antimicrobial agents do, however, play an important role in the overall treatment regimen of infection stones. Preoperative and perioperative antibiotics are essential for preventing sepsis associated with surgical manipulation of the stone *(4)*. Unfortunately, the results of urine cultures obtained preoperatively do not always correspond to the organism isolated from the stone obtained at the time of surgery *(32)*. Preoperative treatment with antimicrobial agents directed at culture-documented organisms and that provides broad-spectrum coverage as well, particularly against common urease-producing bacteria, is advisable and should be initiated 1–2 wk before planned surgical intervention.

Even patients without documented bacteriuria may develop bacteremia, endotoxemia and enhanced release of tumor necrosis factor after endourologic manipulation for stone removal, placing them at risk for sepsis syndrome *(34)*. A recent report of death due to sepsis in a child undergoing percutaneous stone removal for a staghorn calculus was attributed to severe endotoxemia even though bacterial colony counts from the urine obtained in the immediate post-operative period were remarkably low *(35)*.

In the long term, antimicrobials may be used to reduce the severity of urinary infection despite the persistence of the organism. In addition, culture-specific antibiotics can be effective against those organisms that are present in the urine and on the surface of the stone, which comprise the majority of bacteria. This treatment leads to a significant reduction in colony count, and, since the production of urease is directly proportional to the number of organisms present, the quantity of urease decreases accordingly. A reduction in colony count from 10^7 to 10^5 per milliliter reduces urease production by 99%, thereby limiting the rate of stone growth (2).

In patients rendered stone free by surgery, suppressive antibiotics should be administered in order to maintain sterile urine, thereby preventing the morbidity of recurrent infection and further stone formation. One group of investigators recommended prophylactic treatment until the urine is confirmed sterile by monthly cultures for three consecutive months (4). Long-term, low-dose, culture-specific suppressive antibiotics may also be the best course of therapy for those patients who are not considered surgical candidates (4).

Urease Inhibitors

Ureolysis catalyzed by urease is essential for the production of struvite stones in humans. As such, inhibition of urease should abolish the conditions that promote struvite stone formation. Although there is ample clinical and experimental evidence demonstrating the effectiveness of urease-inhibiting drugs such as acetohydoxamic acid, widespread use of urease-inhibitors has not occurred in clinical practice due to the high incidence of side effects including hemolytic anemia, deep venous thrombosis, neurological symptoms (headache, malaise, and nervousness/tremulousness), gastrointestinal symptoms (anorexia, diarrhea, nausea, and vomiting), alopecia, muscle aches, rash, and leg pain or swelling (36). Even with strict compliance, urease inhibitors only reduce the size of the stone rather than completely eliminate the stone. In light of this information these agents should be viewed as palliative rather than therapeutic.

The molecular structure of the R-CONHOH group, which characterizes the hydroxamic acids, is similar to that of urea. This molecular similarity leads to specific inhibition of urease at low concentrations (37). Aromatic hydroxamic acids inhibit urease competitively, whereas fatty acyl hydroxamic acids inhibit noncompetitively (3). Among the four simplest aliphatic compounds, potency decreases and side effects increase as the carbon chain (R-) lengthens; consequently, acetohydoxamic acid, with its short carbon chain, has the greatest pharmacologic potential (38). Phosphotriamide derivatives have been reported to be most effective against urease derived from plants and bacteria (39–41).

Although many urease inhibitors have been evaluated, no single agent has been shown to inhibit urease within bacterial cells where the vast majority of urease is found and also to have a high renal clearance and a favorable long-term safety profile (3). Currently, the only two FDA-approved urease inhibitors are acetohydroxamic acid (AHA) and hydroxyurea (10). Hydroxyurea has been shown in vitro to be less effective than AHA as a urease ihhibitor. Although hydroxyurea is an irreversible urease inhibitor, a fraction of urease enzyme activity persists in the presence of hydroxyurea, unlike the case with AHA (42). In addition, hydroxyurea is broken down by urease thereby liberating ammonia, while AHA is inactive as a substrate (43).

AHA is the most commonly used and best-studied urease inhibitor. It has been shown to effectively lower urinary pH and ammonia levels and to cause stone dissolution (44,45). AHA has also been shown to retard stone growth in a placebo-controlled trial. In a randomized, double-blind study of 37 patients with actively growing stones (18 receiving AHA and 19 controls), none of the AHA patients and seven control patients demonstrated a doubling in size of the stone. However, nine patients receiving drug, compared with only one receiving placebo, required a decrease in dosage or cessation of treatment because of adverse medication effects *(46)*.

When administered orally, AHA is readily absorbed from the gastrointestinal tract and reaches peak serum levels after approximately 1 hour *(47)*. Although a portion of the orally administered drug is metabolized to carbon dioxide and acetamide, 20–48% is excreted intact in the urine *(48)*. The recommended dosing regimen for AHA is an initial dose of 250 mg twice daily by mouth for 3–4 wk, and if tolerated, an increase in the dosage to 250 mg three times daily *(36)*. AHA is contraindicated in patients with renal insufficiency (serum creatinine greater than 2 mg/dL) because therapeutic urinary concentrations are unlikely to be achieved and the risk of toxicity is increased *(7)*. Use of AHA is also contraindicated in pregnant women as AHA has been shown to be teratogenic in animals *(49)*. Use of AHA is relatively contraindicated in patients with poor function in the stone-bearing kidney because of potential increased excretion of AHA on the contralateral side and sub-therapeutic levels within the kidney requiring treatment *(50)*.

Use of AHA and urease inhibitors in general is limited because of toxicity. Major side effects including hemolytic anemia, deep venous thrombosis, gastrointestinal symptoms, headache, tremulousness, hallucinations, loss of taste, and teratogenesis have been reported *(4)*. Although these side effects are transient and resolve upon discontinuation of treatment, they occur in 20–30% of patients *(36)*. Consequently although AHA may serve a palliative role in a select patients, urease-inhibitors play a relatively limited overall role in clinical practice.

Urinary Acidification

Because the formation of struvite stones depends on an alkaline urinary environment, urinary acidification has the potential to increase urinary solubility of struvite and carbonate apatite, thereby preventing stone formation and potentially dissolving existing stones. A variety of acidification agents have been investigated for their dissolution or preventative potential. Ascorbic acid has been used in an attempt to decrease urinary pH, but this has not been successful clinically. In a two-phase, randomized, placebo-controlled, cross-over trial, 12 normal subjects and 12 calcium stone formers received 2 g of ascorbic acid or placebo daily for 6 d while maintained on a controlled metabolic diet. No difference in urinary pH was found between the placebo and ascorbic acid phases in either the normal subjects (6.02 vs 6.02, respectively) or stone formers (6.0 vs 6.0, respectively) *(51)*.

Ammonium chloride has been noted to successfully lower urine pH immediately after initiation, but after 6 d of treatment urinary ammonia excretion increases, counteracting the acidification effect *(52)*. Ammonium sulfate and ammonium nitrate used in combination were shown to be more effective than ammonium chloride for urinary acidification in 24 patients treated over 2 yr *(53)*. Combination-treated patients experienced a reduction in urinary saturation of calcium phosphate and stone formation. However, ammonium sulfate is poorly tolerated due to its cathartic effect, and ammonium nitrate is potentially explosive. As such, neither drug achieved widespread use in Europe or the United States *(4)*.

Lavage Chemolysis

The concept of dissolving a stone *in situ* was particularly attractive when open stone surgery offered the only treatment option for stone removal. With current minimally invasive and non-invasive treatment modalities, the morbidity of surgical stone removal has been greatly reduced and reliance on chemolysis has substantially decreased. Chemolysis is now primarily used in patients who are not considered surgical candidates or as an adjunct to surgical treatment to eliminate small residual fragments *(54)*.

In the 1930s initial attempts at lavage chemolysis for phosphate-containing calculi involved urinary antiseptics and acidifying agents, typically citric acid *(55,56)*. At acid pH, primary and secondary citrates of calcium are formed that are weakly dissociated, resulting in a reduction of free calcium ions in solution *(3)*. Although effective in vitro, dissolution therapy in vivo was successful in only one of four patients during early treatment attempts *(56)*. Moreover, citric acid was found to be irritating to bladder mucosa. The later addition of magnesium ions reduced mucosal irritation, and led to the formulation of what is currently known as Suby's solution G. Direct renal irrigation with solution G resulted in partial or complete dissolution of phosphate-containing stones in all six patients treated in the initial report by Suby and Albright *(57)*.

In vitro dissolution of struvite stones was later accomplished with hemiacidrin (Renacidin), a citric acid and magnesium solution similar to solution G *(58)*. Early clinical use of Suby's G solution and hemiacidrin were associated with frequent cases of hypermagnesemia, with four reported deaths caused by magnesium toxicity *(59,60)*, prompting the Food and Drug Administration to remove these solutions from clinical use at that time. However, other investigators attributed these deaths to urosepsis caused by infusion into the infected collecting system, rather than due to the direct effects of the irrigating solution itself, and they suggested that irrigating solutions should only be used in culture-verified sterile urine with close monitoring of intra-renal pressures *(61)*. With these precautions, they noted no complications and successfully treated stones with hemiacidrin irrigation in eight patients.

Recent use of citric acid (also known as Solution R) irrigation for the treatment of refractory infection stones has also been reported *(62)*. Among 23 patients treated, however, six required termination of irrigation because of complications. Overall, 7 patients were radiographically cleared of stone with irrigation alone and 13 patients were rendered stone free after irrigation in combination with surgical intervention such as PCNL and ureteroscopy. At a mean follow-up of 2.4 yr, however, only 4 of the 23 patients remained free of stones.

Current recommendations for the use of irrigating solutions include the following: (1) maintain sterile urine, (2) ensure unobstructed renal inflow and outflow, (3) maintain intrapelvic pressure below 30 cm H_2O, (4) confirm absence of extravasation, and (5) frequently monitor serum magnesium levels during treatment *(7)*.

Despite limited success with chemolysis for treatment of infection stones, the procedure is rarely used in clinical practice today because of the prolonged treatment times and lengthy hospital stays associated with this therapy. Indeed, Tiselius and colleagues treated 118 patients with infection staghorn calculi with shockwave lithotripsy (SWL) followed by chemolysis via a percutaneous nephrostomy tube with Renacidin or THAM solution (tri-hydroxylmethyl-aminomethan) and achieved a stone free rate of only 60%, with a mean of 3.4 SWL treatments per patient, an average hospital stay of 32 days and a 4.2% incidence of sepsis *(63)*. With effective minimally invasive surgical therapy that is associated with high stone free rates, low complication rates and short hospital stays, the role of chemolysis even for treatment of residual calculi has been relegated to historical interest only.

SURGICAL MANAGEMENT

Before 1980, open surgical stone removal, in conjunction with antibiotics and possibly irrigation with chemolytic agents, constituted the optimal therapy for infection stones. Conservative, nonoperative therapy was advocated by some *(64)*, but evidence suggested that this approach was best reserved for poor surgical candidates due to the high risk of renal failure, sepsis and death. In a retrospective review of patients with staghorn stones treated from 1927 to 1940, the survival rate among 234 patients with unilateral stones was 81% for those undergoing surgical treatment vs 41% for those managed conservatively *(65)*. Likewise, Blandy and Singh compared 60 patients managed conservatively with 125 treated surgically and found a 10-yr mortality rate in the conservative group of 28% vs 7.2% in the surgical group *(66)*. Rous and Turner also reported a 30% mortality rate due to stone-related complications in 95 consecutive patients hospitalized with staghorn stones and managed conservatively *(16)*. Thus, conservative management of staghorn calculi is discouraged in all but the highest risk surgical candidates.

Achieving a stone-free state presents a significant challenge even when open surgical treatment is employed. The AUA Nephrolithiasis Clinical Guidelines Panel reviewed 110 articles containing abstractable data regarding the management of staghorn calculi and found a median stone free rate of 81.6% (95% confidence interval 56.6–95.7%) for open surgical treatment *(67)*. Based on their findings, they deemed that open surgery should not constitute first line therapy for treatment of these stones because of a higher morbidity compared with less invasive treatment approaches. However, open surgery is an appropriate treatment alternative in unusual circumstances where a struvite staghorn calculus is not expected to be expeditiously treated within a reasonable number of percutaneous and/or SWL procedures.

Percutaneous Nephrolithotomy (PCNL)

The introduction of percutaneous endoscopic techniques for stone removal provided a less invasive alternative to the often morbid open stone procedures such as anatrophic nephrolithotomy for treatment of staghorn calculi. Snyder and Smith compared 75 patients treated with percutaneous nephrolithotomy (PCNL) with 25 patients undergoing anatrophic nephrolithotomy for staghorn calculi and found a superior stone free rate in the open group (100% vs 86.7%, respectively), but at the expense of higher morbidity and longer convalescence compared with the PCNL group *(68)*. On the other hand, Patterson and associates reported a 91% stone free rate after PCNL in 74 patients with struvite stones, with 89% of stone free patients remaining free of stones after 3 yr *(69)*. The AUA Nephrolithiasis Clinical Guidelines Panel found a median stone-free rate of 73.3% (95% confidence interval 54.7–87.4%) for PCNL management of staghorn calculi in their meta-analysis, although outcomes were not stratified by infection stones versus metabolic stones *(67)*.

Shockwave Lithotripsy (SWL)

With the advent of SWL investigators turned to this new technology in an effort to reduce the morbidity associated with open surgical treatment of staghorn calculi. Unfortunately, these larger, branched stones were not as readily amenable to SWL treatment as smaller, less complex stones, and success rates were inferior to those seen with the treatment of smaller stones. Published stone-free rates for SWL monotherapy are inconsistent and often unacceptably low, varying from 23–86% *(21)*. Moreover, complication rates and need for secondary procedures are approx 31% and 42%, respectively *(67)*. Beck and Riehle reported a 47% stone free rate after SWL monotherapy in 33 patients (38 kidneys) at a mean follow-up of 27 mo *(70)*. Likewise, Michaels and Fowler achieved a stone free state in 45% of patients and an infection-free rate of 86% in 22 patients treated with SWL monotherapy followed by 2 wk of oral antibiotics *(71)*. The AUA Nephrolithiasis Clinical Guidelines Panel reported a median stone-free rate of 50% (95% confidence interval 25.6–74.4%) for SWL monotherapy of staghorn calculi *(67)*. Ultimately, they recommended that SWL monotherapy should not constitute first-line therapy for staghorn calculi.

Combination Therapy

In an effort to combine the effectiveness of PCNL with the lower morbidity of SWL, combination therapy consisting of initial PCNL debulking followed by SWL treatment of residual stones usually followed by percutaneous retrieval of fragments was introduced. In a series of 90 patients treated with combination therapy, Schulze and colleagues observed a stone-free rate of 76.7% *(72)*. However, after approx 2 yr of follow-up, only 55% of patients remained stone free, which the authors attributed to inadequate medical follow-up. Streem and co-workers evaluated 100 patients with large, extensively branched calculi treated over a 10-yr period and reported a stone free rate of only 63% at 1-mo follow-up. However, among the last 25 patients in the series, a 70% stone free rate was achieved *(73)*. The AUA Nephrolithiasis Clinical Guidelines Panel reported a median stone-free rate of 80.9% (95% confidence interval 67.8–90.5%) for combination therapy, and consequently recommended PCNL, with or without SWL, as first line therapy for struvite staghorn calculi *(67)*. A subsequent prospective, randomized trial comparing SWL monotherapy with combination therapy reinforced this recommendation, demonstrating a significantly greater stone-free rate in the combination therapy group *(74)*. Despite these recommendations, however, there has been a decreasing reliance on adjuvant SWL for treatment of residual fragments after PCNL and an increase in the use of second look flexible nephroscopy to retrieve these small fragments *(75)*.

Ureteroscopy

With recent advances in ureteroscopic instrumentation and ureteroscope design along with the introduction of the Holmium:YAG laser, ureteroscopic treatment of large, complex stones in the kidney has been made possible. In one early study of 34 patients with partial or complete staghorn calculi, a 50% stone free rate was achieved using 10.3–13.3 Fr flexible ureteroscopes *(76)*. A more recent study of 45 patients with large (>2 cm) renal calculi including staghorn stones treated with smaller caliber 7.5–10 Fr ureteroscopes and the Holmium:YAG laser revealed a 76% success rate (stone free or ≤2-mm fragments) with a single procedure and a 91% success rate after second look ureteroscopy in 33% of patients *(77)*. Likewise, El-Anany treated 30 patients with >2-cm renal calculi with ureteroscopy and laser lithotripsy and achieved a success rate (stone free or <2-mm residual fragments) of 77% with a 10% incidence of minor complications *(78)*. These studies demonstrate the feasibility of the ureteroscopic approach to complex stones, although stone-free rates are decidedly lower than those achieved with PCNL. Thus ureteroscopy may be appropriate only in select patients with a modest stone burden who are not suitable candidates for other treatment modalities.

PROGNOSIS

Patients with infection stones remain at high risk for stone recurrence and re-infection even after appropriate surgical treatment because of persistence of the underlying conditions that initially predisposed the patient to infection. Furthermore, the presence of residual fragments after therapy increases the likelihood of continued stone growth and repeated infection. A meta-analysis of the literature from 1924 to 1974 evaluating open surgical treatment of infection stones revealed a 27% incidence of recurrent stones and a 41% incidence of persistent infection within 6.3 yr of treatment, although many of the studies analyzed were completed before the era of widespread antibiotic use (1).

Several investigators have evaluated current long-term stone free and infection-free rates after SWL therapy for infection stones. In a series of 33 patients (38 renal units) treated with SWL monotherapy for staghorn calculi, Beck and Riehle reported an initial stone free rate of 47%. At a mean follow-up of 27 mo, however, 78% of 9 kidneys with large residual fragments and 20% of 20 kidneys initially rendered stone free demonstrated stone re-growth (70). Furthermore, among 16 stone free patients, only one patient experienced a recurrent infection compared with 47% experiencing recurrent infections among the 17 patients with stable or progressive residual fragments. This study emphasizes the importance of a stone free state after surgery to reduce the occurrence of new stone growth and repeated infection.

Interestingly, Michaels and Fowler suggested that prolonged treatment with antibiotics after SWL therapy for struvite stones in patients with preoperative *Proteus mirablis* infection could result in sterilization of the urine despite the presence of residual stone fragments. Indeed 86% of the 22 patients treated remained free of infection despite a stone free rate of only 53%. Among the three patients with recurrent infection, all experienced new or progressive stone growth (71). Likewise, Pode and co-workers found that small infection stones could be treated with SWL with a reasonable likelihood of remaining stone free and infection-free (79). Among 94 patients with stones and recurrent infections treated with SWL, 67% of 59 patients with stones <2 cm in size remained stone free and 76% remained infection free at a mean of 6.4 mo post-SWL. In contrast, only 26% and 35% of patients with stones >2 cm remained free of stones and infections, respectively. Among the 12 patients with staghorn calculi, 42% each remained free of stones and infection.

Despite superior stone free rates with PCNL compared with SWL, Streem and colleagues noted a substantial risk of recurrent stones and infection in 44 patients with infection stones treated with PCNL with or without adjuvant SWL followed for a mean of 42 mo post-treatment (80). With an overall stone free rate of 73%, the authors reported a 28% incidence of recurrent stones: 25% in patients initially rendered stone free and 33% in patients with residual fragments. By Kaplan Meier estimation, the 5-yr recurrence rate after aggressive endourological treatment for infection stones was 36.8%. Furthermore, at a mean follow-up of 42 mo, 41% of patients experienced recurrent urinary tract infections. Interestingly, statistical analysis did not show infection to be an independent risk factor for stone recurrence.

Overall, although prolonged antimicrobial use post-treatment may sterilize the small residual fragments associated with SWL, the best chance of remaining stone free and infection free after surgical stone treatment appears to be associated with complete stone clearance at the time of surgery.

CONCLUSIONS

Urinary infection with urease-producing organisms provides unique urinary conditions of alkaline pH and high ammonia levels that promote the crystallization of struvite and the formation of infection stones. Although most commonly associated with *P. mirabilis*, urease can be synthesized by a variety of microorganisms. Although they account for a small fraction of the overall stone population, infection stones, with their high risk of recurrence, are a significant source of morbidity and expense in susceptible patients. These stones may be suspected based on symptoms of renal colic or infection, and the diagnosis is readily apparent with current imaging techniques. Treatment of infection stones remains a challenge; current medical therapies are rarely effective and are often accompanied by significant side effects. Surgical approaches are highly effective for stone removal, and procedure-related morbidity has dropped substantially in recent years. Consequently, the role of chemolysis is limited at best and surgery constitutes first line therapy. However, despite effective initial therapy, recurrent stones and infections are common. The best outcomes are achieved in patients rendered stone free, and prolonged antimicrobial therapy after surgical intervention may improve the outlook for recurrent infection.

REFERENCES

1. Griffith DP. Struvite stones. 1978; Kidney Int 13: 372.
2. Griffith DP, Osborne CA. Infection (urease) stones. Miner Electrolyte Metab 1987; 13: 278.
3. Gleeson MJ, Kobashi K, Griffith DP. Noncalcium nephrolithiasis. Disorders of Bone and Mineral Metabolism, (Coe FI, Favus MJ, eds.). Raven, New York, NY, 1992; p. 801.
4. Wong HY, Riedl CR, Griffith DP. Medical Management and Prevention of Struvite Stones. Kidney Stones: Medical and Surgical Management. Lippincott-Raven, Philadelphia, PA, 1996.
5. Elliot JS, Sharp RF, Lewis L. J Urol 1959; 81: 366–368.
6. Griffith DP, Musher DM, Itin, C. Urease. The primary cause of infection-induced urinary stones. Invest Urol 1976; 13: 346.
7. Wang LP, Wong HY, Griffith DP. Treatment options in struvite stones. Urol Clin North Am 1997; 24: 149.
8. Silverman DE, Stamey TA. Management of infection stones: the Stanford experience. Medicine (Baltimore) 1983; 62: 44.
9. Peacock M, Robertson WC. The Biochemical Aetiology of Renal Lithiasis. Urinary Calculous Disease, (Wickham JEA, ed.). Churchill Livingstone, Edinburgh, 1979; p. 69.
10. Rodman J S. Struvite stones. Nephron 81 Suppl 1999; 1: 50.
11. Sarmina I, Spirnak JP, Resnick MI. Urinary lithiasis in the black population: an epidemiological study and review of the literature. J Urol 1987; 138: 14.
12. Resnick MI. Evaluation and management of infection stones. Urol Clin North Am 1981; 8: 265.
13. Kohri K, Ishikawa Y, Katoh Y, et al. Epidemiology of urolithiasis in the elderly. Int Urol Nephrol 1991; 23: 413.
14. DeVivo MJ, Fine PR, Cutter GR, Maetz HM. The risk of renal calculi in spinal cord injury patients. J Urol 1984; 131: 857.
15. Gettman MT, Segura J W. Struvite stones: diagnosis and current treatment concepts. J Endourol 1999; 13: 653.
16. Rous, S. N. and Turner, W. R.: Retrospective study of 95 patients with staghorn calculus disease. J Urol, 1977; 118: 902.
17. Vargas AD, Bragin SD, Mendez R. Staghorn calculis: its clinical presentation, complications and management. J Urol 1982; 127: 860.

18. Wasserstein AG. Nephrolithiasis: acute management and prevention. Dis Mon 1998; 44: 196.
19. Grenabo L, Claes G, Hedelin H, Pettersson S. Rapidly recurrent renal calculi caused by Ureaplasma urealyticum: a case report. J Urol 1986; 135: 995.
20. Rose GA, Rosenbaum TP. Recurrent infection stones with apparently negative cultures. The case for blind antibacterial treatment. Br J Urol 1992; 69: 234.
21. Segura JW. Staghorn calculi. Urol Clin North Am 1997; 24: 71.
22. Liberman SN, Halpern EJ, Sullivan K, Bagley DH. Spiral computed tomography for staghorn calculi. Urology 1997; 50: 519.
23. Mostafavi MR, Ernst RD, Saltzman B. Accurate determination of chemical composition of urinary calculi by spiral computerized tomography. J Urol 1998; 159: 673.
24. Shorr E. The possible usefulness of estrogens and aluminum hydroxide gels in the management of renal stone. J Urol 1945; 53: 507.
25. Shorr E, Carter AC. Aluminum gels in the management of renal phosphatic calculi. JAMA 1950; 144: 1549.
26. Lavengood RW Jr, Marshall VF. The prevention of renal phosphatic calculi in the presence of infection by the Shorr regimen. J Urol 1972; 108: 368.
27. McCarrison R. Causation of stone in India. BMJ 1931; 1: 1009.
28. Higgins CC. Urinary lithiasis: experimental production and solution with clinical application and end results. J Urol ; 36: 168.
29. Griffith DP, Bragin S, Musher DM. Dissolution of struvite urinary stones. Experimental studies in vitro. Invest Urol 1976; 13: 351.
30. Griffith DP, Moskowitz PA, Carlton CE Jr. Adjunctive chemotherapy of infection-induced staghorn calculi. J Urol 1979; 121: 711.
31. Feit RM, Fair WR. The treatment of infection stones with penicillin. J Urol 1979; 122: 592.
32. Fowler JE Jr. Bacteriology of branched renal calculi and accompanying urinary tract infection. J Urol 1984; 131: 213.
33. Cohen TD, Preminger GM. Struvite calculi. Semin Nephrol 1996; 16: 425.
34. Rao PN, Dube DA, Weightman NC, Oppenheim BA, Morris J. Prediction of septicemia following endourological manipulation for stones in the upper urinary tract. J Urol 1991; 146: 955.
35. McAleer IM, Kaplan GW, Bradley JS, Carroll SF. Staghorn calculus endotoxin expression in sepsis. Urology 2002; 59: 601.
36. Griffith DP, Gleeson MJ, Lee H, Longuet R, Deman E, Earle N. Randomized, double-blind trial of Lithostat (acetohydroxamic acid) in the palliative treatment of infection-induced urinary calculi. Eur Urol 1991; 20: 243.
37. Kobashi K, Hase J, Uehara K. Specific inhibition of urease by hydroxamic acid. Biochem Biophys Acta 1962; 65: 380.
38. Fishbein WN, Daly JE. Urease inhibitors for hepatic coma. II. Comparative efficacy of four lower hydroxamate homologs in vitro and in vivo. Proc Soc Exp Biol Med 1970; 134: 1083.
39. Hase J, Kobashi K, Kawaguchi N, Sakamoto K. Antimicrobial activity of hydroxamic acids. Chem Pharm Bull (Tokyo) 1971; 19: 363.
40. Dixon NE, Gazzola C, Watters JJ, Blakely RL, Zerner B. Inhibition of Jack Bean urease (EC 3.5.1.5) by acetohydroxamic acid and by phosphoramidate. An equivalent weight for urease. J Am Chem Soc 1975; 97: 4130.
41. Kobashi K, Takebe S, Numata A. Specific inhibition of urease by N-acylphosphoric triamides. J Biochem (Tokyo) 1985; 98: 1681.
42. Fishbein WM, Carbone PP. Urease Catalysis: II. Inhibition of the enzyme by hydroxyurea, hydroxylamine, and acetohydroxamic acid. J Biol Chem 1965; 240: 2407.
43. Fishbein WN, Winter TS, Davidson JD. Urease Catalysis: I. Stoichiometery, Specificity, and Kinetics of a second substrate: Hydroxyurea. J Biol Chem 1965; 240: 202.
44. Griffith DP, Moskowitz PA, Carlton CE Jr. Adjunctive chemotherapy of infection-induced staghorn calculi. J Urol 1979; 121: 711.
45. Martelli A, Buli P, Cortecchia V. Urease inhibitor therapy in infected renal stones. Eur Urol 1981; 7: 291.
46. Williams JJ, Rodman JS, Peterson CM. A randomized double-blind study of acetohydroxamic acid in struvite nephrolithiasis. N Engl J Med 1984; 311: 760.

47. Putcha L, Griffith DP, Feldman S. Disposition of 14C-acetohydroxamic acid and 14C-acetamide in the rat. Drug Metab Dispos 1984; 12: 438.

48. Putcha L, Griffith DP, Feldman S. Pharmacokinetics of acetohydroxamic acid in patients with staghorn renal calculi. Eur J Clin Pharmacol 1985; 28: 439.

49. Bailie NC, Osborne CA, Leininger JR, et al. Teratogenic effect of acetohydroxamic acid in clinically normal beagles. Am J Vet Res 1986; 47: 2604.

50. Rosenstein I. Therapeutic applications of urease inhibitors. J Antimicrob Chemother 1982; 10: 159.

51. Traxer O, Adams-Huet B, Pak CYC, Pearle MS. Risk of calcium oxalate stone formation with ascorbic acid ingestion (abstract). J Urol 2001; 165: 243.

52. Rector FC, Seldin DW, Copenhaver JH. The mechanism of ammonia excretion during ammonium chloride acidosis. J Clin Invest 1955; 34: 20.

53. Pizzarelli F, Peacock M. Effect of chronic administration of ammonium sulfate on phosphatic stone recurrence. Nephron 1987; 46: 247.

54. Rodman JS, Vaughn JED. Chemolysis of urinary calculi. AUA Update Series 1992; 11: 1.

55. Hellstrom J. The significance of staphylococci in the development and treatment of renal and ureteric stones. Br J Urol 1938; 10: 348.

56. Albright F, Sulkowitch HWCR. Nonsurgical aspects of the kidney stone problem. JAMA 1939; 113: 2049.

57. Suby HI, Albright F. Dissolution of phosphatic urinary calculi by the retrograde introduction of citrate solution containing magnesium. N Engl J Med 1943; 228: 81.

58. Mulvaney WP. A new solvent for certain urinary calculi: a preliminary report. J Urol 1959; 82: 546.

59. Kohler FP. Renacidin and tissue reaction. J Urol 1962; 87: 102.

60. Fostvedt GA, Barnes RW. Complications during lavage therapy for renal calculi. J Urol 1963; 80: 329.

61. Nemoy NJ, Staney TA. Surgical, bacteriological, and biochemical management of "infection stones". JAMA 1971; 215: 1470.

62. Joshi HB, Kumar PV, Timoney AG. Citric acid (solution R) irrigation in the treatment of refractory infection (struvite) stone disease: is it useful? Eur Urol 2001, 39: 586.

63. Tiselius HG, Hellgren E, Andersson A, Borrud-Ohlsson A, Eriksson I. Minimally invasive treatment of infection staghorn stones with shock wave lithotripsy and chemolysis. Scand J Urol Nephrol 1999; 33: 286.

64. Libertino JA, Newman HR, Lytton B, Weiss RM. Staghorn calculi in solitary kidneys. J Urol 1971; 105: 753.

65. Priestly JT, Dunn JH. Branched renal calculi. J Urol 1949; 61: 194.

66. Blandy JP, Singh M. The case for a more aggressive approach to staghorn stones. J Urol 1976; 115: 505.

67. Segura JW, Preminger GM, Assimos DG, et al. Nephrolithiasis Clinical Guidelines Panel summary report on the management of staghorn calculi. The American Urological Association Nephrolithiasis Clinical Guidelines Panel. J Urol 1994; 151: 1648.

68. Snyder JA, Smith AD. Staghorn calculi: percutaneous extraction versus anatrophic nephrolithotomy. J Urol 1986; 136: 351.

69. Patterson DE, Segura JW, LeRoy AJ. Long-term follow-up of patients treated by percutaneous ultrasonic lithotripsy for struvite staghorn calculi. J Endourol 1987; 1: 177.

70. Beck EM, Riehle RA Jr. The fate of residual fragments after extracorporeal shock wave lithotripsy monotherapy of infection stones. J Urol 1991; 145: 6; discussion 9–10.

71. Michaels EK, Fowler JE Jr. Extracorporeal shock wave lithotripsy for struvite renal calculi: prospective study with extended followup. J Urol 1991; 146: 728.

72. Schulze H, Hertle L, Kutta A, Graff J, Senge, T. Critical evaluation of treatment of staghorn calculi by percutaneous nephrolithotomy and extracorporeal shock wave lithotripsy. J Urol 1989; 141: 822.

73. Streem SB, Yost A, Dolmatch B. Combination "sandwich" therapy for extensive renal calculi in 100 consecutive patients: immediate, long-term and stratified results from a 10-year experience. J Urol 1997; 158: 342.

74. Meretyk S, Gofrit ON, Gafni O, et al. Complete staghorn calculi: random prospective comparison between extracorporeal shock wave lithotripsy monotherapy and combined with percutaneous nephrostolithotomy. J Urol 1997; 157: 780.

75. Lam HS, Lingeman JE, Mosbaugh PG, et al. Evolution of the technique of combination therapy for staghorn calculi: a decreasing role for extracorporeal shock wave lithotripsy. J Urol 1992; 148: 1058.

76. Aso Y, Ohta N, Nakano M, Ohtawara Y, Tajima A, Kawabe K. Treatment of staghorn calculi by fiberoptic transurethral nephrolithotripsy. J Urol 1990; 144: 17.

77. Grasso M, Conlin M, Bagley D. Retrograde ureteropyeloscopic treatment of 2 cm. or greater upper urinary tract and minor Staghorn calculi. J Urol 1998; 160: 346.

78. El-Anany FG, Hammouda HM, Maghraby HA, Elakkad MA. Retrograde ureteropyeloscopic holmium laser lithotripsy for large renal calculi. BJU Int 2001; 88: 850.

79. Pode D, Lenkovsky Z, Shapiro A, Pfau A. Can extracorporeal shock wave lithotripsy eradicate persistent urinary infection associated with infected stones? J Urol 1988; 140: 257.

80. Streem SB. Long-term incidence and risk factors for recurrent stones following percutaneous nephrostolithotomy or percutaneous nephrostolithotomy/extracorporeal shock wave lithotripsy for infection related calculi. J Urol 1995; 153: 584.

18 Cystine Stone Disease

Bijan Shekarriz, MD

CONTENTS

Key Words: Cystinuria; urolithiasis; calculus; urinary; stone; genetic.

INTRODUCTION

Cystinuria is an autosomal recessive disease characterized by defects in renal and intestinal transport of dibasic amino acids including cystine, ornithine, lysine, and arginine *(1)*. The relative insolubility of cystine results in supersaturation of urine with cystine and recurrent stone formation, which is the hallmark of the disease.

Recent advances in molecular biology have greatly improved our understanding of the pathophysiology of this disease. However, current medical management is often disappointing and many patients continue to suffer from recurrent stone formation despite adequate medical management. Fortunately, with the introduction of minimally invasive techniques, the role of open surgery for management of cystine stones has significantly decreased.

The correct diagnosis and an understanding of the pathophysiology and clinical features of cystinuria are important for therapeutic decision making. In the following, we

From: Current Clinical Urology, *Urinary Stone Disease:*
A Practical Guide to Medical and Surgical Management
Edited by: M. L. Stoller and M. V. Meng © Humana Press Inc., Totowa, NJ

first review the epidemiology and pathophysiology of cystinuria followed by a discussion on genetic aspects of the disease. Unique clinical aspects of this disorder and management issues are presented.

HISTORY

It is interesting that the first cystine calculus was discovered in the bladder by Wollaston in 1810 *(2)*. He called it "cystic oxide" referring to the origin of the stone from the bladder (kystis in Greek) *(3)*. Berzellius *(4)* recognized that the compound was not an oxide, but he also thought that the material originated from the bladder and he named it cystine. The definitive chemical structure was described by Friedman *(5)* in 1902. Garrod *(6)* referred to cystinuria as an inborn error of metabolism of sulfur-containing amino acids in his lecture in 1908. This erroneous belief continued until the middle of the 20th century. Subsequent studies by Dent and Rose *(7)* demonstrated that excretion of dibasic amino acids is abnormally high in cystinuria while the serum levels of these amino acids are normal. Harris and colleagues *(8)* described the genetic basis of cystinuria, including its autosomal recessive inheritance. Crawhall et al. *(9)* described the use of penicillamine as drug therapy for cystinuria in 1963.

Our understanding of the pathogenesis of this disease has improved by the recent molecular developments triggered by discovery of a transporter molecule named rBAT and the localization of the gene to chromosome 2p *(10,11)*. Mutation in the rBAT gene was found to be responsible for type I cystinuria and was first reported in 1994, initiating discovery of multiple additional mutations for both type I and non-type I cystinuria *(10)*.

EPIDEMIOLOGY

Cystinuria has a wide range of incidence worldwide. Newborn screening programs have estimated the disease frequency at 1:2000 in England, 1:4000 in Australia, 1:1900 in Spain, and 1:15000 in the United States. However, this frequency may be an overestimation due to the inclusion of non-type I heterozygotes *(11)*. A much higher frequency of the disease has been noted in Libyan Jews living in Israel, with an estimated frequency of 1:2500. In a school screening student program, 4% of Libyan Jewish students had heterozygote levels of urinary cystine *(12)*. Caucasians are affected more frequently; men and women are affected equally *(13)*.

Cystine stones account for 2% of urinary calculi in adult patients and 6–8% in children *(14)*. The peak age of onset of urinary stone disease is during the third decade of life. The only known clinical presentation of cystinuria is urolithiasis.

RENAL AND INTESTINAL TRANSPORT
OF CYSTINE AND DIBASIC AMINO ACIDS

Under normal circumstances, amino acids are freely filtered at the glomerulus and reabsorbed almost completely at the proximal convoluted tubule. Some amino acids such as L-histidine and L-glycine have a higher fractional excretion at 6% and 3.5%, respectively. Fractional excretion of most amino acids is less than 1%, resulting in a low urinary concentration of amino acids *(15)*. The fractional excretion of cystine is 0.4%. Microperfusion studies have demonstrated that the proximal convoluted tubule is the primary site for amino acid reabsorption *(17)*.

The reabsorption of amino acids, including cystine in the proximal tubule, involves active and passive processes. Amino acids are reabsorbed from the tubular lumen into the proximal cell via the brush border membrane and exit the cell via the basolateral membrane (16). Several protein transporters mediate amino acid movement to transport across the mammalian cell membrane. These transporters recognize and bind amino acids and shuttle them between the intracellular and extracellular compartments.

For most organic solutes filtered through the glomerulus, including cystine, two renal transport systems have been described (17). It is thought that 80–90% of the filtered load is reabsorbed by a high-capacity, low-affinity system, while the remaining 10–20% is extracted by a high-affinity lower capacity system. The high affinity system is shared between dibasic amino acids (18). Functional studies have demonstrated that the low-affinity transport is located in the proximal convoluted tubules (S1 and S2 segments) whereas the high-affinity transport system is located in the proximal straight tubule (S3 segment) (19). The high affinity transporter has a low maximum rate of transport and is competitively inhibited by other dibasic amino acids. The low affinity transporter has a high maximum capacity and is only inhibited by arginine. Furthermore, only the high affinity transporter is sodium independent. These two transport systems participate equally in the reabsorption of cystine under normal filtered cystine loads. Classic cystinuria (type I) results from a defect in the high affinity transport of cystine through epithelial cells of the intestinal tract and renal tubules, which is also shared by cationic amino acids (20).

In the small intestine, amino acids and oligopeptides are end products of protein ingestion after digestion by pancreatic enzymes. There are two specific transport mechanisms responsible for the transepithelial transport of amino acids. Amino acids are carried by the specific transport mechanism located at the intestinal brush border of intestinal epithelial cells. Another transport system then translocates the amino acids across the basolateral membrane into the blood. In vitro studies of mucosal biopsies from cystinuric patients have demonstrated that only a single intestinal transport system for cystine exists (21).

MOLECULAR AND GENETIC BASIS OF CYSTINURIA

Cystinuria is characterized by defects in the renal and intestinal transport of dibasic amino acids (cystine, ornithine, lysine, and arginine). In the proximal tubule, the high-affinity transporter transports all the dibasic amino acids. Therefore, this system has been postulated to be involved in classic cystinuria.

Traditionally, cystinuria has been classified into three types based on the observation of the intestinal mucosal biopsies in homozygotes and urinary cystine excretion in heterozygotes (22). All homozygotes demonstrate high levels of aminoaciduria. Type I heterozygotes show normal aminoaciduria whereas types II and III heterozygotes show high and moderate levels of cystine and other dibasic amino acid excretion, respectively. The oral cystine load test results in an increase in plasma cystine concentration in type III, but no change in types I and II. The intestinal active transport of cystine, arginine, lysine or ornithine is absent in homozygotes type I and II, while it is normal in type III [Table 1]. The proposed defect in renal and intestinal transport of cystine and other dibasic amino acids was initially believed to be related to a single gene encoding for both transport systems (23). Different phenotypic expressions in the intestinal transport of cystine and dibasic amino acids in cystinurics were therefore explained by allelic

Table 1
Classification of Cystinuria: Phenotypic–Genotypic Correlations

Harris et al. [8]	Completely recessive	Incompletely recessive	
Rosenberg et al. [24]	Type I	Type II	Type III
Molecular	Type I	Non-Type I	
• Urinary cystine (heterozygotes)	Normal	Highly elevated (10-fold)	Elevated (2-fold)
• Plasma cystine (oral load test)	No change	No change	Increase
• Intestinal transport (homozygotes)	Absent	Reduced	Reduced
• Protein	rBAT	$b^{0,+}$AT (BAT1)	
• Amino acid transport system	$b^{0,+}$	$b^{0,+}$	
	Heteromeric rBAT/$b^{0,+}$	$b^{0,+}$ Heteromeric rBAT/$b^{0,+}$ AT	
• Localization in proximal tubule	S3 > S1-S2 Pars recta	S1-S2 > S3 Pars convoluta	
Transporter characteristic	High affinity, low capacity [a]	Low affinity, high capacity [b]	
• Gene involved	SLC3A1	SLC7A9	
• Chromosome	2p16.3-21	19q13.1	
• No. of mutations	>60	35	
• Clinical symptoms			
○ Homozygotes	Symptomatic	Most symptomatic (90%)	
○ Heterozygotes	Asymptomatic	Few symptomatic (13%)	

[a] High affinity, low capacity transporter accounts for 10% of total cystine reabsorption.
[b] Low affinity, high capacity transporter accounts for 90% of total cystine reabsorption.
Data from References *13, 26, 27.*

mutations of the same gene *(24).* However, early studies demonstrated that type I cystinuria is inherited in an autosomal recessive manner whereas types II and III are inherited in an incompletely recessive manner, indicating different genes involved for type I and the other two types *(23).*

The traditional classification does not differentiate between the sub-types based on the clinical symptoms and presentation. Type I heterozygous patients have normal urinary excretion of cystine and remain asymptomatic. In contrast, some type II and III heterozygotes present with symptoms indistinguishable from the homozygotes with significant overlap in urinary cystine excretion *(13).* Most homozygotes are symptomatic, but some may never develop stones (Table 1).

This classification correlates poorly with current molecular data and has been modified as type I and non-type I (divided clinically as type II and III) cystinuria *(25).* Type I and nontype I cystinuria differ clinically on the basis of the urinary cystine and dibasic amino acid concentrations in heterozygotes. While the type I heterozygotes are clinically silent with normal urinary cystine levels, the non-type I heterozygotes may present with a wide range of elevated urinary cystine levels. Abnormal urinary cystine excretion is not always associated with clinical stone disease. The term "acalculus cystinuria" describe a group of patients with abnormal urinary cystine and no evidence of urolithiasis *(26).*

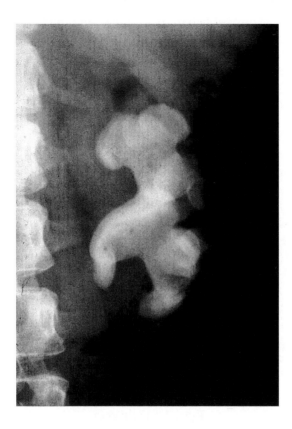

Fig. 1. Plain radiographs demonstrating large cystine stone with complete staghorn configuration.

During the last two decades, several mammalian cell membrane transport systems have been identified. The identification and cloning of a type II membrane glycoprotein, rBAT, was a breakthrough in our understanding of molecular basis of cystinuria. rBAT was associated with a $b^{0,+}$ -like activity of membrane transport *(22,29)*. The membrane transport system $b^{0,+}$ was first described in mouse blastocytes and is a high affinity, sodium independent transport system for cationic and zwitterionic (neutral) amino acids *(30)*. It was demonstrated that rBAT induces a sodium independent $b^{0,+}$-like membrane transporter activity in *Xenopus* oocytes with transport of cystine and other dibasic aminoacids *(10)*. When rBAT was first identified, analysis of its amino acid structure suggested a type II membrane glycoprotein with a cytoplasmic N-terminus and extracellular carboxyl (C) terminus; two to four membrane-spanning domains and a bulky cytoplasmic tail were described *(31)*. However, further studies revealed that it has only a single transmembrane domain *(26,29)*. The structure of rBAT does not make it a suitable candidate for a transport molecule, with the expected multimembrane-spanning transport protein, which would result in a suitable polar environment for amino acid passage through the plasma membrane. Furthermore, rBAT did not transport amino acids when induced in COS-7 cells. Thus, it was apparent that rBAT served as a transport activator or co-transporter and there were other molecules involved in the transport system for cystine.

The discovery of a family of heteromeric amino acid transporters from the plasma membrane of mammaliam cells has given us insight into the molecular events involved in cystinuria *(27)*. Heteromeric amino acid transporters are comprised of two subunits, a heavy subunit (rBAT and 4F2hc) and a corresponding light subunit (LAT-1, LAT-2, asc-1, y$^+$LAT-1,y$^+$LAT-2, xCT, and b$^{0,+}$AT) linked by a disulfide bridge *(27)*. Sequence analysis of the rBAT gene shows it to be 30% homologous to 4F2hc. Co-expression of these heavy and light subunits results in various amino acid transport systems. For instance, co-expression of 4F2hc and y$^+$LAT-1 induces system y$^+$L amino acid transport, which is responsible for the sodium-independent efflux of dibasic amino acids from cells, whereas co-expression of rBAT and b$^{0,+}$ amino acid transport, which is responsible for the renal reabsorption of cystine and dibasic amino acids at the brush border of epithelial cells *(29)*. In the kidney and intestine, it is postulated that rBAT forms heterodimers through disulfide linkages to the (b$^{0,+}$AT) to a light subunit of a 40–50 kDa protein allowing the proper configuration to act as a transporter *(32)*.

Lysine intolerance and cystinuria are examples of recessive disorders associated with mutations of these heteromeric transport systems. As mentioned, 4F2hc/y$^+$LAT-1 complex accounts for the y$^+$L system (catonic amino acid transport system at the basolateral surface of intestinal and renal proximal tubular cells). Mutations of y$^+$LAT-1 gene (SLC7A7) on chromosome 14q11-13 cause the recessive disease *(27)*. Similarly, mutations in rBAT(SLC3A1) or b$^{0,+}$AT (SLC7A9) genes will result in alteration of the b$^{0,+}$ amino acid transport (responsible for the renal reabsorption of cystine and dibasic amino acids at the brush border membrane) causing genetically distinct types of cystinuria.

Type I Cystinuria

The b$^{0,+}$ system type activity associated with rBAT expression in the brush border of the renal and intestinal epithelial cells made this molecule a candidate for the cystinuria gene. In 1992, the first gene involved in cystine and dibasic amino acid transport was cloned in the rabbit, rat and later in humans *(10,33–35)*. Using an expressional cloning approach, a 2.3 kilobase complementary DNA segment was isolated. When expressed in Xenopus oocytes, this DNA segment induced sodium independent transport of cystine and other dibasic amino acids. The clones isolated from rat kidneys were referred to as NAA-Tr and D2, while that isolated from rabbit kidney cortex were referred to as rBAT. Subsequently, the human cDNA, also 2.3 kilobases, was isolated and sequenced using the same technique. The human cDNA, referred to as D2H and rBAT, also induced dibasic amino acid transport when expressed in Xenopus oocytes *(10,34)*. The genome data base nomenclature committee designated this gene solute carrier family 3, member 1, which is abbreviated as SLC3A1 *(36)*. The human rBAT homologue is a 45-kb, ten exon human gene, transcribed into a 2.3 kilobases mRNA, encoding a 685 amino acid glycoprotein with one putative membrane-spanning domain. The SLC3A1 (rBAT) gene was mapped to the short arm of human chromosome 2 (2p21) *(11)*. Calonge et al. *(12)* reported the first rBAT mutation and concluded that it was associated with type I cystinuria. At present, over 60 distinct mutations including nonsense, missense, splice site, frameshift, and large deletions have been reported in the rBAT gene of patients with type I cystinuria *(27)*. It has been demonstrated that these mutations inhibit the transport of cystine and dibasic amino acids in Xenopus oocytes. All known rBAT mutations, whether missense or large gene deletions, are thought to cause loss of transport function in some fashion and are fully recessive. Thus, family members who are heterozygous for rBAT mutation excrete cystine in the normal range (<100 mg/24 h), while affected patients may excrete 350 mg/24 h.

The rBAT gene product is similar to the 4F2 heavy chain (4F2hc) that is involved in other amino acid transport. It is believed that rBAT and 4F2hc are not transporters, but rather they represent specific guidance and activator molecules for selected amino acid transporters.

The majority of amino acid reabsorption (80–90%) occurs in the pars convoluta (S1, S2). However, rBAT is mainly expressed in the parts recta (S3) of the proximal tubule (Table 1). Patients who are homozygous for rBAT mutations may excrete up to 100% of the filtered cystine load. One explanation for this finding may be the contribution of tubular back-leak along the S3 segment. It has been postulated that patients with two defective rBAT genes are unable to handle this back leak in addition to the portion of the filtered load that escapes the convoluted segment *(37)*. In contrast, rBAT heterozygotes have adequate transport activity to ensure normal excretion of cystine and dibasic amino acids.

Non-Type I Cystinuria

It has been long recognized that there is a wide range of phenotypic differences among patients presenting with cystinuria. Linkage analysis and genotype-phenotype correlation data have demonstrated the presence of genetic heterogeneity in cystinuria. Calonge and associates *(38)* performed linkage analysis with the rBAT gene in families with type I or type III cystinuria or both, and found that only type I cystinuria was attributable to mutations in the rBAT gene, whereas other loci could be responsible for types II and III cystinuria. Similarly, using linkage analysis, Biceglia and colleagues *(39)* reported that type III cystinuria locus was on chromosome 19(19q13) between D19S414 and D19S220. In 1999, the SLC7A9 (BAT1) gene was isolated. The gene encodes a 487-amino acid protein and was mapped to chromosome 19 (19q13) with a location identical to that predicted by linkage analysis.

Mutations in the SLC7A9 gene cause nontype I cystinuria. Data has demonstrated several mutations of this gene in associaton with non-type I cystinuria. Data from the International Cystinuria Consortium demonstrated 35 mutations accounting for 79% of the carrier chromosomes in 61 non-type I patients *(40)*. The G105R was the main non-type I cystinuria allele (25%). Missense mutation G105R, V170M and R33W resulted in a severe phenotype in heterozygotes with complete loss of transport activity. Other mutations such as A182T demonstrated the lowest excretion rate of cystine and dibasic amino acids in heterozygotes. These data collectively provide an explanation for the phenotype variability among heterozygotes and it has been shown that mutations affecting small side chains (glycine, serine, or alanine) in the transmembrane domains of $b^{0,+}$ AT are associated with severe phenotype in heterozygotes.

The SLC7A9 product is a membrane protein with 12 membrane-spanning regions. This protein was termed $b^{0,+}$ AT for $b^{0,+}$ amino acid transporter. The dominant hypothesis is the rBAT and $b^{0,+}$ AT are subunits of $b^{0,+}$ amino acid transporter. As noted earlier, Palacin et al. *(41)* postulated that these heterodimers constitute the functional units of the $b^{0,+}$ transporter in renal and intestinal brush border membranes. The membrane spanning protein encoded by SLC7A9 conforms to the properties of a typical transport channel and strongly supports this hypothesis. A recent study investigated the localization and functional properties of human cystinuria related transporter hBAT1/$b^{0,+}$AT *(42)*. The cDNA encoding hBAT1 was isolated from human kidney and mapped to the human chromosome locus 19q12-13.1 using in situ hybridization. Tissue distribution and expression was analyzed using northern blot and immunohistochemistry. They found that hBAT1 message was predominantly expressed in the kidney and the protein was localized to the apical membrane of the proximal tubule. Similar to previous data from rat and mouse, hBAT1 when co-expressed with a type II glycoprotein rBAT in COS-7 cells exhibited transport activity with the characteristic of the amino acid transport system $b^{0,+}$, which transports cystine as well as basic and neutral amino acids in a sodium-independent manner.

Although this data supports that rBAT and $b^{0,+}$AT are subunits of the $b^{0,+}$ amino acid transporter, this hypothesis is challenged by the different local expression of these molecules in the proximal renal tubules. The rBAT protein is located predominantly in the brush border membrane of pars recta (S3 segment) of proximal tubule with a decreasing gradient toward the pars convoluta (S1 segment) while the opposite is true for $b^{0,+}$AT, which has the maximal expression in S1 segment of the proximal convoluted tubule (Table 1) *(32,43)*. This may explain the differences between the severity of clinical presentation in patients with heterozygosity for rBAT or $b^{0,+}$AT mutations. High expression of $b^{0,+}$AT in the pars convoluta (S3) corresponds to high capacity, low affinity transport system responsible for 90% of cystine reabsorption *(21)*. This would explain cystinuria in heterozygotes with $b^{0,+}$AT mutations.

Furthermore, the partial co-localization of these proteins indicates that additional light subunit heterodimers for rBAT or heavy subunit heterodimers for $b^{0,+}$AT may exist *(44)*. Further investigation and identification of these proteins may provide us with a better understanding of the molecular basis of cystinuria and the differences between SLC3A1 and SLC7A9 mutations.

In our laboratories, we have recently developed a murine knockout model for type I cystinuria. The targeted mutation of rBAT was based on a severely affected patient. This patient and his father were genotyped by sequencing each exon and were found to have two mutations in exon 10 that caused the missense mutations M618L and R663K. The murine rBAT (counterpart of the human SLC3A1) gene was isolated from a Sal I mouse genomic DNA library screen. Targeted deletions in this gene eliminated cystine transport. This construct was used to produce mice in whom the endogenous SLC3A1 gene had this truncation. The hypothesis is that mice with a targeted deletion of rBAT will serve as an appropriate model of cystine nephrolithiasis and will exhibit features of urinary stone disease. The preliminary data demonstrate a stone-forming clone. This model provides us with the opportunity to perform biochemical, pathological and molecular studies to investigate multiple steps involved in cystine stone formation. Furthermore, medical inhibition of cystine crystallization using inhibitors can be performed in vivo. Finally, this model allows us to investigate the effect of various medical interventions on stone formation in vivo to develop more effective treatment for recurrent stone formation.

CLINICAL PRESENTATION

Patients present with symptoms related to nephrolithiasis. The clinical presentation is undistinguishable from the more common calcium oxalate calculi. Therefore, a family history is an important clue in the initial diagnosis. Recurrent and multiple stones are common in cystinuria. Furthermore, cystine calculi may develop a large burden in a "staghorn" configuration. Traditionally, this terminology was chosen when the calculus fills the collecting system and the shape resembles the antlers of a male elk (Fig. 2).

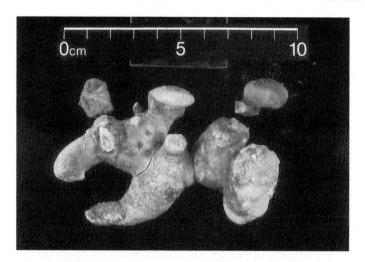

Fig. 2. Surgically removed staghorn cystine calculus.

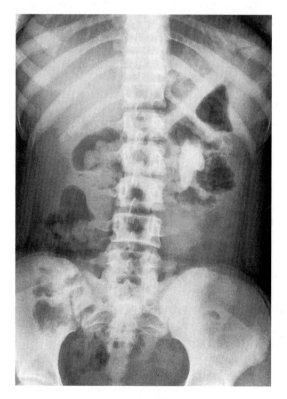

Fig. 3. Plain radiograph of a large partial cystine stone in a 12-yr-old child with noncompliance with medical management.

By definition, staghorn calculi fill the majority of the collecting system including renal pelvis and branches into the majority of calyces *(45)*.

Aside from the similarities in clinical presentation of cystine and calcareous calculi, mixed stones can account for up to half of the stones in cystinuria *(46)*. Patients with homozygous cystinuria may have stones with calcium oxalate as the major and cystine as the minor component. The presence of associated physiological defects such as hypercalciuria (5.3–18.5%), hyperuricosuria (7–22%), and hypocitraturia in the cystinuric population has been demonstrated (25,47). An association between cystinuria and hyperuricemia and uric acid nephrolithiasis has also been reported (48). Therefore, metabolic evaluation should be considered in all patients with cystine or mixed calculi (47).

Other conditions associated with excessive cystine excretion such as Fanconi syndrome and Wilson's disease should be considered (25). Furthermore, cystinuria has been associated with several genetic diseases including mongolism, retinitis pigmentosa, muscular dystrophy, hereditary pancreatitis and hemophilia (49). Infants younger than 6 mo may have increased cystine excretion due to immaturity of renal tubules (50). Urinary tract infections have been reported in up to 34% of patients with cystine calculi (51,52).

DIAGNOSIS

The diagnosis of cystine stones should be suspected in any patient with a history of renal stones in childhood, recurrent episodes of nephrolithiasis, a strong family history of stone disease, or amber colored calculi.

Normal urinary cystine excretion is less than 20 mg/d. The upper limit of solubility of cystine under physiological urinary pH is 300 mg/L. By definition, a urinary cystine concentration of above 150–250 mg/d is abnormal in adults. Stone forming children may excrete lower amounts of cystine (75 mg/d). The initial step in the diagnosis of cystine stones involves the examination of fresh urine for characteristic hexagonal cystine crystals. Although pathognomonic, these crystals may be difficult to identify in dilute or alkaline urine. Urinary acidification to a pH of 4.0 with overnight refrigeration before centrifugation has been recommended to avoid infection or a rise in urinary pH. Nevertheless, these crystals are only seen in a minority of cystinuric patients (52).

A qualitative cystine test can be performed on fresh urine using the colormetric cyanide nitroprusside test. A purple red color after addition of sodium nitroprusside and sodium cyanide suggests a cystine excretion in excess of 75 mg/L. A false positive test may occur in patients with homocystinuria and acetonuria. Furthermore, due to high sensitivity of this test, heterozygous, asymptomatic patients may present with positive results. The use of sulfur-containing drugs may also result in a false positive test due to a nonspecific binding of nitroprusside complex with sulfide groups (16).

A positive qualitative test suggests the diagnosis of cystinuria. Therefore, if the nitroprusside test is positive, urinary cystine excretion should be quantitated. Quantitative cystine excretion can be determined by ion-exchange chromatography. The total cystine excretion in a 24-h urine collection determines the basis for a clinical diagnosis of cystinuria. A urinary cystine excretion above 250 mg/g creatinine usually indicates homozygous cystinuria. The definitive diagnosis is made by stone analysis.

On routine flat-plate radiographic examination, cystine stones are radiopaque (ground glass appearance) owing to the density of the sulfur atoms (Fig. 3). They are less radiopaque than calcium stones (53). However, there is significant variability in the radiodensity of cystine stones due to frequent mixed composition (16). Structurally, cystine stones are generally homogenous without striations and are more rounded in appearance. Ultrasonography may be used for diagnosis of renal, ureteral, and bladder cystine calculi

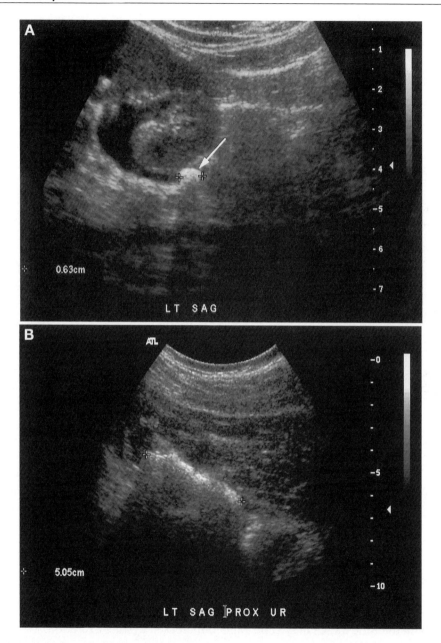

Fig. 4. Ultrasonographic diagnosis of ureteral (**A**), renal (**B**), and bladder (**C**) cystine calculi *(see next page)*. Stones are echogenic with typical posterior acoustic shadowing. Note hydronephrosis associated with large proximal ureteral stone (**A**).

(Fig. 4A–C). This modality will also provide information with regard to the presence and degree of urinary obstruction, which may require more acute intervention. Similar to other stone types, other imaging modalities, which can provide functional information, include intravenous pyelogram and computerized tomography (CT). Intravenous pyelogram was used commonly in the past and has been replaced by CT scan for acute diagnosis of obstructing stones in most institutions.

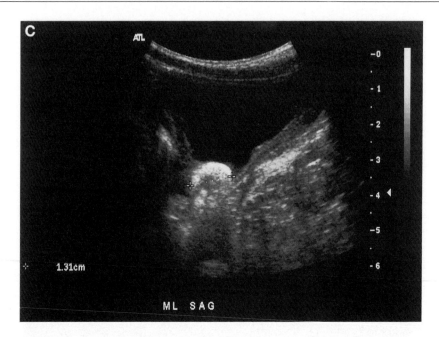

Fig. 4. *(Continued)* Ultrasonographic diagnosis of bladder **(C)** cystine calculi.

MANAGEMENT

Acute management of cystinuria includes measures to resolve the acute stone crisis, which is identical to other stone types. Pain management and hydration are the initial steps. In the chronic phase, the goal of treatment is to decrease the urinary concentration of cystine to below 150 mg/L. This goal can be achieved by non-specific measures or more specific medications designed for cystinuria.

Medical Management of Cystinuria

The goal of medical management is prevention of new stone formation. This can be achieved by the reduction of the cystine concentration in urine or increasing the urinary cystine solubility (Table 2).

Dietary modification is an integral part of treatment. Previous studies have reported that high methionine intake may contribute to increased cystine excretion. Methionine is a precursor of cystine and is contained in essentially all meat products and other high protein foods such as eggs, soy, and wheat. Clearly, a dietary restriction of all methionine-containing products is not practical and patient compliance is a limiting factor. Moreover, only a small proportion of methionine is excreted as cystine and the majority is incorporated into proteins. In current medical practice, therefore, patients are advised to maintain a balanced diet and avoid high protein intake. Cystine excretion is influenced by dietary salt intake *(54)*. A reduction in dietary sodium of 150 mEq/d results in a decrease in urinary cystine concentration of 650 mmol/d *(55)*.

The effect of sodium restriction is, however, limited. Furthermore, similar to methionine restriction, a rigid dietary sodium restriction is difficult *(25)*. A reduction in salt intake to <2g/d has been recommended *(47)*.

Table 2
Medical Management of Cystine Calculi

Dietary	• Moderate protein intake
	• Low salt intake (<2 g/d)
	• Hydration (specific gravity <1.010
Urinary alkalinization	• PH 6.5–7
	• Sodium bicarbonate
	• Potassium citrate
Thiol derivatives	• D-Penicillamine
	• Alpha mercaptoproprionylglycine
	• Bucillamine
ACE inhibitor	• Captopril

ACE, angiotensin-converting enzyme.

The most important, general dietary measure to reduce urinary cystine concentration is hydration. The upper limit of cystine solubility is 400 mg/L. Adequate hydration to keep the urinary cystine concentration below this limit is effective. Hydration has been shown to decrease urinary stone formation in as many as 67% of patients with cystinuria. Adequate hydration can be monitored by checking the specific gravity of urine. A specific gravity of 1.010 has been recommended (16). In a recent study from France, a daily urinary volume of >3.1 liters was recommended (56). This urinary volume was associated with a significant decrease in new stone formation over a long period of time. Furthermore, the appearance of crystalluria in the first morning urine associated with a specific gravity of 1.010 or greater was predictive of stone formation and growth (56). Nocturnal hydration is important to decrease urinary supersaturation during sleeping hours. A bedtime fluid intake of 500 mL has been suggested (50). Various types of fluid can be used. The use of fruit juice, such as orange, is beneficial since they increase the alkali load and subsequently the urinary pH (25).

Urinary alkalinization increases cystine solubility. Although theoretically simple, a limitation of oral alkali therapy is the relative high cystine pKa of 8.5. Therefore, in order to achieve a clinically significant increase in cystine solubility, a urinary pH of >7.5 is desirable. There are two limitations for oral alkali therapy. First, to achieve and maintain a urinary pH above 7.5 is difficult and not practical. Secondly, a high urinary pH will predispose to calcium phosphate stone formation. Considering these limitations, the goal of alkali therapy is to maintain a pH in the 6.5–7.0 range.

Various agents have been used for urinary alkalinization. Sodium bicarbonate is effective but associated with a sodium load, which may not be desired in patients with associated medical conditions, such as hypertension. Furthermore, sodium has the adverse effect of promoting cystine excretion. Potassium citrate is currently the medication of choice for urinary alkalinization. The starting dose is 60–80 mEq/d in divided doses to maintain a constant pH level (15). Patients should be given pH paper to monitor their urinary pH and to titrate their medication dose as needed.

Unfortunately, general measures with hydration and urinary alkalinization are commonly ineffective to control recurrent stone formation and more specific treatment is required. Glutamine intake was once reported to reduce the cystine excretion rate (57).

However, others could not duplicate this finding and currently there is no role for this treatment.

Thiol derivatives are chelating agents. They contain a sulfhydryl group, which can undergo a thio-disulfide exchange with cystine; the disulfide bond of cystine therefore is challenged resulting in more soluble complexes incorporating cystine monomers. Therefore, these medications may result in dissolution of existing stones when other general measures have failed and help prevent stone recurrences.

D-Peniciliamine was the first chelating agent *(9)*. It can produce complexes 50 times more soluble than cystine. D-Penicillamine has been associated with frequent side effects including gastrointestinal disturbances, allergic reactions with fever and rash, arthralgia, leukopenia, thrombocytopenia, proteinuria with nephrotic syndrome, and polymyositis *(58)*. Frequent side effects may occur in as many as 50% of patients after long-term therapy. D-Penicillamine may result in pyridoxine (vitamin B6) deficiency. Therefore, prophylactic medication with vitamin B6 (50 mg/d) is recommended *(50)* and this combination is frequently responsible for discontinuation of the medication.

Alphamercaptopropionylglycine (αMPG) is a second generation chelating agent, which is structurally related to D-penicillamine and has a similar mechanism of action with significantly reduced side effects. In an early report, after long-term treatment with αMPG, one third of stones were dissolved and new stone formation was prevented in 85% of patients. αMPG was found to be 50% more effective than D-penicillamine in reducing free cystine levels and increasing the amount of cystine disulfide in the urine *(59)*. In a multicenter trial, 67% of patients discontinued D-penicillamine due to significant side effect compared to 31% of those taking αMPG *(60)*. This treatment reduced the stone formation rate by 81–94% with a remission rate of 63–71% in 66 patients *(60)*.

It appears that αMPG is a more effective agent for cystinuric patients with reduced severity of side effects compared to D-penicillamine. Therefore, αMPG is currently the medication of choice in most centers. The starting dose is 400 mg/d in divided doses. This dose can be increased to 800–1200 mg/d. Bucillamine (Rimatil) is a third generation chelating agent; Rimatil is theoretically more effective since it is a dithiol compound. Clinical experience with Rimatil is limited. However, a lower toxicity with similar efficacy has been reported *(25)*.

Captopril, an angiotensin-converting enzyme inhibitor, has been reported to decrease the urinary cystine concentration *(61)*. The mechanism of action is similar to thiols. Captopril contains a free sulfhydryl group, which can compete the disulfide bond in cystine and result in formation of cystine-captopril complex, which is 200 times more soluble than cystine. However, studies on the efficacy of captopril have been inconclusive. Some centers have reported a role for captopril especially in patients with hypertension who require antihypertensive medications or those patients who failed standard treatment for cystinuria *(62)*. Conversely, others did not find a significant effect from captopril treatment *(56,63,64)*.

Surgical Management of Cystine Stones

Patients with cystinuria typically have frequent recurrences of multiple stones despite medical management. Management of large volume calculi requires surgical intervention. Due to the natural history of the disease, current surgical management is directed by means of minimally invasive endourological techniques. This includes extracorporeal and intracorporeal lithotripsy using ureteroscopic or percutaneous approaches.

A limitation of extracorporeal shock wave lithotripsy (SWL) is the fact that cystine stones are recalcitrant to cracking and relatively hard to break. This modality is usually reserved for stones smaller than 1.5 cm in diameter *(47)*. Based on the results with SWL, two different crystal structures for cystine stones have been proposed *(65)*. In this study, the rough calculi were composed of large, organized hexagonal crystals that form good cleavage planes for fragmentation. Smooth calculi, however, were made of smaller, disorganized poorly formed crystals and were much more difficult to fragment. Another study reported that SWL of cystine calculi resulted in large fragments compared to other stone types *(53)*. Medical treatment before SWL may result in easier fragmentation by promoting the formation of apatite in cystine calculi *(66)*. Conversely, SWL may be used initially to improve the results of medical chemolysis by increasing the exposed stone surface *(67)*.

The principles of ureteroscopic management are similar to other stone types. The best available modalities of intracorporeal lithotripsy include the lithoclast and holmium-yttrium-aluminum-garnet laser. The Swiss Lithoclast delivers mechanical pneumatic fragmentation generated by compressed air similar to the jackhammer principle *(68)*. Holmium-yttrium-aluminum-garnet laser generated pulsed light at a wavelength of 2100 nm to induce both fragmentation and vaporization *(69)*. In our experience, laser lithotripsy of cystine stones produces a sulfur odor during the procedure, which is harmless and likely related to release of sulfur gas from the stone surface. The introduction of these two modalities have facilitated stone fragmentation and improve stone free rate after ureteroscopic procedures. Both modalities have the advantage of fragmenting all stone types and are equally effective *(68,69)*. However, laser produces smaller fragments and less retrograde stone migration *(47)*.

Larger renal stones or proximal ureteral stones are best managed with percutaneous nephrolithotomy. This modality offers the advantage of large endoscopes and the use of ultrasonic lithotripsy, which can easily fragment cystine stones. Other modalities such as the use of lithoclast and laser can also be employed *(70)*. Another advantage of the percutaneous approach is the direct access for stone chemolysis. If residual fragments persist after the percutaneous approach, chemo-dissolution of residual fragments can be attempted. Various solutions including *N*-acetylcysteine, tris-hydroxymethyl aninomethane (THAM-E), and alkali agents have been successfully utilized *(16)*.

We utilize the percutaneous tube and an indwelling ureteral access catheter for continuous irrigation with alkali solutions. A limitation of percutaneous chemolysis is the need for hospital admission, careful monitoring of intrapelvic pressure, and hence an associated high cost. Therefore, direct chemolysis is mainly used in conjunction with other modalities when ureteroscopic and percutaneous procedures remain unsuccessful in eradicating all stone fragments.

Acceptable stone free rates can be achieved using these modalities. In a recent study of 61 renal units, a stone free rate of 87% has been reported using various modalities, which was not influenced by the initial stone burden or the type of initial management selected *(71)*.

It is important to keep in mind that patients with cystinuria present with early and frequent recurrences after surgical procedures despite medical treatment. Therefore, contrary to other stone types, the primary goals of surgical treatment are relief of symptoms associated with renal obstruction and preservation of renal function rather than achieving a complete stone free status.

FUTURE PERSPECTIVES

Recent advances in molecular biology have provided new insights into the pathophysiology and genetics of cystinuria. However, the new knowledge has not translated into a more effective medical treatment for cystinuria to date. Current modalities for medical treatment of cystinuria with urinary alkalinization and chelating agents have limited effectiveness for prevention of frustrating recurrent calculi. It is expected that future development will be based on molecular and gene therapy. Until that time, the treatment of cystinuric patients remains a difficult task and the goal should be prevention of recurrences and the use of minimally invasive surgery to preserve renal function.

REFERENCES

1. Rosenberg LE, Durant JL, Holland JM. Intestinal absorption and renal extraction of cystine and cystine in cystinuria. N Engl J Med 1965; 273: 1239.
2. Wollston WH. A new species of urinary calculi. Trans R Soc London 1810; 100: 223.
3. Milne MD. Cystinuria, 1810–1965. Sci Basis Med Annu Rev 1967; 227.
4. Berzellius J. Calculus urinaries. Traite Chem 1833; 7: 424.
5. Friedman E. Der Kreislauf des Schwefels in der organischen. Nature Ergeb Physio 1902; 1: 15.
6. Garrod AE. Inborn error of metabolism. Lancet 1908; 2: 1.
7. Dent CC, Rose GA. Amino acid metabolism in cystinuria. Q J Med New Series 1951; 20: 205.
8. Harris MU, Robson EB, Warren FL. Phenotypes and genotypes in cystinuria. Ann Hum Genet 1955; 20: 57.
9. Crawhall SE, Watts RW. Effect of penicillamine on cystinuria. MBJ 1963; 588: 588.
10. Bertran J, Werner A, Chillaron J, et al. Expression cloning of a human renal cDNA that induces high affinity transport of L-cystine shared with dibasic amino acids in Xenopus oocytes. J Bio Chem 1993; 268: 14,842.
11. Pras E, Arber N, Aksentijevich I, et al. Localization of a gene causing cystinuria to chromosome 2p. Nat Genet 1994; 6: 415.
12. Calonge MJ, Gasparini P, Chillaron J, et al. Cystinuria caused by mutations in rBAT, a gene involved in the transport of cystine. Nat Genet 1994; 6: 420.
13. Pras E. Cystinuria at the turn of the millennium: clinical aspects and new molecular developments. Mol Urol 2000; 4: 409.
14. Weinberger A, Sperling O, Rabinovitz M, et al. High frequency of cystinuria among Jews of Libyan origin. Hum Hered 1974; 24: 568.
15. Pak C. Cystinuria. In: Urolithiasis-A Medical and Surgical Reference, (Resnick PC, Park CYC, eds.). WB Saunders, Philadelphia, PA, 1990, p. 133.
16. Rutchik SD, Resnick MI. Cystine calculi. Diagnosis and management. Urol Clin North Am 1997; 24: 163.
17. Cusworth D. Renal clearance of amino acids in normal adults and in patients with aminoaciduria. Biochem J 1960; 74:550.
18. McNamara PD, Pepe LM, Segal S. Cystine uptake by rat renal brush-border vesicles. Biochem J 1981; 194: 443.
19. Segal S, McNamara PD, Pepe LM. Transport interaction of cystine and dibasic amino acids in renal brush border vesicles. Science 1977; 197: 169.
20. Schafer JA, Watkins ML. Transport of L-cystine in isolated perfused proximal straight tubules. Pfluger Arch 1984; 401: 143.
21. Sibernagl S. The renal handling of amino acids and oligopeptides. Physio Rev 1988; 68: 911.
22. Palacin M. A new family of proteins (rBAT and 4F2hc) involved in cationic and zwitterionic amino acid transport: a tale of two proteins in search of a transport function. J Exp Biol 1994; 196: 123.
23. Thier S, Fox M, Segal S, and Rosenberg LE. Cystinuria: in vitro demonstration of a intestinal transport defect. Science 1964; 143: 482.
24. Rosenberg LE, Downing S, Durant JL, et al. Cystinuria: biochemical evidence for three genetically distinct diseases, J. Clin Invest 1966; 45: 365.

25. Sakhaee K, Sutton RAL. Pathogenesis and Medical treatment of cystinuria. In: Kidney Stones: Medical and Surgical Management, (Coe FL, Favus MJ, Pak CYC, Parks JH, Preminger GM, eds.). Lippincott-Raven, Philadephia, PA, 1996; pp. 1007–1017.

26. Ito H, Egoshi K, Mizoguchi K, et al. Advances in genetic aspects of cystinuria. Mol Urol 2000; 4: 403.

27. Palacin M, Borsani G, Sebastio G. The molecular bases of cystinuria and lysinuric protein intolerance. Curr Opin Genet Dev 2001; 11: 328.

28. Stoller ML, McDonald MW, Gentle DL, et al. Acalculous cystinuria. J Endourol 1997; 11: 233.

29. Palacin M, Fernandez E, Chillaron J, et al. The amino acid transport system b(o,+) and cystinuria. Mol Membr Biol 2001; 18: 21.

30. Van Winkle LJ, Campione AL, Gorman JM. Na+ independent transport of basic and zwitterionic amino acids in mouse blastocysts by a shared system and by processes which distinguish between these substrates. J Biol Chem 1988; 263: 3150.

31. Gasparini P, Calonge MJ, Bisceglia L, et al. Molecular genetics of cystinuria: identification of four new mutations and seven polymorphisms and evidence for genetic heterogeneity. Am J Hum Genet 1995; 57: 781.

32. Pfeiffer R, Loffing J, Rossier G, et al. Luminal heterodimeric amino acid transporter defective in cystinuria. Mol Bio Cell 1999; 10: 4135.

33. Bertran J, Werner A, Moore ML, et al. Expression cloning of a cDNA from rabbit kidney cortex that induces a single transport system for cystine and dibasic and neutral amino acids. Proc Natl Acad Sci USA 1992; 89: 5601.

34. Lee WS, Wells RG, Sabbag RV, et al. Cloning and chromosomal localization of a human kidney cDNA involved in cystine, dibasic and neutral amino acid transport. J Clin Invest 1993; 91: 1959.

35. Tate SS, Yan N, Udenfriend S. Expression cloning of a Na (+) independent neural amino acid transport from rat kidney. Proc Natl Acad Sci USA 1992; 89: 1.

36. Gitomer WL, Pak CY. Recent advances in the biochemical and molecular biological basis of cystinuria. J Urol 1996; 156: 1907.

37. Goodyer P, Boutros M, Rozen R. The molecular basis of cystinuria: an update. Exp Nephrol 2000; 8: 123.

38. Calonge MJ, Volpini V, Bisceglia L, et al. Genetic heterogeneity in cystinuria: the SLC3A1 gene is linked to type 1 but not to type III cystinuria. Proc Natl Acad Sci USA 1995; 92: 9667.

39. Bisceglia L, Calonge MJ, Totaro A, et al. Localization, by linkage analysis, of the cystinuria type III gene to chromosome 19q13.1 Am J Hum Genet 1997; 60: 611.

40. Font MA, Feliubadalo L, Estivill X, et al. Functional analysis of mutations in SLC7A9 and genotype-phenotype correlation in non-type I cystinuria. Hum Mol Genet 2001; 10: 305.

41. Palacin M, Estevez R, Zorzano A, et al. Cystinuria calls for heteromultimeric amino acid transporters. Curr Opin Cell Biol 1998; 10: 455.

42. Mizoguchi K, Cha SH, Chairoungdua A, et al. Human cystinuria-related transporter: localization and functional characterization. Kidney Int 2001; 59: 1821.

43. Kanai Y, Stelzer MG, Lee WS, et al. Expression of mRNA (D2) encoding a protein involved in amino acid transport in S3 proximal tubule. Am J Physio 1992; 263: F1087.

44. Palacin M, Estevez R, Bertran J, et al. Molecular biology of mammalian plasma membrane amino acid transporters. Physio Rev 1998; 78: 969.

45. Segura JW, Preminger GM, Assimos DG, et al. Nephrolithiasis Clinical Guidelines Panel summary report on the management of staghorn calculi. The American Urological Association Nephrolithiasis Clinical Guidelines Panel. J Urol 1994; 151: 1648.

46. Their So, Halperin EC. Cystinuria. In: Nephrolithiasis, (Coe FL, ed.). Churchill Livingstone, New York, NY, 1980; pp. 208–230.

47. Ng CS, Streem SB. Contemporary management of cystinuria. J Endourol 1999; 13: 647.

48. Vergis JG, Walker BR. Cystinuria, hyperuricemia and uric acid nephrolithiasis. Case report. Nephron 1970; 7:577.

49. Their So SS. Cystinuria. (Sanbury JB, ed.). 1972.

50. Milliner DAS. Cystinuria. Endocrinol Metab Clin North Am 1990; 19: 889.

51. Dahlberg PJ, Van Den B, Kurtz SB, et al. Clinical features and management of cystinuria. Mayo Clin Proc 1977; 52: 533.

52. Evans WP, Resnick MI, Boyce WH. Homozygous cystinuria—evaluation of 35 patients. J Urol 1982; 127: 707.

53. Dretler SP. Stone fragility—a new therapeutic distinction. J Urol 1988; 139:1124.

54. Norman RW, Manette WA. Dietary restriction of sodium as a means of reducing urinary cystine. J Urol 1990; 143: 1193.

55. Jaeger P, Portmann L, Saunders A, et al. Anticystinuric effects of glutamine and of dietary sodium restriction. N Engl J Med 1986; 315: 1120.

56. Barbey F, Joly D, Rieu P, et al. Medical treatment of cystinuria: critical reappraisal of long-term results. J Urol 2000; 163: 1419.

57. Miyagi K, Nakada F, Ohshiro S. Effect of glutamine on cystine excretion in a patient with cystinuria. N Engl J Med 1979; 301: 196.

58. Halperin EC, Their SO, Rosenberg LE. the use of D-penicillamine in cystinuria: efficacy and untoward reaction. Yale J Bio Med 1981; 54: 439.

59. Harbar JA, Cusworth DC, Lawes LC, et al. Comparison of 2-mercaptopropionylglycine and D-penicillamine in the treatment of cystinuria. J Urol 1986; 136: 146.

60. Pak CY, Fuller C, Sakhaee K, et al. Management of cystine nephrolithiasis with alpha-mercaptopropionylglycine. J Urol 1986; 136: 1003.

61. Sloand JA, Izzo JL, Jr. Captopril reduces urinary cystine excretion in cystinuria. Arch Intern Med 1987; 147: 1409.

62. Cohen TD, Streem SB, Hall P. Clinical effect of captopril on the formation and growth of cystine calculi. J Urol 1995; 154: 164.

63. Aunsholt NA, Ahlbom G. Lack of effect of captopril in cystinuria. Clin Nephrol 1990; 34: 92.

64. Dahlberg PJ, Jones JD. Cystinuria: failure of captopril to reduce cystine excretion. Arch Intern Med 1989; 149: 713.

65. Bhatta KM, Prien EL, Jr, Dretler SP. Cystine calculi-rough and smooth: a new clinical distinction. J Urol, 1989; 142: 937.

66. Koide T, Yoshioka T, Yamaguchi S, et al. A strategy of cystine stone management. J Urol 1992; 147: 112.

67. Schmeller NT, Kersting H, Schuller J, et al. Combination of chemolysis and shock wave lithotripsy in the treatment of cystine renal calculi. J Urol 1984; 131: 434.

68. Schulze H, Haupt G, Piergiovanni M, et al. The Swiss Lithoclast: a new device for endoscopic stone disintegration. J Urol 1993; 149: 15.

69. Razvi HA, Denstedt JD, Chun SS, et al. Intracorporeal lithotripsy with the holmium: YAG laser. J. Urol 1996; 156: 912.

70. Denstedt JD. Use of Swiss Lithoclast for percutaneous nephrolithotripsy. J Endourol 1993; 7:477.

71. Chow GK, Streem SB. Contemporary urological intervention for cystinuric patients: immediate and long-term impact and implications. J Urol 1998; 160: 341.

19 Urinary Stones of Unusual Etiology

Patrick S. Lowry, MD *and Stephen Y. Nakada,* MD

Key Words: Nephrolithiasis; xanthine; antiretroviral medication; ammonium.

INTRODUCTION

The vast majority of urinary stones are composed of calcium oxalate, calcium phosphate, struvite, uric acid, or cystine. Enumerable studies analyzing over 45,000 total calculi have shown urinary stones to be composed of "other" constituents only 0.5–3.5% of the time. Although uncommon, these stones can be challenging to both diagnose and to treat. In many cases, accurate diagnosis is necessary for proper treatment. This challenge begins with routine stone analysis, especially in the case of radiolucent stones that do not clinically fit the uric acid picture, or that recur despite appropriate therapy with strict urinary alkalinization and xanthine oxidase inhibition.

Some types of rare stones are caused by ingestion of inappropriately large doses of medications, and treatment requires merely cessation of the medication to prevent further stone episodes. Other stones are genetic disorders of metabolism, which require a more complex medical decision-making process. Although commonly a fortuitous discovery made through stone analysis, good knowledge of the patient history and an increased awareness of the conditions that predispose to formation of unusual stones will heighten clinical suspicion which may lead to the diagnosis of an unusual stone. Only by understanding the metabolic pathways leading to the formation of these stones, and

From: Current Clinical Urology, *Urinary Stone Disease:*
A Practical Guide to Medical and Surgical Management
Edited by: M. L. Stoller and M. V. Meng © Humana Press Inc., Totowa, NJ

Table 1
Types of Unusual Stones

Metabolic stones
    2,8-Dihydroxyadenine stones
    Ammonium acid urate steones
    Primary xanthine stones
Medication-related stones
    Ephedrine stones
    Guaifenesin stones
    Indinavir stones
    Nelfinavir stones
    Oxypurinol stones
    Silicate stones
    Sulfa stones
    Topimarate-induced stones
    Triamterene stones
    Xanthine stones[a]
    Ammonium acid urate stones[a]
Pediatric stones
    Stones in low-birth-weight premature infants
    Stones in children and adolescents/endemic bladder stones

[a]Caused by both medications and metabolic abnormalities.

applying this knowledge to clinical practice, can we avoid confusing rare calculi with more common stone entities, avoid needless recurrence of stone episodes, and prevent deterioration of renal function.

The goal of this chapter is to present information that will help urologists diagnose and treat unusual urinary stones (Table 1).

METABOLIC STONES

2, 8-Dihydroxyadenine Stones

In purine metabolism, the breakdown of adenine into adenine monophosphate involves the enzyme adenine phosphoribosyl transferase (APRT). Deficiency of the APRT enzyme prevents adenine from entering the salvage pathway, and consequently, adenine is converted by xanthine oxidase into 2, 8-dihydroxyadenine (2,8-DHA) (Fig. 1) (1). 2,8-DHA is highly insoluble in the urine and patients have resulting crystalluria, often with nephrolithiasis (2). APRT deficiency is inherited as an autosomal recessive trait (3), and patients must be homozygotes or compound heterozygotes with a null allele for the patient to have APRT deficiency (1).

Two types of APRT deficiency have been described. Type I predominantly affects Caucasians, and has almost no APRT activity, as measured by the level of enzyme activity in erythrocytes (4). Until recently, type II APRT deficiency was found only in Japan, but is now described in patients of Polish ancestry (5). In type II disease, mutations exist in both genes, yet residual APRT activity (10–25% activity) remains (1).

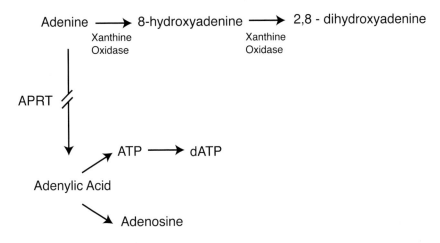

APRT - adenine phosphoribosyl transferase

Fig. 1. Pathway of purine metabolism leading to 2,8-dihydroxyadenine.

2,8-DHA excretion into the urine follows a circadian rhythm, with increased elevation during the late night and early morning *(6)*. Owing to usual sleeping habits, this is the time when most people have the lowest fluid intake, and the most concentrated urine, resulting in a circadian dependent risk of 2,8-DHA stone formation.

2,8-DHA urinary stones were first described in 1974 *(7)*, yet likely went misdiagnosed before that as uric acid stones. Interestingly, deposition of 2,8-DHA crystals in renal tubular lumen were reported by Joost et al in 1898 *(8)*. Like uric acid stones, 2,8-DHA calculi are radiolucent, although they can be seen on CT scans. 2,8-DHA stones are also difficult to distinguish from uric acid stones from an analysis standpoint. 2,8-DHA appears indistinguishable from uric acid in biochemical analysis (murexide test for urate; phosphotungstate or phosphomolybdate for uric acid) *(1,3)*. Ultraviolet testing may also fail to distinguish the two, if performed in alkaline solution *(2)*. Only infrared spectroscopy, X-ray diffraction, and properly performed UV testing will distinguish the two *(1,2,6)*. Gross appearances should suggest a difference between the two when closely examined; uric acid stones have a smooth, yellow, hard surface, whereas dried 2,8-DHA calculi are rough, gray, and friable *(1)*.

Another confounder to prevent recognition of 2,8-DHA stones is the treatment. To prevent crystallization of 2,8-DHA in the urine, the production must be stopped. Allopurinol inhibits xanthine oxidase, preventing the conversion of adenine to 2,8-DHA, and is very effective for stone prophylaxis *(1)*. The patients misdiagnosed with uric acid stones will likely be placed on allopurinol at some point as their stones recur. This will aid in the prevention of further stone formation from either uric acid or 2,8-DHA.

Early recognition of APRT deficiency and proper diagnosis of stone type is necessary to prevent decline of renal function. In a series of 17 APRT deficient patients, 8 presented with renal insufficiency, 25% of which progressed to renal failure or died from uremic complications *(1)*. Renal damage occurs because of deposition of crystalline material in tubular lumen and within epithelial cells *(9)*. Failure of transplanted kidneys in patients with undiagnosed, and consequently, untreated 2,8-DHA lithiasis has been reported *(10,11)*. In one report, the patient presented with renal failure, and after appropriate acute stone management and initiation of allopurinol, the renal failure resolved (11). In the other report, the patient was undiagnosed until after transplanted organ was rejected and removed; the failure may have been prevented on appropriate therapy (10). In fact, both patients had multiple previous surgeries for stone recurrence before renal failure and transplantation. If 2,8-DHA had been properly diagnosed to begin with, these patients may not have progressed to renal failure. When managed with proper medication, transplantation of these patients is successful (4).

Additionally, the formation of 2,8-DHA stones may be exacerbated during pregnancy. A pregnant patient with APRT deficiency, who had stopped allopurinol therapy on the advice of her obstetrician, presented with a 2,8-DHA steinstrasse. She was managed conservatively with chronic ureteral stent changes until delivery, after which the stones were removed. She experienced renal insufficiency, and her creatinine never returned to normal (12). Females with APRT should be adequately counseled about the potential fetal effects of allopurinol, as well as the possible risks to the mother associated with discontinuation of allopurinol. Should patients continue through pregnancy, fluid intake and urine output should be carefully monitored, especially at night when circadian patterns increase risk of 2,8-DHA crystals in the urine.

Diagnosis may be accomplished with infrared spectroscopy. Quantitative 2,8-DHA measurement of urine and determination of APRT activity in erythrocytes confirm existence of APRT deficiency. Quantitative 24 h 2,8-DHA measurements may also be used to monitor treatment.

Treatment of 2,8-DHA calculi may be accomplished via any surgical modality, including shock-wave lithotripsy (1). Prevention is accomplished with allopurinol therapy (300 mg/d) and maintenance of urine output of at least 2.5 L/d (6). Dietary control has shown little potential benefit (1,6), likely because the majority of adenine does not come from the diet. However, a reported case described a child presenting in renal failure who was from a commune where the primary diet was adenine rich lentils, grains, and vegetables. This report could implicate high adenine intake as detrimental. Consequently, mild purine restriction may be beneficial (4). Urinary alkalinization has no role; it has been described as decreasing solubility of 2,8-DHA (11,13), although at physiologic urinary pH ranges, is probably not detrimental, only ineffective at changing 2,8-DHA solubility (4).

2,8-DHA calculi should be suspected in all children with radiolucent stones, especially if presumed uric acid stones do not respond appropriately to treatment, or if coexisting renal insufficiency develops. Brown smudges in diapers and small, yellowish-brown, round urinary crystals suggest APRT deficiency. Suspicion, however, cannot be limited to the pediatric population, as age presentation ranges from several months old to the seventh decade (1).

Ammonium Acid Urate Stones (Fig. 2)

Stones composed primarily of ammonium acid urate (AAU) are rarely seen in North American patients, and account for less than 1% of urinary stones (14). In multiple studies, the prevalence of predominantly AAU stones has been shown to be in the range of 0.3 % (14–16). In third world countries, endemic AAU lithiasis, predominantly in the form of pediatric bladder calculi, is more common. Navajo Indians in the United States and aboriginal children in Australia have also been identified with AAU calculi (17–19). Pure AAU stones are radiolucent, but usually these stone types have a secondary component which may make them faintly radiopaque.

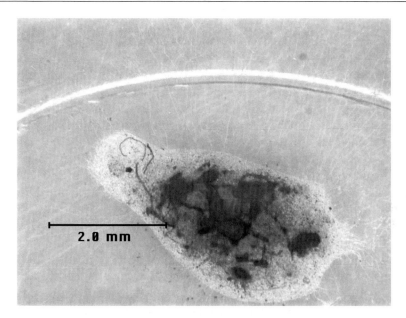

Fig. 2. Ammonium acid urate calculus (Courtesy of Mission Pharmacal, San Antonio, Texas).

Risk factors for the formation of AAU stones include decreased urine volume, hyperuricosuria, stasis (for bladder stones), and the moderate elevation in ammonium excretion associated with low phosphorus intake or phosphorus malabsorption. Other risk factors include high urinary ammonium levels (a result of the alkaline urine of existing infection, or acidic urine owing to diet), hypokalemia, dehydration, or starvation states *(14)*. Commonly, more than one of these risk factors coexist. Dehydration decreases urine output and can result in acid urine, and a diet with excessive meat causes hyperuricosuria and acidic urine. Conditions that predispose to uric acid stones and struvite stones also lead to AAU precipitation.

AAU stones seen in third world countries are postulated to be multifactoral. The combination of an acidic diet high in purines but low in phosphorus (perhaps owing to dependence on breast milk), low fluid intake, and frequent diarrhea predisposes to a urine with elevated concentrations of uric acid and ammonium, leading to AAU precipitation *(20,21)*. The secondary components in AAU calculi are generally uric acid or calcium oxalate, but in the face of urinary infection with urea splitting organisms, the urine alkalinization will support struvite formation as the secondary component (*see* section on pediatric stones).

Pichette et al. analyzed 1346 stones and found 43 with some percentage of AAU, but in only 3 of the 43 was AAU the dominant component (>50%) *(14)*. They also observed that the most common associated components were struvite (41%) and uric acid (35%). Additionally, it was noted that in 75% of stones, the AAU was found as discrete deposits, either intercrystalline or peripheral, mixed in with other stone constituents. The remaining 25% of AAU was diffusely mixed with other stone components. Comparatively, Soble et al. found that in 3400 stones, AAU was present in 44. In 11 of the 44, AAU was the main component (mean of 44%). The most common secondary components were uric acid (91%), calcium oxalate (63%), calcium phosphate (50%), and struvite (31%).

The cohort was examined for risk factors: 41% were obese (BMI >30), 36% had recurrent urinary tract infections, 25% had inflammatory bowel disease, 13% were laxative abusers, and 9% had a history of recurrent uric acid stones. These population groups of AAU stone formers are consistent with the risk factors for AAU stone formation.

AAU formation in patients with laxative abuse has been well characterized by Dick et al. *(21)*. Eleven patients with documented laxative abuse were identified at two institutions. They were metabolically tested with serum studies and 24-h urine analysis. Three of the patients had 24-h urine studies while taking laxatives and after a 1-mo hiatus from laxatives. Serum electrolytes revealed normal parameters, except magnesium and potassium, which were at the lower limit of normal, and bicarbonate, which was low in five patients. Twenty-four-hour urine studies showed decrease in volume, sodium, potassium, magnesium, phosphorus, uric acid, and citrate. In the three patients who submitted a repeat study while not taking laxatives for a month, all values normalized. Laxative abuse may cause metabolic acidosis, or alkalosis, depending on how long term and regular the usage occurs and the amount of subsequent bicarbonate loss. Laxative abuse produces a state similar to that of the endemic stone formation; low urine output, diarrhea and resulting gastrointestinal (GI) electrolyte losses, sterile urine, and decreased phosphorus in the urine. The GI water and electrolyte loss produces a volume-contracted state with potassium depletion and an intracellular acidosis, leading to low urine volume, sodium, potassium, and citrate. Increased ammonia in the urine interacts with the urate, which, because of the low urine sodium, becomes ammonium acid urate instead of the usual soluble sodium urate *(22)*.

HIV infected patients represent an additional group that is more predisposed to AAU stone formation *(23)*. In a small series of 11 stones formed by patients taking indinavir, 2 (18%) were composed of AAU. In a manner similar to that of laxative abusers, the mechanism of AAU formation is thought to be related to the chronic diarrhea and malnutrition.

Although the exact mechanisms for formation of AAU stones are not known, the renal physiology surrounding AAU stone formation is well characterized. The pH at which a minimum concentration of AAU will crystallize occurs at 6.2–6.3 *(24)*. As the pH increases, a higher concentration of AAU is required for stone crystals to form. At the level of the nephron, ammonia is produced in the proximal convoluted tubule (PCT). Ammonia is used by the kidney as an acid buffer. Increased amounts of ammonium are excreted in states of metabolic acidosis, as well as potassium depletion, which is a form of intracellular acidosis *(25)*. Uric acid, which comes from urate in the serum, is freely filtered at the glomerulus, and 99% reabsorbed in the PCT. Fifty percent of the original filtered load is then secreted by the PCT, and all but 10% gets reabsorbed. After leaving the nephron, the form of urate is pH dependent. At its dissociation constant, a pKa of 5.7, uric acid and urate exist in a 50:50 ratio. As the pH increases, the urate predominates, usually in the form of sodium urate.

Uric acid stone formers with urinary tract infections from urea splitting organisms are at risk for AAU formation. When these patients have sterile urine, normal ammonium, hyperuricosuria, and any pH, AAU will not form. However, in the face of urinary infection with urea splitting organisms, the increased pH and elevated ammonium make AAU formation (with struvite) likely if enough urate is present *(14,21)*. This situation must be considered in patients with urinary tract infections who are afflicted with the Lesch–Nyhan syndrome, as these patients are uric acid stone formers. Some may treat Lesch–

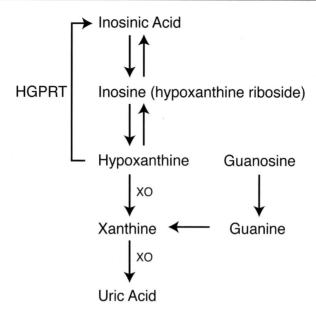

HGPRT - hypoxanthine guanine phosphoribosyl transferase
XO - xanthine oxidase

Fig. 3. Uric acid metabolism.

Nyhan patients with urinary tract infections with temporary allopurinol to decrease the amount of urate, lowering the chance of AAU stone formation *(26)*.

Treatment of these stones, after elimination of existing stones, is aimed at prevention. Acute stones may be successfully treated with SWL, although slow dissolution with cessation of laxatives and proper fluid intake has been described *(21)*. After initial treatment, risk factors must be identified for preventive counseling and treatment. Patients should have follow-up with multiple twenty-four urine studies to ensure adequate treatment and compliance. Patients with diarrhea from ileostomies must maintain proper urine volume and electrolyte replacement, and must be followed with 24-h urine studies. Recurrent urinary infections must be eliminated, especially in patients who form uric acid stones. Uric acid stone patients need treatment with alkalinization, volume and if hyperuricosuric, dietary restriction and allopurinol. Ammonium acid urate stones are rare, and occur in discrete situations. Stone analysis provides definitive diagnosis. Awareness of the conditions that predispose their formation will prevent confusion with other radiolucent stone types.

Xanthine Stones

Primary xanthine stones are found only in patients with hereditary xanthinuria. Xanthinuria is a metabolic disorder of purine metabolism, which is passed on in an autosomal recessive pattern. This disorder is characterized by a deficiency of xanthine oxidase, which prevents the conversion of hypoxanthine to xanthine, and further prevents xanthine from being converted into uric acid (Fig. 3). Serum and urine uric acid levels are extremely low (serum 0.8–1.0) *(27,28)*, and the uric acid precursors, xanthine and hypoxanthine, are elevated. After being excreted, xanthine precipitates in the urine to form stones. Hypoxanthine, being more soluble, does not form stones. Stone formation is the primary manifestation of this disease, and occurs in approximately one-third of affected patients (27).

Xanthine stones are radiolucent, but can be detected by using computed tomography (CT) (29). Usual excretion of xanthine and hypoxanthine is between 10 and 20 mg/24 h, but during allopurinol therapy, these amounts may exceed 150 mg. However, in patients with excess production of urate, the values can be as high as 700 mg/24 h (30). The solubility of xanthine increases from a concentration of 5 mg/100 mL at a pH of 5 to 13 mg/100 mL at a pH of 7 (31). This relatively moderate increase in solubility places more importance on increased urinary output and dietary purine restriction, rather than on pH modulation as the primary therapy for prevention of xanthine stones. Analysis of xanthine stones have revealed stones of xanthine mixed with oxypurinol in patients treated with xanthine oxidase inhibitors (32) and stones made of almost pure xanthine (27). They are described as faintly radiopaque (27,32).

Secondary xanthine stones are also formed under several specific circumstances. Patients with Lesch–Nyhan syndrome have a deficiency of the enzyme hypoxanthine guanine phosphoribosyl transferase (HGPRT), which is important in the purine salvage pathway (Fig. 1). Without HGPRT, hypoxanthine cannot be taken back into the salvage pathway, and is consequently metabolized by xanthine oxidase (XO) to uric acid, the end product of the pathway. As a result, Lesch-Nyhan patients are hyperuricemic and hyperuricosuric. These metabolic abnormalities are treated with urinary alkalinization and allopurinol, which inhibits xanthine oxidase, lowering the uric acid production and decreasing the incidence of uric acid stone formation. However, in rare cases, the inactivation of xanthine oxidase by allopurinol may lead to the formation of stones by an excess of xanthine, the precursor to uric acid (30,32). Attempts at dissolution of allopurinol induced xanthine stones with alternating acidic and basic solutions has been described in vitro, but has not been developed into clinical treatment (32). Some have used high dose allopurinol in the face of urinary tract infection for Lesch–Nyhan patients to decrease the risk of ammonium acid urate stones, and have reported xanthine stones as an effect of this therapy (33). To date, the optimal prevention of xanthine stones in Lesch–Nyhan patients on allopurinol therapy is achieved by continuing allopurinol, but placing added emphasis on their hydration and alkalinization.

Another situation in which secondary xanthine stones have been described is with the use of allopurinol to treat the state of hyperuricemia seen in hematopoetic malignancies. The urate overproduction seen in hematopoetic malignancies comes from cell breakdown, which result in uric acid excretion up to four-times normal, especially during the rapid cell lysis associated with chemotherapy or radiotherapy (34). The side effects of nausea and vomiting can interfere with proper fluid intake, or worse cause dehydration, further increasing the risk of stone formation in this patient population. Rarely, the use of allopurinol for inhibition of XO to decrease the uric acid in these patients will result in excess xanthine accumulation and xanthine stone formation.

The formation of xanthine stones in the hematopoetic malignancy patient population is through a similar mechanism by which the Lesch–Nyhan patients form xanthine stones. Unlike Lesch–Nyhan patients, who fail to properly metabolize uric acid precursors via the purine salvage pathway, the metabolic abnormality in patients with hematopoetic malignancies is urate overproduction. The excess urate overloads the purine salvage pathway, leading to uric acid production as the method of ridding the body of the excess by-products released by the malignancy. The massive uric acid excretion places these patients at risk for uric acid urolithiasis, and to prevent this, patients are prophylactically treated with allopurinol, alkalinization, and increased diuresis (3000 mL/d) before the initiation of chemotherapy *(35)*. Paradoxically, the allopurinol used to prevent uric acid stones can lead to excess accumulation of xanthine, leading to xanthine urolithiasis. These stones rarely form when patients adhere to recommended fluid intake.

Formation of xanthine stones has been described in patients with uric acid nephrolithiasis or gout who are treated with allopurinol *(36)*. Certainly, with the administration of allopurinol, the excess xanthine and hypoxanthine will be excreted in the urine. However, allopurinol does not completely inhibit XO at usual doses. Consequently, one will rarely see serum urate levels drop below 3 mg/dL or urinary urate levels below 250 mg/d. Xanthine stones are not likely to form at these levels *(28)*. Patients with uric acid nephrolithiasis or gout on allopurinol therapy can further decrease their risk by adhering to recommended fluid intake.

Acute stone episodes should be managed in the usual manner to control symptoms. If operative therapy is required, xanthine stones may be treated endourologically or by shockwave lithotripsy (SWL)*(37)*. Outside of the patient population with hereditary xanthinuria, xanthine stones are quite rare, even in the specific instances, described here, which increase the risk of secondary xanthine stones. Primarily, preventive therapy is achieved through adequate intake of fluids. Urine alkalinization also increases xanthine solubility in the urine.

MEDICATION-RELATED STONES

Ephedrine Stones

Ephedrine and its metabolites, pseudoephedrine and norephedrine, have recently been shown to be capable of forming urinary calculi *(38)*. This initial report resulted from a patient who chronically abused ephedrine containing medication, and ingested up to 120 ephedrine containing tablets daily (25 mg/tablet). Subsequent reports outline small series of patients with ephedrine stones, many of whom abuse the medication for stimulatory effects *(39,40)*. Often a history of drug or alcohol abuse may be elicited. Claims of euphoria, increased energy, heightened sexual tension, weight reduction, and addition of muscle mass are justification given by those abusing ephedrine *(39)*. Some patients receive ephedrine in drugs made for bronchodilating effects, which become less noticed after long term use. Patients then increase the dosage, leading to the high doses that cause calculi *(39)*.

Ephedrine stones are radiolucent, but may be visualized by CT. They are easily fragmented with SWL *(39)*. To improve diagnosis, attention must be given to obtaining a proper drug history and social history for previous substance abuse. Treatment is aimed at reduction of ephedrine intake, and increase of urinary output.

Substance abuse counseling is recommended for abusers of ephedrine or users with a history of substance abuse not only to prevent further stone episodes, but also to avoid more serious sequelae of ephedrine abuse. The potential for major complications exist, including but not limited to death, myocardial infarction, stroke, respiratory depression, seizure, hypertension, cardiac arrhythmia, and headache. Over 100 ephedrine stones were identified at a single stone analysis company (L. Herring) between January 1996 and June 1997, out of over 166,000 samples *(40)*. Although the incidence was only 0.064%, one must believe that this represents only a small portion of the ephedrine abusers who form stones.

Guaifenesin Stones

Approved by the FDA for over the counter use in 1989, guaifenesin is a common component of cough/cold medications, which often contain ephedrine *(41)*. Guaifenesin containing urinary calculi were first noted in 1999 *(42,39)*. Specifically, the guaifenesin metabolite, β-(2-methoxyphenoxy)-lactic acid, is the component found in the calculi *(42)*. The majority of the affected patients were abusers of the offending medications (refer to the section on ephedrine stones). Many were abusing the medication for the effect of the ephedrine. Because the FDA, in 1994, limited the amount of pure ephedrine that may be contained in medication *(43)*, abusers take larger amounts of predominantly guaifenesin containing preparations for the effect of the minor component, ephedrine *(42)*. Some, however, were taking customary doses of the medications, but were simultaneously taking numerous preparations that contained guaifenesin, resulting in excessive guaifenisin intake *(42)*.

Patients using prescribed amounts as directed by the manufacturer for the treatment of colds, coughs, or allergies are at almost no risk of forming stones composed of guaifenesin. Like ephedrine stones, guaifenesin stones are radiolucent, but can be seen on CT scanning. They are easily fragmented with SWL *(39)*.

Indinavir Stones (Fig. 4)

Indinavir stones were first described in 1995 *(44–46)*. Used in the treatment of the HIV virus, indinavir competitively inhibits HIV protease and decreases viral load by 90–99%. Indinavir is commonly used with reverse transcriptase inhibitors such as nucleoside analogues and/or nonnucleoside reverse transcriptase inhibitors as part of a multi-drug antiretroviral regimen. Indications for use of antiretroviral therapy in HIV infected individuals include acute HIV syndrome, symptomatic disease, and asymptomatic disease with low CD4+ T cell counts or with elevated HIV titer. Treatment may also be offered to uninfected individuals for the purpose of postexposure prophylaxis following an exposure to HIV *(47)*.

Indinavir is predominantly excreted in the feces after hepatic metabolism. Nineteen percent, however, is excreted in the urine *(48)*. Patients taking this medication may form indinavir crystals in their urine, leading to stone formation. Indinavir crystals are very distinctive, with a fan-shaped or starburst type of appearance. They have been described in 20% of patients on indinavir *(49)*. When examined with microscopy, crystalluria has been reported to occur in over 30% of patients on indinavir therapy *(50)*. Indinavir stones were first thought to have an incidence of 2–12 % *(51–53)*; however, much higher rates of over 40% have also been reported *(54)*. In populations of patients on indinavir therapy, the average time to stone episodes has varied from 21 wk (range 6–50) *(55)* to 11 mo (range 4–19) *(56)*.

The etiology of stones among patients taking indinavir was examined in a group of 11 patients who passed a stone that underwent analysis *(23)*. Of these 11, only 4 patients (36%) had stones with indinavir as a detected component; the remainder was composed of calcium oxalate (3), calcium phosphate (1), ammonium acid urate (2), and uric acid

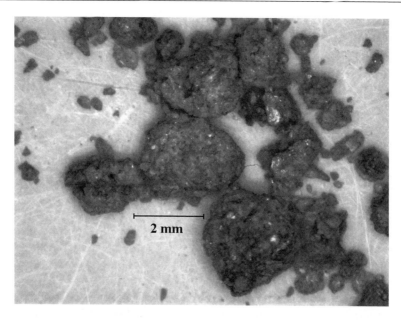

Fig 4. Indinivir calculus (Courtesy of Mission Pharmacal, San Antonio, Texas).

(1). Additionally, nine patients taking indinavir underwent 24-h urine testing, which revealed hypocitraturia (3), hyperoxaluria (2), hypomagnesuria (2), hypercalciuria (1), and hyperuricosuria (2). Although previous stone history was not discussed and the patient numbers were limited, this series reveals abnormal urine testing and the formation of stones primarily from components other than indinavir. This data suggests that stone formation by patients on indinavir therapy may have a substantial metabolic component, in addition to the effects of urinary indinavir excretion.

Indinavir crystals form at a pH of 7 (57) and are soluble at a pH of 4.5 in vitro (56). Although such an acidic pH is difficult to obtain in vivo, short term acidification of 2–3 d for treatment of stone episodes has been suggested (51) to help partially dissolve stones to facilitate passage. Acidification may result in deposition of uric acid crystals (56), further exacerbating episodes, although risk is small in the short term. The metabolic acidosis and hypocitraturia caused by urinary acidification may also result in calcium oxalate supersaturation (58). Increasing the intake of citrate containing fluids (lemonade) may decrease the risk of stone calcification. Concern has been raised regarding the hypothetical risk of virus mutation and subsequent development of resistance during temporary cessation of indinavir (47), but no evidence exists to support this.

Pure indinavir calculi are radiolucent and are unique in that they are not visualized on spiral CT scanning (59). On gross appearance, pure indinavir stones are brown and have a pliable, puttylike consistency.

Conservative management successfully treats most stone episodes. Treatment consists of hydration, analgesics, and temporary withdrawal of indinavir (60–62). Temporary urinary acidification may be considered. One must keep a low threshold for emergent stent placement, as these patients may be dangerously immunosuppressed. After resolution of a stone episode, indinavir may be restarted and increased oral hydration may be initiated (61).

If conservative measures fail, indinavir stones may be fragmented and removed endoscopically. Shock wave lithotripsy has been used to successfully treat indinavir stones *(56)*.

It is not understood why some patients taking indinavir form urinary crystals and stones whereas others do not. Risk factors for the formation of indinavir stones are unknown. At this time, adequate hydration, 2 L daily, is the best prevention *(54,64)*. To minimize recurrence, patients with stones of mixed composition or with a history of stones may benefit from metabolic evaluation. HIV patients need continuation of indinavir for optimal treatment of their disease, and because almost 10% of patients have discontinued the use of indinavir because of nephrolithiasis, maximal effort must be given to prevention of stones in this patient population.

Nelfinavir Stones

The most recent medication to cause stone formation is nelfinavir, a protease inhibitor used for the treatment of the HIV virus. Before 2002, nephrolithiasis owing to protease inhibitors as an etiology had only been described with indinavir. However, stones composed of nelfinavir have now been reported *(65)*.

Similar to indinavir stones, those composed of nelfinavir are radiolucent. However, in contrast to indinavir calculi, nelfinavir stones are visible on CT scan *(65)*. Nelfinavir stones are successfully fragmented with SWL, or may be treated with other forms of stone ablation.

In one report, a patient had a short course of indinavir therapy and changed to nelfinavir because of intolerable side effects. Subsequently, the patient developed a large renal pelvis calculus. The stone composition was 99% nelfinavir and 1% indinavir. As only 1–2% on nelfinavir is excreted in the urine, compared to 20% of indinavir, it was postulated that indinavir crystals may have provided the nidus for nelfinavir stone formation *(65,66)*.

Patients on other lithogenic medications and patients with a history of nephrolithiasis who also have a need for nelfinavir may benefit from metabolic evaluation and surveillance to keep stone episodes minimized.

Oxypurinol Stones

Oxypurinol was an early xanthine oxidase inhibitor, but was abandoned in favor of allopurinol, in part owing to the improved urinary solubility of allopurinol. Oxypurinol is the primary metabolite of allopurinol and is excreted via the kidneys. Although allopurinol is broken down into an oxypurinol component, about half is excreted as allopurinol, keeping the oxypurinol excretion lower than if oxypurinol were the only drug administered *(67)*. The presence of oxypurinol has been detected in stones produced by patients with the Lesch–Nyhan syndrome who were on allopurinol therapy *(68)*. Oxypurinol as a primary stone constituent, mixed with xanthine (increased excretion owing to the xanthine oxidase inhibitor) and uric acid, has also been described in patients on high dose allopurinol (600 mg/d) for prophylaxis of uric acid stones *(69)*. These stones are described as radiolucent *(69)*. Oxypurinol has not been described as a constituent with calcium stones. In fact, there is no interaction between oxypurinol and either calcium or oxalate at oxypurinol concentrations expected with therapeutic doses of allopurinol *(70)*.

The presence of oxypurinol as a stone constituent is primarily seen in patients using high dose (600 mg/d) allopurinol. Patients with oxypurinol as a stone constituent may benefit from a decrease in the allopurinol dosing, although, because these stones are uncommonly rare, the risks and benefits in modification of allopurinol dosing should be carefully considered. Metabolic studies of 24-h uric acid excretion will reveal how much of an advantage, if any, exists with increased doses of allopurinol. This can be compared to the increased oxypurinol excretion resulting from increased allopurinol dosing; approximately half of an allopurinol dose is excreted as oxypurinol. One report *(69)* showed, with constant diet, uric acid excretion falling from 481 to 346 to 334 mg/d on 0, 300, and 900 mg allopurinol daily. On the same respective allopurinol doses, oxypurinol excretion increased from 0 to 243 to 440 mg/d, and xanthine excretion increased from 6 to 47 to 145 mg/d. The patient identified in this report showed only a minute benefit in uric acid excretion with an allopurinol increase of 300 to 900 mg/d, yet the daily excretion of oxypurinol and xanthine increased by over 80% and 200% respectively. In this instance, the 3% decrease in uric acid excretion must be weighed against the 80% increase in oxypurinol excretion in this patient who produced stones made of oxypurinol (major constituent) and xanthine.

If high allopurinol doses reveal a treatment advantage as seen with 24-h urine analysis, a decrease of the allopurinol dose might place the patient at risk for other clinical problems. Increasing urine output to dilute urinary oxypurinol concentration may better serve the patient. Twenty-four hour urine studies will help guide therapy on an individual basis. Continued radiolucent stone formation while on allopurinol therapy should raise suspicion to other types of stones, and oxypurinol must be considered as a possibility. For accurate stone analysis, special notation should be made on analysis requests to reflect this suspicion.

Silicate Stones

Silicate urinary calculi occur exclusively in patients taking large amounts of magnesium silicate antacids. In 1912, silica stones were first found in cattle living in sandy areas *(71)*. The first human patient with silicate stones was reported in 1953 *(72)*. This patient had gastric ulcers and ingested 2 g daily of magnesium trisilicate, an antacid. Subsequently, other reports of silicate stones have been presented, all involving patients with a history of silicate abuse *(73–76)*. Invariably, sufferers of silicate stones also have associated upper gastrointestinal disease such as esophagitis, gastric ulcers, gastritis, or hiatal hernia, prompting them to abuse magnesium trisilicate antacids.

No report exists linking an episode of silicate stones to any source other than silicate antacids. The only report suggesting another etiology was regarding a patient who died in the months before establishment of silicate antacids as an etiology. This patient's family reported no knowledge of abdominal pain or antacid use; this is the only reported case of silicate stones in a patient not on silicate antacid therapy *(77)*. It has also been postulated, although never reported, that methyl polysiloxane, or dimethicone, used for prevention of flatulence, may be a source of urinary silica *(77)*.

As in other unusual stones, failure to suspect silicate stones leads to a delay in diagnosis and prevention. A 1973 report outlines a 5-yr delay in diagnosis in a patient with multiple stone passages; part of the explanation for the delay was poor quality of stone analysis *(74)*. The gross appearance of silica stones can resemble the gross appearance of calcium oxalate jackstones. Electron microscopy, however, reveals the subtle difference of the spikes blending into the body in silica, whereas they appear more demarcated from the body on calcium oxalate jackstones *(78)*. This reinforces the value of quality stone analysis. The potential delay in diagnosis also reinforces the need to send the stones for analysis. We recommend that all radiolucent stones be analyzed in new patients, as well as patients who fail alkalinization therapy.

Silicate stones are generally described as faintly calcified, similar to cysteine *(74–76)*, or radiolucent uric acid stones *(73)*. Urine studies of human volunteers ingesting 5 g of magnesium trisilicate daily revealed that about 5% of the ingested silica was excreted in the urine *(79)*. After ingestion of silicate, exposure to hydrochloric acid causes the formation of a soluble colloid made of silica. Further exposure to alkali propagated other silica compounds that were more soluble and absorbable *(79)*. In canines with silicate urolithiasis, pH varied from acidic to basic.

The treatment of silicate stones is straightforward. Acute stone management proceeds with no deviation from standard protocol. After stone passage or SWL *(80)*, cessation of the magnesium trisilicates prevents further episodes.

One might expect that silica stones may become historical as a result of decreased usage of magnesium trisilicates and awareness of potential stone formation. More importantly, improved therapy for gastric ulcers and dyspepsia (H2 blockers, proton pump inhibitors) results in decreased usage of magnesium trisilicates. However, a new case report was published out of Spain in 2000 *(81)*. Silicate stones are among the rarest of the unusual stones, and are always linked to a history of antacid abuse, specifically those containing magnesium trisilicates.

Sulfa Stones

One of the oldest examples of medication related urinary lithiasis came after use of sulfa containing drugs around the time of World War II. Despite improved solubility in the urine, present day sulfa compounds, such as acetylsulfamethoxazole, acetylsulfasoxazole, acetylsulfaguanadine, and sulfadiazine may precipitate in the urine *(82)*. Stones composed of not only sulfamethoxazole, but trimethoprim as well, have also been described *(83)*. Most patients formed stones within 1–4 wk of initiating sulfa therapy.

Primary metabolism of sulfa medication occurs by acetylation in the liver, followed by excretion via the kidneys. The crystals are formed with the relatively insoluble acetylated sulfa metabolites *(85)*. The main factors that are involved with formation of sulfa crystals are drug concentration in the urine, degree of acetylation of the drug, urinary stasis, urine pH, and temperature of the urine *(85,86)*. Higher dosage and longer duration of treatment also increase the risk of stone formation *(85)*. However, small dosages, in either single or repeated doses, can lead to crystal formation, especially in patients with infection or obstruction *(85)*.

Acetylsulfapyridine, the acetylated metabolite of sulfasalazine, which is used in the treatment of ulcerative colitis, has caused rare instances of urinary stone formation *(84)*. Exacerbations of inflammatory bowel disease, leading to prolonged episodes of diarrhea can leave these patients in a state of dehydration with low urine output. This increases the concentration of acetylsulfapyridine in the urine, and increases the risk of stone formation. Acetylsulfapyridine stones are described as faintly calcified, but visible on X-rays. A large series of sulfa stones, which included 35 stones analyzed by a research laboratory, revealed that most were found in the bladder *(85)*.

Treatment of sulfa stones, or suspected sulfa stones may benefit from urinary alkalinization, as sulfa crystals are more soluble at higher a pH. If the patient is anuric or oliguric, evaluation to rule out medical renal disease is in order as sulfonamides have a long history of causing renal toxicity, especially in patients with preexisting or acute renal insufficiency *(87)*. When surgical intervention is warranted, these calculi may be successfully treated with SWL *(84)*.

The primary prevention of sulfa containing stones is increased urinary volume. Patients with a history of urinary stone formation may benefit from alternative antibiotics.

Topiramate Induced Stones

Topiramate, an anticonvulsant used to treat refractory partial seizures in adults, is associated with a 1–2% increased risk of urinary stone formation *(88,89)*. Stones are primarily calcium phosphate in nature, and consequently are radiopaque. Current information on this medication does not reflect content of topiramate or a metabolite as a stone constituent. The proposed mechanism for stone formation is via an inhibition of carbonic anhydrase by topiramate, which can cause urinary alkalinization and hypocitraturia. Observed urinary effects were similar to that seen during acetazolamide therapy *(90)*.

Although the increased risk of stone formation in patients who take topiramate is small, one may reconsider usage of this medication in patients with other predisposing factors for stone formation *(89)*. On the other hand, patients with refractory neurologic disease requiring such medication might be better served with multidisciplinary treatment to add input from urology or nephrology to existing neurology care. This could help provide a continuation of topiramate and the neurologic benefit of its effects, while concurrently offering stone prophylaxis via citrate supplementation and close monitoring of their metabolic risk factors.

Triamterene Stones

Triamterene is a potassium sparing diuretic that has been used commercially since the 1960s. Triamterene acts in the distal tubule, inhibiting the reabsorption of sodium ions in exchange for potassium and hydrogen ions. Triamterene is used for the treatment of hypertension, usually in combination with hydrochlorothiazide. Triamterene is initially metabolized in the liver, with a half-life of 90–120 min *(91)*. The metabolites, as well as about 20% of unchanged triamterene, are then excreted in the urine *(92)*. Triamterene containing urinary calculi were first described in 1979 *(93)*.

In 1980, fifty-thousand stones analyzed by a commercial company (Herring, Orlando, FL) revealed 180 with a triamterene component. This corresponds to an annual incidence of 1/1500 patients taking triamterene *(94)*. Unless the stone has large calcium components, triamterene calculi are radiolucent. Triamterene stones are, however, detectable with CT scanning *(95)*. Triamterene is most commonly seen as a secondary component of calcium oxalate or uric acid stones, and has been described as a nidus for secondary stone formation *(94)*.

Triamterene is excreted through the kidneys in 3 components: unchanged triamterene, hydroxytriamterene, and hydroxytriamterene sulfate. Triamterene is soluble in urine with concentrations below 36 μg/mL, and hydroxytriamterene sulfate is soluble below concentrations of 30μg/mL. Urinary pH has no effect on the solubility of triamterene and its metabolites. Although triamterene sulfate is the primary metabolite seen in serum and urine, unchanged triamterene is the predominant constituent of calculi *(96)*. Triamterene spherules resembling a Maltese cross may be seen under polarized light microscopy, and are pathognomonic for triamterene *(97)*. On average, triamterene stone content is followed in descending order by hydroxytriamterene sulfate and hydroxytriamterene, but considerable variation exists between individual stones (one stone was reported to be composed of >99% hydroxytriamterene) *(96)*. Most triamterene-containing stones are comprised of less than 5% total weight of triamterene and its metabolites.

Patients with a history of liver disease may benefit from avoiding triamterene. One series of 1500 analyzed stones revealed that of the three patients who formed triamterene stones, two had chronic active hepatitis and the third had macronodular hepatic cirrhosis *(97)*. No studies exist on this patient population that examine the urine or serum for increased levels of the drug, however, stone analysis of these three patients revealed the presence of porphyrins. This could be due to increased excretion of porphyrin metabolites in patients with hepatic dysfunction, and it is postulated that the increased urinary porphyrin could act as a lithogenic cofactor in the crystallization of triamterene *(97)*.

Special notation should be made when submitting stone analyses of patients who take triamterene. Patients on triamterene therapy who pass a triamterene stone, or any other stone, should discontinue the medication in favor of other antihypertensives *(98)*. Initiation of triamterene therapy should be made with caution in patients with a history of stone passage. Because most of the stones have only small amounts of triamterene, and the mechanism of formation is not clearly understood, one must consider the potential risk of adding the lithogenic agent that drives a patient from a nonstone-forming state to a stone-forming state.

Triamterene stones may be treated with SWL, or with endourologic surgery. After the stone has been removed, triamterene should be discontinued in favor of a nonlithogenic antihypertensive.

PEDIATRIC STONES

Pediatric stones may be categorized into two groups; stones in premature low birth-weight infants and stones in children and adolescents.

Nephrocalcinosis in Premature Low Birth-Weight Infants

Nephrocalcinosis in premature low birth-weight infants is thought to be from the hypercalciuric effects of the furosemide used to treat the lung problems seen in the premature patient population. Commonly, these patients require lengthy periods of immobility and mechanical ventilation, extended courses of furosemide, and restriction of fluid. In these patients, the incidence of nephrolithiasis is 48–65% *(99–101)*. Nephrocalcinosis has also been seen in premature infants who did not receive furosemide *(102–104)*, and hypercalciuria has been shown to be present in virtually all premature births *(105,106)*.

Other metabolic abnormalities may also lead to stone formation in premature low birth weight infants. Acidosis may lead to hypocitraturia, and vitamin D supplementation or steroid administration may also increase urinary calcium *(107)*. Furthermore, when these patients are treated with hyperalimentation, urinary oxalate excretion is elevated *(108,109)*. Finally, compared to term infants, premature infants had higher urinary oxalate levels *(109)*.

Approximately 50% of the premature infants with nephrocalcinosis will have spontaneous resolution of their stones with withdrawal of the furosemide *(110)*. The only factor identified that reveals increased risk of persistent nephrocalcinosis is an increased serum calcium to creatinine ratio at diagnosis while on furosemide therapy; average value for patients who showed resolution was 0.38 whereas average value for patients who had persistent nephrocalcinosis was 2.23 *(110)*. The use of thiazide diuretics has been reported to stop or reverse the nephrocalcinosis seen in premature infants.

Acute problems include gross hematuria, sepsis from urinary tract infection, ureteral obstruction, and acute renal failure *(111,112)*. Long-term significance is debated. Although studies have shown no long-term adverse effects in kidneys with nephro-calcinosis *(113,114)*, conflicting studies suggest a potential for diminished renal growth and renal function *(102,115)*. Consequently, these patients need metabolic workup and diligent followup to insure stability of renal function and existing stones.

Stones in Children and Adolescents

Studies from pediatric urologic centers reveal structural abnormalities with an incidence of 32-35% in children with nephrolithiasis *(116–118)*. A high association with urinary tract infection, up to 75%, was also noted *(117)*. In children without anatomical abnormality, underlying metabolic abnormalities are present 90% of the time.

Children do not present with the classic renal colic seen in adults. Most are found during a urinary tract infection workup. Most other symptoms are hematuria and abdominal pain. Presenting symptoms vary with age, as well. Preschool age children are more likely to present with urinary tract infection, whereas older children more commonly present with pain as a chief complaint. Patients present with the classic renal colic less than 15% of the time *(117)*. Average age of presentation usually occurs between 8 and 10 yr of age, with a male:female pattern of 1.5:1 *(117)*.

Diagnosis may be made with IVP, spiral CT, or ultrasound. If IVP is performed, genitalia and gonads need protection, and the IVP may be modified to minimize radiation exposure. The pediatric population requires surgical therapy more often than adults, about two-thirds of the time *(119,120)*. After resolution of the stone, complete workup is mandatory. Numerous genetic diseases (Dent's disease, primary hyperoxaluria, cystinuria, APRT deficiency, orotic aciduria, xanthinuria, familial hyperuricosuria) cause pediatric nephrolithiasis, and should be discovered early so that preventative treatment can be started. If no genetic diagnosis is revealed, then a metabolic work up is mandatory. Attention must be given to age-adjusted normal values, because oxalate, citrate, uric acid, and calcium excretion is much higher in the first 2 yr of life. Diet must be considered; infants fed human breast milk have the highest calcium excretion, whereas those fed soy milk have the lowest calcium excretion *(121)*. For school age children, calcium excretion is less than 4 mg/kg/d, uric acid is less than 0.56 mg/dL GFR, oxalate is less than 50 mg/1.73m^2/d, citrate is greater than 400 mg/g creatinine, and urinary volume should be over 20 mL/kg/d *(122)*. Serum studies should include creatinine, uric acid, bicarbonate, phosphorus, and calcium.

In children, the most common metabolic abnormality is idiopathic hypercalciuria *(116,123)*. This should be confirmed with a 24-h urine collection, as random collections are affected by food intake *(124)*. Twenty-four hour calcium to creatinine ratio should be determined; if the value is less than 0.2, further work-up is not necessary *(122)*. Values are higher in younger patients; normal calcium to creatinine ratio for infants to 6 mo of age is 0.8, and 0.6 from 6 mo to 1 yr of life *(125)*. Urinary citrate should be obtained, as low citrate excretion needs further work-up to rule out distal renal tubular acidosis. Serum calcium and phosphate values will rule out hyperparathyroidism. However, if calcium is elevated or if phosphate is decreased, then intact PTH levels should be obtained.

Table 2
Characteristics of Various Unusual Calculi: Are They Successfully Treated With Shock-Wave
Lithotripsy? Are They Seen On CT Scan? Are They Radiolucent On KUB?

	SWL	CT	KUB[a]
2, 8-DHA	Yes	Yes	No
AAU	Yes	Yes	No
Silicate	Yes	Yes	No/sometimes faint
Triamterene	Yes	Yes	No
Topiramate (Ca Phosphate)	Yes[b]	Yes	Yes
Ephedrine	Yes	Yes	No
Guafenesin	Yes	Yes	No
Oxypurinol	No data[c]	Yes	No
Xanthine	Yes	Yes	Faint
Indinavir	Yes	**No**	No
Nelfinavir	Yes	Yes	No
Sulfa	Yes	Yes	Faint

As they are commonly a constituent of a mixed stone, rare stones are likely to respond to SWL, as the varying components throughout the mixed stone provide differences in impedance for SWL forces.

[a]If pure; however, often stones are mixed (or nidus), which may be radiopaque.

[b]Some Ca Phosphate stones may be resistant to SWL.

[c]Oxypurinol stones have been described as components mixed with xanthine and uric acid, which are both treatable with SWL.

Additionally, endemic bladder stones are seen in foreign countries in which the pediatric diet is low in phosphorus (breast milk, polished rice). Low dietary phosphorus results in high ammonia excretion, leading to formation of ammonium acid urate (AAU) crystals (see section on AAU). Oxalate containing vegetables may exacerbate the effects of the low phosphorus diet. Finally, high protein diets decrease citrate excretion. As third world diets are not always balanced, children eating otherwise healthy foods in unbalanced quantities may become predisposed to formation of stones.

All pediatric stone formers need comprehensive work-up for the etiology of their stones. If recurrent or radiolucent, consideration should be give to the possibility of rare metabolic origin (2, 8-DHA, xanthine).

CONCLUSIONS

Although the definitive diagnosis of the unusual stone is via stone analysis, an increased awareness of the pathways effecting formation of these stones leads to heightened clinical awareness and improved treatment outcomes. If pure in composition, most rare stones are radiolucent (Table 2), however, many rare stones are mixed with other components. For example, heterogeneous nucleation may allow calcium or struvite to collect on rare crystals that might otherwise remain insignificant. Likewise, uric acid may act as a nidus for xanthine or AAU stones. These examples illustrate that unusual stone components may represent only a portion of the overall stone problem.

Radiolucent stones in the pediatric population should raise high suspicion for existence of unusual stones. Whether their stones are lucent or opaque, we believe pediatric stone forming patients should undergo comprehensive work-up.

In general, treatment of unusual stones varies depending on the individual stone type. Often, patients cannot withdraw safely from lithogenic medications, such as indinavir or topiramate; consequently, adequate hydration to maintain dilute urine becomes especially important. Patients with unusual stones will require close, long-term monitoring of their particular risk factors. Some relatives of metabolic stone patients will benefit from genetic screening, especially relatives of those with 2,8-dihydroxyadenine calculi, as that can present with renal insufficiency. When surgical therapy is necessary, all endourological forms of stone treatment may be employed. In most instances, SWL successfully fragments unusual stones (Table 2).

Although relatively rare, the diagnosis and treatment of unusual stones represents an important challenge to urologists.

REFERENCES

1. Edvardsson V, Palsson R, Olafsson I, Hjaltadottir G, Laxdal T. Clinical features and genotype of adenine phosphoribosyltransferase deficiency in Iceland Am J Kidney Dis 2001; 38: 473–480.
2. Simmonds HA, Van Acker KJ, Cameron JS, Snedden W. The identification of 2,8-dihydroxyadenine, a new component of urinary stones. Biochem J 1976; 157: 485-487.
3. Gault MH, Simmonds HA, Snedden W, Dow D, Churchill DN, Penney H. Urolitiasis due to 2,8-dihydroxyadenine in an adult, NEJM 1981; 305: 1570.
4. Sahots AS, Tirshfield JA, Kamatani N, Simmonds HA. Adenine phosphoribosyl transferase deficiency and 2,8-dihydroxyadenine lithiasis. In: Scriver CR, Beaudet AL, Sly WS, Valle D, eds. *The Metabolic and Molecular Basis of Inherited Disease*. 8th ed. McGraw-Hill, New York, 2001: 2571–2584.
5. Deng L, Yang M, Frund S, et al. 2,8-dihydroxyadenine urolithiasis in a patient with considerable residual phosphoribosyl transferase activity in cell extracts but with mutations in both copies of *APRT*. Mol Genet Metab 2001; 72: 260–264.
6. Hesse A, Miersch WD, Classen A, Thon A, Doppler W. 2,8-dihydroxyadeninuria: laboratory diagnosis and therapy control, Urol Int 1988; 43: 174–178.
7. Cartier P, Hamet M. Une nouvelle maladie metabolique: le deficit complet en adenine-phosphoribosyl-transferase avec lithiase de 3,8-dihydroxyadenine. Cemptes rendus hebdomadaires des séances de l'Academie des sciences, Serie D, Sciences Noevrelles 1974; 279: 883–886.
8. Joost J, Doppler W. 2,8-dihydroxyadenine Stones in Children, Urology 1982; 20: 67–70.
9. Simmonds HA. 2,8-dihydroxyadeninuria, or when is a uric acid stone not a uric acid stone, Clin Nephrol 1979; 12: 195.
10. DeJong DJ, Assman JJ, De Abreu RA, Monnens LA, Van Liebergen JH. 2,8-dihydroxyadenine stone formation in a transplant recipient due to adenine phosphoribosyltransferase deficiency. J Urol 1996; 156: 1754, 1755.
11. Glicklich D, Gruber HE, Matas AJ, Tellis VA, Karwa G. 2,8-dihydroxyadenine urolithiasis: report of a case first diagnosed after renal transplant, Quart J Med 1988; 69: 785–793.
12. Wagner K, et al. 2,8-dihydroxyadenine urolithiasis with acute renal failure as a complication of pregnancy. Submitted for publication.
13. Martin T, Barratt TM. Urinary calculi: disorders of purine metabolism. In: Holliday MA, Barratt TM, Avner ED, Kogan BA, eds. *Pediatric Nephrology* 3rd ed., Williams and Wilkins, 1994: 1077.
14. Pichette V, Bonnardeaux A, Cardinal J, Houde M, Nolin L. Ammonium acid urate crystal formation in adult North American stone-formers. Am J Kid Dis 1997; 30(2): 237.
15. Herring LC. Observations on the analysis of ten thousand urinary calculi. J Urol 1962; 88: 545.
16. Soble JJ, Hamilton BD, Streem SB. Ammonium acid urate calculi: A reevaluation of risk factors. J Urol 1999; 161: 869.

17. Borden TA, Dean WM. Ammonium acid urate stones in navajo indian children. Urology 1979; 14: 9.

18. Wisniewski ZS, Brochios JG, Ryan GD. Urinary bladder stones in aboriginal children. Aust NZ J Surg 1981; 151: 292.

19. Thambi Dorai CR, Dewan PA, Boucaut HA, Ehrlich J. Urolithiasis in Australian aboriginal children. Aust N Z J Surg 1994; 64(2): 99.

20. Klohn M, Bolle JF, Reverdin NP, Susini A, Baud CA. Ammonium urate urinary stones. Urol Res 1986; 14(6): 315.

21. Dick WH, Lingeman JE, Preminger GM, Smith LH, Wilson DM. Laxative abuse as a cause for ammonium acid urate renal alculi. J Urol 1990; 143: 244.

22. Werness PG, Brown CM, Smith LH, Finlayson B. EQUIL2: a basic computer program for the calculation of urinary saturation. J Urol 1985; 134: 1242.

23. Nadler RB, Rubenstein JN, Eggener SE, Loor MM, Smith ND. The etiology of urolithiasis in HIV infected patients. J Urol 2003; 169: 475.

24. Bowyer RC, McCulloch RK, Brockis JG, Ryan GD. Factors affecting the solubility of ammonium acid urate. Clin Chem Acta 1979; 95: 17.

25. Tannen RL, McGill J. Influence of potassium on renal ammonia production. Amer J Physiology 1976; 231: 1178.

26. Oka T, Utsunomiya M, Ichikawa Y, Koide T, Takaha M. Xanthine calculi in the patient with the Lesch-Nyhan syndrome associated with urinary tract infection. Urol Int 1985; 40: 138.

27. Yokoyama M, Suzuki T, Aso Y, Akaoka I. A xanthine stone in a xanthinuric boy: a biochemical case study. J Urol 1977; 118: 651.

28. Pak CY. Miscellaneous stones. In: Pak CY, Resnick MI, eds., *Urolithiasis, A Medical and Surgical Reference.* WB Saunders, Philadelphia, 1990: 146–147.

29. Federle MP, McAninch JW, Kaiser JA, Goodman PC, Roberts J. Computed tomography of urinary calculi. Am J Roentgenol 1981; 136(2): 255.

30. Kranen S, Keough D, Gordon RB, Emmerson BT. Xanthine containing calculi during allopurinol therapy. J Urol 1985; 133: 658.

31. Klinenberg JR, Goldfinger SE, Seegmiller JE. The effectiveness of xanthine oxidase inhibitor allopurinol in the treatment of gout. Ann Int Med 1965; 62(4): 639.

32. Brock WA, Golden J, Kaplan GW. Xanthine calculi in the Lesch-Nyan syndrome. J Urol 1983; 130:157.

33. Ogawa A, Watanaba K, Minejima N. Renal xanthine stone in the Lesch-Nyan sundrome treated with allopurinol. Urology 1985; 26(1): 56.

34. Band PR, Silverberg DS, Henderson JF, Ulan RA, Wensel RH. Xanthine nephropathy in a patient with lymphosarcoma treated with allopurinol. NEJM 1970; 283(7): 354.

35. Morris JC, Holland JF. Tumor lysis syndrome. In: Holland JF, Bast Jr, RC, Morton DL, Frei III, E, Kufe DW, Weischelbaum RR. *Cancer Medicine*, vol 2, 4th ed., Williams and Wilkins, Philadelphia, 1997: 3361–3363.

36. Seegmiller JE, Laster L, Howell RR. Biochemistry of uric acid and its relationship to gout. N Engl J Med 1968; 268: 712.

37. Morino M, Shiigai N, Kusuyama H, Okada K. Extracorporeal shock wave lithotripsy and xanthine calculi in Lesch-Nyhan syndrome. Pediatr Radiol 1992; 22(4): 304.

38. Blau JJ. Ephedrine nephrolithiasis associated with chronic ephedrine abuse. J Urol 1998; 160: 825.

39. Assimos DG, Langenstroer P, Leinbach RF, et. al. Guaifenesin- and ephedrine-induced stones. J Endourol 1999; 13(9): 665.

40. Powell T, Hsu FF, Turk J, Hruska K. Ma-Huang strikes again: ephedrine nephrolithiasis. Am J Kid Dis 1998; 32(1): 153.

41. Federal Register 21 CFR Part 341. Cold, Cough, Allergy, Bronchodilator, and Antiasthmatic Drug Products for OTC Human Use; Expectorant Drug Products for Over-the-Counter Human Use; Final Monograph; Final Rule. Volume 54, 1989, pp 8454–8509.

42. Pickens CL, Milliron AR, Fussner AL, et.al. Abuse of guaifenesin-containing medications generates an excess of a carboxylate salt of beta-(2-methoxyphenoxy)-lactic acid, a guaifenesin metabolite, and results in urolithiasis. Urology 1999; 54(1): 23.

43. Federal Register 21 CFR Parts 1310 and 1313. Elimination of Threshold for Ephedrine. Volume 59, 1994, p 51365.

44. Chodakewitz J, Duetsch P, Leavitt R. Preliminary evidence of the long term safety& retroviral activity exerted by CRIXIVAN (MK-639), an oral HIV protease inhibitor. Readings of the European Conference on Clinical Aspects and Treatment of HIV infection, Copenhagen, p.7, 1995.

45. Massari F, Stazewshi S, Berry P. A double blind randomized trial of indinavir (MK-639 anole or with zidovudine (ADV) vs. zidovudine alone in zidovudine-niave patients. Read at Interscience Conference on Antimicrobial Agents and Chemotherapy, California, 1995.

46. Mellors J, Steigbigel R., Gulick R. Antiretroviral activity of the oral protease inhibitor MK-639, in P-24 antigen… HIV-1 infected patients with <500 CD4/mm3. Read at Interscience Conference on Antimicrobial Agents and Chemotherapy, California, 1995.

47. Fauci AS, Lane HC. Human Immunodeficiency Virus (HIV) Disease: AIDS and Related Disorders. In: Braunwald E, Fauci AS, Isselbacher KJ, et al., eds., *Harrison's Principles of Internal Medicine*. Chapter 309, 14th ed., McGraw-Hill, New Jersey, 1998.

48. Indinavir package insert

49. Kopp JB, Miller KD, Mican JA, et al: Crystalluria and urinary tract abnormalities associated with indinavir. Ann Intern Med 1997; 127: 119.

50. Hortin GL, King C, Miller KD, Kopp JB. Detection of indinavir crystals in urine: dependence on method of analysis. Arch Pathol Lab Med 2000; 124(2): 246.

51. Lerner LB, Cendron M, Rous SN. Nephrolithiasis from indinavir, a new human immunodeficiency virus drug. J Urol 1998; 159: 2074.

52. Eron JJ, Hirsch MS: Antiviral therapy of human immunodeficiency virus infection. In: Holmes KK, Sparling PF, Mardh PA, et al., eds., *Sexually Transmitted Diseases*, 3rd ed., McGraw-Hill, New York, 1999: 1009–1029.

53. Hermieu J, Prevot M, Ravery V, et. al. Urolithiasis and the protease inhibitor indinavir. Eur Urol 1999; 35(3): 239.

54. Saltel E, Angel JB, Futter NG, et.al. Increased prevalence and analysis of risk factors for indinavir nephrolithiasis. J Urol 2000; 164: 1895.

55. Bach MC, Godofsky EW. Indinavir nephrolithiasis in warm climates. J Acquir Immune Defic Syndr Hum Retrovirol 1997; 14: 296.

56. Sunduram CP, Saltzman B. Urolithiasis associated with protease inhibitors. J Endourol 1999; 13(4): 309.

57. Krieger JN, Corman J.MAIDS and related conditions. In: Walsh PC, Retik AB, Vaughn ED, Wein AJ., eds., *Campbell's Urology* 8th ed., vol 1, WB Saunders, Philadelphia, 2002: 693–714.

58. Bruce RG, Munch LC, Hoven AD, et al. Urolithiasis associated with the protease inhibitor indinavir. Urology 1997; 50: 513.

59. Schwartz BF, Schenkman N, Armenakas NA, Stoller ML. Imaging characteristics of indinavir calculi. J Urol 1999; 161: (4)1085.

60. Hermieu J, Prevot M, Ravery V, et. al. Urolithiasis and the protease inhibitor indinavir. Eur Urol 1999; 35(3): 239.

61. Kohan AD, Armenekas NA, Fracchia JA. Indinavir urolithiasis: an emerging cause of renal colic in patients with huuman immunodeficiency virus. J Urol 1999; 161: 1765.

62. Hug B, Naef M, Bucher HC, Sponagel L, Lehmann K, Battegay M. Treatment for human immunodeficiency virus with indinavir may cause relevant urological side-effects, effectively treatable by rehydration. BJU 1999; 84: 610.

63. Clayman RV. Crystalluria and urinary tract abnormalities associated with indinavir. J Urol 1998; 160(2): 633.

64. Reiter WJ, Schon-Pernerstorfer H, Dorfinger K, Hofbauer J, Marberger M. Frequency of urolithiasis in individuals seropositive for human immunodeficiency virus treated with indinavir is higher than previously assumed. J Urol 1999; 161: 1082.

65. Engeler DS, John H, Rentsch KM, Ruef C, Oertle D, Suter S. Nelfinavir urinary stones. J Urol 2002; 167(3): 1384–1385.

66. Physician's Desk Reference, 56th Ed. Medical Economics, Montvale, NJ, 2002.

67. Landgrebe AR, Nyhan WL, Coleman M. Urinary-tract stones resulting from the excretion of oxypurinol. N Engl J Med 1975; 292(12): 626.

68. Kranen S, Keough D, Gordon RB, Emmerson BT. Xanthine containing calculi during allopurinol therapy. J Urol 1985; 133: 658.

69. Stote RM, Smith LH, Dubb JW, et al. Oxypurinol nephrolithiasis in regional enteritis secondary to allopurinol excretion. Ann Int Med 1980; 92: 384.

70. Finlayson B, Burns J, Smith A, Du Bois L. Effect of oxiourinol and allopurinol riboside on whewellite crystallization. Invest Urol 1979; 17(3): 227.

71. Law J. Special report on the diseases of cattle. USDA, Washington DC, 1912.

72. Hammarsten G, Helldorff I, Magnuson W, Rilton T. Dubbelsidiga njurstenar av kiselsyra efter bruk av silikthaltigt antacidum. Swensk Latartid 1983; 50: 1242.

73. Rapado A, Traba ML, Caycho C, Cifuentes-Delatte L. Drug-induced renal stones: incidence, clinical expression and stone analysis. Contrib Nephrol 1987; 58: 25.

74. Joerkes AM, Rose GA, Sutor J. Multiple renal silicate calculi. BMJ 1973; 1: 146.

75. Lee MH, Lee YH, Hsu TH, Chen MT, Chang LS. Silica stone-development due to long time oral trisilicate intake. Scand J Urol Nephrol 1993; 27(2): 267–269.

76. Farrer JH, Rajfter J. Silicate Urolithiasis. J Urol 1984; 132: 739.

77. Haddad FS, Kouyoumdjian A. Silica stones found in humans. Urol Int 1986; 41: 70.

78. Levison DA, Banim S, Crocker PR, Wallace DMA. Silica stones in the urinary bladder. Lancet 1982; 1(8274): 704.

79. Page RC, Heffner RR, Frey A. Urinary excretion of silica in humans following oral administration of magnesium trisilicate. Am J Dig Dis 1941; 8: 13.

80. Inahara M, Amakasu M, Nagata M, Yamaguchi K. Silicate calculi: report of four caes. Hinyokika Kiyo 2002; 48(6): 359.

81. Cruz Guerra NA, Gomez Garcia MA, Lovaco Castellano F, Saez Garrido JC, Garcia Cuerpo E, Escudero Barrilero A. Silica urolithiasis: report of a new case. Actas Urol Esp 2000; 24(2): 202.

82. Drach GW. Secondary and miscellaneous stones. Urol Clin North Am 2000; 27: 269–273.

83. Seigel WH: Unusual complication of therapy with sulfamethoxazole-trimethoprim. J Urol 1977; 117: 397.

84. Erturk EM, Casamento JB, Guertin KR, Kende AS. Bilateral acetylsulfapyridine nephrolithiasis associated with chronic sulfasalazine therapy. J Urol 1994; 151: 1605–1606.

85. Albala DM, Prien EL, Galal HA. Urolithiasis as a hazard of sulfonamide therapy. J Endo 1994; 8: 401–403.

86. Barnes AW, Kawaichi GK. Factors influencing the formation of sulfonamide urinary concretions. J Urol 1943; 49: 324.

87. Vilter CF, Blankenhorn MA. The toxic reactions of the newer sulfonamides. JAMA 1944; 126: 691.

88. Wasserstein AG, Rak I, Reife RA. Nephrolithiasis during treatment with topiramate. Epilepsia 1995; 36(3): s153.

89. Markind JE. Topiramate: a new antiepileptic drug. Am J Health Syst Pharm 1998; 55(6): 554.

90. Wasserstein AG, Rak I, Reife RA. Investigation of the mechanistic basis for topiramate-associated nephrolithiasis: examination of the urine and serum constituents. Epilepsia 1995; 36(3): s153.

91. Grundberg RW, Silberg SJ. Triamterene-induced nephrolithiasis. JAMA 1981; 245(24): 2494.

92. Carr MC, Prien EL, Babayan RK. Trimaterene nephrolithiasis: renewed attention is warrented. J Urol 1990; 144: 1339.

93. Ettinger B, Weil E, Mandel NS, Darling S. Triamterene-induced nephrolithiasis. Ann Int Med 1979; 91: 745.

94. Ettinger B, Oldroyd NO, Sorgel F. Triamterene nephrolithiasis. JAMA 1980; 244(21): 2443.

95. Guevara A, Springman KE, Drach GW, Hillman BJ. Triamterene stones and computerized axial tomography. Urology 1986; 27(2): 104.

96. Sorgel F, Ettinger B, Benet LZ. The true composition of kidney stones passed during triamterene therapy. J Urol 1985; 134: 871.

97. Rapado A, Traba ML, Caycho C, Cifuentes-Delatte L. Drug-induced renal stones: incidence, clinical expression and stone analysis. Contrib Nephrol 1987; 58: 25.

98. Dickstein ES, Loeser WD. Triamterene calculus. J Urol 1985; 133: 1019.

99. Jacinto JS, Modanlou HD, Crade M, Strauss AA, Bosu SK. Renal calcification incidence in very low birth weight infants. Pediatrics 1988; 81: 31.

100. Robinson CM, Cox MA. The incidence of renal calcifications in low birth weight (LBW) infants on lasix for bronchopulmonary dysplasia (BPD). Ped Res 1986; 20: 359.

101. Short A, Cooke RW. The incidence of renal calcification in preterm infants. Arch Dis Child 1991; suppl 66: 412.

102. Ezzedeen F, Adelman RD, Ahlfors CE. Renal calcification in preterm infants: pathophysiology and long-term sequelae. J Ped 1988; 113: 532.

103. Glasier CM, Stoddard RA, Ackerman NB, McCurdy FA, Null DM, deLemos RA. Nephrolithiasis in infants: association with chronic furosemide therapy. AJR 1983; 140: 107.

104. Jacinto JS, Modanlou HD, Crade M, Strauss AA, Bosu SK. Renal calcification incidence in very low birth weight infants. Pediatrics 1988; 81: 31.

105. Short A, Cooke RW. The incidence of renal calcification in preterm infants. Arch Dis Child 1991; suppl 66: 412.

106. Langman CB, Moore ES. Hypercalciuria in clinical pediatrics. A review. Clin Ped 1984; 23: 135.

107. Menon M, Resnick M. Urinary lithiasis: etiology, diagnosis, and medical management. In: Walsh PC, Retik AB, Vaughn ED, Wein AJ, eds., *Campbell's Urology*. 8th ed., vol 4, WB Saunders, Philadelphia, 2002: 3289–3292.

108. Polinsky MS, Kaiser BA, Baluarte HJ, Gruskin AB. Renal stones and hypercalciuria. Adv Pediatr 1993; 40: 353.

109. Campfield T, Braden P, Flynn-Valone P, Clark N. Urinary oxalate excretion in premature infants: effects of human milk versus formula feeding. Pediatrics 1994; 94: 674.

110. Pope JC, Trusler LA, Klein AM, Walsh WF, Yared A, Brock JW. The natural history of nephrocalcinosis in premature infants treated with loop diuretics. J Urol 1996; 156: 709.

111. Glasier CM, Stoddard RA, Ackerman NB, McCurdy FA, Null DM, deLemos RA. Nephrolithiasis in infants: association with chronic furosemide therapy. AJR 1983; 140: 107.

112. Noe HN, Bryant JF, Roy S, Stapleton FB. Urolithiasis in pre-term infants associated with furosemide therapy. J Urol 1984; 132: 93.

113. Adams ND, Rowe JC. Nephrocalcinosis. Clin Perinatol 1992; 19: 179.

114. Jacinto JS, Modanlou HD, Crade M, Strauss AA, Bosu SK. Renal calcification incidence in very low birth weight infants. Pediatrics 1988; 81: 31.

115. Downing GJ, Thomas MK, Daily DK, Alon U. Nephrocalcinosis associated renal function impairment in furosemide treated VLBW infants at 1 year of age. Ped Res 1991; 29: 1252.

116. Choi H, Snyder HM 3rd, Duckett JW. Urolithiasis in childhood: current management. J Pediatr Surg 1987; 22(2): 158.

117. Diamond DA, Rickwood AM, Lee PH, Johnston JH. Infection stones in children: a twenty-seven-year review. Urology 1994; 43(4): 525.

118. Malek RS, Kelalis PP. Pediatric nephrolithiasis. J Urol 1975; 113(4): 545.

119. Steele BT, Lowe P, Rance CP, Hardy BE, Churchill BM. Urinary tract calculi in children. Int J Pediatr Nephrol 1983; 4(1): 47.

120. Diamond DA, Menon M, Lee PH, Rickwood AM, Johnston JH. Etiological factors in pediatric stone recurrence. J Urol 1989; 142(2 Pt 2): 606, discussion 619.

121. Hillman LS, Hoff N, Salmons S, Martin L, McAlister W, Haddad J. Mineral homeostasis in very premature infants: serial evaluation of serum 25-hydroxyvitamin D, serum minerals, and bone mineralization. J Pediatr 1985; 106(6): 970.

122. Stapleton FB. Current approaches to pediatric stone disease. AUA Update Series 2000; 19(40): 314.

123. Milliner DS, Murphy ME. Urolithiasis in pediatric patients. Mayo Clin Proc 1993; 68(3): 241.

124. Stapleton FB, Noe HN, Jerkins G, Roy S 3rd. Urinary excretion of calcium following an oral calcium loading test in healthy children. Pediatrics 1982; 69(5): 594.

125. Sargent JD, Stukel TA, Kresel J, et al. Normal values for random urinary calcium to creatinine ratios in infancy. J Pediatr 1988; 112: 864.

III PRESENTATION AND EVALUATION

20 Imaging of Urinary Stone Disease

Richard S. Breiman, MD *and Fergus V. Coakley,* MD

CONTENTS

BACKGROUND
GENERAL CONSIDERATIONS IN THE IMAGING
  OF URINARY STONE DISEASE
SPECIFIC IMAGING MODALITIES IN URINARY STONE DISEASE
FUTURE TRENDS
SUMMARY
REFERENCES

Key Words: Computed tomography; urogram; radiograph; obstruction.

BACKGROUND

Acute flank pain, with or without hematuria, is a common complaint and urolithiasis is the primary consideration in many of these patients. Clinical findings are often non-specific and may overlap other conditions. Imaging plays an important role in both diagnosis and subsequent management of urinary stone disease. Radiological imaging of urinary stones dates back to 1897, the year after Roentgen's discovery of X-rays. Early attempts at opacification of the urinary tract included retrograde placement of ureteral intraluminal wires and opaque catheters, air, colloidal silver, and sodium iodide [1]. Iodinated contrast agents that were excreted by the kidneys and could be administered intravenously were developed in the 1920s. For the next 70 yr, intravenous pyelography or excretory urography, including a preliminary noncontrast scout view, was the primary modality for imaging urinary stones. Computed tomography (CT) was introduced in the mid-1970s. Early CT scanners could sometimes visualize urinary calculi, but CT was not a reliable method to confidently exclude stones because these slower nonhelical scanners were plagued by misregistration between sequential images. Stones present in these nonvisualized gaps could escape detection. If seen, stone size was frequently under-estimated if only the top or bottom edge of the stone was included in the slice. For these

From: Current Clinical Urology, *Urinary Stone Disease:*
A Practical Guide to Medical and Surgical Management
Edited by: M. L. Stoller and M. V. Meng © Humana Press Inc., Totowa, NJ

reasons, nonhelical CT was unsuitable for the primary work-up of suspected urolithiasis. The introduction of helical CT scanners in the early 1990s revolutionized the imaging of urinary stone disease. With these more rapid helical CT scanners, large anatomic regions could be scanned during a single breath hold with thin slices and no misregistration. Multislice helical scanners, introduced in the late 1990s, led to the ability to obtain even thinner slices in less time, allowing the detection of smaller, less dense calculi and reducing the likelihood of false-negative scans. In most centers, nonenhanced CT has replaced the intravenous urography (IVU) as the modality of choice for the imaging of urinary stones.

The selection of the appropriate imaging modalities remains complex, with patient-specific issues influencing the imaging work-up of urinary calculi. Currently, radiographs and noncontrast CT are the cornerstones of the imaging assessment of most patients with suspected stone disease. IVU, ultrasonography (US), magnetic resonance imaging (MR), scan projection radiography (SPR), radionuclide scintigraphy, retrograde and antegrade pyelography, cystography, and tomography are available as alternative or supplemental modalities as needed.

GENERAL CONSIDERATIONS IN THE IMAGING OF URINARY STONE DISEASE

Goals of Imaging

The primary goal of imaging in urolithiasis is the detection of all urinary stones in the urinary tract. The accuracy of stone detection by the various modalities is discussed in the subsequent section. Other secondary goals include stone characterization, surveillance of stone evolution or migration, guidance and monitoring of therapy, such as endoscopy and lithotripsy, diagnosis of underlying anatomic variants predisposing to stone formation, such as ureteropelvic junction obstruction or caliceal diverticulum, detection of obstruction and other complications, such as atrophy and pyelonephritis, evaluation of the opposite kidney and collecting system, and detection of other conditions that may present with flank pain and mimic renal colic such as appendicitis or diverticulitis. As all imaging techniques have some limitations or may be contra-indicated in certain patients, a combination of examinations is often necessary.

Stone Characterization by Imaging

Imaging features that reflect stone composition and formation include morphology, internal structure, and density.

STONE MORPHOLOGY

Most stones are small and round, which is relatively nonspecific. Pure calcium oxalate stones are often homogenous, dense, and smooth. Mixed calcium oxalate stones may be irregular in shape, inhomogeneous, and may have dendritic projections. Staghorn calculi are so called because they develop in the pelvicaliceal system, and in advanced cases have a branching configuration that resembles the antlers of a stag (Fig. 1). Staghorn calculi are typically composed of magnesium ammonium phosphate (struvite), which forms in urine that has abnormally high pH (above 7.2). However, large uric acid and cystine stones also can have a staghorn configuration, and staghorn calculi in children or young adults with no history of infection are frequently composed of cystine. Radio-

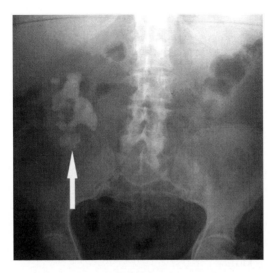

Fig. 1. Plain abdominal radiograph showing a staghorn calculus (arrow) in the right kidney. Such calculi are so called because they develop within the pelvicaliceal system, and advanced cases have a branching configuration that conforms to the shape of the pelvicaliceal system and therefore resembles the antlers of a stag.

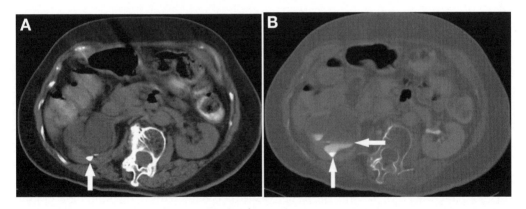

Fig. 2. (A) Nonenhanced CT in a patient with longstanding right-sided ureteropelvic junction obstruction. A small faceted stone (arrow) is seen within the dilated pelvicaliceal system. **(B)** Delayed post-contrast CT (shown at bone windows) confirms the stone (vertical arrow) is within a dilated pelvicaliceal system, because layering contrast (horizontal arrow) can be seen superior to the stone.

graphically, struvite stones are relatively low density. Low-density struvite stones may not be appreciated on plain radiographs, but can be readily detected by US or CT. IVU or retrograde pyelography may also be used to demonstrate the typical branching appearance of staghorn calculi. Faceted stones are usually multiple and have arisen in a small cavity, such as a renal pelvis above an ureteropelvic junction obstruction or in a caliceal diverticulum (Fig. 2), where the stones are minimally mobile but in contact with each other.

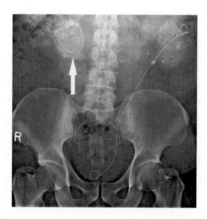

Fig. 3. Plain abdominal radiograph in a patient with bilateral partial staghorn calculi. Such stones are often composed of struvite, and may have a laminated appearance as demonstrated in the stone (arrow) in the right kidney.

INTERNAL STRUCTURE

Most stones are homogeneously dense. Struvite stones may have a laminated appearance, with alternating dense and relative lucent layers (Fig. 3).

DENSITY

In the IVU era, stones were traditionally divided into radiopaque (calcium and struvite stones) and radiolucent (pure cystine, urate, and matrix or mucoprotein stones) (Fig. 4). This division was not precise, because so-called lucent stones could become secondarily calcified and become at least partially opaque. More importantly, the distinction between radiopaque and radiolucent stones has become obsolete in the CT era. Because of the exquisite sensitivity of CT to even small amounts of calcium, all stones appear opaque (i.e., white) on CT. The only common exception to this statement is the occurrence of indinavir stones in HIV-infected patients. These "lucent" stones may still be detectable due to secondary calcification (2–5) or to signs of ureteral obstruction in the setting of an HIV patient with flank pain. Stone density affects detectability on plain radiographs; a 1–2 mm pure calcium stone may be detectable, whereas pure cystine or urate stones may not be detectable until they are 3–10 mm in size (6,7). On CT, the threshold size for stone detection varies with composition but ranges from 0.8 to 1.3 mm. These threshold sizes increase by 8–17% if low radiation dose parameters are selected (8).

The ability to predict stone fragility is of great interest to urologists, as lithotripsy could be avoided in patients with shock-wave resistant stones. Stones composed of a greater amount of calcium are harder and denser. These stones create more X-ray attenuation, and are therefore associated with a higher CT number or Hounsfield unit (HU). Uric acid and cystine stones create relatively less X-ray attenuation compared with stones composed of other materials, with attenuation coefficients ranging from 100 to 300 HU. Stones that contain significant calcium are often associated with CT numbers of 600 HU or greater, occasionally exceeding 1000 HU. Several studies have assessed stone density based on CT attenuation coefficients and have suggested that denser stones are more resistant to shock wave, particularly when CT numbers are greater than 1000 HU. However, stone density characterization is currently more accurate in vitro than in vivo (9–11).

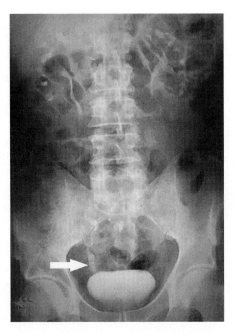

Fig. 4. Twenty-minute film from an IVU demonstrating radiolucent stones (arrow) in the distal right ureter of a patient with cystinuria. In the IVU era, stones were traditionally divided into radiopaque and radiolucent stones. Cystine stones, as in this patient, were among the stone types that could be radiolucent.

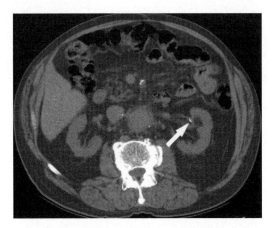

Fig. 5. Nonenhanced CT showing the typical curvilinear and perivascular appearance of arterial calcification (arrow), which is frequently seen in the renal hilum of older or diabetic patients.

Noncalculous Renal Calcifications

It is important to be aware that not all calcifications in the kidney are urinary stones. Arterial calcification is frequently seen in the renal hilum of older or diabetic patients, and has a characteristic curvilinear and perivascular appearance (Fig. 5). Dystrophic renal calcification may be a result of infection, tumors, or prior hemorrhage. Nephrocalcinosis (deposition of calcium in the renal parenchyma) is commonly a result of renal tubular acidosis, hyperparathyroidism, or medullary sponge kidney (Figs. 6 and 7).

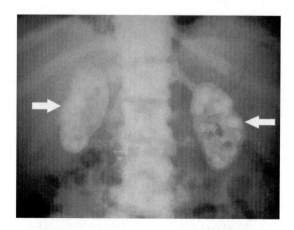

Fig. 6. Plain abdominal radiograph showing widespread nephrocalcinosis in both kidneys (arrows), which in this patient was caused by renal tubular acidosis.

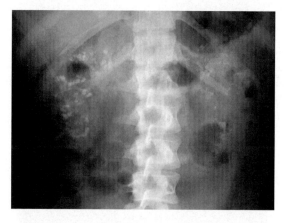

Fig. 7. Bilateral nephrocalcinosis in a patient with medullary sponge kidney. Note that in this case the calcifications are more discreet and correspond to the locations of the medullary pyramids, where these calcifications form.

Other causes include hypercalciuria, primary hyperoxaluria (oxalosis, Fig. 8), acute cortical necrosis, chronic glomerulonephritis, and renal transplant rejection. It should be noted that some of these conditions, such as hypercalciuria and hyperoxaluria, can cause both urinary calculi and nephrocalcinosis. It has been suggested that stones may begin as calcified deposits in the subepithelial portion of the renal papilla, with subsequent extrusion into and growth within the collecting system. This hypothesis is supported by the finding that papillary calcifications are common at high-resolution radiography of pathology specimens. These so-called Randall's plaques have also been shown to be more common in stone formers than nonstone formers, particularly in association with calcium oxalate and phosphate stones *(12)*. In vivo, these plaques are too small to be detected by any imaging examination except high-resolution noncontrast CT, where they may be mistaken for renal calculi (Fig. 9). Detection of these papillary calcifications may be important in identifying individuals at increased risk for stone disease *(13)*.

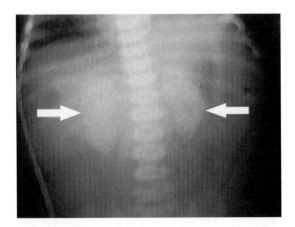

Fig. 8. Plain abdominal radiograph in a child demonstrating the characteristic nephrocalcinosis (arrows) seen in children with primary hyperoxaluria (oxalosis).

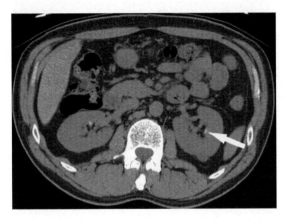

Fig. 9. Nonenhanced CT showing a thin curvilinear calcification at the expected location of a medullary pyramid in the left kidney. The appearance suggests this may be a Randall's plaque in the parenchyma rather than a true stone in the collecting system.

Impact of Stone Location on Management

The location of a stone within the urinary tract is an important factor in determining management, because it is related to the likelihood of spontaneous passage and to the choice of therapeutic approach. Coll et al. found the rate of spontaneous stone passage to be 48% for stones in the proximal ureter, 60% for mid ureteral stones, 75% for distal stones, and 79% for ureterovesical junction stones *(14)*. For example, lithotripsy may not be as successful in treating stones in the lower pole calyx if the angle between the lower pole infundibulum and renal pelvis is acute, because this anatomic arrangement could impede the passage of small stone fragments. Ultrasound or fluoroscopy can be used for guidance during percutaneous nephrostomy, needed to relieve obstruction caused by stone impaction or for the placement of an endoscopic lithotripsy device. Imaging, particularly CT, may be helpful in planning of a safe route for nephrostomy, in an effort to avoid injury to adjacent organs, such as the spleen or bowel *(15)*. CT, with the patient in the prone position used for percutaneous nephrostomy, can demonstrate the effect of

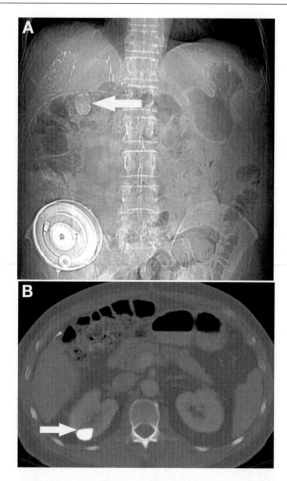

Fig. 10. (A) Plain abdominal radiograph showing a 2-cm calcific density (arrow) projected over the right kidney. The radiographic appearances are suggestive of a stone. A hepatic artery chemotherapy infusion reservoir and catheter are also evident, as are surgical clips related to prior right hepatectomy, in this patient being treated for metastatic colorectal cancer. (B) Axial CT image through the level of the calcific density demonstrates that it is caused by milk of calcium within a caliceal diverticulum. Layering of milk of calcium results in a characteristic fluid level (arrow).

gravity on the position of bowel or spleen relative to the kidney in the patient position used during intervention. Imaging demonstrating the presence of ureteropelvic junction obstruction may also influence the choice of therapy, as stone fragments created by lithotripsy may not pass.

Urinary Tract Anomalies Associated With Stone Formation

Most urinary calculi form in the collecting system as a consequence of metabolic disturbances. Occasionally, stones form because of anatomic anomalies in the urinary tract that result in stasis or infection. Caliceal diverticula are associated with stasis and often result in stone formation. The resultant stones are frequently small and seed-like or faceted. Diverticula may be associated with milk of calcium, a fine colloidal suspension of calcium carbonate (Fig. 10). Diverticula occur in 0.2–0.4% of the population but stones occur in 9.5–39% of diverticula *(16,17)*. Diverticular stones may be related to scarring, frequently associated with adjacent focal atrophy. Calculi rarely escape diverticula through their narrow neck. Milk of calcium may appear to represent a stone on a supine frontal film. The margins of a collection of milk of calcium may fade gradually rather than demonstrate the sharp defined margins of a stone. A fluid-calcium level may be visible on upright or decubitus views, or on CT and US. On post intravenous contrast excretory films, the diverticulum fills with contrast and the milk of calcium is no longer visible. No filling defect is seen within the opacified diverticulum. High echogenicity is often seen on US with milk of calcium and occasionally shadowing, with layering and shifting of the material with changes in patient position. Milk of calcium can develop in less than 12 mo. Although it is most frequently seen in calyceal diverticula, milk of calcium may be encountered with chronic dilation of a renal pelvis or calyx, as well as within cysts. Anatomic anomalies that may result in primary ureteral calculi include acquired or congenital megaloureter, ureteral stricture or obstruction, ureteral stump, blind ended or bifid ureter, or ureteral foreign body. Stones occur in a higher frequency with anatomic variations such as a horseshoe kidney, an ectopic kidney with a high insertion of ureters in the bladder, congenital UPJ stenosis with stasis and in polycystic kidneys. There is an increased incidence of stone formation within megalocalyces or megaloureters. Ureteral reflux is often associated with stasis and infection leading to an increased frequency of stone formation.

Medullary sponge kidney is an anatomic condition associated with stone formation. Dilatation of the collecting ducts of Bellini in the renal papilla leads to ductal urine stasis, increasing the risk of stone formation. Half of patients with medullary sponge kidney develop calcifications in the medulla and 12% develop urinary calculi *(18)*. Calcifications as well as calculi are often bilateral in patients with medullary sponge kidneys, but may be unilateral, frequently segmental or even localized to a single papilla. Calcifications related to most other entities are usually diffuse. Stones associated with medullary sponge kidney may vary from tiny to large. They are often clustered in a triangular shape corresponding to the configuration of a papilla (Fig. 7).

Pathophysiology of Ureteral Obstruction

Calculous obstruction of the ureter results in an abrupt rise in intraluminal pressure from the usual 6–12 mmHg to 50–70 mmHg or more *(19–21)*. The luminal pressure depends on the rate of urine flow and the degree of spasm. Ureteral spasm or more active peristalsis may be associated with an increase in colicky pain. In the first sixty to ninety minutes, a paradoxical increase in renal blood flow occurs associated with an increase in afferent arteriolar dilatation, in an attempt to prolong glomerular filtration. One and a half to five hours following ureteral obstruction, there is a decrease in renal blood flow secondary to vascular constriction of afferent arterioles. Ureteral pressure is maintained as tubular filtration continues. Edema occurs in the perinephric soft tissues with increased lymphatic resorption, resulting in prominent perinephric lymphatics *(22,23)*. Edema and distended lymphatics contribute to thin wispy opacities in perinephric fat on CT, referred to as fat stranding, usually associated with a loss of definition of renal contours (Fig. 11). Perinephric edema appears as high T2-weighted signal intensity on MRI. Increased volume of urine is associated with collecting system and ureteral dilatation. Persistent high luminal pressure may result in calyceal or forniceal rupture with perinephric fluid collections representing extravasated urine (Fig. 12). Prolonged elevated luminal pressures may eventually result in a decrease in collecting system

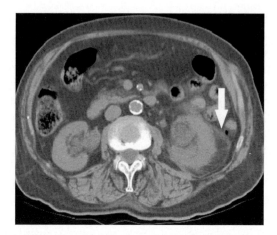

Fig. 11. Perinephric fat stranding (arrow) around the left kidney caused by a distal obstructing stone (not shown). Perinephric fat stranding in this setting reflects edema and distended lymphatics, and is often associated with a loss of definition of renal contours.

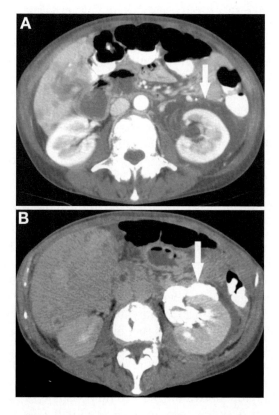

Fig. 12. (A) Contrast enhanced CT in a patient with metastatic breast cancer and acute left sided flank pain. Images at a lower level (not shown) showed a 5 mm stone in the left ureterovesical junction. Note the presence of fluid (arrow) around the left kidney. **(B)** CT image obtained 15 mins later. Excreted contrast is seen to pass from the left pelvicaliceal system into the left perirenal space (arrow), confirming the diagnosis of forniceal rupture secondary to calculous obstruction.

peristalsis, with a potential paradoxical decrease in pain. Complete obstruction lasting 4–7 d or partially for 14 d may result in various degrees of irreversible decrease in renal function *(24,25)*.

SPECIFIC IMAGING MODALITIES IN URINARY STONE DISEASE
Overview: Imaging Evaluation of Acute Flank Pain

The primary diagnostic consideration in a patient with acute flank pain is an obstructing ureteral stone. Consequently, studies investigating imaging algorithms typically use identification of a ureteral stone as the end-point. This obscures the fact that the radiological evaluation of acute flank pain should answer two related but distinct questions— is urinary obstruction present and, if so, what is the level and cause of obstruction? The presence or absence of ureteral obstruction is a functional question, whereas cause and level are anatomic issues. Many imaging tests are primarily anatomic or functional in nature. The apparently conflicting views on appropriate imaging in acute flank pain often reflect a conceptual failure to distinguish these two issues. US and noncontrast enhanced CT (NCCT) use the anatomic findings of hydronephrosis and hydroureter as indirect indicators of obstruction, but do not provide direct functional assessment. Only contrast-enhanced CT and IVU provide direct functional information. Plain radiographs provide no meaningful evaluation of obstruction, but can directly demonstrate the cause and level of obstruction, if obstruction is a result of a radiographically demonstrable calculus. US rarely directly visualizes the cause of obstruction. CT can depict the cause and level of obstruction in nearly all cases.

Plain Radiography

In the past the first imaging study requested in patients with acute flank pain was frequently a plain radiograph (also known as a conventional abdominal film, abdominal flat plate, or KUB; the latter refers to inclusion of the kidneys, ureters, and bladder in the field of view). Detectability of stones on conventional radiographs depends on size and composition as well as factors relating to technique, patient body habitus and overlying structures, such as bowel contents. In theory 90–95% of stones are sufficiently radiopaque to be visible by plain radiography *(26)*. In practice, the plain radiograph is limited in the evaluation of renal colic because multiple radiodensities can mimic stones (e.g., gallstones, costochondral calcifications, bone islands, and fecal densities) and stones may be easily missed (e.g., radiolucent stones, and stones obscured by bowel content or bone) (Fig. 13). Bowel preparation has been traditionally thought to improve detection of stones, but a recent randomized study failed to confirm this hypothesis *(27)*. These limitations are illustrated by the reported accuracy of plain radiographs for renal colic. In a study of 51 patients, using IVU as the gold standard, the sensitivity was 29% and specificity was 73% *(28)*. In a study of 49 patients, using stone passage or retrieval as the gold standard, plain radiography had a sensitivity of 68% and a specificity of 96% *(29)*. In another study of 40 patients, using stone passage or retrieval as the gold standard, plain radiography had a sensitivity of 54% and a specificity of 67% *(30)*. The sensitivity of a plain radiograph for the detection of urinary calculi ranges from 45 to 58% when NCCT is used as the standard *(31–36)*. The addition of nephrotomography improves radiographic sensitivity by 30–40%, but patient radiation dosage is increased significantly and overall accuracy remains well below NCCT *(35)*. Plain radiographs remain useful in the planning and the guidance of shock-wave lithotripsy (SWL) and in moni-

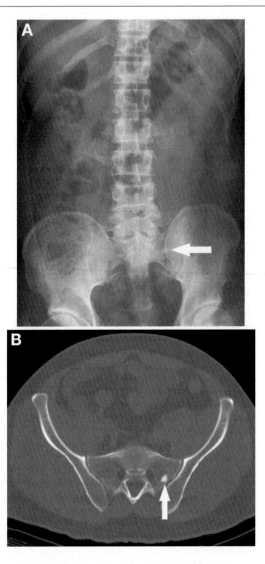

Fig. 13. (A) Plain abdominal radiograph in a patient with left flank pain. A small calcific density (arrow) is seen projected over the left sacroiliac joint, and was initially interpreted as suggestive of a ureteral calculus. **(B)** Axial CT image (shown at bone windows) through the level of the density seen in (A) shows that the appearance is caused by a bone island (arrow) in the left side of the sacrum. This example illustrates the known limitations of plain radiography in the assessment of flank pain, because there are multiple causes of both false positive and false negative results.

toring the progress of a stone treated conservatively or stone fragments after lithotripsy, provided the stone can be seen on plain radiographs and has been confirmed by CT.

In some centers, digital radiographs (DR) or computed radiographs (CR), and scanned projection radiographs (SPR), including CT scout radiographs, serve as an alternative to conventional film screen-based radiographs for stone detection and follow-up. The scout radiograph, obtained at the time of a diagnostic CT, may be used as a baseline study in those patients to be followed with plain radiographs and may help in predicting the success of radiographs for monitoring the progress of stone passage and whether stone opacity is adequate to allow radiographic or fluoroscopic guidance of lithotripsy planning *(32)*. Digital scout radiographs may also help predict stone composition, as a large stone seen on CT but not evident on the scout view likely contains little calcium and a high concentration of uric acid or xanthine *(32)*. The resolution of digital radiographs is slightly less than that of conventional radiography. Averch *(37)* showed the accuracy of these modalities to be similar for detection of stones, whereas Assi *(31)* demonstrated a significantly lower sensitivity of the scout radiograph compared with conventional radiography, particularly for stones 3 mm or less in diameter.

Intravenous Urography

Until the advent of spiral CT, the excretory or intravenous pyelogram or IVU was the gold standard for the evaluation of urolithiasis for over 70 yr (Fig. 14). It is a relatively safe and accurate means of diagnosing and characterizing urinary calculi, yielding information on renal function as well as anatomy. The IVU is particularly useful in documenting complex or subtle abnormalities of the urinary tract that may lead to stone formation or complicate management. Nonopaque radiolucent stones can be detected as filling defects within the collecting system, ureters or bladder. An IVU can usually differentiate renal calcifications and calculi from extrarenal calcifications but may not always be able to differentiate renal parenchymal calcifications from calculi. The location and size of a calculus, the precise relationship of a renal calculus to the renal collecting system, and the degree of resultant obstruction can be assessed with an IVU. Underlying anatomic abnormalities predisposing to stone formation, or affecting the choice of therapy, can be assessed as well. A logistical disadvantage of IVU is that a physician must be present because of the risk of contrast reactions. This may limit the availability of IVU in small departments with fewer personnel or off-site coverage. Another disadvantage is that the study may be protracted in patients with obstruction, when delayed images may be required several hours after injection of contrast for complete assessment. The emergence of NCCT as the primary test in patients with flank pain also exposes physicians who still request or perform IVU for this indication to medicolegal liability in the event of a contrast reaction. In a case where an emergency IVU resulted in a fatal contrast reaction, the subsequent settlement distributed 90% of the responsibility to the performing radiologist and 10% to the ordering urologist, despite an attempt by the radiologist to convince the urologist that a noncontrast CT had become the community standard. Criminal manslaughter charges were also pressed, but were eventually dropped *(38)*.

Although the IVU for flank pain is rapidly passing into history, the imaging findings of urolithiasis on IVU remain of interest. Following calculous ureteral obstruction, the nephrogram may initially be normal, but later becomes dense and associated with delayed excretion as tubular filtration decreases (Fig. 14). Fine striations related to dilated tubules may be present in the area of the renal pyramids. Opacification of the obstructed collecting system may take as long as 24 h when the obstruction is severe. As excreted contrast is heavier than unopacified urine, a change in patient position may be helpful in opacifying previously unopacified portions of the collecting systems or ureters. Radiolucent stones may be identified as filling defects on an IVU (Fig. 4). If a stone is similar in density to excreted contrast, it may not be recognized on excretory films, and may be only visible on the precontrast scout radiograph. An IVU may be helpful in differentiating intra- from extraluminal opacities. A stone impacted at the

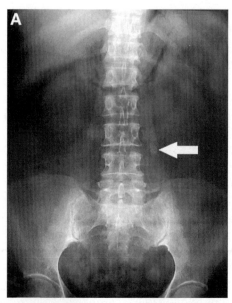

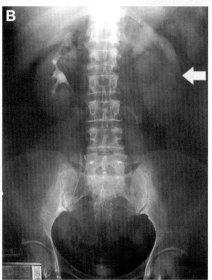

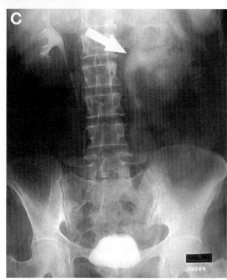

Fig. 14. (A) Scout radiograph from an IVP shows a 2 cm calcific density (arrow) at the left L3/4 disc space. **(B)** Five-minute film shows asymmetry of the upper tracts. The right nephrogram and pelvicaliceal system are unremarkable, whereas the left kidney is enlarged with a dense nephrogram and delayed excretion. These findings are typical of obstruction. **(C)** Thirty-minute film shows contrast excretion into a dilated left pelvicaliceal system (arrow) and ureter, to a level of the previously noted calcific density. The findings confirm the diagnosis of an obstructing ureteral calculus.

ureterovesical junction may create an apparent bladder wall mass on an IVU. This pseudomass is most frequently associated with stones lodged in the ureterovesical junction. Edema surrounding an impacted UVJ stone may create a pseudoureterocele. Nodular bladder wall edema may simulate a bladder neoplasm. Overall, although IVU reliably demonstrates obstruction, the cause is not always clearly delineated. In a series of 46 patients with calculous ureteral obstruction, the stone was not visible at IVP in 6 (13%) *(39)*. The six missed stones were confirmed by retrograde pyelography, ureteroscopy, or spontaneous passage. In two other series, obstructing stones were missed by IVU in 12 of 28 and 6 of 11 patients *(30,40)*. The emergence of NCCT probably accounts for the apparent drop in IVU sensitivity for stone identification. In the past, an IVU showing mild hydroureteronephorosis but no stone was often reported as "possible recent stone passage." It is possible that many of these cases were caused by small, urographically occult stones.

Persistent urinary obstruction may result in forniceal rupture. The resultant decrease in pressure from the forniceal rupture may result in symptomatic relief and be mistaken for stone passage. A forniceal rupture of short duration and in the absence of infected urine is usually of no clinical significance. Perinephric fluid resulting from a forniceal rupture is important to differentiate from perinephric edema and fat stranding in a patient with infected urine, however, as prophylactic antibiotic treatment may be administered to avoid perinephric abscess formation. Other findings of acute ureteral obstruction include an enlarged ipsilateral kidney (nephromegaly), and hydronephrosis or hydroureter.

Intravenous iodinated contrast may be required for IVU or CT urography (CTU), so a brief discussion of safety is warranted. Contrast reactions range from mild hives with pruritis to bronchospasm, hypotension and anaphylactic reaction or death. Low osmolality nonionic contrast agents, available since the late 1980s, have reduced the risk of severe reactions by approx 80%. The risk of fatal anaphylaxis following intravenous contrast is approx 0.9/100,000 with both high and low osmolality contrast *(41)*. Premedication regimens including steroids and both histamine-1 and histamine-2 blockers reduce the risk of contrast reactions, but have not been shown to specifically reduce the risk of death. Nephrotoxicity is the other major adverse effect of intravenous contrast. Strategies to reduce the frequency of nephrotoxicity, particularly in high-risk patients such as those with diabetes or renal impairment, include hydration, premedication with acetylcystine, or use of iso-osmolar dimeric contrast media *(41–43)*.

Ultrasound

US may be used to directly depict stones, to identify hydronephrosis in calculous ureteral obstruction, or to guide therapy such as percutaneous nephrostomy tube placement, SWL, and percutaneous nephrolithotomy. The advantages of US include safety (no iodinated contrast or ionizing radiation), availability, and lower cost relative to CT. The disadvantages are related to limited accuracy, and will be discussed in greater detail.

Calculi reflect sound creating echogenic, bright foci with acoustic shadowing deep to the calculus (Fig. 15). Calculi that have a high percentage of matrix rather than calcium may be echogenic without acoustic shadowing. Small stones, less than 5 mm, may be difficult for US to confidently diagnose, as they are less likely to cast an acoustic shadow. The use of a higher frequency transducer, 5–10 MHz, increases the echogenicity of small stones and accentuates shadowing, but is associated with decreased beam penetration, which often limits its application particularly in medium sized to large patients. Renal parenchymal calcifications and focal echogenic renal sinus fat may be difficult to distinguish from stones by US. The difficulty in depicting small echogenic stones against a background of echogenic renal sinus fat should not be underestimated, and represents

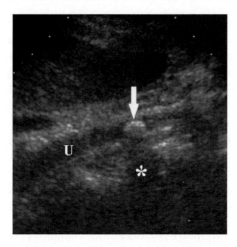

Fig. 15. Ultrasound image in a patient with right-sided flank pain. The right ureter (U) is dilated to the level of an echogenic stone (arrow) that is casting a characteristic acoustic shadow (asterisk).

a major limitation of sonography for diagnosis of renal calculi. In a recent study using nonenhanced CT as the gold standard, US only detected 24 of 101 calculi, with a specificity of 90% *(44)*.

US is used to identify obstruction by demonstration of hydronephrosis rather than by direct visualization of a stone (although an obstructing calculus may sometimes be seen high in the ureter through the acoustic window for the kidney, or in the distal ureter through the bladder). Bowel and bone limit acoustic access to the rest of the ureter in the retroperitoneum. The main drawback of US is that not all obstructed kidneys have dilated pelvicaliceal systems, either because dilatation has not yet developed, the upper tract has decompressed by forniceal rupture *(45)*, or the upper tract is noncompliant. In addition, the diuretic effect of intravenous contrast likely explains why dilatation is occasionally absent at US but present at IVU *(45)*. Reports of the false negative rates for US include absence of dilation in (1) 8 of 21 (38%) patients with a delayed nephrogram on IVU *(29)*; (2) 7 of 20 (35%) patients with clinically proven obstruction *(45)*; (3) 3 of 53 (6%) patients with IVU-proven obstruction *(39)*; and (4) 5 of 14 (36%) patients with IVU-proven obstruction *(46)*.

The false negative rate of 6–38% for US in acute renal colic represents a major limitation. Doppler US has been advocated as a method of identifying nondilated obstructed kidneys, based on the increased vascular resistance in obstructed kidneys. However, this is not widely used because the results have been disappointing and the technique is operator dependent *(46)*. The addition of forced diuresis has been suggested *(47)*, but is not in common use. Color flow Doppler may be useful in assessing ureteral jets in the bladder. On average, 1–12 jets of urine arising from the ureteral orifices will be observed per minute in an asymptomatic patient (Fig. 16). Ureteral jets are usually symmetric in appearance. Asymmetry of visible ureteral jets on color flow Doppler or asymmetric flow velocity on pulsed Doppler may suggest ureteral obstruction on the side of reduced flow. For this sign to be most useful, the patient must be well hydrated. As some nonobstructed patients demonstrate variability in the pattern and symmetry of ureteral jets, this technique is felt to be of limited usefulness.

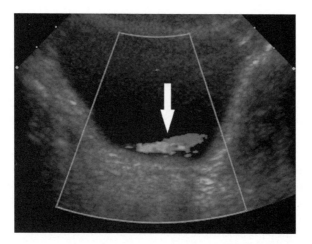

Fig. 16. Axial Doppler ultrasound image of the bladder demonstrating a right ureteral jet (arrow). On average, 1–12 jets of urine arising from the ureteral orifices will be observed per minute in a normal person.

Combined Plain Radiography and Ultrasound

Given the limitations of KUB and US individually, there is no good reason to believe that the combination is superior to either modality alone. This is generally supported by the literature, with the exception of one paper that claimed that the combination was 100% sensitive and specific (100%), because all stones missed by US were fortuitously visible on KUB *(48)*. A more plausible study reported a sensitivity of 80% and a specificity of 58% for a combination of both tests *(29)*.

Computed Tomography

Although many stones are radiolucent on plain radiographs, essentially all stones are sufficiently dense to be visible on CT. The only exceptions are the urinary stone/sludge formation associated with indinavir *(49)* and the very rare pure matrix stone composed of mucous and debris *(50)*. Therefore, the terms radiopaque and radiolucent are only appropriate for plain radiography, and should not be used in the context of CT. The volumetric capability of spiral CT allows rapid acquisition of overlapping thin slices without the possibility of missing small stones between slices. The advent of spiral CT has revolutionized the imaging of urinary stone disease, and noncontrast spiral CT has emerged as a highly accurate modality for the identification of ureteral calculi. In a comparative study of IVU and noncontrast CT in 40 patients with flank pain, 28 with stones proven by retrieval or passage, IVU had a sensitivity and specificity of 64% and 92%, compared to 100% and 92% for noncontrast CT, respectively *(30)*. Another study of stone detection by noncontrast CT reported a sensitivity of 97% and a specificity of 96% *(51)*. False positives and negatives are still possible because stones may be mistaken for phleboliths or vascular calcifications, and vice versa. Contrast can be administered in difficult cases to resolve any doubts. Other advantages of CT include better stone characterization and anatomic localization, improved depiction of nonstone pathology, and speed. CT allows examination of the entire abdomen and pelvis in a single breath hold in most patients on modern multi-slice helical scanners. NCCT acquisition times are less than a minute and usually less than 20 s on multislice CT scanners, approx 10 s with 16 slice helical scanners. Because contrast is not required, NCCT is particularly useful in patients with contrast allergy or impaired renal function. As intravenous iodinated contrast is not administered, NCCT does not require a physician or nurse in attendance during scanning, increasing the accessibility of the examination after hours. NCCT for urinary stones has been criticized as lacking a functional component, as compared to IVU, because contrast is not administered. This may limit the ability to depict obstruction based on an asymmetric nephrogram or delayed excretion. However, the assessment of the chronicity and severity of obstruction may not significantly contribute to management decisions or to the success of therapy. With respect to the radiation dose delivered by CT, the risks of low dose radiation are controversial; there is general agreement that the lowest reasonable dose that allows a diagnostic study should be used (52).

COMPUTED-TOMOGRAPHY TECHNIQUE

In our institution, we scan patients on single, 4, 8, and 16 slice helical scanners. We select an mA in a range of 100–450, commensurate with the size of the patient, 240 mA on average, with a higher mA selected for larger patients. Automatic modulation of mA is available on some CT scanners. This modulates the mA on a scan-by-scan basis as needed to achieve a preset level of image quality, accounting for the thickness and X-ray attenuating characteristics of the tissues present in the area included in the slice volume. The mA (and radiation dose) would be lower through the upper abdomen, which include the lung bases (which attenuate relatively little X-ray), than through the pelvis, which includes the iliac bones (which greatly attenuate X-rays), for example. Reduction of mA helps lower radiation dose, without compromising stone detection (52). When using a 16 slice scanner, we obtain 3 mm contiguous scans with the patient in the prone position, with a pitch of 0.9, a rotation time of 0.75 s per rotation and 120 kVp. No intravenous or oral contrast is initially administered. Patients are scanned prospectively in the prone position to aid in distinguishing a bladder stone from a stone impacted in the interureteric ridge portion of the ureterovesical junction, which may simulate a bladder stone on a supine image (53) (Fig. 17). In our institution, noncontrast scans obtained to search for urinary calculi are performed prospectively in the prone position, avoiding the need to rescan with the associated reduction in radiation dose, prolongation of the examination, or need to recall the patient if the need for prone images was not recognized while the patient was still in the department.

With multi-slice helical CT scanners, it is also possible to retrospectively create thinner slices from the original standard thicker source images. Retrospective targeted high-resolution reconstructions decreasing pixel size and increasing spatial resolution may also supplement routine scans when needed (Fig. 18). These retrospective reconstructions can be performed without the physical presence of the patient, as long as source image raw data is still available. On newer scanners, raw data is usually available for 12–36 h, depending on the number of patients scanned and the complexity of their examinations. As mentioned previously, multiplanar reformations (MPR) may also be helpful in resolving diagnostic dilemmas. MPRs and three-dimensional reformations require only image data and not raw source data, allowing manipulation years after the original examination, presuming digital data has been archived.

Delayed post intravenous contrast excretory phase CT scans may, on occasion, be necessary to further delineate small ureteral stones and to differentiate them from phleboliths in close proximity to the ureter or to assess unexpected renal parenchymal

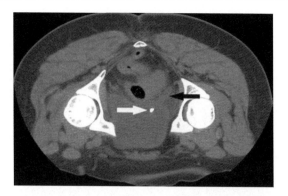

Fig. 17. Nonenhanced CT image demonstrating the advantage of prone positioning in the evaluation of urinary stones. The distal right ureter (black arrow) is dilated to the level of a small stone (white arrow) impacted in the ureterovesical junction. With a scan obtained in the supine position, it could be difficult to distinguish a stone in the ureterovesical junction protruding into the bladder from a stone that has passed from the ureter and was lying freely within the bladder.

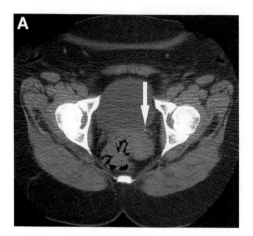
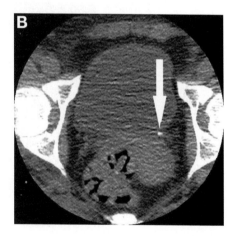

Fig. 18. (A) Nonenhanced 5–mm-thick CT section obtained on a multidetector CT scanner showing a questionable calcific density (arrow) in the left ureterovesical junction. **(B)** Thin section small field-of-view image reconstructed from the same dataset confirms a small stone (arrow) in the left ureterovesical junction. The ability to retrospectively create such targeted high-resolution reconstructions (while the raw data remains available) is one of the advantages of multidetector CT scanners.

abnormalities suspected on initial noncontrast scans. As with an IVU, a dense nephrogram associated with delayed excretion of contrast and dilatation of the collecting system is often associated with ureteral obstruction on post-contrast scans.

COMPUTED-TOMOGRAPHY SIGNS OF UROLITHIASIS AND OBSTRUCTION

Ureteral obstruction is associated with secondary signs on CT. These include unilateral hydroureter and/or hydronephrosis. Subtle degrees of collecting system distention or perinephric fat stranding are most easily recognized in or about the upper or lower poles of the kidney. Perinephric or periureteral fat stranding may also be encountered

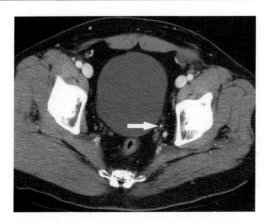

Fig. 19. CT image showing a small stone (arrow) in the distal left ureter. A thin surrounding rim of tissue is visible, representing the edematous ureteral wall. This so-called ureteral rim sign helps to differentiate a ureteral calculus from a phlebolith.

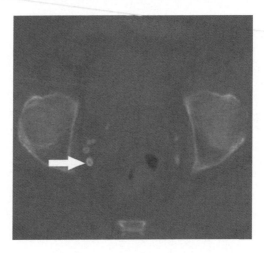

Fig. 20. Nonenhanced CT image (filmed at bone windows) demonstrating numerous pelvic phleboliths. The characteristic central lucency is evident within the largest phlebolith (arrow).

(Fig. 11). Fat stranding represents edema, as well as engorged lymphatics, attempting to drain increased renal interstitial fluid, secondary to post obstructive elevation of collecting system pressure. The presence of both of these signs is associated with 99% positive predictive value and 95% negative predictive value for ureteral obstruction *(54)*.

A calculus lodged in a ureter is often associated with thickening of the ureteral wall resulting from edema, the ureteral rim sign, which may be helpful in differentiating a ureteral calculus from a phlebolith (Fig. 19). A ureteral rim sign is noted in 76–77% of calculi, but less than 10% of phleboliths *(54,55)*. It is detected in as many as 91% of ureteral stones 4 mm or less in size, but larger stones may obscure the ureteral rim sign.

COMPUTED-TOMOGRAPHY PITFALLS

Phleboliths are usually round with smooth contours and often contain a central lucency (Fig. 20) *(54)*. Phleboliths increase in number with age. Many phleboliths lie below a line

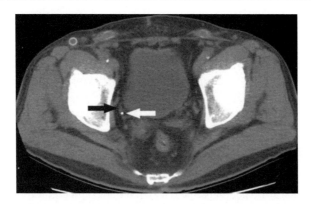

Fig. 21. Nonenhanced CT showing a pelvic phlebolith (white arrow). A linear strand of tissue (black arrow) is seen extending from the phlebolith. This tissue strand is believed to represent the atretic vessel within which the phlebolith formed, and this so-called "comet-tail" sign is another finding that may help distinguish stones and phleboliths.

drawn between the iliac spines, and are more lateral than the bladder and distal ureters. A pelvic phlebolith may be associated with a comet tail sign, representing a noncalcified thrombus adjacent to a calcified component (55–58) (Fig. 21). Boridy et al demonstrated a sensitivity of 65% and a specificity of 100% for a calcified phlebolith when the comet tail sign was detected; no calculi were associated with a comet tail (57). Bell also demonstrated 100% specificity for a phlebolith when a comet tail was noted (55). However, Guest et al. demonstrated poor observer agreement on whether the comet tail sign was present in patients with pelvic opacities, and the sign frequently was related to a ureteral calculus (58). If problems persist in differentiating a phlebolith from a distal ureteral calculus following a noncontrast CT, the use of intravenous contrast with excretory phase images may be helpful for a definitive diagnosis. A gonadal vein phlebolith may mimic a ureteral stone. It is important to carefully follow the course of the ureters and periureteral vascular structures on each sequential image to avoid errors in interpretation. Arterial calcifications may lie in the vicinity of the renal collecting system or a ureter and simulate a stone, particularly on X-rays.

INCIDENTAL NONSTONE PATHOLOGY DETECTED ON COMPUTED TOMOGRAPHY

Among the advantages of noncontrast CT as the primary modality in the assessment of suspected urinary stone disease is the ability of CT to visualize extraurinary tract abnormalities. These findings may be incidental, but in some cases may represent the etiology of the patient's clinical presentation. In one study, unsuspected findings that could affect acute patient care were observed at 5.9% of unenhanced CT examinations (59). Extraurinary tract conditions most often mimicking renal colic include; appendicitis (Fig. 22), diverticulitis (Fig. 23), adnexal pathology including tubo-ovarian abscess, retroperitoneal hemorrhage or infection, and retroperitoneal neoplasm, secondarily involving a ureter (Fig. 24). CT performed to assess suspected stone disease may detect occult urinary and extra-urinary tract pathology, unrelated to the acute clinical presentation, but potentially clinically significant. As with screening CT, these findings include abdominal aortic aneurysm, gallstones, lymphadenopathy, organomegaly and occult malignancy (Fig. 25).

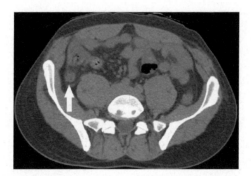

Fig. 22. Nonenhanced CT in a patient suspected of having a right ureteral calculus. The appendix (arrow) is thickened with surrounding fat stranding. The radiological diagnosis of acute appendicitis was confirmed at surgery.

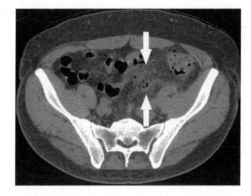

Fig. 23. Nonenhanced CT image obtained in a patient with acute left sided flank pain. The scan was requested by the emergency department to evaluate for possible urinary stone. Small bubbles of free air and associated infiltration within the sigmoid mesocolon (arrows) were caused by unsuspected perforated diverticulitis.

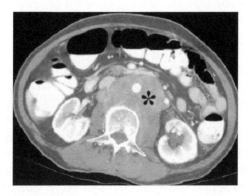

Fig. 24. Contrast-enhanced CT performed in a patient with left flank pain, after an initial nonenhanced study (not shown) had failed to demonstrate urinary stones but did show a retroperitoneal mass. Enhancing soft tissue (asterisk) is seen encasing the aorta and displacing the inferior vena cava. The left kidney is mildly hydronephrotic. A diagnosis of lymphoma was established at biopsy.

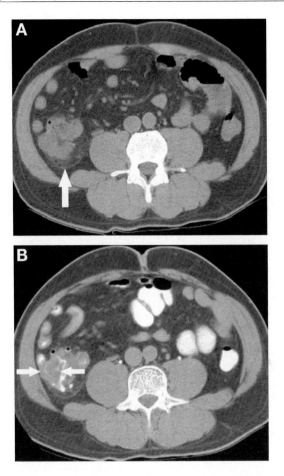

Fig. 25. (A) Nonenhanced urinary stone CT performed to assess right flank pain. Fat stranding (arrow) is present around the cecum, and the cecal wall appears thickened. **(B)** Subsequent CT performed after oral contrast confirms circumferential cecal wall thickening. Cecal carcinoma was proven at resection.

Magnetic Resonance Imaging

Noncontrast CT is currently the modality of choice for the evaluation of acute flank pain, but MR may be helpful in select patients, particularly in pregnancy when avoidance of ionizing radiation is a priority. Most reports advocate the use of heavily T2-weighted sequences for the MR assessment of the urinary tract. HASTE (half Fourier acquisition single shot turbo spin echo) and RARE (rapid acquisition with relaxation enhancement) sequences have been shown to be particularly useful in creating an MR urogram *(60–63)*. Maximum intensity projection (MIP) reconstructions in coronal and sagittal projections may be helpful. Stones are identified as a filling defect (signal void) within the abundant bright signal of the urine filled collecting system, ureter or bladder on a T2-weighted sequence (Fig. 26) *(60,64,65)*, although MR imaging is generally insensitive to urinary stones (Fig. 27) and the primary use of this modality is in the demonstration of hydronephrosis and hydroureter.

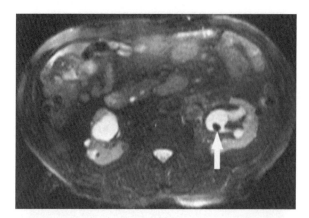

Fig. 26. Fat-saturated T2-weighted axial MR image demonstrates the characteristic appearance of a urinary stone, which appears as a filling defect (arrow) within the fluid filled collecting system. Fluid is bright on T2-weighted imaging, facilitating stone identification.

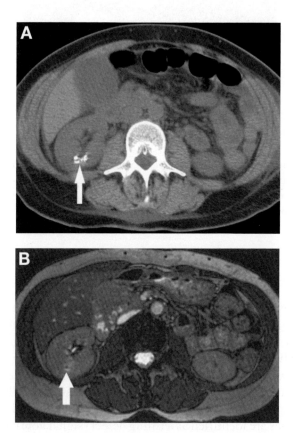

Fig. 27. (A) Nonenhanced axial CT image showing a cluster of small stones (arrow) within the parenchyma of the lower pole of the right kidney. **(B)** Gradient echo axial T2-weighted MR image at the same level. The cluster of stones (arrow) is difficult to appreciate. In general, MR imaging is inferior to CT in the evaluation of stones, and is therefore rarely used for this indication.

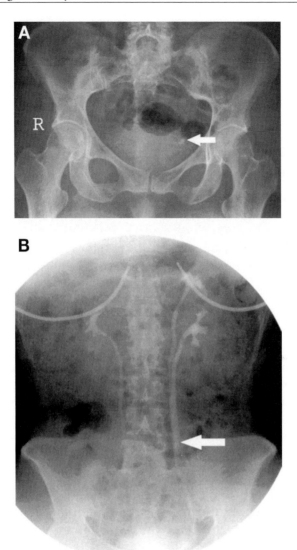

Fig. 28. (A) Plain radiograph showing a stone (arrow) in the distal left ureter. **(B)** Retrograde pyelogram performed after laser lithotripsy of the stone shows the left ureter (arrow) to be stone free. A duplicated left upper tract is also demonstrated.

Retrograde Pyelography

Retrograde pyelography may be helpful in azotemic patients and others in whom opacification of the urinary tract is desirable but intravenous iodinated contrast is contraindicated or produced insufficient luminal opacification (Fig. 28). For example, a patient with multiple pelvic opacities in close proximity to the distal ureters in whom a distal ureteral calculus can not be excluded by other examinations because of contraindications for intravenous contrast or insufficient contrast excretion. A retrograde pyelogram may be helpful when other examinations are unsuccessful in detecting a urinary stone in a patient with a strong clinical suspicion of stone disease.

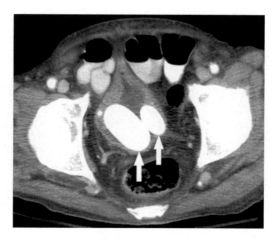

Fig. 29. Axial CT image in an elderly man with chronic bladder outlet obstruction. Large bladder stones (arrows) are present within the bladder. Bladder wall thickening and a Foley catheter can also be seen.

Retrograde pyelography is occasionally used in association with SWL to locate a faintly visible stone. The ureteral catheter used at retrograde pyelography may be helpful as a reference for targeting a stone at lithotripsy. Dilute contrast is used with fluoroscopy to prevent over distension and extravasation. If infection exists proximal to obstruction the patient is at risk for sepsis, possibly life-threatening infection or irreversible renal failure. Retrograde placement of a ureteral catheter above the level of obstruction under fluoroscopic guidance, may provide adequate drainage of the infected upper tract.

IMAGING BLADDER AND URETHRAL CALCULI

Primary bladder calculi are usually a manifestation of underlying pathology, including voiding dysfunction, foreign bodies, infection, parasites, migrant renal calculi, bladder outlet obstruction, and neurogenic bladder (Fig. 29). Foreign bodies in the bladder include chronic indwelling Foley catheters or double J ureteral catheters. Bladder infection may serve as a nidus for stone formation, as it does in the kidney. Post infection bladder calculi are most common in males and are usually associated with a urea splitting organism or a parasitic infection. Most bladder calculi are solitary, but multiple calculi can be seen. Bladder calculi are most often composed of ammonium urate, uric acid, or calcium oxalate. Uric acid stones are often radiolucent in the bladder on a radiograph, as they are elsewhere, and may be identified as filling defects on an IVU. Bladder calculi may be detected or confirmed with US as even radiolucent stones are echogenic on a sonogram and usually cast an acoustic shadow. Stone mobility is easily demonstrated with US when a patient changes position during scanning, aiding in the differentiation of nonmobile calculi impacted at the ureterovesical junction, particularly the inter-ureteric ridge portion of the distal ureter, from mobile bladder calculi.

Various structures may mimic bladder calculi on imaging studies, particularly X-ray based procedures such as plain films and an IVU. These include: a punctate collection of rectal contrast, dense impacted stool, phleboliths, an appendicolith, calcified fibroids or adnexal masses, post inflammatory, hemorrhagic or infectious calcifications, and

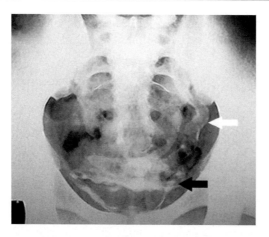

Fig. 30. Plain abdominal radiograph in a patient with urinary schistosomiasis. Calcification of the bladder (black arrow) and of the distal left ureter (white arrow) are evident.

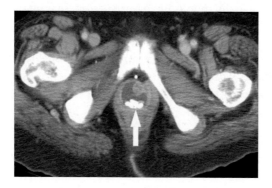

Fig. 31. Axial CT image in an elderly woman showing stones (arrow) within a urethral diverticulum. The appearance of the diverticulum is characteristic.

calcifications related to amyloidosis. Schistosomiasis is the most common cause of bladder calcification (Fig. 30) where the disease is endemic in the Middle East and Africa. Calcifications secondary to Schistosomiasis may also involve the distal ureters. Calcifications related to tuberculosis may involve the bladder wall, seminal vesicles, vas deferens and epididymis. However bladder calculi are rare in patients with tuberculosis.

Prostatic and seminal vesicle calcifications, including calcified amylacea of the prostate in older males, may mimic bladder calculi on radiographs. Prostatic calcifications are rarely associated with prostatitis. Seminal vesicle stones are often smooth, round and may rarely be associated with hematospermia. They may be mistakenly attributed to tuberculous infection.

Urethral calculi arise from the bladder and rarely from the upper tracts. Most ureteral calculi pass unimpeded through the urethra. Urethral calculi may be secondary to urinary stasis in a diverticulum or related to a stricture, possibly in the region of previous surgery. In males, urethral stones are most commonly in the prostatic and bulbar portions and are usually solitary. Urethral calculi are rare in females, secondary to a short urethra. Urethral calculi may be secondary to diverticula, particularly in females (Fig. 31). Symptoms secondary to urethral calculi are similar to those of bladder stones, including intermittent interruption of the urinary stream, dribbling, terminal hematuria, infection and pain.

IMAGING FLANK PAIN IN PREGNANCY

Ultrasound is often the initial modality used to search for suspected urinary stones in a pregnant patient. If an obstructing calculus is identified, no further imaging may be necessary. If US does not yield an explanation of the patient's clinical presentation, a KUB may be helpful. A KUB may be the initial examination when a ureteral calculus is suspected in the second or third trimester of pregnancy. If an IVU is felt necessary during the second or third trimester, a limited examination consisting of a single film 20 min post-IV contrast infusion may yield important additional information, while limiting radiation. Most stones pass spontaneously in this population, but intervention may be required for persistent pain, sepsis, progressive or high-grade hydronephrosis or obstruction of a solitary kidney. If necessary, the workup may proceed to a retrograde pyelogram with stent placement to relieve obstruction, leaving an offending stone to be addressed postpartum. Hydronephrosis of pregnancy or over distention syndrome is often encountered as an incidental finding on second and third trimester obstetric US, but may be difficult to differentiate from an occult stone with ureteral distension sonographically. Simple hydronephrosis of pregnancy is not usually associated with an elevated resistive index, as occurs with obstruction secondary to a stone.

SUMMARY

The management of urinary stone disease benefits from a multidisciplinary approach, combining traditional and high tech clinical and imaging approaches. Imaging plays a pivotal role in the diagnosis, characterization and follow-up of calculi, often providing crucial information contributing to the successful management of urinary stones. Goals of imaging include not only the detection of stones but equally important, characterization of stones and the urinary tract. This information contributes to a determination of prognosis and to the selection of an appropriate management plan, selection and guidance of therapy, as well as the assessment of the success of management and a determination of timing and selection of alternative therapies. Important imaging data includes size, shape, composition, (hardness) of stones, as well as information relating to the urinary tract, including: anatomic condition leading to stasis and stone formation, presence, level, and degree of obstruction, resultant presence and degree of complications, such as atrophy or infection. Imaging is often important to the selection and design of appropriate therapy, in monitoring the success of treatment and in detecting complications. Noncontrast CT has become the initial modality in the assessment of suspected nephroureterolithiasis and urinary tract obstruction as it is accurate, readily available, and does not usually require the use of intravenous iodinated contrast, avoiding the potential risks of contrast in most patients. Other modalities still play a role in the management of stone disease, particularly plain films and US.

ACKNOWLEDGMENT

The authors wish to acknowledge the contribution of Xia Wang, MD to the research of the literature and selection and preparation of case material for this chapter.

REFERENCES

1. Smith RC, Varanelli M. Diagnosis and management of acute ureterolithiasis. AJR 2000; 175: 3–6.
2. Reiter WJ, Schon-Pernerstorfer H, Dorfinger K, Hofbauer J, Marberger M. Frequency of urolithiasis in individuals seropositive for human immunodeficiency virus treated with indinavir is higher than previously assumed. J Urol 1999; 161: 1082–1084.
3. Schwartz BF, Schenkman N, Armenakas NA, Stoller ML. Imaging characteristics of indinavir calculi. J Urol 1999; 161: 1085–1087.
4. Bruce GR, Munch LC, Hoven AD, et al. Urolithiasis associated with the protease inhibitor indinavir. Urology 1997; 50: 513–518.
5. Blake SP, McNicholas MM, Raptopoulos V. Nonopaque crystal deposition causing ureteric obstruction in patients with HIV undergoing indinavir therapy. AJR 1998; 171: 717–720.
6. Leroy AJ. Diagnosis and treatment of nephrolithiasis: Current perspectives. AJR 1994; 163: 1309–1313.
7. Amis ES, Newhouse JH. Urinary stone disease. In: *Amises*, Newhouse JH eds., Essentials of Uroradiology. Boston, Little, Brown, 1991: 213–231.
8. Tublin ME, Murphy ME, Delong DM, Tessler FN, Kliewer MA. Conspicuity of renal calculi at unenhanced CT: Effects of calculus composition and size and CT technique. Radiology 2002; 225: 91–96.
9. Motley G, Dalrymple N, Kessling C, Fischer J, Harmon W. Hounsfield unit density in the determination of urinary stone. Urology 2001; 58 (2): 170–173.
10. Williams JC Jr, Saw KC, Monga AG, Chua GT, Lingeman JE, McAteer JA. Correction of helical CT attenuation values with wide beam collimation: in vitro test with urinary calculi. Acad Radiol 2001; 8 (6): 478–483.
11. Joseph P, Manda AK, Singh SK, Mandal P, Sankhwar SN, Sharma SK. Computerized tomography attenuation value of renal calculus: can it predict successful fragmentation of the calculus by extracorporeal shock wave lithotripsy? A preliminary study. J Urol 2002; 167: 1968–1971.
12. Low RK, Stoller ML. Endoscopic mapping of renal papillae for Randall's plaques in patients with urinary stone disease. J Urol 1997; 158: 2062–2064.
13. Evan AP, Lingeman JE, Coe FL, et al. Randall's plaque of patients with nephrolithiasis begins in basement membranes of thin loops of Henle. J Clin Invest 2003; 111: 607–616.
14. Coll DM, Varanelli MJ, Smith RC. Relationship of spontaneous passage of ureteral calculi to stone size and location as revealed by unenhanced helical CT. AJR 2002; 178: 101–103.
15. Tuttle DN, Yeh BM, Meng MV, Breiman RS, Stoller ML, Coakley FV. Risk of injury to adjacent organs at lower pole fluoroscopically-guided percutaneous nephrostomy: Evaluation by prone, supine and multiplanar reformatted CT. J Vasc Interv Radiol. 2005; 16(11): 1489–1492.
16. Middleton AW Jr, Pfister RC. Stone containing pyelocaliceal diverticulum: Embroyogenic, anatomic, radiologic and clinical characteristics. J Urol 1974; 111: 2–6.
17. Timmons JW, Malek RS, Hattery RR, Deweerd JH. Caliceal diverticulum. J Urol 1975; 114: 6–9.
18. Ginalski JM, Portmann L, Jaeger PH. Does medullary sponge kidney cause nephrolithiasis? AJR 1990; 155: 299–302.
19. Rose JG, Gillenwater JY. Pathophysiology of ureteral obstruction. Am J of Physiol 1973; 225: 830–837.
20. Michaelson G. Percutaneous puncture of the renal pelvis, intrapelvic pressure, and the concentrating capacity of the kidney in hydronephrosis. Acta Med Scand 1974; 559(Suppl): 1–26.
21. Gillenwater JY. The pathophysiology of urinary tract obstruction. In: Campbell's Urology, 6th Ed., (Walsh PC, Retik AB, Stamey TA, Vaughn ED, eds.). Saunders, Philadelphia, PA, 1992, p. 509.
22. Holmes MJ, O'Morchoe PJ, O'Morchoe CC. Morphology of the intrarenal lymphatic system: capsular and hilar communications. Am J Anat 1977; 149: 333–337.
23. Heney NM, O'Morchoe PJ, O'Morchoe CC. The renal lymphatic system during obstructed urine flow. J Urol 1971; 106: 455–462.
24. Leahy AL, Ryan PC, McEntee GM, Nelson AC, Fitzpatrick JM. Renal injury and recovery in partial ureteric obstruction. J Urol 1989; 142: 199–203.

25. Kerr WS. Effect of complete ureteral obstruction for one week on kidney function. J Appl Physiol 1954; 6: 763.

26. Thornbury JR, Parker TW. Ureteral calculi. Semin Roentgenol 1982; 17: 133–138.

27. Schuster GA, Nazos D, Lewis GA. Preparation of outpatients for excretory urography: is bowel preparation with laxatives and dietary restrictions necessary? AJR Am J Roentgenol 1995; 164: 1425–1428.

28. Boyd R, Gray AJ. Role of the plain radiograph and urinalysis in acute ureteric colic. J Accid Emerg Med 1996; 13: 390, 391.

29. Svedstrom E, Alanen A, Nurmi N. Radiologic diagnosis of renal colic: The role of plain films, excretory urography, and sonography. Eur J Radiol 1990; 11: 180–183.

30. Niall O, Russell J, MacGregor R, Duncan H, Mullins J. A comparison of noncontrast computerized tomography with excretory urography in the assessment of acute flank pain. J Urol 1999; 161: 534–537.

31. Assi Z, Platt JF, Francis IR, Cohan RH, Korobkin M. Sensitivity of CT scout radiography and abdominal radiography for revealing ureteral calculi on helical CT: implications for radiologic follow-up. AJR 2000; 175: 333–337.

32. Chu G, Rosenfield AT, Anderson K, Scout L, Smith RC. Sensitivity and value of digital CT scout radiography for detecting ureteral stones in patients with Ureterolithiasis diagnosed on unenhanced CT. AJR 1999; 173: 417–423.

33. Levine JA, Neitlich J, Verga M, Dalrymple N, Smith RC. Ureteral calculi in patients with flank pain: correlation of plain radiography with unenhanced helical CT. Radiology 1997; 204: 27–31.

34. Jackman SV, Potter SR, Regan F, Jarrett TW. Plain abdominal X-ray versus computerized tomography screening: sensitivity for localization after nonenhanced spiral computerized tomography. J Urol 2000; 164: 308–310.

35. Goldwasser B, Cohan RH, Dunnick NR, Andriani CC, Carsen CC 3rd, Weinerth JL. Role of linear tomography in evaluation of patients with nephrolithiasis. Urology 1989; 33: 253–256.

36. Ahn SH, Mayo-Smith WW, Murphy BL, Reinert SE, Cronan JJ. Acute nontraumatic abdominal pain in adult patients: Abdominal radiography compared with CT evaluation. Radiology 2002; 225: 159–164.

37. Averch TD, O'Sullivan D, Breitenbach C, Beser N, Schulam PG, Moore RG, Kavoussi LR: Digital radiographic imaging transfer: comparison with plain radiographs. J Endourol 1997; 11: 99–101.

38. Eisenberg RL, Berlin L When does malpractice become manslaughter? AJR 2002; 179: 331–335.

39. Juul N, Brons J, Torp-Pedersen S, Fredfeldt KE. Ultrasound versus intravenous urography in the evaluation of patients with suspected obstructing urinary calculi. Scand J Urol Nephrol 1991 (Suppl); 137: 45–47.

40. Smith RC, Rosenfield AT, Choe KA, et al. Acute flank pain: Comparison of non contrast-enhanced CT and intravenous urography. Radiology 1995; 194: 789–794.

41. Caro JJ, Trindade E, McGregor M. The risks of death and of severe nonfatal reactions with high- vs low- osmolality contrast media: a meta-analysis. AJR 1991;156: 825–832.

42. Tepel M, van der Giet M, Schwarzfeld C, Laufer U, Liermann D, Zidek W. Prevention of radio-graphic-contrast-agent-induced reductions in renal function by acetylcysteine. N Engl J Med 2000; 343: 180–184.

43. Aspelin P, Aubry P, Fransson SG, Strasser R, Willenbrock R, Berg KJ. Nephrotoxicity in High-Risk Patients Study of Iso-Osmolar and Low-Osmolar Non-Ionic Contrast Media Study Investigators. Nephrotoxic effects in high-risk patients undergoing angiography. N Engl J Med. 2003; 348: 491–499.

44. Fowler KAB, Locken JA, Duchesne JH, Williamson MR. US for detecting renal calculi with nonenhanced CT as a reference standard. Radiology 2002; 222: 109–113.

45. Laing FC, Jeffrey RB, Wing VW. Ultrasound versus excretory urography in evaluating acute flank pain. Radiology 1985; 154: 613–616.

46. Rodgers PM, Bates JA, Irving HC. Intrarenal Doppler ultrasound studies in normal and acutely obstructed kidneys. Brit J Radiol 1992; 65: 207–212.

47. Mallek R, Bankier AA, Etele-Hainz A, Kletter K, Mostbeck GH. Distinction between obstructive and nonobstructive hydronephrosis: Value of diuresis duplex Doppler sonography. AJR 1996; 166: 113–117.

48. Hill MC, Rich JI, Mardiat JG, Finder CA. Sonography versus excretory urography in acute flank pain. AJR 1985; 144: 1235–1238.

49. Schwartz BF, Schenkman N, Armenakas NA, Stoller ML. Imaging characteristics of indinavir calculi. J Urol 1999; 161: 1085–1087.

50. Olcott EW, Sommer FG, Napel S. Accuracy of detection and measurement of renal calculi: in vitro comparison of three-dimensional spiral CT, radiography, and nephrotomography. Radiology 1997; 204: 19–25.

51. Smith RC, Verga M, McCarthy S, Rosenfield AT. Diagnosis of acute flank pain: Value of unenhanced helical CT. AJR 1996; 166: 97–101.

52. Heneghan JP, McGuire KA, Leder RA, DeLong DM, Yoshizumi T, Nelson RC. Helical CT for nephrolithiasis and ureterolithiasis: comparison of conventional and reduced radiation-dose techniques. Radiology. 2003; 229: 575–580.

53. Levine J, Neitlich J, Smith RC. The value of prone scanning to distinguish ureterovesical junction stones from ureteral stones that have passed into the bladder: leave no stone unturned. AJR 1999; 172: 977–981.

54. Smith RC, Verga M, Dalrymple N, McCarthy S, Rosenfield AT. Acute ureteral obstruction: value of secondary signs of helical unenhanced CT. AJR 1996; 167: 1109–1113.

55. Bell TV, Fenlon HM, Davison BD, Ahari HK, Hussain S. Unenhanced helical CT criteria to differentiate distal ureteral calculi from pelvic phleboliths. Radiology 1998; 207: 363–367.

56. Heneghan JP, Dalrymple NC, Verga M, Resenfield AT, Smith RC. Soft-tissue "rim" sign in the diagnosis of ureteral calculi with use of nonenhanced helical CT. Radiology 1997; 202: 709–711.

57. Boridy IC, Nikolaidis P, Kawashima A, Goldman SM, Sandler CM. Ureterolithiasis: value of the tail sign in differentiating phleboliths from ureteral calculi at nonenhanced helical CT. Radiology 1999; 211: 619–621.

58. Guest AR, Cohan RH, Korobkin M, et al. Assessment of the clinical utility of the rim and comet-tail signs in differentiating ureteral stones from Phleboliths. AJR 2001; 177: 1285–1291.

59. Gottlieb RH, La TC, Erturk EN, et al. CT in detecting urinary tract calculi: influence on patient imaging and clinical outcomes. Radiology 2002; 225: 441–449.

60. Sudah M, Vanninen R, Partanen K, Heino A, Vainio P, Ala-Opas M. MR urography in evaluation of acute flank pain. AJR 2001; 176: 105–112.

61. O'Malley ME, Hahn PF, Yoder IC, Gazelle GS, McGovern FJ, Mueller PR. Comparison of excretory phase, helical computed tomography with intravenous urography in patients with painless haematuria. Clin Radiol 2003; 58: 294–300.

62. Sudah M, Vanninen RL, Partanen K, et al. Patients with acute flank pain: comparison of MR urography with unenhanced helical CT. Radiology 2002; 223: 98–105.

63. Regan F, Bohlman ME, Khazan R, Rodriguez R, Schultze-Haakh H. MR urography using HASTE imaging in the assessment of ureteric obstruction. AJR 1996; 167: 1115–1120.

64. Rothpearl D, Frager D, Subramanian A, et al. MR urography: technique and application. Radiology 1995; 194: 125–130.

65. Roy C, Saussine C, Jahn C, et al. Fast imaging MR assessment of ureterohydronephrosis during pregnancy. Magn Reson Imaging 1995; 13: 767–772.

21 Physician Safety

Ronald M. Yang, MD *and Gary C. Bellman,* MD

Key Words: Radiation; fluoroscopy; safety; infection control.

INTRODUCTION

Percutaneous nephrolithotomy is a well-established procedure of proven safety and efficacy. According to Bass et al., nearly 90% of target stones can be successfully removed in the community center *(1)*, whereas almost 100% of stones may be treated in tertiary care centers *(2–4)*. The benefit of low early morbidity *(5,6)* and early return to work and recreational activities *(7–10)* has popularized this approach for treatment of renal calculi. Central to the success of any percutaneous procedure is the establishment of a safe and reliable access into the renal collecting systems. As with any interventional procedure, the creation of a percutaneous access tract into the renal collecting system requires imaging equipment for guidance. The availability of high-quality C-arm configuration fluoroscopy equipment allows fluoroscopic monitoring essential for introduction of complex intrarenal catheters and guidewire manipulation. Although the advent of real-time diagnostic ultrasonography *(10,11)* and CT guidance *(12)* provides alternative guidance systems for urinary tract intervention, primary fluoroscopic guidance for percutaneous nephrostomy placement is still the preferred technique for most percutaneous stone therapies. The use of fluoroscopic guidance has increased the exposure of the urologists to the possible deleterious effects of radiation. In addition, risks of infection with deadly pathogens always exist in any surgical procedure. In this chapter, we will discuss the aspects of physician safety in the treatment of urinary stone disease, including radiation and infectious precautions.

From: Current Clinical Urology, *Urinary Stone Disease:*
A Practical Guide to Medical and Surgical Management
Edited by: M. L. Stoller and M. V. Meng © Humana Press Inc., Totowa, NJ

RADIATION SAFETY GUIDELINES
Radiation Effects

Ionizing radiation refers to forms of electromagnetic radiation and particulate matter that can impart sufficient energy to break ionic and chemical bonds in the matter that interact with them. X-rays and gamma rays are the most common agents used for diagnostic imaging. The standard international unit (SI) used to measure units of ionizing radiation is the gray (Gy). Each gray is the quantity of energy (1 Joule) being absorbed by 1 kg of mass. An older form of classification is the rad (radiation absorbed dose), which is equivalent to .01 Gy (1 Gy = 100 rad).

To comprehensively describe the deleterious effects of ionizing radiation is beyond the scope of the chapter. We will attempt to briefly review the biologic basis of radiation effects and provide recommendations for methods the surgeon can use for self-protection. The mechanisms by which ionizing radiation produces biologic damage can be broadly divided into either "direct action" effects vs "indirect action" effects. Direct action effects refer to ionization of chemical bonds in essential biomolecules such as DNA. The most deleterious effect of damage includes single- and double-strand breakage, deletion of a base, and chemical crosslinking of two strands. This damage is amplified during DNA proliferation as the chromosome mismatches accumulate over multiple cell replication cycles. These mistakes in the genome ultimately manifest clinically as cell death or carcinoma. Other host factors can indirectly affect the clinical manifestation of the DNA damage. Factors such as the cell mitotic rate, cell death rate, nutrient supply, hormonal status, immunocompetence, DNA mismatch repair mechanisms, and presence of other toxic substances such as chemicals or drugs can determine whether or not the damage is clinically expressed (13). The whole body lethal dose of X-ray is approx 5 Gy, and the yearly maximum permissible dose equivalent for occupation exposure in any one year for the combined whole body is 5 rems as recommended by the National Commission on Radiation Protection (NCRP). Rem is equal to the number of rads multiplied by a quality factor ranging from 1 to 20 that represents the degree of biologic insult for equal amounts of difference types of ionizing radiation.

Radiation Protection Recommendations

With recent technological advancement and technical improvements, urologists are using the help of different radiation imaging equipment for urologic procedures, including percutaneous nephrolithotomies for renal stone extraction. Fluoroscopic devices are central to the development of this endourologic technique. Despite this familiarity, the urologist usually has little formal protective equipment other than the standard lead aprons and thyroid shield.

The radiation dose necessary to produce skin injury is variable and depends on several factors. Typical threshold doses include 300 rads for temporary depilation of skin and 600 rads for erythema to be visible in the skin. The consequences of receiving radiation doses in the range of 1500–2000 rads include epidermal desquamation, dermal necrosis, and secondary ulceration (14). Because the deleterious effects of radiation exposure is well known (15), the endourologist should protect himself/herself and patients from radiation exposure by using a dose that is as low as reasonably achievable (ALARA) with no concurrent loss of image quality to minimize the radiation exposure.

Lead aprons and thyroid shields are the basic form of protection to the urologist. They provide up to 99% of radiation protection to the thorax, abdominal, and genital region.

Currently all hospitals in United States have lead aprons and shields available for all operators of radiation equipment in the operating room. They are easy to use and provide effective protection for the surgeon. One needs to remember to wear the lead aprons and shields under the operative gown to maintain sterile continuity during the surgical procedure. Though lead aprons and thyroid shields provide effective protection to the thyroid, thorax, and genital regions, scatter radiation to the forehead of the urologist are often not protected by this equipment. Radiation entering the patient is usually absorbed, scattered, or transmitted as a function of the density of the tissue it encounters. Though only 0.1% of incident beam is scattered in a 90° angle to the incident radiation, contribution from tube leakage, scatter from machine components, and scatter from the patient comprises the secondary radiation field *(16)*. Though it is often difficult to objectively compare the secondary radiation field exposure in different operative theater settings, in our experience using fluoroscopic guidance for percutaneous access, the secondary radiation field can measure as high as 187 mrad an hour 25 cm from the source of the radiation and 51 mrad an hour 50 cm from the source *(17)*. Numerous new radiation shields that were originally used to shield urologists during cystoscopies to further protect the urologist from the deleterious effect of radiation are now available for percutaneous stone procedures *(18)*.

In order for an effective radiation shield to be used in percutaneous procedures, the shield should be able to be easily installed on the standard operative table and not significantly hamper the surgeon's view or access to the operative field (Fig. 1). Similar shielding instruments have been described in the literature for use during gastrointestinal *(19)* and interventional radiology procedures *(20)*. Usually such shields are constructed from 0.5 mm lead-equivalent vinyl-coated lead sheeting, and can be easily installed onto a standard operating table using clamps that fasten onto steel supporting beams that hold the shield onto the side of an operating table. The entire assembly takes less than 5 min in experienced hands. The shield height can be adjusted to fit the urologist to provide an optimal view and access to the operative field. These shields have been shown to reduce an average of 96.1% of the radiation at a distance of 25 cm and 71.2% at a distance of 50 cm from the source of the radiation when used *(17)*.

The NCRP states that the maximum permissible dose equivalent for occupation exposure in any one year for the combined whole body is 5 rems. Given the experience of the urologist, the number of cases performed per year, the difficulty in establishing the percutaneous access, and the amount of intraoperative imaging required for each endourologic procedure, an urologist may be exposed to a significant amount of radiation. The radiation shield is an effective means of reducing that source of radiation.

The best method of reducing radiation exposure to the patient and urologist is to reduce the amount of time spent near a radiation field and to shorten the time that a fluoroscopy unit is used. As the deleterious effects of radiation is cumulative and results in increase risk of DNA damage and cancer, the ALARA principal should be strictly respected *(15)*. In cases where the time is minimized and the maximal allowable distance is employed, shielding is the most effective method of protection for the urologist. Lead aprons and thyroid shields with an equivalent lead thickness of 0.5 mm should be used by everyone exposed to the radiation field. In addition to the usage of lead aprons, the urologist should also consider use of a mounted radiation shield such as the one used in our study at the tableside to further minimize the radiation exposure owing to the close proximity to the radiation source. The image intensifier should also be positioned above the table with the radiation sources placed below the table to allow the table to act as a shield and further reduce scattered radiation.

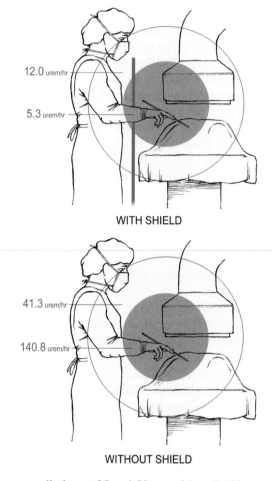

Fig. 1. Exposure to radiation at 25 and 50 cm with and without radiation shield.

As new generations of equipment, designed to reduce the dose of radiation delivered to the patient and surgeon, such as the pulsed fluoroscopy and digital imaging fluoroscopy unit becomes available, the combined method of shielding coupled with minimal fluoroscopic usage time will minimize the deleterious effects of radiation to the urologist and patient.

Conclusion

As technology advances, continuing efforts to reduce the radiation exposure of the patient and urologist involved in endourologic procedures and improving imaging quality will be the ultimate goal for all parties involved. The use of basic, common sense ALARA concepts, which include minimal fluoroscopic usage, maximal allowable distance from source of radiation, and implementation of effective shielding can provide a significant reduction in radiation to both urologist and patient. The radiation shields can also be one more step in the goal of reducing the amount of radiation exposure to the urologist. Other methods such as the establishment of effective dose-minimizing imaging protocols and the adaptation of equipment optimized in reduction of radiation exposure are important steps toward the formation of a safer endourologic environment for both the urologist and patient.

INFECTION-CONTROL PRACTICES
Introduction

With the advent of the AIDS epidemic, much attention has been focused on the prevention of infectious disease transmission in the health-care setting. According to the CDC, an exposure-prone invasive procedure is defined as "surgical entry into tissues, cavities, or organs or repair of major traumatic injuries" associated with "an operating or delivery room, emergency department, or outpatient setting, including both physician' and dentists' offices *(21)*." All procedures performed in endourology certainly qualify as such and universal precautions should be strictly followed to minimize the risk of exposure. In this chapter, we will briefly review the principles of universal precautions, then embark on a discussion of the three most significant pathogens that can be transmitted, namely HIV, hepatitis B, and hepatitis C. In the following discussion, let us keep in mind that although the our discussion focuses on prevention of disease transmission from the patient to the health care worker (HCW), universal precautions are equally effective in preventing transmission of disease from the HCW to the patient.

Universal Precautions

In 1987, the Center for Disease Control published an article in the Morbidity and Mortality Weekly Report that was titled "Recommendations for prevention of HIV transmission in health-care settings *(1)*." The recommendations included in the article have since been known as "Universal Blood and Body Fluid Precautions." By applying the universal precaution principles, HCWs circumvent the need for extensive HIV testing or specific HIV labeling of specimens or other materials *(22)*. The basic tenant of washing hands and wearing gloves, gowns, and masks is elementary to the practice of modern sterile surgical technique. Eye protection using glasses, goggles, or face shields should be stressed in all operative settings. Disposal of sharp instruments in special puncture-resistant containers along with proper disposal of contaminated material and sterilization techniques are other standard principles of the universal precautions. One of the less implemented recommendations is to double-glove for all invasive procedures. The benefit of this practice has consistently been shown to reduce the number of needle sticks and cutaneous exposures during surgery *(23)*. Given that a 25–60% occult-glove perforation rate during surgery was documented in studies by vascular surgeons and otolaryngologists, the additional layer offered by the second pair of gloves can be very reassuring *(24,25)*. It is also theorized that the amount of viral inoculum exposed to the surgeon is also reduced to a minimum with the use of double gloves as the two layers of latex literally wipes blood away from the penetrating instrument as it passes though the layers of latex *(26)*.

Whereas the practice of universal precautions focuses on what HCWs can do actively to reduce infectious exposure risks, numerous innovations in equipment design have been created to improve safety. Syringes that do not allow the user to recap the needle and needles that have a recap guard, which can be slid on after usage, are a few of the new safety measures employed on sharp instruments. Hospitals should actively encourage their material management departments to procure these instruments as allowed by the budget.

As for surgeons, one should weigh the benefit of replacing individual sharp instruments with newly designed pieces that offer more protection. For example, the shielded double-skin hook tenaculum can be used instead of the traditional double hook to provide exposure. Of course, the individual preference and ease of use for a particular instrument in a particular situation can only be decided by the experience and preference of each individual.

The operating room staff and scrub nurses should also adapt new techniques to minimize risks. A no-pass technique should be used to avoid injury to either surgeon or scrub nurse by avoiding direct handing off of instruments. Instead, instruments are passed to and from the surgeon using a kidney basin as a neutral zone. Magnetic pads can also be used to prevent instruments from slipping off the surgical field, reducing the impulse to quickly grab for a potentially sharp instrument. Bovie and bipolar coagulators instead of scalpels should be considered for soft tissue dissection to reduce possible blade injury (7).

Among thoroughly educated health care professionals, universal precautions have been demonstrated to show a decrease in body fluid exposure incidents. A study of 900 HCWs in a tertiary hospital showed that the blood contact rate was halved when universal precautions were implemented (27). It is simple and easy to implement. The mainstay of infection prevention in endourology and any field of medicine should be focused on adequate education of health care workers regarding universal precautions and actively encouraging the strict adherence to them.

Blood-Borne Pathogens

To truly appreciate the infectious risk of any surgical procedure, one needs to understand the nature of the disease. Of all the possible infectious pathogens that can be transmitted during endourological cases, HIV, hepatitis B, and hepatitis C remain the most feared. We will review each of the three diseases in detail and provide a more clear understanding of the risks involved.

Hepatitis B Virus (HBV)

Of the three pathogens, hepatitis B is the only virus that health care workers can be effectively vaccinated against. It is a double-stranded DNA virus that has been a known to cause occupational infection since the 1940s (28). The method of transmission closely parallels that of HIV: exposure to blood and other body fluids and sexual contact (29). In the 1991 surveillance data published by the Center for Disease Control and Prevention, 5100 health care workers who reported frequent blood contacts developed occupationally acquired HBV infection in the United States. Based on the natural history of the disease, 255 (5%) of these individuals will eventually be hospitalized for their illness in the acute period and 5 (0.1%) of those individuals would die of fulminant hepatic failure. After the acute phase of the disease, 510 (10%) of the individuals would become chronic carriers and 107 (21%) of the chronic carriers would succumb to cirrhosis or hepatocellular carcinoma (30). Indeed, Hepatitis B is a deadly disease that will claim the lives of a quarter of its victims.

One of the biggest risk factors associated with hepatitis B transmission from patients to health care workers is the seroprevalence of the virus among the patients. Multiple factors determine the seroprevalence of a particular disease, including ethnicity, country of origin, intravenous drug use, and sexual contact with infected individuals. From a sample of four studies, the prevalence ranged between 0.9 and 6% in hospitalized and emergency room patients *(31–34)*. For health care workers, the mode of transmission of hepatitis B virus is through blood contact from a sharp object injury. In any given case of exposure, the risk of acquiring HBV infection is correlated to the e-antigen positivity of the source patient. In other words, the higher the concentration of circulating HBV e antigen in the blood, the higher the risk of infection. The risk of acquiring infection from a single percutaneous exposure to e-antigen positive blood is approx 30% *(30)*.

Vaccination for hepatitis B virus is an effective means of preventing infection with HBV. A random testing of 3239 orthopedic surgeons in 1990 revealed that 90% of those 20–29 yr of age had been effectively vaccinated against the HBV, whereas only 35% of those older than 60 yr reported vaccination *(35)*. Another study of 770 hospital-based surgeons in general surgery, gynecology, and orthopedics who were tested in 1992 sero-survey in 21 hospitals showed that only 424 (55%) surgeons reported receiving at least three doses of hepatitis B vaccine. In the same study, 225 (22%) of the 770 surgeons were still susceptible to HBV infection based on their sero profile. Of these 225 individuals, 62 had reported receiving at least one dose of vaccine, but either were nonresponders or had antibody levels that could not be detected *(36)*. The findings above suggests that although an effective means of prevention against HBV is available to most individuals, many are still not utilizing them.

Hepatitis B prophylaxis after percutaneous injury centers on usage of hepatitis B immunoglobulin (HBIG) and HBV vaccination sequence if the individual has not been previously vaccinated. If the individual has been vaccinated and the antibody titer adequate, no further precautions are required. If the titer is inadequate, the health care worker should be given HBIG and a hepatitis B vaccine booster *(29)*.

Hepatitis C Virus (HCV)

Of the three pathogens that are being discussed in detail, hepatitis C virus is probably the least understood. It is a RNA virus that is transmitted the same way as hepatitis B virus. Of the individuals infected, approx 20% will develop a clinically recognizable acute infection. About half of those will progress to chronic active hepatitis and 20% of those with chronic active hepatitis will develop cirrhosis *(37)*. It is felt that owing to the lower level of viremia associated with HCV infection (up to 10 trillion virion per milliliter blood for HBV infection vs 100–1000 virions/mL blood for HCV infection) the risk of transmission for each percutaneous exposure is approx 2.7–10% *(38)*.

Data regarding the sero prevalence of HCV among patients is limited. The first-generation tests for antibody to HCV has only been commercially available since 1990. A random sample of 2523 patients from an urban hospital in Baltimore collected in 1991 showed that 454 (18%) individuals were seropositive *(31)*. A separate Toronto region study that included 3000 patients admitted to a teaching hospital revealed the seroprevalence to be 0.5% *(39)*. Thus the actual prevalence of HCV may vary greatly based on the particular patient population that the surgeon interacts with.

Owing to the fact that no vaccination currently exists for HCV and treatment for the virus is not 100% effective, it is considered a much deadlier disease compared to HBV. Immediate post exposure prophylaxis requires topical disinfection with providone-iodine solution. There is insufficient evidence for use of immunoglobulin after a needlestick injury and it is currently not indicated for acute exposure. Antiviral agents are also not recommended for lack of effectiveness *(40)*. Treatment with interferon has been shown to reduce the liver inflammation, but the drug is only effective in approx 50% of patients.

In addition, the improvement is sustained only in 50% of those patients that responded to interferon after cessation of treatment. Coupled with the poor effectiveness with the multiple side effects that plague the patients during treatment, HCV should be considered a much more significant occupational hazard for surgeons.

HUMAN IMMUNODEFICIENCY VIRUS (HIV)

Although the clinical syndrome caused by the HIV virus known as acquired immunodeficiency syndrome (AIDS) has only been described in the literature within the past 20 yr, AIDS and HIV have captured the attention of the public like no other infectious pathogens. HIV is a RNA retrovirus that uses its outer envelope protein gp-120 to bind host cells that express the cell surface protein CD4. Once attached to the cell surface, HIV invades the cell and integrates its DNA into the host cell chromosome via the enzyme reverse transcriptase. After successful integration, the proviral DNA directs the production and assembly of progeny virus, eventually leading to cell lysis and death (29). Clinical latency averages 10 yr in the adult population. The CD4 cell population gradually declines over the course of the disease eventually leading to the immunocompromised state manifested by AIDS-related complex and AIDS. HIV infection is a terminal disease, which will eventually claim the lives of its victims. A full discussion of the disease process is beyond the scope of this chapter, but we will focus on the important risk factors for transmission and preventive measures to minimize exposure in the health care setting.

Epidemiological studies have reported that approx 1.1–1.5 million Americans are infected with HIV. The seroprevalence differs greatly depending on the population surveyed (inner city vs suburban vs intravenous drug users) and generally range from 0.2% to 14% (41). The highest risk for HIV transmission for surgeons is due to percutaneous injury or mucocutaneous contact between breached skin barriers and blood. The risk of percutaneous injury during operative procedures is related to the length of surgery, amount of blood loss, and emergent nature of procedure (42). The rate for mucocutaneous exposure is not as well documented compared to the rate of percutaneous exposure, but is believed to be higher compared to percutaneous exposure owing to the higher incidence of exposure (29).

The rate of HIV infection per exposure to HIV-infected blood via hollow-bore needles is estimated at about 0.3% (30). For solid-bore suture needles, the transmission rate is significantly lower owing to the lower inoculum of blood delivered by the solid-bore needles. Another important factor in infectivity rate is the titer of HIV in the patient's blood (43).

In addition to potential percutaneous exposure, a theoretical risk of aerosolized transmission of HIV via the respiratory route was a concern in the last decade. However, no current biologic or epidemiologic evidence support fears that transmission of aerosolized HIV particles occurs through the respiratory route in vivo (29).

All health care institutions in the United States must have medications available to health care workers within an hour of exposure to possible HIV infection based on CDC guidelines. Institutions may provide "starter packs" through the institutional pharmacy and may dispense them immediately upon approval by the exposure counselor. Before releasing the medication, the exposure counselor should ascertain from the health care worker whether there are underlying medical conditions, allergies to medications, or other reasons the antiretroviral medication should not be administered. Most programs have traditionally offered 4–6 wk of zidovudine prophylaxis based on the CDC's recommendation *(44)*. The health care worker should undergo a complete clinical evaluation by a clinician familiar with the use of antiretroviral agents and the management of exposed health care workers within 72 h of exposure. Baseline blood should be drawn for HIV serology, hepatitis serology and vaccination status. In addition, liver enzymes and chemistry should be evaluated to facilitate the long-term treatment plan of the health care worker. Blood from the source patient should also be evaluated if the patients are willing to donate them. On the occasion that the patient refuses to provide blood samples, available options differ from state to state in these cases. Some states have consent laws in which the patient is deemed to have provided consent by virtue of presenting for care at an institution, whereas other states clearly allow no testing in the absence of written informed consent from the patient. Health care workers should be monitored with HIV antibody testing 6 wk, 3 mo, and 6 mo following exposure. Other more sensitive tests such as PCR for HIV RNA may also be performed, and can provide evidence of infection up to 9 d before the appearance of HIV-specific antibodies *(45)*. Most health care workers who seroconvert following an exposure do so within 3 mo, and all reported cases have occurred within 6 mo *(46)*. Because the treatment with antiretroviral medication during the acute phase of HIV infection has been shown to decrease the risk of disease progression, the health care worker along with clinicians should not delay the diagnosis and the treatment *(47)*.

Conclusion

The most important factor in the prevention of infectious pathogens in endourological procedures is the surgeon's own attitude. Although the lifetime risk of HIV, hepatitis B, and hepatitis C is small, the incapacitating disease these pathogens cause should never be underestimated. The universal precautions have been shown to be an effective and practical technique to minimize the risk to the surgeon and the staff. Each of us will need to compare the benefit to the inconvenience of preventive methods such as wearing eye protection and double gloving. Only then can one make an informed decision to make our work environment the safest possible for ourselves.

REFERENCES

1. Bass RB Jr, Beard JH, Looner WH, Mosley BR, Pond HS, Rutherford CL Jr. Percutaneous ultrasonic lithotripsy in the community hospital. J Urol 1985; 133: 586.
2. Reddy PK, Hulbert JC, Lange PH, et al. Percutaneous removal of renal and ureteral calculi: Experience with 400 cases. J Urol 1985; 134: 662.
3. Segura JH, Patterson DE, LeRoy AJ, et al. Percutaneous removal of kidney stones: Review of 1000 cases. J Urol 1985; 134: 1077.
4. Lee WJ, Smith AD, Cubelli V, Vernace FM. Percutaneous nephrolithotomy: Anaylsis of 500 consecutive cases. Urol Radiol 1986; 8: 61.
5. LeRoy AJ, Segura JW, Williams JH Jr, Patterson DE. Percutaneous renal calculus removal in an extracorporeal shockwave lithotripsy practice. J Urol 1987; 138: 703.
6. Carson CC, Danneberger JE, Weinerth JL. Percutaneous lithotripsy in morbid obesity. J Urol 1988; 139: 243.
7. Preminger GM, Clayman RV, Hardeman SW, Franklin J, Curry T, Peters PC. Percutaneous nephrolithotomy vs. open surgery for renal calculi: A comparative study. JAMA 1985; 254: 1054.
8. Brannen GE, Bush WH, Correa RJ, Gibbons RP, Elder JS. Kidney stone removal: Percutaneous versus surgical lithotomy. J Urol 1985; 133: 6.
9. Burns JR, Hamrick LC, Keller FS. Percutaneous nephrolithotomy in 86 patients: Analysis of results and costs. South Med J 1986; 79: 975.

10. Brown MW, Culley CC, Dunnick NR, Weinerth JL. Comparison of the costs and morbidity of percutaneous and open flank procedures. J Urol 1986; 135: 1150.

11. Charton M, Vallancien G, Veillon B, Brisset JM. Urinary tract infection in percutaneous surgery for renal calculi. J Urol 1986; 135: 15.

12. Marberger M, Stackl W, Hruby W. Percutaneous litholopaxy of renal calculi with ultrasound. Eur Urol 1982; 8: 236.

13. Putman CE, Ravin CE. Textbook of Diagnostic Imaging. WB Saunders, Philadelphia, PA, 1998.

14. Wagner LK, Eiffel PJ, Geise RA. Potential biological effects following high x-ray dose interventional procedures. J Vasc Intervent Radiol 1994; 5: 71.

15. FDA Public Health Advisory. Avoidance of serious x-ray-induced skin injuries to patients during fluoroscopically guided procedures. United States Government Printing Office, Washington, DC, 1994.

16. Castaneda W and Espenan G. How to protect yourself and others from radiation. In: Smith AD, Badlani GH, Badlu, DH et al., eds. Smith's Textbook of Endourology. Quality Medical Publishing, St. Louis, MO, 1996, pp. 21–28.

17. Yang RM, Bellman G. Radiation protection during percutaneous nephrolithotomies utilizing a newly designed urologic surgery radiation shield. In Press.

18. Giblin JG, Rubenstein J, Taylor A, Pahira J. Radiation risk to the urologist during endourologic procedures, and a new shield that reduces exposure. Urology 1996; 48: 624–627.

19. Miotto D, Feltrin G, Calamosca M. A radiation protection device for use during percutaneous transhepatic examinations. Radiology 1984; 151: 799.

20. Faulkner K. Radiation protection in interventional radiology. Br J Radiol 1997; 70: 325.

21. Center for Disease Control. Recommendation for prevention of HIV transmission in health-care settings. Morbidity and Mortality Weekly Report 1987; 36 (Suppl. 2S): 6S–7S.

22. Center for Disease Control. Guidelines for prevention of transmission of human immunodeficiency virus and hepatitis B virus to health-care and public safety workers. MMRW 1989; 38 (S6): 1–37.

23. Bennett B, Duff P. The effect of double gloving on frequency of glove perforations. Obstetrics and Gynecology 1991; 78(6): 101–122.

24. Aarino P, Laine T. Glove perforation rate in vascular surgery – a comparison between single and double gloving. VASA 2001; 30:122–124.

25. Godlin MS, Lavernia CJ, Harris JP. Occult surgical glove perforations in otolaryngology-head and neck surgery. Arch Otolaryngology and Head Neck Surg 1993; 108 (1): 91–95.

26. Murr AH, Lee KC. Universal Precautions for the Otolaryngologist: Techniques and Equipment for Minimizing Exposure Risk. ENT Journal 1995; 74(5): 338,341–346.

27. Kristensen MS, Wernberg NM, Anker-Moller, E. Healthcare workers' risk of contract with body fluids in a hospital: the effect of complying with the universal precautions policy. Infection Control and Hospital Epidemiology 1992; 13(12): 719–724.

28. Fry DE. Occupational risks of infection in the surgical management of trauma patients. Am J Surg 1993; 165 (2A Suppl): 26–33.

29. Chou L, Reynolds MR, Esterhai JL. Hazards to the orthopaedic trauma surgeon: occupational exposure to HIV and viral hepatitis (a review article). J Orthopedic Traumas 1996; 10(4): 289–296.

30. Short LJ, DM Bell. Risk of occupational infection with blood-borne pathogens in operating and delivery room settings. Am J Infection Control 1993; 21(6): 343–350.

31. Kelen GD, Green GB, Purcell RH, et al. Hepatitis B and Hepatitis C in emergency department patients. NEJM 1992; 326: 1399–1404.

32. Mahoney JP, Richman AV, Teague PO. Admission screening for hepatitis B surface antigen in a university hospital. South Med J 1978; 71: 624–628;637.

33. Handsfield HH, Cummings MJ, Swenson PD. Prevalence of antibody to human immunodeficiency virus and hepatitis B surface antigen in blood samples submitted to a hospital laboratory. JAMA 1987; 258: 3395–3397.

34. Gordin FM, Gilbert C, Hawley HP, Willoughby A. Prevalence of human immunodeficiency virus and hepatitis B virus in unselected hospital admissions: implications for mandatory testing and universal precautions. J Infect Dis. 1990; 11: 14–17.

35. Tokars JI, Chamberland ME, Shapiro C. Infection with hepatitis B virus, hepatitis C virus, and human immunodeficiency virus among orthopedic surgeons [abstract 22]. Second Annual Meeting of the Society for Hospital Epidemiology of America, Baltimore, MD, 1992.

36. Panlilio AL, Chamberland ME, Shapiro C, et al. Human immunodeficiency virus, hepatitis B virus, and hepatitis C virus serosurvey among hospital based surgeons. [abstract 31] Infect Control Hosp Epidemiol 1993; 14: 419.

37. Regnier SJ. ACS/CDC meeting explores risks of blood-born pathogens. Am Coll Surg Bull 1994; 79: 30–38.

38. Kiyosawa E, Sodeyama T, Tanaka E, et al. hepatitis C in hospital employees with needle stick injuries. Ann Intern Med 1991; 115: 367–369.

39. Louie M, Low DE, Feinman SV. Prevalence of bloodborne infective agents among people admitted to a Canadian hospital. Can Med Assoc J 1992; 146: 1331–1334.

40. McGrory BJ, Kilby AE. Hepatitis C virus infection: review and implications. Am J Orthop 2000; 29(4): 261–266.

41. Janssen RS, St. Louis ME, Satten GA, et al. HIV infection among patients in US acute care hospitals. NEJM 1992; 327: 445–452.

42. Tokar JL, Bell DM, Culver DH, et al. Percutaneous injuries during surgical procedures. JAMA 1992; 267: 2899–1904.

43. Mast S, Woolwine JD, Gerberding JL. Efficacy of gloves in reducing blood volumes transferred during simulated needle stick injuries. J Infect Dis 1993; 168: 1589–1592.

44. Centers for Disease Control and Prevention. Update: Investigations of persons treated by HIV-infected health care workers—United States. MMWR 1993;42: 329–331.

45. Busch MP, Herman SA, Henrard DR, et al. Time course and kinetics of HIV viremia during primary infection [abstract 38]. Third National Conference of Human Retroviruses and Related Infections, Washington, DC, 1996.

46. Henderson DL. HIV-1 in the health care setting. In: Principles and Practice of Infectious Diseases, (Mandell GL, Douglass Jr RG, Bennett JE, eds.). Churchill Livingstone, New York, NY, 1995, pp. 104–117.

47. Wheeler DA. Human immunodeficiency virus in the health care setting. Occupational Medicine 1997; 12(4): 741–756.

22

Treatment of Acute Renal Colic

Albert M. Ong, MD and Thomas W. Jarrett, MD

CONTENTS

Key Words: Renal colic; nephrolithiasis; pain; ureter; hematuria.

PRESENTATION

Acute renal colic presents as paroxysmal severe flank pain with or without radiation to the ipsilateral groin. It is caused by partial or complete acute renal obstruction. Like other obstructed hollow visceral organs, renal colic is frequently associated with nausea and vomiting. Because of the characteristically poor localization of visceral abdominal pain, the pain from renal colic can be confused with pain arising in other abdominal organs, leading to a broad differential diagnosis *(1)* (Table 1). It is a common ailment— it is estimated that 2–3% of the Western population will suffer an attack of renal colic in their lifetime. In the United States, it is estimated that 12% of the population will develop kidney stones by the age of 70 *(2)*.

The pain owing to renal colic is traditionally thought to arise from stretching or distension of the ureter or renal pelvis caused by violent contraction of the ureteral musculature around an obstructing lesion *(1)*. Recent studies suggest that lactate production from prolonged muscular contraction owing to disrupted peristalsis irritates type A and C nerve fibers in the ureteral walls. These nerves send afferent signals through the

From: Current Clinical Urology, *Urinary Stone Disease:*
A Practical Guide to Medical and Surgical Management
Edited by: M. L. Stoller and M. V. Meng © Humana Press Inc., Totowa, NJ

Table 1
Differential Diagnosis of Renal Colic

Peritonitis
- Local
  (diverticulitis, early appendicitis, PID)
- Generalized

Vascular
- Abdominal aortic aneurysm
- Renal artery aneurysm
- Splenic artery aneurysm
- Autoimmune (vasculitis)
- Bowel ischemia/mesenteric ischemia
- Renal artery/vein thrombosis
- Retroperitoneal hematoma
- Loin pain/hematuria syndrome

Gynecologic
- Ectopic pregnancy
- PID
- Endometriosis
- Ovarian torsion
- Tubo-ovarian abscess

Psychiatric
- Malingering

Metabolic derangement
- Ketosis
- Lead colic
- Intermittent porphyria

Infectious
- Pyelonephritis
- Renal abscess
- Psoas abscess
- Fitz-Hugh-Curtis Syndrome

Cardiac
- Cardiac ischemia

Pulmonary
- Lower lobe pneumonia

Musculoskeletal pain (radicular pain)

Other obstructed viscous organs
- Biliary colic
- Early appendicitis
- Bowel obstruction
- Incarcerated inguinal hernia

visceral sympathetics to the dorsal root ganglia at T11-L1 levels of the spinal cord and are interpreted as pain *(3)*.

Depending on the level of renal obstruction, the typical pattern of pain consists of a constant ache located at the costovertebral angle with episodes of intermittent, severe pain, which does not improve with changes in position. The patient may frequently be observed to be pacing the room or changing positions frequently in an attempt to "escape" the pain *(1,3,4)*.

The patient may give a history of migrating pain gradually moving from the flank to the umbilicus and then to the ipsilateral groin. Rarely, the pain may occur contralateral to the side of the actual pathology *(3)*. The patient may complain of urinary frequency and urgency accompanying the movement of pain. If the obstruction is very proximal (stone obstructing a renal calyx), the pattern of pain may instead be constant and not paroxysmal. Occasionally, patients with urine extravasation may present with symptoms simulating an acute abdomen *(5)*.

As with any patient presenting with abdominal pain, the evaluation of a patient with suspected renal colic requires a thorough history and physical examination. The history should seek risk factors for renal obstruction and exclude other disease processes that can simulate renal colic. A previous history of kidney stones, metabolic abnormalities, chronic urinary tract infection, urothelial cancer, chronic analgesic abuse, family history of stone formation, or sickle cell trait can be suggestive of renal colic. A review of systems should also be performed to exclude other diagnostic possibilities.

Coexistent medical conditions, which may complicate or alter therapy, should also be considered. These include the presence of a solitary kidney, pregnancy, immunosuppression, diabetes, pulmonary or cardiac disease, and patient age. Other disorders, which may predispose to stone formation, such as chronic diarrhea, history of inflammatory bowel disease, history of urinary or fecal diversion, and sarcoidosis should also be considered. A complete medication history, including coumadin, nonsteroidal analgesics, and retroviral protease inhibitors may also be helpful.

Hyperesthesia of the associated dermatome may be present; however the patient should not have rebound or other signs of peritonitis. Careful abdominal palpation should be performed to exclude the presence of a pulsatile abdominal mass. Pressure applied by the examiner's hand to the abdomen should not worsen the pain. A rectal exam should be performed to exclude acute prostatitis, which often presents with bilateral flank pain. In women, a complete pelvic exam with bimanual palpation should be performed to exclude gynecologic processes, which can simulate renal colic. Auscultation of the abdomen and chest should be performed as part of the physical exam to rule out absent or high-pitched bowel sounds, abdominal bruits, signs of congestive heart failure, or pneumonia.

One of the most important parts of the physical examination is the careful evaluation of the patient's vital signs and overall clinical picture. Patients who are afebrile, who are not tachycardic, and show no signs of sepsis may be managed more expectantly than patients who are febrile, tachycardic, hypotensive, or moribund. Any evidence of systemic infection in the setting of flank pain demands urgent evaluation and therapy, as obstructed pyelonephritis is a true medical emergency.

In particular, any episode of hypotension in the setting of severe abdominal or back pain, particularly in elderly patients with vascular disease or history of tobacco use, should warrant an immediate search for a ruptured intra-abdominal aneurysm. A retrospective, multi-institution study published by Marston et al. found that initial misdiagnosis of ruptured abdominal aortic aneurysms occurred in 30% of referred cases. Of these cases, renal colic was the most frequent incorrect diagnosis (6). Aneurysms in other locations with similar presenting symptoms have been reported with near-fatal outcomes (7).

MUNCHAUSEN'S SYNDROME

In some cases, the stated symptom of pain may be factitious in origin. Moldwin suggests that renal colic is an ideal disorder for malingering patients to simulate, because it is treated with narcotic analgesics on the basis of reported symptoms (8). Malingering is part of a spectrum of somatoform disorders, which also includes Munchausen's syndrome and conversion disorders. They may be distinguished from each other based on the patient's awareness of gain and presence of conscious symptom production. It is a psychiatric disease that presents with physical symptoms. Symptom diaries of patients with somatization disorders suggest that these patients develop one new symptom per week (9).

Malingering can be differentiated as either "pure" or "partial" based on the existence of actual symptoms. Partial malingering is the gross exaggeration of existing physical symptoms for secondary gain. Pure malingering is the fraudulent presentation of completely nonexistent symptoms. There is a strong association with antisocial personality disorder with both types of malingering *(8,9)*.

Conversion disorders are the subconscious expression of physical complaints as a manifestation of underlying psychiatric disorders. In this disorder, the conversion process occurs in the subconscious, and the patient may not be aware of this process, or of potential secondary gain resulting from the manufacture of symptoms *(8)*.

In Munchausen's syndrome, patients attempt to maintain the "sick role" with their complaints. Unlike malingering patients, whose secondary gain is to miss work, obtain narcotics, or obtain sympathy, patients with Munchausen's syndrome will not attempt to avoid painful or dangerous procedures. Individuals with this disorder report physical complaints as a means to deal with stressful situations exceeding the individual's ability to cope. Some authors suggest that the hospital environment provides a sense of stability in patients with this disorder *(9,10)*.

Reich et al. found that the prevalence of factitious disorders presenting as renal colic in two Philadelphia hospitals was 0.6%. This rate is lower than the rate observed by Gault et al., who determined a malingering rate of 2.6% by examining the composition of renal stones submitted by patients for analysis. They found that 2.6% of the patients in their study submitted stones that were nonphysiologic (mineral) in nature and could not have possibly been from renal stones. Other fields may report even higher numbers—a study from the National Institute of Allergy and Infectious Disease found that 9.3% of patients referred for evaluation of fever of unknown origin were eventually diagnosed with factitious disorder after a complete workup *(11,12)*.

Riech and Hanno suggest that the diagnosis of malingering should be one of exclusion, and a formal work-up should be done to rule out serious disorders. In their series, patient characteristics associated with malingering were male sex, recurrent urologic complaints, history of radiolucent stones, and contrast allergy. A high proportion of these patients underwent unnecessary testing, which was estimated to cost $3100 more than patients with legitimate renal colic. Thirty nine percent (39%) of malingering patients left the hospital against medical advice. Most of this cost arose from unnecessary retrograde pyelography and hospitalization. It is likely that this cost could be reduced by routine use of noncontrast CT imaging *(11)*.

This is similar to the report of Gluckman and Stoller, who reported on the characteristics of three patients with Munchausen's syndrome presenting with renal colic in San Francisco area hospitals. They found that all the patients in their series had a history of bizarre past experiences, history of travel, and a willingness to accept potentially dangerous operative procedures. They suggest that it is difficult to treat the underlying psychiatric condition causing this behavior because these patients tend to leave when confronted *(13)*.

Although many physicians are familiar with these disorders in a medical setting, many members of the legal profession and lay public are not. The public generally assumes that the patient and physician work together as a team to uncover a pathological condition that causes the patient harm. This is not true with malingering patients. However, it is important to remember that the diagnosis of factitious disorder can coexist with a real episode of renal colic. Alternatively, hard to diagnose renal disorders such as intermittent hydronephrosis may have symptoms that sound suspiciously like malingering *(8,14,15)*.

Other clues to the presence of a factitious disorder include accurate prediction of a worsening disease course by the patient, failure to reach a diagnosis despite care by multiple physicians at multiple institutions, and unusually high number of disease recurrences. In many cases, patients with this disorder come from a medical background. Patients with complaints arising from factitious disorder may be unaware of the true origin of their symptoms because this disease process takes place on a subconscious level *(15)*.

DIFFERENTIAL DIAGNOSIS

In cases of true renal colic, the differential diagnosis includes nephrolithiasis, upper tract transitional cell carcinoma (TCC), renal papillary necrosis, clot obstruction, and extrinsic ureteral compression. Of these, nephrolithiasis is the most common disease entity on the differential diagnosis, and has a lifetime incidence of 12% in the United States *(2)*.

Because the ureters are adjacent to many different organs, pain arising from the ureters may initially be confused with different disease entities, particularly when stones become impacted. There are several anatomic areas where stones may become impacted. The first is the infundibulum of the renal calyx. Stones in this area tend to generate dull, nonparoxysmal pain. The second site is at the ureteropelvic junction. Stones in this area will present with renal colic if the obstruction is acute. The third location is the point where the ureter crosses the iliac vessels at the lower to mid-ureter. These stones may be mistaken for appendicitis when in the right ureter and diverticulitis when on the left. Finally, stones may become impacted at the ureterovesical junction. Stones in this location will present with frequency and dysuria, and is known as "tunnel syndrome" *(1,3,4)*.

Clot obstruction from a bleeding tumor, arteriovenous malformation, or patients with sickle cell trait after papillary necrosis occurs more rarely. Upper tract TCC consists only of 5% of all cases of TCC. It presents with clot obstruction in 10–40% of cases *(16)*. Treatment of upper tract TCC consists of stenting, ureteroscopy, biopsy and fulguration with pathologic diagnosis, followed by staging CT scan *(16,17)*. Percutaneous nephrostomy is avoided unless the tumor is known to be of low grade by biopsy *(16,18, 19)*. Diagnosis and treatment of a bleeding renal arteriovenous malformation consists of emergent urinary decompression with a nephrostomy tube followed by angiographic embolization *(20)*.

LABORATORY EVALUATION

Laboratory testing in cases of suspected renal colic should aim to exclude other etiologies of abdominal pain before the diagnosis of renal colic is made. Therefore, we recommend a complete metabolic panel, including liver enzymes and serum calcium (SMA-20), as well as a complete blood count, urinalysis, and urine culture. Coagulation parameters may be helpful in patients on anticoagulation therapy. Other laboratory tests, such as testing for sickle cell trait, may be ordered as clinically indicated. For patients with recurrent nephrolithiasis, a urine stone risk profile is recommended as an outpatient *(21)*.

Despite a meticulous history and physical examination, review of the patient's vital signs, combined with laboratory testing and plain abdominal films, the diagnosis of acute renal colic by these criteria alone may be unreliable. A retrospective review by Chen et al. on 380 patients with suspected renal colic by clinical criteria and plain radiography found that only 14% of these patients had pain attributable to urinary obstruction when evaluated by intravenous urography (IVU). Of this 14%, ureteral obstruction caused by stones or edema was diagnosed in 94% of cases *(22)*. The use of plain abdominal radiographs as a screening tool for renal stones was reported by Mutgi et al. in a study of 85 patients presenting with symptoms consistent with renal colic. They found a sensitivity of 58% and a specificity of 69% for stone detection in this population when plain abdominal radiographs were compared with intravenous pyelogram or stone retrieval. Based on these results Mutgi et al. concluded that plain abdominal radiographs are not useful when used as a screening test *(2)*. However, once discovered by other imaging modalities, plain abdominal radiography may be used as a follow-up study for patients with renal stones.

RADIOLOGICAL EVALUATION

The goal of imaging in the setting of renal colic and suspected renal stone is to secure the diagnosis of nephrolithiasis and to rule out obstructive nephrolithiasis. Before 1995, the standard for evaluation of patients with suspected renal colic was IVU, or retrograde pyelography if the patient had a contrast allergy. Spiral non-contrast computed tomography became the gold standard after a study by Smith et al. demonstrated the superiority of noncontrast CT over intravenous pyelography. This group compared the sensitivity and specificity of noncontrast helical CT scan with IVU in 22 patients with acute flank pain *(23)*. They concluded that noncontrast CT imaging has significant advantages to IVU, including faster study time (3–5 min), no requirement for intravenous contrast, and ability to diagnose other etiologies for abdominal pain. In their series, one patient with suspected renal colic was diagnosed instead with ovarian torsion and treated accordingly.

Their findings are supported by several other authors. Miller and Kane reported a series of 106 patients with suspected acute renal colic who underwent noncontrast spiral CT scan followed by IVU. They found a sensitivity of 96% and specificity of 100% for noncontrast CT scans, and a sensitivity of 87% and specificity of 94% for IVU. This corresponded to a positive and negative value of 100% and 91% for noncontrast computed tomography, and 97% and 41% for IVU. IVU was unable to detect stones in 13% of patients with calculi found on noncontrast CT scan *(24)*.

In their study, 71% of the referred patients were found to have urinary tract calculi. Of the patients without stones, the most frequent diagnosis was nonspecific abdominal pain, followed by prostatitis and renal or pelvic mass. They correlated their findings with the presence or absence of hematuria, and found that of the patients with renal stones, 93% had more than 5 RBC/HPF, compared with 61% of patients without urinary tract calculi *(24)*.

A retrospective review by Katz et al. on 1000 consecutive noncontrast CT scans for suspected renal colic found that 62.4% of patients undergoing noncontrast spiral CT scan for suspected renal colic had evidence of either ureteral calculi (55.7%) or evidence of recent passage of ureteral calculi (6.7%). Significant alternative diagnoses were present in 7.5% of cases without evidence of ureteral calculi and in 2.6% of patients with concomitant ureteral calculi. The most frequent alternative diagnosis in this series was an adnexal or pelvic mass, which comprised 2.5% of cases without any evidence of urinary calculi. The second most frequent diagnosis was colonic or gastrointestinal pathology, and accounted for another 2.2% of patients without evidence of urinary calculi, followed by pyelonephritis. There was one case of aortic dissection. In patients with urinary calculi, significant additional findings were observed in 2.5% of cases. No correlation was made with the presence or absence of hematuria *(25)*. This is similar to the result seen by Abramson et al., who found that 18% of patients with clinically suspected renal colic had other diagnoses as the cause of their symptoms (26).

Luchs and Perlmutter reported the results of a retrospective analysis of 950 patients with renal colic and suspected nephrolithiasis. All patients underwent unenhanced helical CT scan following urinanalysis. Sixty-two percent of patients were found to have nephrolithiasis as the etiology of their pain. Thirty-eight percent had negative examinations. Significant alternative diagnoses were found in 7% of patients in their series. The most common alternative diagnoses were adnexal or ovarian pathology, followed by diverticulitis and pyelonephritis (27).

The added benefit of computed tomography is faster time to diagnosis owing to the speed and widespread availability of CT scans. Rekant et al. examined the average waiting time in the emergency room for patients. Patients receiving noncontrast CT scan as an initial screening test for renal colic waited an average of 119 min less than patients receiving an IVU (28).

Surprisingly, many groups have found that the presence or absence of hematuria has insufficient predictive value to predict the presence or absence of nephrolithiasis. Overall, the results of various series have shown that hematuria is absent in up to 40% of cases of renal colic caused by nephrolithiasis. There does not appear to be any correlation between the degree of obstruction and the presence or absence of hematuria (29).

Luchs et al. found that in their series of patients with nephrolithiasis as the etiology for their renal colic, hematuria was absent in 10% of cases, and was present in 54% of patients with an alternative diagnosis. Using the criteria of <10 RBC/HPF, they found that the sensitivity of hematuria in the diagnosis of nephrolithiasis was 84%, with a specificity of only 48%. In their study population, the positive predictive value of hematuria was 72%, and the negative predictive value was 65%. The use of a more stringent cutoff of >10 RBC/HPF changed these numbers only slightly, raising specificity to 52% and dropping sensitivity to 81%. Because of this, the authors suggest that the presence or absence of blood on routine urinalysis should not be used to determine which patients should undergo imaging (27).

Bove et al. published similar results in a retrospective review of 183 patients with acute flank pain referred for unenhanced spiral CT scan. They found that 11% of patients with ureteral calculi did not have hematuria, and that 35% had fewer than 5 RBC/HPF. Setting the criteria of hematuria as 1 RBC/HPF, hematuria only had a sensitivity of 81% for ureterolithiasis. Twenty-six percent of patients with flank pain and a negative microscopic examination of the urine were diagnosed with ureterolithiasis by noncontrast CT scan. The specificity of hematuria was also poor; using a value of 1 RBC/HPF, 40% of patients with hematuria did not have ureterolithiasis. Increasing the cutoff to 5 RBC/HPF, 35% of patients with hematuria did not have calculi (30). These results are similar to those published by Li et al. Their group found that up to 9% of patients diagnosed with urinary tract calculi in the setting of acute flank pain did not have hematuria (31).

However, hematuria is a useful test when used in a population with a very high pretest probability of having nephrolithiasis. In the study by Abramson et al., all patients with a previous history of stones and hematuria had nephrolithiasis detected on noncontrast computed tomography (Table 2).

It is important to remember that noncontrast spiral CT scan is an anatomic study and provides no information about the degree of renal obstruction. A study by Sfakianakis et al. comparing 99Tc-MAG3 renal scan with various noncontrast CT found that noncontrast CT imaging had a positive predictive value of only 56% for renal obstruc-

Table 2
Hematuria and Ureteral Calculi

Study	No. of patients	Sensitivity	Specificity
Luchs 2002	950	84%	48%
Bove 1999	183	81%	40%
Abramson 2000	83	64%	55%

tion, however this was higher than the positive predictive value for clinical criteria alone (35%) or plain abdominal films (32%) *(32)*.

A subsequent study by Bird et al. in a series of 77 patients undergoing both noncontrast CT imaging and 99Tc-MAG3 diuretic scintirenography for flank pain, found that noncontrast CT is unable to determine the severity of renal obstruction. However, positive CT findings were able to differentiate patients without obstruction compared to patients with any degree of obstruction. Findings on CT imaging associated with urinary obstruction were perinephric and periureteral fat stranding, with odds ratios of 4.21 and 4.08, respectively *(33)*.

Noncontrast CT imaging tends to overestimate stone size in the craniocaudal dimension. In a review of 39 patients who underwent noncontrast CT imaging as well as plain abdominal radiography, Narepalem et al. report that craniocaudal stone size measured by conventional abdominal films was 0.8 mm smaller than the size estimated on CT imaging. Noncontrast CT imaging was performed using 5 mm slices, and the size difference was attributed to volume averaging. The authors concluded that finer collimation or thinner cuts would improve the size estimate *(34)*. The authors suggest a combination of plain abdominal radiography, IVU, as well as noncontrast CT imaging to plan treatment.

A study by Olcott et al. comparing linear nephrotomography, abdominal radiography, and noncontrast CT imaging with three-dimensional reconstruction, found that with three-dimensional reconstruction and thin cuts (3 mm collimation and 2 mm reconstructions), the linear dimensions of stone size were estimated to within 3.6% of the actual size measured by plain abdominal imaging. The estimated volume was correct to within 4.8%. However, three-dimensional reconstructions are not usually performed at our institution for renal stones owing to the increased time and expense associated with generating a three-dimensional reconstruction *(35)*.

Once a diagnosis of nephrolithiasis as the cause of flank pain has been established, plain abdominal films are used to follow patients after they are discharged from the hospital. Although some groups advocate noncontrast CT imaging without plain abdominal radiography *(36)*, it is difficult to correlate stone location and size on plain abdominal radiography to the scout film of a noncontrast CT scan. Jackman et al. found that the scout view of the noncontrast CT scan has a sensitivity of only 17%, compared with plain abdominal radiography, which has a sensitivity of 48%. They found that plain abdominal radiographs at the initial patient presentation facilitated patient follow-up and obviated the need for more complicated imaging studies *(37)*.

Corroborating these results, Assi et al. found that plain abdominal films had better sensitivity (60%) than the scout film of noncontrast CT imaging (49%). When they stratified the sensitivity of detection for stone size larger than 3 mm, the rates increased to 86% for plain radiography and 81% for scout CT imaging. They conclude that plain abdominal radiography is superior to CT scout radiography for the detection of renal calculi, particularly for proximal and mid-ureteral calculi *(38)*.

Work by Zagoria et al. suggests an influence of both stone size and density on the visualization of stones on plain abdominal films. In their series, they found that 78% of stones larger than 5 mm, and only 36% of stones smaller than 5 mm were detected on plain films. When they examined stone detection vs stone density, they found that 95% of stones with a density equal to 300 Hounsfield units (HU) or greater were visualized. Only 0.6% of stones with a density of 200 HU or less were visualized on plain films. Only 28% of stones with densities between 200–300 HU were visualized on plain films. Based on these findings, they propose a treatment algorithm in which patients with stone densities >300 HU would be followed with plain radiography. If the stones are less then 200 HU in density, noncontrast CT imaging is required to follow stone passage. For stones in the indeterminate area between 200–300 HU, the patient may require unenhanced CT scan to confirm plain abdominal films when clinically indicated *(39)*.

The duration of obstruction is also important in the diagnostic accuracy of noncontrast computed tomography. In patients with renal obstruction, there is an increase in frequency of secondary signs on ureteral obstruction with increasing duration of obstruction. These signs include perinephric and periureteral stranding, ureteral dilation, and collecting system dilation. Varanelli et al. found that ureteral dilation was the most sensitive—in patients with duration of renal obstruction less than 2 h, the presence of ureteral dilation was only 84%. This increases to 97% of patients with obstruction lasting longer than 8 h. The presence of perinephric stranding was 75% and did not increase in prevalence with time of obstruction. However, in patients who had stranding, the severity was worse with time *(40)*.

PREGNANCY

Although fast and accurate, CT imaging is associated with a relatively high dose (6.6 mSv) of ionizing radiation as compared to IVU, which has a dose of 2.4 mSv. This is of concern for patients who are pregnant or those who require a large number of serial imaging studies. Because of this, alternative low-dose noncontrast CT protocols have been developed, and CT imaging is avoided in pregnant patients whenever possible. In patients with a relatively low body to mass index, low radiation noncontrast CT protocols have comparable sensitivity and specificity relative to standard radiation dose noncontrast CT imaging *(41)*.

Renal colic complicating pregnancy offers a unique diagnostic and therapeutic challenge. Renal colic caused by nephrolithiasis occurs in as many as 1 in 715 pregnancies, and is the most common cause of nonobstetric abdominal pain *(42,43)*. Some authors have found that the incidence of stones increases with the number of pregnancies *(44)*. Because the anatomic relationships of retroperitoneal organs are not distorted by pregnancy, the symptoms of renal colic are similar in gravid and nongravid patients. However, the relationship of abdominal organs is distorted by the gravid uterus, and an erroneous diagnosis of appendicitis, diverticulitis, placental abruption, or premature labor may be made in 28% of patients *(45)*. As in other cases of suspected renal colic, it is necessary to make a rapid diagnosis to exclude many more serious conditions.

Additionally, the presence of renal colic alone in the absence of infection increases the risk of premature labor and fetal loss.

Physiologic dilation of the collecting system is seen in 90% of all pregnancies and is unrelated to the number of previous gestations. This dilation gradually resolves over 8 wk postpartum. Early in pregnancy, ureteral dilation may be caused by hormonal effects on the ureter. Hydronephrosis seen later in gestation is most likely caused by the compressive effects of the fetal head, and is more severe on the right side. The left ureter is thought to be protected by the sigmoid colon. This makes imaging more complicated, because the clinician must differentiate physiologic obstruction from pathologic obstruction (46).

In pregnant patients, exposure to ionizing radiation is associated with an increase in the rate of fetal cancer induction as well as of spontaneous abortion. The amount of damage induced by radiation depends on both the dosage as well as the stage of pregnancy. Epidemiologic studies suggest a 40% overall excess risk of childhood malignancies associated with 10 mSv of radiation exposure during pregnancy, which is the radiation dose associated with obstetric X-rays (47). Exposure to diagnostic radiation increases the risk of childhood leukemia from a background rate of 1:3000 to 1:2000.

Oxford survey data on British women receiving obstetric radiographs from 1943 to 1965 suggests that the fetus is particularly susceptible for the first 8 wk after conception (relative risk = 4.60), followed by the first trimester (relative risk = 3.19). The relative risk of malignancy is similar for exposure during the second and third trimesters (relative risk 1.29 and 1.30, respectively). Based on this data, the British National Radiogical Protection Board has concluded that there is a 6% excess risk of malignancy before the age of 15 yr for each Sv of radiation exposure *in utero*. Forty percent of this increased risk ratio is the result of an increase in childhood leukemia (47).

Although data from the atom bomb survivors shows no association between fetal irradiation and childhood cancers, the Oxford data is corroborated by animal experiments, which demonstrate an increased risk of malignancy in beagles exposed to high-dose ionizing radiation *in utero* (48).

There appears to be a threshold value of 100 mSv below which there does not appear to be any increased risk of fetal damage. Exposure of the fetus to radiation doses in this range or higher is a strong indication for a therapeutic abortion (49). The majority of diagnostic procedures do not approach this level, even with repeated exposures (50). A causal association between radiation and birth defects is difficult to establish scientifically, because 5–10% of all children with no history of radiation exposure have a detectable congenital anomaly (51).

In spite of this, there have been several lawsuits following the birth of a child with multiple birth defects after exposure to low-dose radiation *in utero*. Because of these concerns, it is prudent to avoid ionizing radiation whenever possible in the diagnosis and treatment of pregnant patients with suspected renal colic. MRI has been suggested as an alternative to CT imaging owing to its lack of ionizing radiation. The National Radiological Protection Board does not recommend routine use of this imaging technique during the first trimester owing to the unknown effects of magnetic fields on fetal development (49). However, it has been used safely for the routine evaluation of maternal pelvic masses and fetal growth restriction later during gestation, and for MR urography (52).

Ultrasound (US) is the imaging technique recommended by the ACOG as long as the energy delivered by the ultrasound falls below 94 mW/cm^2 (49). However, this imaging method may be of limited use, because the sensitivity of ultrasound ranges from 35–95% (46).

A study by Fowler et al. comparing US to noncontrast CT imaging for stones in the renal parenchyma and pelvis in a series of 123 patients found that US had a sensitivity of only 24% and a specificity of 90% for stones in these locations. US frequently missed renal stones less than 3 mm in size (53). Patlas et al. examined the sensitivity of US compared to noncontrast CT imaging for ureteral stones. In their study, US had a sensitivity of 93% and specificity of 95% when compared to noncontrast CT examination. US was most effective in detecting the presence of a stone in the setting of hydoureterone-phrosis secondary to nephrolithiasis. The sensitivity of US is better for the detection of ureteral stones than renal parenchymal or pelvic stones (54).

A prospective study by Irving and Burgess comparing a two-film IVU and US in 15 women with flank pain presenting at 32 wk of pregnancy found that all women in the study presented with hydronephrosis ipsilateral to the symptoms when screened with US. Of these patients, 14 out of 15 were found to have delayed excretion, and 3 out of 15 were found to have obstructing stones. The authors suggest that IVU should be the imaging method of choice, because it gives both anatomic and functional information (55). They conclude that ultrasound may not be useful to screen for hydronephrosis, because the majority of pregnancies are associated with upper tract dilation by term, and may be seen as early as 6 to 10 wk of gestation.

Variations on the technique of US, such as looking for evidence of ureteral jets, imaging the full length of ureter, or examining the renal resistive index may add extra sensitivity to US. The renal resistive index is calculated by (peak systolic velocity - peak diastolic velocity) / peak systolic velocity. Values less than 0.7 are considered as normal in the nonobstructed kidney. Values >0.7 are considered as suggestive of an obstructed system (46).

Work in animal models demonstrates changes in renal hemodynamic parameters accompanying renal obstruction, and suggests a role for Doppler US in the diagnosis of complete or partial obstruction (56,57). This has not been shown to be reproducible in clinical trials. Cronan et al. found that only 30–37% of patients with obstruction could be diagnosed with acute obstruction using published guidelines for the change in renal resistive index. In this series, the duration of obstruction was uncertain, and many patients had received nonsteroidal analgesics before radiographic evaluation. They conclude that the use of Doppler US is highly operator-dependent, and should be reserved to centers experienced in this technique (58). The sensitivity of this index may be dependent on the duration of obstruction and is most sensitive after 3–4 h, although patients have presented with a complete obstruction and a completely normal renal resistive index (55).

This contrasts with the results of Shokeir et al., who published the results of a prospective study of 109 patients that compared noncontrast CT with Doppler US and IVU in the setting of renal colic. They found that the change in renal resistive index ($\Delta RI \leq 0.04$) had a sensitivity of 90%, specificity of 100%, and diagnostic accuracy of 95%, for the diagnosis of renal obstruction, which is comparable to the accuracy of noncontrast CT imaging. In their series, patients with unilateral obstruction had an observed increase in renal resistive index of 0.059 ± 0.01 ($p < 0.0001$) in the obstructed side. Patients were imaged using US before administration of nonsteroidal analgesics, and while the patient was still experiencing pain. Shokeir suggests that the routine use of nonsteroidal anti-inflammatory drugs before US imaging may decrease the diagnostic accuracy of Doppler ultrasound *(59)*.

If therapeutic intervention is required in pregnant patients, a number of authors have published techniques that exploit the potential of US for real-time imaging *(60)*. If radiographic imaging is unavoidable, judicious use of fluoroscopy during stent placement to mark the ureteral orifice and confirm stent placement is associated with a radiation exposure of only 2.5 mSv. Irving and Burgess advocate nephrostomy tube placement under US guidance late in gestation, with double-J stent placement earlier in pregnancy. In light of the higher rate of ureteral stent encrustation during pregnancy, and the high rate of discomfort associated with percutaneous nephrotomy, other authors suggest definitive removal of the stones using holmium laser lithotripsy and ureteroscopy. In experienced hands, this treatment is safe and avoids numerous procedures for stent changes as well as the discomfort associated with percutaneous nephrostomy *(61,62)*. Extracorporeal shock-wave lithotripsy is absolutely contraindicated in all pregnant patients.

Magnetic resonance urography is a relatively new technique, which is able to accurately visualize fluid within closed spaces without the need for contrast. This imaging method is particularly well suited for the pediatric population, and is more sensitive than either US or IVU for the detection of congenital anomalies *(63)*. There is a report of HASTE-MR urography used for the determination of the cause of hydronephrosis in a pregnant patient, whose fetus was also found to have hydronephrosis *in utero (64)*. However, MR urography may not be as sensitive for the detection of ureteral stones. Blandino et al. suggest that some ureteral stones may be missed without careful scrutiny of the MR study because ureteral stones appear as an area of signal void *(74)*. It is possible for these areas to be obscured by the surrounding high-intensity signal arising from fluid or urine. Roy suggests an emerging role for MR urography as a second-line relatively noninvasive diagnostic test when the US study is nondiagnostic *(65)*.

URINARY EXTRAVASATION

The presence of urinary extravasation as demonstrated by IVU is estimated to be 0.1% in normal individuals, but may be as high as 25% in patients with ureteral obstruction receiving high-dose intravenous contrast *(66)*. Urinary extravasation may occur in either peripelvic or perirenal locations. Peripelvic extravasation is much more common and arises from microscopic tears in the urothelium of the calyceal fornices or by transflow of urine through mucosa in the setting of increased hydrostatic pressure. The normal resting pressure of the renal pelvis is 5–15 cm water. Pyelosinus backflow (lymphatic backflow) occurs at pelvic pressures of 30 cm water, and forniceal rupture at 50–100 cm water *(67)*. Extravasation is a natural mechanism of renal decompression and is usually managed conservatively, although urinoma and abscess formation have been reported following urine extravasation *(68)*.

Radiologic findings suggestive of this etiology are "hornlike" extension of contrast from a calyceal fornix, peripelvic opacification, parallel translucent lines around the ureteric wall, and demarcation of the lateral psoas border *(69)*. The presence of a dense nephrogram in the setting of perirenal contrast extravasation helps to confirm the diagnosis *(70)*. Retrograde pyelography is contraindicated in this setting, as it is thought that it may worsen the extravasation or enlarge the forniceal tear *(67)*. In the rarer form of perirenal extravasation, of which there are two reported cases, it is thought that urine extravasation takes place directly across the renal parenchyma *(71)*.

This entity may also occur in patients without obstruction of the collecting system, and is termed spontaneous obstruction. As with extravasation following renal obstruction, excellent results are obtained with conservative management *(72,73)*. Significant fibrosis may result from urinary extravasation and may be confused with idiopathic retroperitoneal fibrosis *(68)*.

Other entities that may be confused with forniceal rupture are spontaneous rupture of the pelvis and rupture of calyceal diverticula, both of which are managed operatively with decompression and repair *(75)*. Decompression is also indicated in cases of forniceal extravasation with persistent pain, fever, or leukocytosis.

TREATMENT

Patients initially present in the emergency room with acute renal colic and are given pain medications before any urologic consult. The emergency medicine literature has found intravenous ketorolac is more effective than intravenous opioids for the relief of flank pain caused by renal obstruction. There is a theoretical increase in ureteral smooth muscle tone accompanying many opioid analgesics, and this may exacerbate the degree of ureteral spasm associated with renal stones.

Sandhu et al. compared ketorolac to meperidine in a prospective double-blinded randomized study in patients with renal colic. In this study, a single dose of ketorolac 30 mg or meperidine 100 mg was administered to patients. They found that 56% of patients receiving ketorolac required repeat analgesia within 24 h, as compared to 80% of patients receiving meperidine. They also observed a faster onset of pain relief and lower incidence of side effects in the group of patients treated with ketorolac when compared to the group receiving meperidine *(76)*.

This agrees with the results found by Oosterlink et al., who conducted a randomized, double-blinded trial comparing ketorolac with meperidine. This group found that ketorolac in the 90 mg dose was superior to both meperidine 100 mg and ketorolac 10 mg for pain control. Fewer patients in the high-dose ketorolac group required subsequent medication (17%) for pain control as compared to patients in the meperidine 100 mg arm (47%), or ketorolac 10 mg (39%). This group also found a dose-dependent effect for ketorolac and perceived pain intensity, with the results favoring the ketorolac 90 mg dosage. There was no statistically significant difference between the ketorolac 10 mg group and the meperidine 100 mg group in terms of efficacy of pain control or durability of pain relief. The incidence of adverse effects, especially vomiting, was lower in the ketorolac groups than in the meperidine group *(77)*.

Aggressive hydration in the setting of renal colic may help to pass the renal stones. However, this may also increase patient discomfort and require ureteral stenting. Patients suffering from renal stones are advised to ingest 2–3 L of fluid per day *(78)*. However, it is interesting to note that patients who are encouraged to drink more fluids only increased their daily urine output by only 0.3 L/d. Accompanying this increase in urine volume was an increase in the filtered sodium load, which in turn increases calcium excretion and can increase the risk of recurrent stone disease *(79)*.

Hospitalization for potential decompression is indicated for patients unable to tolerate oral hydration, have no relief of pain with oral analgesics, or have a concomitant urinary tract infection in the setting of urinary obstruction. More aggressive management is also indicated in patients with a solitary kidney with renal colic or symptoms of renal obstruction. Patients with symptoms refractory to a trial of intravenous hydration and analgesics should be strongly considered for stent placement. Stenting or urinary tract decompression is also indicated in patients with an impacted calculus >6 mm in diameter, or who fail to pass a stone after 4 wk (79).

URINARY DECOMPRESSION

Depending on the clinical setting, there is some debate over the most appropriate method of decompression in the setting of obstructed pyelonephritis. To date, there is no conclusive study that demonstrates superiority of one technique over the other. A randomized prospective study by Pearle et al. comparing retrograde ureteral stenting with percutaneous nephrostomy found no significant difference in efficacy or time to recovery between the two groups. The only significant difference was that percutaneous nephrostomy was more cost-effective in their center than retrograde ureteral stenting. Interestingly, they had one failed percutaneous nephrostomy that was salvaged by retrograde ureteral stenting. There was no incidence of unsuccessful retrograde stenting in their study. The rate of positive urine cultures was also higher in the percutaneous nephrostomy group, suggestive of better urinary drainage than retrograde ureteral stenting (80).

This is similar to the results of Joshi et al., who found no statistically significant difference in clinical outcome between double-J stenting and percutaneous nephrostomy in a nonrandomized prospective trial. The authors suggest that percutaneous nephrostomy tube placement is a less invasive procedure than ureteral stenting, and may be associated with a lower rate of urosepsis, although this was not seen in their study (81).

This contrasts with the findings of a randomized controlled trial by Mokhmalji comparing ureteral stenting with percutaneous nephrostomy in a series of 40 patients. This study approached but did not reach statistical significance. They found that percutaneous nephrostomy was associated with less postoperative pain, less radiation exposure, and was successful in every case. In their study, double-J stent placement had a success rate of 80%, and was found to have a 20% conversion rate to percutaneous nephrostomy. Unsuccessful cases were attributed to lack of adequate sedation in half of the patients and benign prostatic hypertrophy in the remainder. There was no incidence of failed percutaneous nephrostomy tube placement; however, up to 40% of patients with proximal ureteral stones and 10% of patients with distal ureteral stones required revision of the nephrostomy tube the following day (82).

Though not statistically significant, there was a statistical trend in the same study suggesting that the duration of diversion, amount of administered analgesic, and length of antibiotic therapy with a percutaneous nephrostomy were consistently less than with a ureteral stent, suggesting that percutaneous nephrostomy was more efficient at draining the obstructed kidney. The same findings also showed that males and patients less than 40 yr of age tolerated nephrostomy tubes better than indwelling stents. The authors conclude that a percutaneous nephrostomy should be preferred to ureteral stent placement in cases of infected hydronephrosis or upper ureteral stones (82).

Both studies found a statistically significant, though not clinically significant, difference in the amount of fluoroscopy time required for placement of retrograde ureteral stents versus percutaneous nephrostomy tubes. It is interesting to note, however, that the success of percutaneous nephrostomy is dependent on the number of cases performed by the radiologist per year. Lee et al. found that the success rate is close to 100% for radiologists performing more than 20 cases/yr. This rate drops to 83% for those performing fewer than 10 procedures/yr, and may play a factor in the decision between retrograde ureteral stent placement and percutaneous nephrostomy placement *(83)*.

Disadvantages of nephrostomy tube placement are patient discomfort with an indwelling tube, tube dislodgement, leakage, and potential to introduce infection. Advantages include potentially better drainage, the ability to perform antegrade studies without intravenous contrast, and the ability to perform the procedure under regional or local anesthesia. When appropriately placed, the nephrostomy tube tract may also be used for definitive stone removal. If retrograde stenting is chosen as a method of decompression, the operative success rate may be improved with general anesthesia instead of intravenous sedation.

REFERENCES

1. Manthey DE, Teichman J. Nephrolithiasis, Emerg Med Clin North Am 2001; 19(3): 633–653.
2. Mutgi A, Williams JW, Nettleman M. Renal colic: utility of the plain abdominal roentenogram. Arch Int Med 1991; 151: 1589–1592.
3. Clark AJ, Norman RW. Mirror pain as an unusual presentation of renal colic. Urology 1998; 51(1): 116–118.
4. Manthey DE, Teichman J. Nephrolithiasis. Emerg Med Clin North Am 2001; 19(3): 633–654, viii.
5. Paajanen H, Kettunen J, Tainio H, Jauhiainen K, Spontaneous Peripelvic Extravasation of Urine as a Cause of Acute abdomen Scan J Urol Nephrol 1993; 27: 333–336.
6. Marston WA, Ahlquist R, Johnson G, Meyer AA. Misdiagnosis of ruptured abdominal aortic aneurysms. J Vasc Surg 1992; 16: 17–22.
7. Power RE, Winter DC, Kelly CJ. A near fatal case of renal colic. J Urol 2001; 165: 1987.
8. Moldwin R, When renal colic is really malingering. Postgrad Med 1987; 82(7), 49–52.
9. Walker EA. Medically Unexplained Physical Symptoms. Clin OB Gyn 1997; 40(3): 589–600.
10. LoPiccolo CJ, Goodkin K, Baldewicz TT. Current issues in the diagnosis and management of malingering, Ann Med 1999; 31: 166–174.
11. Reich JD, Hanno PM. Facticious Renal Colic, Urology 1997; 50(6): 858–862.
12. Gault MH, Campbell NRC, Aksu AE. Spurious Stones Nephron 1988; 48: 274–279.
13. Gluckman GR, Stoller M. Munchausen's syndrome: manifestation as renal colic. Urology 1993; 42: 347–350.
14. Lowenstein LF. Recent research into dealing with the problem of malingering. Medico–Legal J 2002; 70(Pt. 1): 38–49.
15. Eisendrath SJ. When Munchausen becomes malingering: facticious disorders that penetrate the legal system. Bull Am Acad Psychiatry Law 1996; 24(4): 471–481.
16. Jarrett TW, Sagalowsky AI. Management of urothelial tumors of the renal pelvis and ureter. In: Campbell's Textbook of Urology, 8th Ed. Saunders, PA, 2002, pp. 2845–2873.
17. Murphy DP, Gill IS, Streem SB. Evolving management of upper-tract transitional-cell carcinoma at a tertiary-care center. J Endo 2002; 16(7): 483–487.
18. Goel MC, Mahendra GV, Roberts JG. Percutaneous management of renal pelvic urothelial tumors: long-term followup. J Urol 2003; 169: 925–930.
19. Smith AD, Orihuela E Crowley AR. Percutaneous management of renal pelvic tumors: a treatment option in selected cases J Urol 1987; 137l: 852.
20. Savastano S, Feltrin GP, Miotto D, Chiesura-Corona M. Renal aneurysm and arteriovenous fistula. Management with transcatheter embolization. Acta Radiol 1990; 31: 73–76.
21. Pak CY, Peterson R, Poindexter JR. Adequacy of a single stone risk analysis in the medical evaluation of urolithiasis. J Urol 2001; 165: 378–381.
22. Chen MY, Zagoria RJ, Dyer RB. Radiologic findings in acute urinary tract obstruction. J Emerg Med 1997; 15: 339–343.

23. Smith RC, Rosenfield AT, Choe KA, et al. Acute flank pain: comparison of non-contrast-enhanced CT and intravenous urography. Radiology 1995; 194: 789–794.

24. Miller OF, Rineer SK, Reichard SR, et al. Prospective comparison of unenhanced spiral computed tomography and intravenous urogram in the evaluation of acute flank pain. Urology 1998; 52(6): 982–987.

25. Katz DS, Scheer M, Lumerman JH, Mellinger BC, Stillman CA, Lane MJ. Alternative or additional Diagnoses on unenhanced helical computed tomography for suspected renal colic: experience with 1000 consecutive examinations. Urology 2000; 56(1): 53–57.

26. Abramson S, Walders N, Applegate KE, Gilkeson RC, Robbin MR. Impact in the emergency department of unenhanced CT on diagnostic confidence and therapeutic efficacy in patients with suspected renal colic: a prospective survey. 2000 ARRS President's Award, American Roentgenol Ray Society. Am J Roentgenol 2000; 175(6): 1689–1695.

27. Luchs JS, Katz DS, Lane MJ, et al. Utility of hematuria testing in patients with suspected renal colic: correlation with unenhanced helical CT results. Urology 2002; 59(6): 839–842.

28. Rekant EM, Gilbert CL, Counselman FL. Emergency department time for Evaluation of patients discharged with a diagnosis of renal colic: unenhanced helical computed tomography versus intravenous Urography. J Emerg Med 2001; 21(4): 371–374.

29. Stewart DP, Kowalski R, Wong P, Krome R. Microscopic hematuria and calculus–related ureteral obstruction. J Emerg Med 1990; 8(6): 693–695.

30. Bove P, Kaplan D, Dalrymple N, et al. Reexamining the value of hematuria testing in patients with Acute flank pain. J Urol 1999; 162: 685–687.

31. Li J, Kennedy D, Levine M, Kumar A, Mullen J. Absent hematuria and expensive computerized tomography: case characteristics of emergency nephrolithiasis. J Urol 2001; 165: 782–784.

32. Sfakianakis GN, Cohen DJ, Braunstein RH, et al. MAG3-F0 scintigraphy in decision making for emergency intervention in renal colic after helical CT positive for a urolith. J Nucl Med 2000; 41(11): 1813–1822.

33. Bird VG, Gomez-Marin O, Leveillee RJ, Sfakianakis GN, Rivas LA, Amendola MA. A comparison of unenhanced helical computerized tomography findings and renal obstruction determined by furosemide 99 Tc-MAG3 diuretic scintirenography for patients with acute renal colic J Urol 2002; 167: 1597–1603.

34. Narepalem N, Sundram CP, Boridy IC, Yan Y, Heiken JP, Clayman RV. Comparison of helical computed tomography and plain radiography for estimating stone size. J Urol 2002; 167: 1235–1238.

35. Olcott EW, Sommer FG, Napel S. Accuracy of detection and measurement of renal calculi: in vitro comparison of three-dimensional spiral CT, radiography, and nephrotomography. Radiology 1997; 204(1): 19–25.

36. Levine JA, Neitlich J, Verga M, Dalrymple N, Smith RC. Ureteral calculi in patients with flank pain: correlation of plain radiography with unenhanced helical CT. Radiology 1997; 204(1): 27–31.

37. Jackman SV, Potter SR, Regan F, Jarrett TW. Plain abdominal X-ray versus Computerized tomography screening: sensitivity for stone localization after nonenhanced spiral computed tomography. J Urol 2000; 164: 308–310.

38. Assi Z, Platt JF, Francis IR, Cohan RH, Korobkin M. Sensitivity of CT scout radiography and abdominal radiography for revealing ureteral calculi on helical CT: implications for radiologic follow-up. Am J Roent 2000; 175: 333–337.

39. Zagoira RJ, Khatod EG, Chen MYM. Abdominal radiography after CT reveals urinary calculi: a method to predict usefulness on the basis of size and CT attenuation of calculi. Am J Roent 2001; 176: 1117–1122.

40. Varanelli MJ, Coll DM, Levine JA, Rosenfeld AT, Smith RC. Relationship between duration of pain and secondary signs of obstruction of the urinary tract on unenhanced helical CT, Am J Roent 2001; 177:325–330.

41. Meagher T, Sukmar VP, Collingwood J, et al. Low dose computed tomography in suspected acute renal colic. Clin Radiol 2001; 56: 873–876.

42. Parulkar, BG, Hopkins TB, Wollin MR, Howard PJ Jr. Renal colic during pregnancy: a case for conservative treatment. J Urol 1998; 159(2): 365–368.

43. Folger GK. Pain and pregnancy. Obstet Gynecol 1955; 5(4): 513–518.

44. Grenier N, Pariente JL, Trillaud H, Soussotte C, Douws C. Dilatation of the collecting system during pregnancy: physiologic vs obstructive dilatation. Eur Radiol 148(5):1383–1387.

45. Stothers L, Lee LM. Renal colic in pregnancy. J Urol 1992; 148(5): 1383–1387.

46. Grenier N, Pariente JL, Trillaud H, Soussotte C, Douws C. Dilatation of the collecting system during pregnancy: physiologic vs obstructive dilatation. Eur Radiol 2000; 10(2): 271–279.

47. Doll R, Wakeford R. Risk of childhood cancer from fetal irradiation. Brit J Radiol 1997; 70: 130–139.

48. Benjamin SA, Lee AC, Angleton GM, et al. Neoplasms in young dogs after perinatal irradiation. J Natl Cancer Inst 1986; 77(2): 563–571.

49. ACOG Opinion – Guidelines for diagnostic imaging during pregnancy. Int J Gyn Ob 1995; :288–291.

50. Hellawell GO, Cowan NC, Hold SJ, Mutch SJ. A radiation persepctive for treating loin pain in pregnancy by double pigtail stents. B J Urol Int 2002; 90: 801–808.

51. Berlin L. Malpractice issues in radiology: radiation exposure and the pregnant patient. Am J Roentgenol 1996; 167:1377–1379.

52. Roy C, Saussine C, Jahn C, LeBras Y, Steichen G, Delepaul B. Campos M, Fast MR Assessment of Ureterohydronephrosis During Pregenancy, Mag Res Imagaing 1995; 13(6): 767–772.

53. Fowler KAB, Locken JA, Duchesne JH, Williamson MR. US for detecting renal calculi with nonenhanced CT as a reference standard. Radiology 2002; 222(1): 109–113.

54. Patlas M, Farkas A, Fisher D, Zaghal I, Hadas-Halpern I. Ultrasound vs CT for the detection of ureteric stones in patients with renal colic. Br J Radiol 2001; 886: 901–904.

55. Irving So, Burgess NA, Managing Severe loin pain in pregnancy. Br J Obstet Gynecol 2002; 109: 1025–1029.

56. Yokoyama H, Tsuji Y. Diuretic Doppler ultrasonography in chronic unilateral partial ureteric obstruction in dogs. Br J Urol Int 2002; 90(1): 100–104.

57. Shokeir AA, Nijman RJ, el-Azab M, Provoost AP. Partial ureteral obstruction: effect of intravenous normal saline and furosemide upon the renal resistive index J Urol 1997; 157(3): 1074–1077.

58. Cronan JJ, Tublin ME. Role of renal resistive index in the evaluation of acute renal obstruction. Am J Roentgenol 1995; 164: 377–378.

59. Shokeir AA, Mahran MR, Abdulaaboud M. Renal colic in pregnant Women: Role of renal resistive index. Urology 2000; 55(3): 345–347.

60. Fabrizio MD, Gray DS, Feld RI, Bagley DH. Placement of ureteral stents in pregnancy using ultrasound guidance. Tech Urol 1996; 2(3):121–125.

61. Watterson JD, Girvan AR, Beiko DT, et al. Ureteroscopy and Holmium:YAG laser lithotripsy: an emerging definitive management strategy for symptomatic ureteral calculi in pregnancy. Urology 2002; 60(3):383–387.

62. Kavoussi LR, Jackman SV, Bishoff JT. Renal colic during pregnancy: a case for conservative treatment. J Urol 1998; 160(3 Pt 1): 837–888.

63. Leppert A, Nadalin S, Schirg E, et al. Impact of magnetic resonance urography on preoperative diagnostic workup in children affected by hydronephrosis: should IVU be replaced? J Ped Surg 2002; 37 (10): 1441–1445.

64. Fradin JM, Regan F, Rodriquez R, Moore R. Hydronephrosis in pregnancy: simultaneous depiction of fetal and maternal hydronephrosis by magnetic resonance urography. Urology 1999; 53(4): 825–827.

65. Roy C, Saussine C, Jahn C, et al. Fast imaging MR assessment of ureterohydronephrosis during pregnancy. Magn Reson Imaging 1995; 13(6): 767–772.

66. Dunnick NR, Long JA, Javadpour N. Perirenal extravasation of urographic contrast medium demonstrated by computed tomography. J Comp Asst Tomog 1980; 4(4): 538–539.

67. Paajanen H, Kettunen J, Tainio H, Jauhiainen K. Spontaneous peripelvic extravasation of urine as a cause of acute abdomen. Scan J Urol Nephrol 1993; 27: 333–336.

68. Harrow BR. Spontaneous urinary extravasation associated with renal colic causing a perinephric abscess. Am J Roentgenol Radium Ther Nucl Med 1966; 98(1): 47–53.

69. Haverson G. Spontaneous peripelvic extravasation of contrast during excretion urography, Br J Radiol 1972; 45: 759–761.

70. Davies P, Price HM, Knapp DR. Two types of pyelosinus extravasation. Clin Radiol 1981; 32: 413–419.

71. Dunnick NR, Long JA, Javadpour N. Perirenal extravasation of urographic contrast medium demonstrated by computed tomography. J Comp Asst Tomog 1980; 4(4): 538–539.

72. Gold IW, Sternbach GL. Spontaneous extravasation following intravenous pyelography, Ann Emerg Med 1982; 11:9: 485–486.

73. Hafiz A, Rodko EA, Extravasation of contrast during excretory pyelography. J Assoc Can Radiol; 1970: 21:46–50.

74. Blandino A, Gaeta M, Minutoli F, et al. MR urography of the ureter. AJR Am J Roentgenol 2002; 179: 1307–1314.

75. Hosomi M, Oka T, Miyake O, Matsumiya K, Takaha M, Pak S. Spontaneous rupture of a pyelocaliceal diverticulum. Urol Radiol 1989; 11: 136–138.

76. Sandhu DPS, Iacovou JW, Fletcher MS, Kaisary AV, Philip NH, Arkell DG. A comparison of intramuscular ketorolac and pethidine in the alleviation of renal colic. Br J Urol 1994; 74: 690–693.

77. Oosterlink W, Philp NH, Charig C, Gilles G, Hetherington JW, Lloyd J. A double-blind single dose comparison of intramuscular ketorolac tromethamine and penthidine in the treatment of renal colic. J Clin Pharmacol 1990; 30: 336–341.

78. Bihl G, Meyers A. Recurrent renal stone disease-advances in pathogenesis and clinical management. Lancet 2001; 358(9282): 651–656.

79. Lingeman JE, Lifshitz DA, Evan AP. Surgical management of urinary lithaisis. In: Campbell's Urology, 8th Ed., (Walsh, PC, ed.). Elsevier Health Sciences, UK, 2002; pp. 3361–3365.

80. Pearle MS, Pierce HL, Miller GL, et al. Optimal method of urgent decompression of the collecting system for obstruction and infection due to ureteral calculi. J Urol 1998; 160(4): 1260–1264.

81. Joshi HB, Obadeyi OO, Rao PN. A comparative analysis of nephrostomy, JJ stent and urgent in situ extracorporeal shock wave lithotripsy for obstructing ureteric stones. Br J Urol Int 1999; 84(3): 264–269.

82. Mokhmalji H, Braun PM, Martinez et al. Percutaneous nephrostomy versus ureteral stents for diversion of hydronephrosis caused by stones: a prospective, randomized clinical trial. J Urol 2001; 165(4): 1088–1092.

83. Lee WJ, Mond DJ, Patel M, Pillari GP. Emergency percutaneous nephrostomy: technical success based on level of operator experience. J Vasc Interv Radiol 1994; 5(2): 327–330.

23 Anatomical Considerations in Urinary Stone Disease

Louis Eichel, MD and Ralph V. Clayman, MD

CONTENTS

URETHRAL ANATOMY
BLADDER ANATOMY
URETERAL ANATOMY
RENAL ANATOMY
IMPACT OF ANATOMY ON SELECTION OF STONE THERAPY
SUMMARY
REFERENCES

Key Words: Kidney; ureter; calyx; anatomy.

URETHRAL ANATOMY

In the urinary tract, all roads lead to the urethra. An understanding of its anatomy, in both the male and female, is important for the successful and safe removal of bladder calculi and for the safe passage of both cystoscopes and ureteroscopes.

The male urethra spans approx 20 cm from the distal meatus to the bladder neck. The urethral meatus can vary greatly in its diameter but in general is the tightest portion of the entire urethra. Occasionally it is necessary to manually dilate the urethral meatus or perform a meatotomy to pass an instrument or to extract a distally lodged stone.

For practical purposes the male urethra is divided into three sections: the pendulous, membranous, and prostatic urethra. The pendulous urethra encompasses the distal penile and more proximal bulbar portions of the urethra, which lie within the corpus spongiosum. The urethra will normally accommodate instruments up to 28 French. As the penile urethra runs directly into the bulbar urethra, its course curves anteriorly and enters the membranous urethra. The membranous urethra is intimately surrounded by the external (voluntary) sphincter. This point of anterior deflection and muscular

From: Current Clinical Urology, *Urinary Stone Disease:*
A Practical Guide to Medical and Surgical Management
Edited by: M. L. Stoller and M. V. Meng © Humana Press Inc., Totowa, NJ

based occlusion is a potential site of trauma where false passages can be made posterior; understandably it is the most common point of stricture formation. It is important for the endoscopist to realize that if a false passage has been made with a catheter or rigid endoscope, that the flexible endoscope may be most helpful as it can be manipulated such that its tip will hug the anterior portion of the urethra and facilitate passage of a guide wire or the endoscope itself into the true urethral lumen. When stone passage is inhibited by short strictures along the course of the urethra, direct vision urethrotomy with retrograde manipulation of the stone back into the bladder can usually be performed followed by cystolitholapaxy. More significant strictures that cannot be easily dilated may require transvesical extraction of a bladder stone followed by urethroplasty (1,2).

The prostatic urethra extends from the male external sphincter in the membranous urethra to the bladder neck (internal sphincter). Here, the urethral lumen is usually at its widest. Under certain pathologic circumstances that cause obstruction of the bladder neck such as prostatic hyperplasia and bladder neck contracture or bladder neck hypertrophy, there can be difficulty passing stones out of the bladder or passing an endoscope into the bladder. Obstruction at this level may require transurethral incision of the prostate or bladder neck.

In females, the urethra is typically 4 cm in length. The female urethra can usually be dilated to 32 Fr to accommodate endoscopes of varying size and for the removal of bladder stones up to 9 mm in diameter. In addition, stones can form inside urethral diverticuli. These are best treated with diverticulectomy and primary repair.

BLADDER ANATOMY

The normal functioning bladder is able to store urine at low pressure and then, in a coordinated fashion with the urethral sphincters, empty to completion. The majority of the bladder wall is composed of large bundles of interconnecting smooth muscle fibers that form a powerful meshwork capable of expansion and contraction depending on the stage of the voiding cycle. These fibers react primarily to cholinergic input. In contrast, the smooth muscle configuration of the trigone and bladder neck is more organized and performs several key functions. The trigonal muscle provides a thick supportive backing for the ureters, which enter the bladder base posterolaterally and travel medially for 1.5–2.5 cm to open into the bladder lumen at the trigone. As the ureter passes through the bladder wall it is compressed and narrowed, which can prevent passage of a stone antegrade or a ureteroscope retrograde. Difficulties with ureteral access can be encountered following ureteroneocystotomy (discussed later in this chapter).

The bladder neck is intimately related to the trigone and the two as a unit act to funnel urine into the urethra during the active phase of micturition. Difficulty with bladder emptying caused by a neurogenic problem, an obstructive process, or poor detrusor function may lead to urinary stasis and increase the risk of infection. Stasis and infection are the two main risk factors for bladder stone formation.

Several other factors can lead to bladder stones. In particular, bladder diverticuli can be a source of urinary stasis and thereby promote stone formation. Foreign bodies such as iatrogenically placed sutures, indwelling Foley catheters, and indwelling ureteral stents can each act as a nidus for vesicolithiasis. Last, in patients who have undergone bladder augmentation or continent urinary diversion, mucous formation and stasis can create a lithogenic environment (3).

URETERAL ANATOMY

The ureter originates from the renal pelvis and transports urine to the bladder in peristaltic waves. The length of the ureter varies from 22 to 30 cm *(4)*. Its course runs from the ureteropelvic junction medially where it travels along the medial border of the psoas muscle just lateral to the transverse processes of the lumbar vertebrae. In the supine position, this is an uphill climb as the ureter travels over the sacral promontory. At the L3-L4 level the ureter is crossed anteriorly by the gonadal vessels. As the ureter passes over the pelvic brim it crosses directly over the bifurcation of the common iliac artery and then proceeds downhill hugging the contour of the pelvis just medial to the internal iliac artery. Once the artery branches, the ureter courses between the inferior vesical artery inferomedially and the superior vesical artery superolaterally. Just before its oblique insertion into the bladder base (the ureterovesical junction), the ureter is coursed anteriorly in males by the vas deferens and in females by the round ligament and then slightly more caudal, laterally by the obliterated umbilical artery (i.e., the medial umbilical ligament).

Stones tend to lodge at four common points of narrowing along the course of the ureter: the ureteropelvic junction, the pelvic brim as the ureter courses over the iliac vessels, the ureterovesical junction, and the ureteral orifice. Among these, the ureterovesical junction is often the narrowest, with a diameter of 2 mm. The combination of these areas of narrowing and the relatively serpiginous course that the ureter takes from the kidney to the bladder, can make passage of guide wires or endoscopes within the ureteral lumen quite challenging. For example, it is sometimes necessary to balloon dilate the intramural portion of the ureter or the ureterovesical junction in order to allow passage of a ureteroscope. In addition, when passing a ureteroscope up the ureter over a guide wire in a supine patient, one must visualize the three dimensional course of the ureter coursing laterally and downward through the bladder wall and then taking a sharp turn upward (anteriorly) and medially as the instrument needs to be guided anterior out of the pelvis and over the iliac vessels. The pulsations of the common iliac artery are clearly transmitted to the ureter at this point. On occasion, it may be difficult to pass a semi rigid ureteroscope over the pelvic brim, especially in the male patient. This is a potential cause of ureteral and/or endoscope damage and can be avoided by changing to a flexible endoscope. Alternatively, this angulation can be modified in the male by manually pushing the suspensory ligament of the phallus posterior thereby helping with the alignment of the urethra toward the ureteral orifice.

The upper ureter can, on occasion, J hook making the passage of a guide wire difficult. This is more common in elderly patients with ptotic kidneys. A variety of endourological methods for overcoming this problem have been described; however, the simplest approach is to place the patient in a steep head down position and proceed to manually push the kidney upward by pressing upward along the upper quadrant of the abdomen subcostally (Mertz maneuver) *(5)*.

After summiting the sacral promontory it is a slightly downhill course along the mid and upper ureter toward the renal pelvis, which usually sits at the level of the second lumbar vertebral body. However, to traverse the ureteropelvic junction, the endoscope usually needs to be guided even more posterior.

The anterior-posterior course of the ureter as described above is reversed if the patient is in the prone position during flexible ureteroscopy. In this position, it is most helpful to first pass a ureteral access sheath to facilitate passage of the flexible ureteroscope.

RENAL ANATOMY

Kidney Position and External Relationships

The kidneys lie in the retroperitoneum on top of the quadratus lumborum and psoas muscles. Each kidney has a thin walled fibrous capsule that is intimately adherent to the parenchyma, which in turn is surrounded by perirenal fat. The perirenal fat is contained by Gerota's fascia, which in turn is surrounded by another layer of fat (i.e., the pararenal fat).

Posteriorly, the superior pole of each kidney rests against the diaphragm and the tips of the 11th and 12th ribs. Deep to this, the underlying pleura attaches to the 11th rib, which must be considered when a superior pole percutaneous approach is planned, especially on the left where the kidney lies higher in the retroperitoneum. The adrenal glands rest on top of the kidneys medially against the cava on the right and aorta on the left.

The anterior surface of the right kidney is associated with the liver superiorly, the curve of the duodenum over the midportion and the ascending colon inferior and medially. On the right side, the colon often covers the lower half of the kidney medially. The anterior surface of the upper pole of the left kidney is covered by the spleen superiorly and just the tail of the pancreas medially as well as by, the splenic flexure of the colon; the anteromedial surface of the entire left kidney is covered by the descending colon. A retrorenal colon can be seen on either side in 1–10% of percutaneous cases depending on patient positioning; it is more common when the patient is in the prone position. However, this condition is usually limited to patients with a markedly redundant colon or patients with a horseshoe kidney *(6)*. Usually the retrorenal colon covers only the lateral most portion or upper pole of the kidney.

For anatomic purposes, the kidney can be divided into anterior and posterior segments. The plane of division for these segments rests 30–50° posterior to the frontal plane of division for the body as a whole owing to the rotation of the renal axis anteriorly by the psoas major muscle (Fig. 1) *(7)*. The psoas muscle also defines the axis of the kidneys in the longitudinal plane so that the upper pole is medial and posterior whereas the lower pole is more lateral and anterior *(6)*. As such, the distance from skin to collecting system is shortest at the upper pole and greatest at the lower pole of the kidney.

Internal Architecture of the Kidney and Collecting System

The glomeruli, proximal tubules, and distal convoluted tubules rest within the renal cortex, which is the outer most layer of the renal parenchyma. The loops of Henle and collecting ducts rest within the renal pyramids, which together comprise the medulla of the renal parenchyma and rest within the center of the kidney. The renal pyramids are separated by incursions of cortical tissue called the columns of Bertin. The collecting ducts within each pyramid cone down to drain into a papilla, which is bordered by the fornix of a minor calyx, the area surrounding the papilla.

Each kidney typically contains 4–14 minor calyces (mean 8) *(6,7)*. The minor calyces comprising the middle pole of the kidney tend to drain single papilla (simple calyx) whereas the polar calyces tend to drain two or three papillae (compound calyx). These papillae may actually be fused to one another in varying degrees. A minor calyx may drain directly via an infundibulum into the renal pelvis or several minor calyces, as in the polar areas, may drain into a major calyx, which in turn drains via a single major infundibulum into the renal pelvis (Fig. 2).

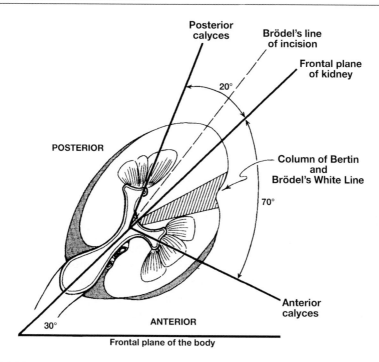

Fig. 1. Left kidney viewed from above showing anterior calyces projecting 70° and posterior calyces 20° from the frontal plane of the kidney, as in a classic Brödel-type kidney. Used with permission from Reference 7.

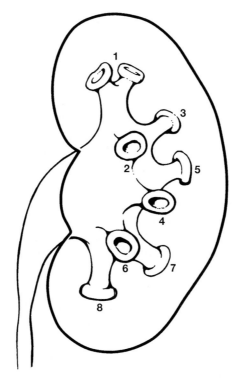

Fig. 2. "Classic" left kidney: compound polar calyces (1); anterior calyces (2, 4, and 6) and posterior calyces (3, 5, and 7). Used with permission from Reference 7.

Sampaio et al. analyzed 140 endocasts of the pelviocaliceal systems of cadaver kidneys and derived from this a descriptive classification system based on polar anatomy *(6)*. Group A kidneys have pelviocaliceal systems comprised of an upper and a lower pole system. The middle pole minor calyces drain into one of these two major divisions. Group B kidneys have pelviocaliceal systems in which the midpole calyceal drainage is independent of the upper and lower pole collecting systems.

The traditional teaching regarding the correlation between the actual anatomy of the pelviocaliceal and the appearance of the collecting system on intravenous pyelography is that on a standard AP view, the anterior calyces appear to be seen in cross section laterally and the posterior calices appear to be more medial and are seen from a cuplike end on point of view. Sampaio et al. studied 40 cadaver kidneys in which retrograde pyelography was correlated with the actual anatomy of the pelviocaliceal system derived from endocasts *(6)*. In actuality, this relationship (where the anterior calices are seen laterally and the posterior calices are seen medially) was only present in 27.8% of the kidneys studied. The posterior calices were more lateral in 19.3% of cases. The largest proportion of kidneys (52.9%) had a mixed pattern. These findings underscore the importance of obtaining high quality imaging studies before planning an operative approach. In the case of IVP or retrograde pyelography this should include lateral and oblique views.

Assessment of the Lower Pole Infundibulopelvic Angle, Infundibular Length, Infundibular Width, and Calyceal Pelvic Height

It is widely accepted among endourologists that lower pole calculi have a poor clearance rate compared to stones in other locations following shockwave lithotripsy (SWL; in our study, lower pole anatomy had no impact on clearance after ureteroscopic lithotripsy). The dependent position of the lower pole is thought to play a major role. Other important anatomical relationships to understand with regard to this phenomenon are the lower pole infundibulopelvic angle (LIP angle), infundibular length (IL), infundibular width (IW), and calyceal pelvic height (CPH). Several studies exist in the literature that either support or refute the importance of these parameters with regard to stone clearance rates and treatment success rates for lower pole stones. When reviewing studies that use the LIP angle as a potential indicator of the odds of treatment success, it is important to remember that the angle can be measured several ways. Figure 3A demonstrates this point. The measurement is calculated using the angle between the central axis of the lower pole infundibulum and one of the following: the ureteropelvic axis, the vertical ureteral axis, or the renal pelvic axis *(8–10)*.

The IL is calculated as the distance from the most distal point at the bottom of the calyx containing the stone to the midpoint of the lower lip of the renal pelvis *(8)* (Fig. 3B). Another similar measurement used to predict odds of stone clearance is the CPH. This is defined as the distance between the lower lip of the renal pelvis the lowermost point of the stone containing calyx *(11,12)* (Fig. 3C). The IW is measured at the narrowest point along the lower pole infundibular axis (Fig. 3D).

Several studies support the theory that lower pole infundibulopelvic anatomy affects stone clearance rates. In his original article on this subject, Sampaio et al. studied endocasts from the collecting systems of 146 cadaveric kidneys. He found three factors that may play a role in lower pole stone clearance: the infundibulopelvic angle (clearance of

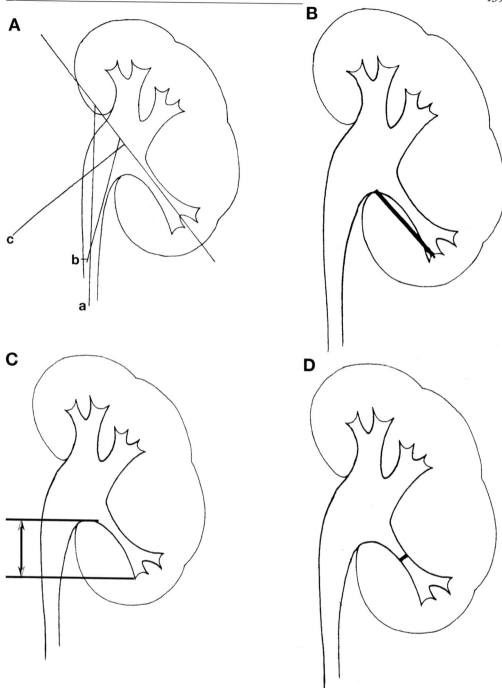

Fig. 3. (A) Different method of determining main axis for measuring lower pole infundibulo-pelvic angle using vertical ureteral axis (a), ureteropelivic axis (b), and renal pelivic axis (c). **(B)** Infundibular length measured as distance from the most distal point at the bottom of calyx containing stone to mid-point of lower lip of the renal pelvis. **(C)** The calyceal pelvic height is measured as the distance between the lower lip of the renal pelvis and the lowermost point of the stone containing calyx. **(D)** Infundibular width is measured at the narrowest point along the lower pole infundibular axis.

74% when the angle is >90° and 26% when the angle is <90°), the infundibular diameter (60% clearance when it is >4 mm and 40% clearance when it is <4 mm), and the inferior pole calyceal distribution (57% clearance when the calyces were multiple and simple vs 43% when the calyces were single and of a compound nature) *(10)*. In a follow up prospective study by Sampaio, 74 patients received SWL for lower pole stones. The stone clearance rates for patients with an LIP angle greater than vs less than 90° was 75% vs 23% respectively *(13)*. Another retrospective study by Elbahnasy et al. reported 21 SWL patients and 13 ureteroscopy patients who were treated for lower pole stones. In the SWL group, the infundibulopelvic angle in the stone free vs residual group was significantly larger (75° vs 51°). There was no difference, however, in the ureteroscopy group (56° vs 49°). Furthermore, in the SWL group, the IL was significantly shorter and the IW greater in the success vs nonsuccess (32 mm vs 38 mm and 9 mm vs 6 mm respectively). Again, there were no significant differences in the ureteroscopy group. These findings were supported in a later study comparing treatment of solitary lower pole stones with SWL, PCNL, and ureteroscopy where SWL was sensitive to lower pole anatomy but PCNL and ureteroscopy were not *(14)*. In this study, they also found that having two or more favorable or unfavorable parameters had a much greater effect than any single parameter alone in terms of clearance. Based on both of these studies, the authors concluded that patients with lower pole stones 17 mm or less who have favorable anatomy (LIP angle >70°, IL <3 cm, and IW >5 mm) are excellent candidates for SWL whereas patients with less favorable anatomy (LIP angle <40°, IL >3 cm, and IW <5mm) would be better served by ureteroscopy or PCNL. In further support of these findings, Keeley et al. retrospectively analyzed the records of 116 patients with lower pole stones between 11 and 20 mm with regard to LIP angle and also found a superior stone free rate among patients with a more obtuse angle *(15)*. Infundibular diameter and calyceal configuration were not found to be significant factors. In the largest study to date, Poulakis et al. reviewed lower pole calculi results in 680 patients (701 renal units) treated on a Piezolith 2500. They, like Elbahnasy, found the critical LIP angle to be 45°. A CPH greater than 15 mm was also found to be a significant variable. In this series all patients with residual fragments had inversion therapy, and the average follow up was 26 mo *(16)*. Interestingly, in another recent study, an infundibular length to diameter ratio of less than 7 and an infundibular diameter of >4mm with a single minor calyx affected in multivariate analysis appeared to be predictive of clearance (85% in 63 patients) *(17)*.

Looking at ureteroscopic treatment for lower pole stones, however, although Elbahnasy et al. did not find the LIP anatomy to be a significant factor, Kumar, Joshi, and Keeley did find a negative impact of an acute LIP angle on stone free rate *(18)*. Thus, some degree of controversy continues regarding this matter.

Even more controversy exists regarding the significance of lower pole anatomy itself. Moody et al. analyzed the 26 patients who underwent SWL from the Lower Pole Study Group with regard to LIP angle, IW, and IL as measured according to Elbahnasy. No significant differences in these parameters were seen with regard to stone free rate. In fact, the only significant factor measured was stone size (mean 9.6 vs 15.3 mm for stone free vs not stone free) *(19)*. However, these few patients were treated at 18 different institutions using 5 different machines. In a retrospective study of 108 patients with lower pole stones, Madbouly et al. also were unable to find any correlation between lower pole anatomy and stone clearance following SWL *(9)*. In this study the only significant factor that affected stone clearance was a history of pyelonephritis. However, again in this study, patients were treated with three different lithotriptors, some patients had multiple lower pole stones, uric acid calculi were included, and over half of the patients underwent multiple SWL treatments. The diversity of the patient population could well have contributed to the authors' inability to identify any significant parameters. More recently, an article by Sorenson and Chandhoke reviewed 190 patients treated on a Doli U/50 with lower pole, single, calcified stones all ≤ 2 cm. These authors found no impact of lower pole anatomy on stone clearance rates. Of note, in this study, all patients had postoperative inversion therapy.

As such, the impact of lower pole anatomy as measured on the intravenous urogram remains controversial. Perhaps, all of these patients should be treated by post-SWL inversion therapy as this maneuver in two separate studies singularly increased the stone free rate from 3% to 40% in one study and from 23% to 88% in another study (20,21).

In the final analysis, in this day and age, the point of lower pole anatomy may well be on its way to becoming moot owing to the demise of the IVP. Indeed, the ability to measure these parameters is becoming increasingly more difficult given that most renal calculi are being diagnosed now by means of CT scan. The CT scan of the kidneys, in its current state, precludes the ability to measure infundibular length, width, and angle. In the future, there may be a resurgence of interest in this topic when 3D reconstruction of the CT scan becomes more commonplace enabling a more reliable and reproducible measurement of these various parameters.

Intrarenal Vascular Anatomy

The pioneering work of Brödel (22) and Graves (23) defined the distinct anatomical segments of the kidney with their individual arterial branches. Although wide variation exists, the renal arteries, in general, originate from the lateral margin of the aorta just below the level of the superior mesenteric artery. They course posterior to the renal vein and branch on the appropriate side of the renal pelvis into an anterior and posterior division. The posterior branch is the first main branch of the renal artery in 50% of cases and supplies the posterior middle segment of the kidney. The anterior segment typically divides into four branches (apical, upper, middle, and lower). Kaye in 1982 described this relationship as a hand (i.e., the main renal artery) grasping a glass (i.e., the renal pelvis) with the thumb branching early and coursing posteriorly (i.e., the posterior segmental artery) and the 4 fingers spreading out over the anterior surface of the glass (i.e., the apical, upper, middle, and lower segmental arteries) (24). The segmental branches, in turn, split to form interlobar arteries that wrap around the superior and inferior poles of the infundibula to form the arcuate arteries. The arcuate arteries, in turn, branch and run between the renal pyramids and columns of Bertin. Small branches of the arcuate arteries perforate the renal cortex to supply blood peripherally. Each individual arterial branch is functionally an end artery and injury to a branch can lead to loss of segmental function owing to infarction (Figs. 4A and B).

In an effort to characterize the renal vascular anatomy more specifically in the context of percutaneous renal surgery, Sampaio and coworkers performed three-dimensional endocasts of renal collecting systems, arteries, and veins in fresh cadavers (25–27). They also studied the extent of vascular injuries sustained from percutaneous punctures of the renal collecting system at various locations (28). They discovered that there is a high likelihood of a significant vascular injury if the collecting system is punctured through an infundibulum or if the renal pelvis is accessed directly because the larger vessels surround these structures. Significant vascular injuries were discovered in 67%, 23%, and 13% of upper pole, middle, and lower pole infundibular punctures respectively.

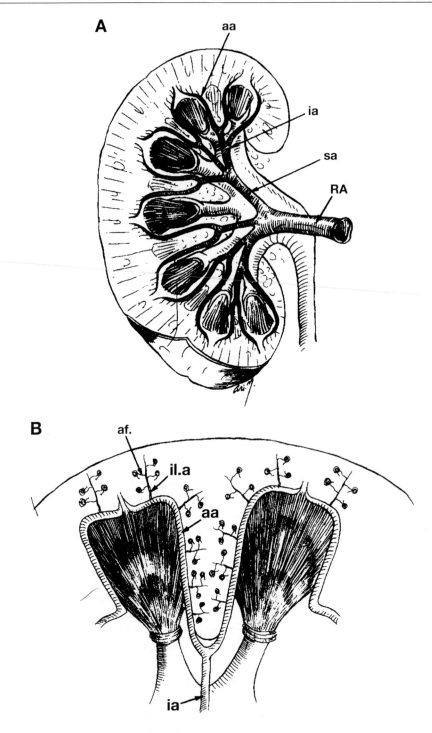

Fig. 4. (A) Anterior view of right kidney showing the branching of the renal arteries and their official nomenclature according to kidney regions. RA, renal artery; sa, segmental artery; ia, interlobar (infundibular) artery; aa, arcuate artery. **(B)** The two adjacent pyramids and minor calices showing the renal vasculature from the level of the interlobar arteries to the glomerular level. Ia, interlobar (infundibular) artery; aa, arcuate artery; il.a, interlobular artery; and af, afferent arteriole of the glomerulus. From ref. *6* with permission.

When testing forniceal punctures, however, there were no arterial injuries and less than an 8% rate of vascular injury. Thus, puncture of the collecting system should always be performed through a fornix or directly into a posterior calyx.

IMPACT OF ANATOMY ON SELECTION OF STONE THERAPY
Obstruction
URETERO-PELVIC JUNCTION OBSTRUCTION

Patients with primary uretero-pelvic junction (UPJ) obstruction have a 16–30% chance of concomitant renal stones *(29)*. Stasis and to a lesser extent metabolic factors are thought to play a role in stone formation in the setting of UPJ obstruction *(30–32)*. Hence, one must consider that even after successful treatment of a UPJ obstruction with endopyelotomy or surgery, these patients may still be at risk for recurrent stone disease and treatable metabolic risk factors should be evaluated and treated. SWL is contraindicated in the setting of UPJ obstruction because distal drainage is required *(33)*. Occasionally, when the stone sits directly at the UPJ, it can be difficult to discern whether or not the UPJ is obstructed primarily or secondarily, from an impacted stone with edema. In this situation, it is best to first treat the stones percutaneously, leave a nephrostomy tube in place albeit well away from the UPJ, wait 2 wk for resolution of edema, and then assess the drainage of the renal collecting system. This can be done using a DTPA or MAG-3 renal scan with furosemide washout or, if the nephrostomy tube has been left in place, a Whitaker test *(29)*.

Open pyelolithotomy and pyeloplasty has long been the gold standard of therapy for UPJ obstruction with renal stones. With the advent of minimally invasive techniques, however, several other effective options for treatment now exist. One well recognized alternative treatment for simultaneous renal stones and UPJ obstruction is to perform percutaneous lithotripsy followed by antegrade percutaneous endopyelotomy. Using these combined techniques patients can be rendered stone free and success rates of up to 94% can be achieved in terms of UPJ patency *(34)*.

Another possible minimally invasive option that blends the benefits of open surgery with the minimally invasive philosophy of percutaneous surgery is laparoscopic pyeloplasty and pyelolithotomy. In one study, Ramakumar et al. performed 20 laparoscopic pyelolithotomies with pyeloplasty and reported an overall long term patency rate of 90% and a stone free rate of 80% at 1 yr *(35)*.

CALYCEAL DIVERTICULI

Caliceal diverticula are nonsecretory outpouchings of the renal collecting system that communicate via a tight neck, usually along the fornix. Up to 50% of patients with calyceal diverticula will have stones within them *(29,36)*. The condition itself does not require treatment. The criteria for treatment are pain and/or infection.

Treatment options include SWL, percutaneous nephrolithotomy and simultaneous calyceal obliteration, retrograde ureteroscopic approach, laparoscopic approach, and open surgery. In general, SWL can provide a reasonable short-term pain free rate (36–75 %) but because it does not address the actual mechanical obstructive process, the stone clearance rate is poor (4–25%) *(37–41)*. In contrast, direct percutaneous stone extraction followed by incision of the diverticular neck and fulguration of the diverticular wall with placement of a nephrostomy tube through the dilated neck provides for both stone extraction and treatment of the primary problem. Using such techniques, stone

clearance rates of 93–100%, symptom free rates of 85–100%, and diverticular obliteration in 73–100% can be achieved (40,42–44).

   With the constant improvement of flexible ureteroscopes and the widely available use
of the holmium laser, a retrograde ureteroscopic approach to calyceal diverticula is also
an attractive option. This entails cannulation of the diverticular neck with a guide wire
under direct vision. Either balloon dilation or incision of the neck can be performed in
the 3 or 9 o'clock positions. This is followed by intracorporeal lithotripsy. In earlier
reports, no attempt was made to obliterate the diverticulum. Using this technique Batter
and Dretler report an immediate treatment success rate of 84% for upper and mid pole
diverticula. The success rate for lower pole diverticula was poor owing to a high rate of
failure to cannulate the diverticulum. The symptom-free rate at a mean follow up of 39
mo was 100% in those treated successfully; however follow-up results regarding the
drainage or disappearance of the diverticulum was not reported (45).

   Another minimally invasive treatment option for a large diverticulum (i.e., ≥ 5 cm),
especially those in an anterior or perihilar position that have poorly accessible necks and
very little overlying parenchyma (i.e., are bulging off of the surface of the normal renal
contour) is laparoscopic stone extraction and marsupialization. This can be done via a
transperitoneal or retroperitoneal approach depending on the circumstances. Intraoperative ultrasound may be necessary to localize a relatively endophytic diverticulum. Several authors report small series of patients treated successfully in this manner with
minimal complications (46–49).

RENAL CYSTS

   Peripelvic cysts are simple cysts that are located within the renal hilus. They comprise
6% of all renal cysts. They are intimately associated with the renal pelvis, calyces, and
major renal vessels and can be single or multiple in number (50). The renal hilum is a
relatively tight space and the cysts can cause obstruction of the renal collecting system
resulting in pain, infection, hypertension, and stone formation (51). Because of their
intimacy with the collecting system and hilar vessels, the historical management of
peripelvic cysts required open surgical decortication (52). There have been anecdotal
reports of treatment with percutaneous drainage and endoscopic marsupialization; however, percutaneous drainage with sclerotherapy is contraindicated for fear of vascular
injury or injury to the collecting system from errant sclerosant (53,54). A growing
number of urologists are now considering laparoscopic cyst ablation for these lesions.
In one series reported by Roberts et al., 11 patients underwent laparoscopic peripelvic
cyst ablation. All patients were treated successfully and the complication rate for his
entire series, which also included parenchymal renal cysts (n = 32), was 13%, much
lower than the rate reported for open cyst decortication (33%) (55). In another case series
by Hoenig et al. involving four patients, three cyst ablations were successful long term
and there were no complications (51). The authors also noted occasional difficulty with
the differentiation between the stretched wall of the renal vein and the blue domed wall
of the cysts. Intraoperative ultrasound was used to distinguish between the two. In both
series it was noted that fulguration of the cyst base is not recommended owing to the risk
of damage to the collecting system or vasculature. They also noted that if a cyst could
not be opened widely, it was prudent to suture a tongue of omentum or pararenal fat
inside the cyst to act as a wick.

   Occasionally, cysts within the parenchyma of the kidney can compress the collecting
system and cause stasis and stone formation proximally. Reports of such cases are

sporadic but Cass *(56)* reported a series of 13 patients of which two had peripelvic cysts, four had autosomal dominant polycystic kidney disease (ADPKD), and seven had simple or multiple cysts. All patients were treated with a Medstone STS lithotriptor under general anesthesia. The stone free rate, not surprisingly, at 3 mo was only 46%. The author attributed the retained fragments to continued obstruction and indicated that PCNL or percutaneous cyst drainage and sclerosis would be a more appropriate option for treatment.

Urolithiasis occurs in 10–36% of patients with ADPKD *(57,58)*. Many of these patients have uric acid stones that can be treated with urinary alkalinization. In general, it is best to avoid instrumentation of polycystic kidneys, if possible, because the cysts once infected are very difficult to penetrate with antibiotics. If, however, this is not possible, SWL, PCNL, or a combination of the two can be performed. Ng et al. reported the Cleveland clinic experience with urolithiasis in patients with ADPKD *(58)*. They found that 6 out of 13 patients could be treated with urinary alkalinization, and 7 out of 13 required subsequent treatment. The average number of procedures per patient was 1.7 indicating that often a second procedure or sandwich therapy (SWL, PCNL, and SWL) is necessary. Overall, the success rate in treated patients was 57% with the remaining patients having "dust." Interestingly, stone analysis revealed uric acid stones in five out of seven treated patients. In another series of 48 consecutive ADPKD patients 15 were found to have stones. The presence of hypertension was not a significant factor. Patients did seem to have a greater number of cysts and larger cysts adding to the proof that anatomic factors (obstructing cysts causing urinary stasis) may play an important role in stone formation. Patients with stones had lower GFR, 24-h urine volume, urinary magnesium, potassium, and phosphate. Stone composition was not noted; however, the urinary uric acid level was similar in stone and non stone formers *(59)*.

Anatomical Variants

Horseshoe Kidney

Horseshoe kidney is a common renal fusion anomaly that occurs in up to 1 in 400 births. In most cases the lower poles of the kidneys are fused. Normal renal ascent is blocked by the inferior mesenteric artery and the inferior longitudinal axis of the kidneys is pulled medially. Rotation of the kidneys is also abnormal such that the pelves and ureters lie anterior to the isthmus and the ureters often insert high on the pelvis. This configuration predisposes to renal calculi, which occur in 21% and potential UPJ obstruction, which has been reported to occur in 15% *(60)*. The unusual location and rotation of the kidney makes management more challenging; however, the options still include SWL, PCNL, retrograde ureteroscopy, and laparoscopy. The biggest problem with these patients is that access to the lower pole is difficult with the ureteroscope and the dependency of the lower pole plus the anterior insertion of the ureter into the pelvis means poor clearance after SWL; hence PCNL is usually the most definitive therapy.

SWL is a valid treatment option for stones in horseshoe kidneys, however patient positioning can be more challenging. Stones in the upper and middle poles can usually be pinpointed in the supine position but lower pole stones often require prone positioning owing to the medial and anterior deviation of that location *(61,62)*. Pearle and Traxler recently reviewed the results of seven stone series treated with the HM 3 and 7 with various electromagnetic lithotripters and noted a 61.9% and a 66.7 % stone free rate among patients with horseshoe kidneys, respectively. They also noted that although the stone free rates come close to those achieved on conventional kidneys, the retreatment rates tend to be higher, most likely secondary to poor drainage (22.5% and 38.1% for the HM 3 and electromagnetic series, respectively) *(29)*.

PCNL is an effective treatment option for stones in horseshoe kidneys, but the technique for establishment of the percutaneous tract must be modified owing to the abnormal anatomy. Janetschek and Kunzel studied the anatomic variations found in cadaver horseshoe kidneys *(63)*. Accessory renal arteries may originate from the aorta, the iliac bifurcation, the common iliac arteries, as well as the middle sacral arteries and insert directly into the isthmus or the poles of the kidneys. Except for vessels going to the isthmus, however, no arteries were found along the dorsal aspect of the kidney. They also noted that the posterior row of calices points more dorsomedially and the ventral row of calices dorsolaterally. In addition to the pelvis lying anterior, they also noted that the calices to the isthmus lie within the coronal plane and point medially.

With the anatomy in mind, puncture of the upper pole posterior calyx provides the shortest and safest access to the rest of the kidney. The position of the puncture is more medial than a typical percutaneous nephrostomy and should traverse the paraspinous muscles. In addition, the nephrostomy tract must travel a longer distance to reach the anteriorly displaced kidney and may be in excess of 20 cm *(64)*. For this reason, longer nephroscopes, or a short semirigid ureteroscope, as well as a flexible nephroscope should be available *(28)*. Among series reporting results of PCNL in horseshoe kidneys, the stone free rates are 75–89% and second procedure rates are 10–70 % *(63,65,66)*. It is also important to remember that PCNL is also very appropriate for the simultaneous treatment of UPJ obstruction and renal lithiasis because lithotripsy and antegrade endopyelotomy can be performed at the same time, even in these patients *(65)*. Ureteroscopy has been reported anecdotally as being successful for upper and middle pole stones but is less effective for lower pole stones *(29)*. In a recent review article, Yohannes and Smith recommend SWL as the first line treatment for small stones in horseshoe kidneys. For larger stones or SWL failures, the authors recommend PCNL *(67)*.

TRANSPLANTED AND PELVIC KIDNEYS

The incidence of renal stone formation in renal transplant recipients is roughly the same as in the population at large estimated as approx 0.4–1% *(68,69)*. Anatomically, transplanted kidneys lie within the pelvis overlying the iliac vessels. They are shielded posteriorly by the sacrum and iliac bones and may have overlying bowel anteriorly. These factors complicate the use of SWL and PCNL as treatment modalities. The ureteral path may be tortuous and most commonly the ureter inserts into the bladder at the dome and, if there are renal calculi, a ureteral stricture may be present. Retrograde instrumentation of the ureter can therefore be difficult. There may also be scar tissue encasing the kidney, which can make percutaneous access and endoscopic manipulation difficult. Because of these potential variations, each individual case must be evaluated with regard to stone size, location, the presence of infection, and the individual renal and ureteral anatomy based on operative report and a comprehensive radiologic evaluation.

The anatomy of the pelvic kidney was well described by Dretler et al. *(70)*. Pelvic kidneys occur with a frequency of 1 in 1000 autopsies and have a 3:2 male to female ratio. Right and left ectopias have an equal frequency; 15% of ectopic kidneys are crossed. These kidneys tend to be smaller and malrotated such that the collecting system faces anteriorly. The pyelocalyceal system may be entirely extrarenal and appear to be dilated because in these kidneys the collecting system is more easily distended with urine. There may be multiple vessels arising from the aorta and common or internal iliac vessels.

Because of the relative rarity of this condition, series reported in the literature are few. SWL has been used successfully for the treatment of small stones in transplanted kidneys. The pelvic location of the kidney necessitates modified positioning: patients, if supine, must be positioned such that the shock waves pass just below the sacrosciatic notch (40), or they can be turned into the prone position (62,71). Furthermore, it is recommended that only stones ≤ 1 cm be treated with SWL because the risk of steinstrasse has much more severe ramifications in this patient population. SWL has also been used for various size stones in ectopic pelvic kidneys. In one series, 11 of 12 stones were cleared at 3 mo (72).

Retrograde ureteroscopy in the transplanted kidney has been reported for stone treatment, retrieval of migrated stents, and evaluation of funguria and abnormal cytology (73). The same issues with potential difficulty accessing the lower pole or negotiating a malrotated kidney apply (29). Only sporadic cases of successful ureteroscopic stone treatment in ectopic pelvic kidneys exist in the literature (73,74).

PCNL is another viable modality of treatment for larger stones in transplant or pelvic kidneys. The anterior position of the transplanted kidney allows excellent visualization of the stone and localization for nephrostomy puncture; however in the congenital pelvic kidney one must contend with overlying bowel. If there is concern over bowel injury, the nephrostomy access has been reported in one case to have been successfully obtained using laparoscopic guidance (75). Cases of PCNL for transplanted kidneys in the literature are sporadic but indicate successful results (76–78).

If SWL is not successful or inappropriate and percutaneous and ureteroscopic techniques are not possible, laparoscopic pyelolithotomy is another potential minimally invasive option in ectopic or pelvic kidneys. Two case reports exist in the literature in which a transperitoneal approach is described (79,80).

REIMPLANTED URETERS

Catheterization of the ureter in patients who have had a cross trigonal reimplantation or post transplantation ureteroneocystotomy can be difficult owing to the abnormal position and configuration of the orifice as well as the abnormal tortuous path of the ureter. If routine retrograde access is not possible, one can use a special deflecting catheter passed retrograde (e.g., Cohen deflecting guide wire and catheter, or Kumpe catheter) or via a suprapubic puncture to cannulate the ureter.

If a retrograde approach is not possible then a guide wire can be retrieved from the bladder following antegrade percutaneous guide wire placement (81). Retrograde passage of a ureteroscope using standard techniques is then possible.

ILEAL CONDUITS

The ileal urinary conduit, popularized by Bricker, has been the standard solution to urinary diversion for the last 50 yr (82). Rates of upper tract stone formation in patients with ileal conduit urinary diversion range from 4.8 to 20% (83–87). In the absence of stricture, the standard Bricker anastomosis as well as the Wallace anastomosis (88) both allow free reflux of urine into the upper urinary tracts. In Dretler's extensive study of this topic, several significant risk factors for stone formation were identified. Infection with urea splitting organisms was found in 91% and previous pyelonephritis was found in

84% of stone formers. Reflux of infected urine likely leads to struvite stone formation; indeed, the overwhelming majority of stones in patients with urinary diversion are struvite stones *(83,89–91)*. Stone formers had a mean residual conduit volume of 30 mL vs 8 mL for nonstone formers. The majority of patients with a high urine residual had a hyperchloremic metabolic acidosis, severe HCO_3^- loss and a high incidence of hypercalciuria. Although it was not measured in this study, these patients often have citrate levels so low they cannot be measured, which may potentiate the stone diathesis affected by a urease splitting infection. It should also be noted that in addition to renal lithiasis, Dretler also noted two freestanding stones within the conduits themselves. Other stones associated with permanent suture material were not included in the analysis but foreign bodies within the urinary tract have long been known to act as a nidus of stone formation within an ileal conduit (e.g., staples).

SWL, ureteroscopy, and PCNL alone and in combination can be used to treat upper tract calculi in patients with ileal loop diversions. When opacification of the collecting system is required for SWL or PCNL, a loopogram can be performed on the treatment table. However, because these are usually infection stones, it is essential that the patient receives appropriate antibiotic coverage and has a sterile urine culture, before proceeding with stone manipulation or even a loopogram. The choice of treatment depends on stone size, location, and the specific anatomic situation that exists. It should be noted that patients with urinary diversions might respond to expectant management of their stone disease *(84)*. In patients who do require treatment, experienced centers *(90)* have found that renal stones less than 2 cm, in the absence of obstruction, can be treated with SWL with an initial expected success rate of 76%. If a secondary SWL is used to clean up residual stones the success rate rises to 92%. PCNL can be used for larger stones with a success rate approaching 100%. For residual stone fragments post PCNL, SWL can be effective. For ureteroscopic access to the upper tracts in patients with intestinal loop diversions, flexible looposcopy can be performed to pass a guide wire up the ureter in question. If this is not possible owing to poor visibility or ureteroenteric stricture, an antegrade approach can be taken via a nephrostomy tract *(16,91)*. In this case, the stone and stricture are treated simultaneously. One caveat is appropriate, in paraplegic or quadriplegic patients, ureteral peristalsis is significantly impaired and hence success with SWL or even ureteroscopic renal procedures may be markedly reduced versus percutaneous stone removal.

Ectopic Continent Neobladders

From the standpoint of stone formation, continent urinary reservoirs can be classified as those that contain exposed foreign body material such as sutures, staples, or mesh (e.g., Kock pouch) and those that do not (e.g., Indiana pouch). The Kock pouch is a nonrefluxing continent catheterizeable urinary reservoir that is fashioned from a 72-cm segment of ileum. The midportion is detubularized and the proximal and distal 20 cm are intussuscepted to form a nonrefluxing afferent and efferent limb. The valve is stapled in three areas that can lead to stone formation on the exposed staples. To re-enforce the limbs, a collar of mesh is placed around the outside. The mesh can erode into the reservoir and also act as a nidus for stone formation *(93)*.

The Indiana pouch is formed from an isolated segment of bowel comprised of the ascending colon, cecum, and 10 cm of terminal ileum. The colon is detubularized and the ureters are reimplanted in a nonrefluxing fashion. The catheterizeable continent limb is formed by reinforcing the ileocecal valve with various imbricating suture techniques.

The catheterizeable limb is tapered into a narrow "Mitrofanoff" like tube that can be brought out to a stoma *(93)*.

Thus, the two main differences between a Kock pouch and an Indiana pouch is the presence or absence of foreign body material and the ability or inability to place a sizeable endoscope through the efferent limb. Infection with urea splitting organisms, urinary stasis, and mucus formation are all lithogenic risk factors common to both types of diversion *(94)*.

Stone formation in the Kock pouch vs Indiana pouch is estimated to occur in 16.7–43% vs 0–12.9% of patients, respectively *(94,95)*. Although these ranges overlap, it is generally believed that the Kock pouch has a higher rate of stone formation because of the presence of exposed staples and mesh. In one study the rate of stone formation was noted to drop significantly after the mesh was changed from permanent to absorbable *(95)*. Furthermore, a significant percentage of the stones that form within the Indiana pouch occur on retained absorbable sutures or debris *(94)*.

With the Kock pouch, the configuration of the efferent limb usually allows the placement of a nephroscope directly through it into the pouch. Lithotripsy and evacuation of debris can be performed with a wide array of devices *(94–97)*. Retrograde ureteroscopic retrieval of stones and retained stents within the afferent limb of the pouch have been described *(96)*. SWL has also been described for treatment of stones both in the pouch and within the afferent limb *(97)* but, in general, SWL for this group of patients is discouraged owing to inability to clear out the fragmented stone debris *(96,97)*. Concerns regarding injury to the continence mechanism of the Kock pouch have been raised; however, a high rate of incontinence after the procedure has not been reported. One author suggests placing a 26-Fr working sheath through the stoma to avoid repeated traumatization *(103)*.

Treatment of stones within the Indiana pouch or within urinary reservoirs with a Mitrofanoff like efferent limb can be more challenging because, at times, the catheterizeable lumen can be narrow and may necessitate the use of a small bore fiber optic scope. Again, SWL has been used to treat stones within these pouches, however other authors advise against this because of difficulty with clearance and irrigation of debris through the small channel and the high risk of recurrence *(96,97)*. One solution is percutaneous pouch lithotripsy. To move overlying bowel out of the path to the pouch, the puncture can be performed under direct vision with a small flexible cystoscope *(100)* or better yet, after retrograde filling with saline under ultrasound guidance *(101)*. The tract is then dilated using standard techniques and pouchoscopy, lithotripsy, and evacuation of debris can be performed.

ORTHOTOPIC NEOBLADDERS

Orthotopic neobladders may be fashioned in multiple configurations but all rely on preservation of the external sphincter mechanism to maintain urinary continence. Because a urethroenteric anastomosis is created, these pouches are accessible transurethrally. Thus, standard methods for cystolitholapaxy are used *(93)*. Neobladders that have exposed staple lines such as the hemi Kock pouch are at a higher risk of stone formation than neobladders without foreign bodies.

SUMMARY

The skilled endoscopist requires a thorough knowledge of both normal and congenital or iatrogenically altered renal, ureteral and bladder anatomy. A clear understanding of this topic enables the astute clinician to effectively select the most appropriate form of therapy.

REFERENCES

1. Sharfi AR. Presentation and Management of Urethral Calculi. Br J Urol 1991; 68: 271.
2. Koga S, Arakaki Y, Matsuoka M, Ohyama C. Urethral Calculi. Br J Urol 1990; 65: 288.
3. Schwartz BF, Stoller ML. The vesical calculus. Urol Clin North Am 2000; 27: 333.
4. Abdel-Razzak OM. Ureteral Anatomy. In: Smith's Textbook of Endourology, Chapter 7, (Smith AD, Badlani GH, Bagley DH, et al., eds.). Quality Medical Publishing, St. Louis, MO, 1996, pp. 388–396.
5. Lingeman JE. Mertz maneuver for catheterizing the tortuous ureter. J Endourol 2: 16, 1987.
6. Sampaio FJB. Surgical anatomy of the kidney. In: Smith's Textbook of Endourology, (Smith AD, Badlani GH, Bagley DH, et al., eds.). Quality Medical Publishing, St. Louis, MO, 1996, pp. 153–184.
7. Kaye KW. Renal anatomy: endourological considerations. In: Techniques in Endourology: A Guide To The Percutaneous Removal of Renal and Ureteral Calculi, Chapter 3, (Clayman RV, Castañeda-Zuñiga W, eds.). Heritage Press, Dallas, TX, 1984, pp. 55–71.
8. Elbahnasy AM, Clayman RV, Shalhav AL, et al. Lower-pole caliceal stone clearance after shock wave lithotripsy, percutaneous nephrolithotomy, and flexible ureteroscopy: impact of radiographic spatial anatomy. J Endourol 1998; 12: 113.
9. Madbouly K, Sheir KZ, Elsobky E. Impact of lower pole renal anatomy on stone clearance after shock wave lithotripsy: fact or fiction? J Urol 2001; 165: 1415.
10. Sampaio FJB, Aragao AHM. Inferior pole collecting system anatomy: its probable role in extracorporeal shock wave lithotripsy. J Urol 1992; 147: 322.
11. Poulakis V, Dahm P, Witzsch U, de Vries R, Remplik J, Becht E. Prediction of lower pole stone clearance following shock wave lithotripsy using an artificial neural network. J Urol 2003;169: 1250–1256.
12. Tuckey J, Devasia A, Murthy L, et al. Is there a simpler method for predicting lower pole stone clearance after shockwave lithotripsy than measuring infundibulopelvic angle? J Endourol 2000; 14: 475.
13. Sampaio FJB, D'Anunciacao AL, Silva ECG. Comparative follow-up of patients with acute and obtuse infundibulum-pelvic angle submitted to extracorporeal shockwave lithotripsy for lower caliceal stones: preliminary report and proposed study design. J Endourol 1997; 11: 157.
14. Elbahnasy AM, Clayman RV, Shalhav AL, et al. Lower-pole caliceal stone clearance after shock wave lithotripsy. J Endourol 1998; 12: 113.
15. Keeley FX, Moussa SA, Smith G, Tolley DA. Clearance of lower-pole stones following shock wave lithotripsy: effect of the infundibulopelvic angle. Eur Urol 1999; 36: 371.
16. Poulakis V, Witzsch U, deVries R, Becht E. Antegrade percutaneous endoluminal treatment of non-malignant ureterointestinal anastomotic strictures following urinary diversion. Eur Urol 2001; 39: 308.
17. Sumino Y, Mimata H, Tasaki Y, et al. Predictors of lower pole renal stone clearance after extracorporeal shock wave lithotripsy. J Urol 2002; 168: 1344.
18. Jumar PVS, Joshi HB, Keeley FX. An acute infundibulopelvic angle: a contraindication to flexible ureteroscopy for lower pole stones. J Endourol 1999; 13: 43A.
19. Moody JA, Williams JC, Lingeman JE. Lower pole renal anatomy: effects on stone clearance after shock wave lithotripsy in a randomized population. J Urol 1999; 161: 378.
20. Pace KT, Tariq N, Dyer SJ, et al. Mechanical percussion, inversion and diuresis for residual lower pole fragments after shock wave lithotripsy: a prospective, single blind, randomized controlled trial. J Urol 2001; 166: 2065.
21. Brownlee N, Foster M, Griffith DP, et al. Controlled inversion therapy: an adjunct to the elimination of gravity-dependent fragments following extracorporeal shock wave lithotripsy. J Urol 1990; 143: 1096.
22. Brödel M. The intrinsic blood vessels of the kidney and their significance in nephrostomy. Johns Hopkins Hosp. Bull 1901; 12: 10.

23. Graves FT. The anatomy of the intrarenal arteries and its application to segmental resection of the kidney. Br J Surg 1954; 42: 132.
24. Kaye KW, Goldberg ME. Applied anatomy of the kidney and ureter. Urol Clin North Am 1982; 9: 3.
25. Sampaio FJB, Aragao AHM. Anatomical relationship between the intrarenal arteries and the kidney collection system. J Urol 1990; 143: 679.
26. Sampaio FJB, Aragao AHM. Anatomical relationship between the renal venous arrangement and the kidney collection system. J Urol 1990; 144: 1089.
27. Sampaio FJB. Renal anatomy: endourologic considerations. Urology 1990; 27: 585.
28. Sampaio FJB, Zanier JFC, Aragao AHM, Favorito LA. Intrarenal access: 3-dimenstional anatomical study. J Urol 1992; 148: 1769.
29. Pearle MS, Traxer O. Renal urolithiasis: therapy for special circumstances, part II, Lesson 40. AUA Update Series, Lesson 40, 2000; 20: 314.
30. Matin SF, Streem SB. Metabolic risk factors in patients with ureteropelvic junction obstruction and renal calculi. J Urol 2000; 163: 1676.
31. Husmann DA, Milliner DS, Segura JW. Ureteropelvic junction obstruction with concurrent renal pelvic calculi in the pediatric patient: a long-term follow-up. J Urol 1996; 156: 741.
32. Bernardo NO, Liatsikos EN, Dinlenc CZ, Kapoor R, Fogarty JD, Smith AD. Stone recurrence after endopyelotomy. Urology 2000; 56: 378.
33. Streem SB. Stone extraction. In: Smith's Textbook of Endourology, vol. 1, Chapter 18, (Smith AD, Badlani GH, Bagley DH, et al., eds.). Quality Medical Publishing, St. Louis, MO, 1996, pp. 239–263.
34. Shalhav AL, Giusti G, Elbahnasy AM, et al. Adult endopyelotomy: impact of etiology and antegrade versus retrograde approach on outcome. J Urol 1998; 160: 685.
35. Ramakumar S, Lancini V, Chan DY, Parsons JK, Kavoussi LR, Jarrett TW. Laparoscopic pyeloplasty with concomitant pyelolithotomy. J Urol 2002; 167: 1378.
36. Yow RM, Bunts RC. Caliceal diverticulum. J Urol 1955; 73: 663.
37. Wilbert DM, Jenny E, Stoeckle M. Calyceal diverticular stones: Is ESWL worthwhile? J Urol 1986; 135: 183A.
38. Psihramis DE, Dretler SP. Extracorporeal shock wave lithotripsy of caliceal diverticular calculi. J Urol 1987; 138: 707.
39. Ritchie AW, Parr NJ, Moussa SA, Tolley DA. Lithotripsy for calculi in caliceal diverticuli. Br J Urol 1990; 66: 1990.
40. Jones JA, Lingeman JE, Steidle CP. The roles of extracorporeal shock wave lithotripsy and percutaneous nephrostolithotomy in the management of pyelocaliceal diverticulua. J Urol 1991; 146: 724.
41. Hendrikx AJ, Bierkens AF, Bos R, Oosterhof GO, Debruyne FM. Treatment of stones in caliceal diverticuli: Extracorporeal shock wave lithotripsy versus percutaneous nephrolitholapaxy. Br J Urol 1992; 70: 478.
42. Monga M, Smith R, Ferral H, Thomas R. Percutaneous ablation of caliceal diverticulum: long-term follow-up. J Urol 2000; 163: 28.
43. Bellman GC, Silverstein JI, Blickensderfer S, Smith AD. Technique and follow-up of percutaneous management of caliceal diverticula. Urology 1993; 42: 21.
44. Shalhav AL, Soble JJ, Nakada SY, Wolf S Jr, McClennan BL, Clayman RV. Long-term outcome of caliceal diverticula following percutaneous endosurgical management. J Urol 1998; 160: 1998.
45. Batter SJ, Dretler SP. Ureterorenoscopic approach to the symptomatic caliceal diverticulum. J Urol 1997; 158: 709.
46. Gluckman GR, Stoller M, Irby P. Laparoscopic pyelocaliceal diverticuli ablation. J Endourol 1993; 7: 315.
47. Ruckle HC, Segura JW. Laparoscopic treatment of a stone filled, caliceal diverticulum: a definitive, minimally invasive therapeutic option. J Urol 1994; 151: 122.
48. Harewood LM, Agarwal D, Lindsay S, Vaughan MG, Cleeve LK, Webb DR. Extraperitoneal laparoscopic caliceal diverticulectomy. J Endourol 1996; 10: 425.
49. Hoznek A, Herard A, Ogiez N, Amsellem D, Chopin DK, Abbou CC. Symptomatic caliceal diverticula treated with extraperitoneal laparoscopic marsupialization fulguration and gelatin resorcinol formaldehyde glue obliteration. J Urol 1998; 160: 352.

50. Amis ES, Cronan JJ, Pfister RC. The spectrum of peripelvic cysts. Br J Urol 1993; 55: 150.
51. Hoenig DM, McDougall EM, Shalhav AL, Elbahnasy AM, Clayman RV. Laparoscopic ablation of peripelvic renal cysts. J Urol 1997; 158: 1345.
52. Johanson KE, Plaine L, Farcon E, Morales P. Management of intrarenal peripelvic cysts. Urology 1974; 4: 514.
53. Hubner W, Pfaf R, Porpacz P. Renal cysts: percutaneous resection with standard urologic instruments. J Endourol 1990; 4: 61.
54. Hulbert JC, Hunter D, Young AT, Castañeda-Zuñiga W. Percutaneous intrarenal marsupialization of a perirenal cystic collection-endocystolysis. J Urol 1988; 139: 1039.
55. Roberts WW, Bluebond-Langner R, Boyle KE, Jarrett TW, Kavoussi LR. Laparoscopic ablation of symptomatic parenchymal and peripelvic renal cysts. Urol 2001; 58: 165.
56. Cass AS. Extracorporeal shock wave lithotripsy for renal stones with renal cysts present. J Urol 1995; 153: 599.
57. Torres VE, Erickson SB, Smith LH, et al. The association of nephrolithiasis with autosomal dominant poycystic kidney disease. Am J Kidney Dis 1988; 11: 318.
58. Ng CS, Yost A, Streem SB. Urolithiasis associated with autosomal dominant poycystic kidney disease: contemporary urological management. J Urol 2000; 163: 726.
59. Grampsas SA, Chandhoke PS, Fan J, et al. Anatomic and metabolic risk factors for nephrolithiasis in patients with autosomal dominant polycystic kidney disease. Am J Kidney Dis 2000; 36: 53.
60. Pitts WR Jr, Muecke EC. Horseshoe kidneys: a 40-year experience. J Urol 1975; 113: 743.
61. Vandeursen H, Baert L. Electromagnetic extracorporeal shock wave lithotripsy for calculi in horseshoe kidneys. J Urol 1992; 148: 1120.
62. Jenkins AD, Gillenwater JY. Extracorporeal shock wave lithotripsy in the prone position: treatment of stones in the distal ureter or anomalous kidney. J Urol 1988; 139: 911.
63. Janetschek G, Kunzel KH. Percutaneous nephrolithotomy in horseshoe kidneys: applied anatomy and clinical experience. Br J Urol 1988; 62: 117.
64. Clayman RV, Castaneda-Zuniga W. Planning the approach: general and specific aspects. In: Techniques in Endourology: A Guide to the Percutaneous Removal of Renal and Ureteral Calculi, (Clayman RV, Castaneda-Zuniga W, eds.). Heritage Press, Dallas, TX, 1984, p. 23.
65. Lingeman JE, Chee SK. Percutaneous operative procedures in horseshoe kidneys. J Urol 1999; 161: 371.
66. Jones DJ, Wickham JEA, Kellett MJ. Percutaneous nephrolithotomy for calculi in horseshoe kidneys. J Urol 1991; 145: 481.
67. Yohannes P, Smith AD. The endourological management of complications associated with horseshoe kidney. J Urol 2002; 168: 5.
68. Rhee BK, Bretan PN, Stoller ML. Urolithiasis in renal and combined pancreas/renal transplant recipients. J Urol 1999; 161: 1458.
69. Hayes JM, Streem SB, Graneto D, Steinmuller DR, Novick AC. Urolithiasis after renal transplantation. Trans Proc 1989; 21: 1960.
70. Dretler SP, Olsson C, Pfister RC. The anatomic, radiologic and clinical characteristics of the pelvic kidney: an analysis of 86 cases. J Urol 1971; 105: 623.
71. Wheatley M, Ohl DA, Sonda LP, Wang SC, Konnak JW. Treatment of renal transplant stone by extracorporeal shock wave lithotripsy in the prone position. Urology 1991; 37: 57.
72. Rigatti P, Montorsi F, Guazzoni G, et al. Multimodal therapy for stones in pelvic kidneys. Urol Int 1991; 46: 29.
73. Del Pizzo JJ, Jacobs SC, Sklar GN. Ureteroscopic evaluation in renal transplant recipients. J Endourol 1998; 12: 135.
74. Fabrizio MD, Behari A, Bagley DH. Ureteroscopic management of intrarenal calculi. J Urol 1998; 159: 1139.
75. Eshghi AM, Roth JS, Smith AD. Percutaneous transperitoneal approach to a pelvic kidney for endourological removal of staghorn calculus. J Urol 1985; 134: 525.
76. Eshghi M, Smith AD. Endourologic approach to a transplant kidney. Urol, 18: 504, 1986.
77. Hulbert JC, Reddy P, Young AT, et al. The percutaneous removal of calculi from transplanted kidneys. J Urol 134: 324, 1985.

78. Francesca F, Felipetto R, Mosca F, Boggi U, Rizzo G, Puccini R. Percutaneous nephrolithotomy of transplanted kidney. J Endourol 2002; 16: 225–227.

79. Harmon WJ, Kleer E, Segura JW. Laparoscopic pyelolithotomy for calculus removal in a pelvic kidney. J Urol 1996; 155: 2019.

80. Chang TD, Dretler SP. Laparoscopic pyelolithotomy in and ectopic kidney. J Urol 1996; 156: 1753.

81. Cho DK, Zackson DA, Cheigh J, et al. Urinary calculi in renal transplant recipients. Transplantation 1988; 45: 899.

82. Bricker EM. Symposium on clinical surgery; bladder substitution after pelvic evisceration. Surg Clin North Am 1950; 30: 1511.

83. Dretler SP. The pathogenesis of urinary tract calculi occurring after ileal conduit diversion: i. clinical study. ii. conduit study. iii. prevention. J Urol 1973; 109: 204.

84. Turk TM, Koleski FC, Albala DM. Incidence of urolithiasis in cystectomy patients after intestinal conduit or continent urinary diversion. World J Urol 1999; 17: 305.

85. Sullivan JW, Grabstald H, Whitmore Jr WF . Complication of ureteroileal conduit with radical cystectomy: review of 336 cases. J Urol 1980; 124: 797.

86. Schmidt JD, Hawtrey CE, Flocks RH, Culp DA. Complications, results and problems of ileal conduit diversion. J Urol 1973; 109: 210.

87. McDougal WS, Kock MO. Impaired growth and development and urinary intestinal interposition. Trans Am Assoc Genitourinary Surg 1991; 105: 3.

88. Kelalis PP. Noncontinent urinary diversion. Chapter 15, in: Atlas of Urologic Surgery (Hinman F, Jr). WB Saunders, Philadelphia, PA, 1998, pp. 623–676.

89. Turk TMT, Koleski FC, Albala DM. The pathogenesis of urinary tract calculi occurring after ileal conduit diversion: i. clinical study. ii. conduit study. iii. prevention. World J Urol 1999; 17: 305.

90. Cohen T D, Streem SB, Lammert G. Long-term incidence and risks for recurrent stones following contemporary management of upper tract calculi in patients with a urinary diversion. J Urol 1996; 155: 62.

91. McDougal WS. Metabolic complication of urinary intestinal diversion. J Urol 1992; 147: 1199.

92. Delvecchio FC, Kuo RL, Iselin CE, Webster GD, Preminger GM. Combined antegrade and retrograde endoscopic approach for the management of urinary diversion-associated pathology. J Endourol 2000; 14: 251.

93. Benson MC, Olsson CA. Continent urinary diversion. In: Campbell's Urology, vol. 3, (Walsh PC, Retik AB, Vaughan ED, Wein AJ, eds.). WB Saunders, Philadelphia, PA, 1996, pp. 3190–3245.

94. Terai A, Ueda T, Kakehi Y, et al. Urinary calculi as a late complication of the Indiana continent urinary diversion: comparison with the Kock pouch procedure. J Urol 1996; 155: 66.

95. Arai Y, Kawakita M, Terachi T, et. al. Long-term follow up of the Kock and Indiana pouch procedures. J Urol 1993; 150: 51.

96. Ginsberg D, Huffman JL, Lieskovsky G, Boyd S, Skinner DG. Urinary tract stones: A complication of the Kock pouch continent urinary diversion. J Urol 1991; 145: 956.

97. Huffman JL. Endoscopic management of complications of continent urinary diversion. Urology 1992; 39: 145.

98. Delvicchio FC, Preiminger GM. Report of the United States cooperative study on extracorporeal shock wave lithotripsy. AUA Update Series, Lesson 19, 2000, 20.

99. Cohen TD, Streem SB. Minimally invasive endourologic management of calculi in continent urinary reservoirs. Urology 1994; 43: 865.

100. Hensle TW, Dean GE. Complications of urinary tract reconstruction. Urol Clin North Am 1991; 18: 755.

101. Roth S, Van Ahlen A, Semjonow B, Von Heyden B, Hertle L. Percutaneous pouch lithotripsy in continent urinary diversions with narrowed Mitrofanoff conduit. J Urol 1994; 73: 316.

IV TREATMENT

24 Conservative Management of Ureteral Calculi

Christopher J. Kane, MD

Key Words: Ureter; calculi; kidney; calcium channel blockers; steroids; β-blockers; obstruction.

INTRODUCTION

Urolithiasis is a common condition affecting up to 12% of the US population *(1)*. The majority of patients initially present with pain or hematuria. Approximately 60–70% of patients presenting to an emergency department with flank pain who undergo imaging will be diagnosed with ureterolithiasis *(2)*. Of those patients with ureterolithiasis, depending on stone size and location, approx 80% will pass the stone spontaneously if given an opportunity *(3)*. The widespread use of shockwave lithotripsy and ureteroscopy has prompted earlier intervention of ureteral calculi with excellent results. However, observation is the most appropriate initial management in the majority of patients with symptomatic urolithiasis because of its noninvasiveness, success, and low cost. This chapter will examine the spontaneous passage of ureteral calculi, factors predictive of

From: Current Clinical Urology, *Urinary Stone Disease:*
A Practical Guide to Medical and Surgical Management
Edited by: M. L. Stoller and M. V. Meng © Humana Press Inc., Totowa, NJ

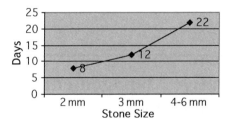

Fig. 1. Average days to stone passage for ureteral stones by size. Adapted from Reference *3*.

successful conservative management, options available for medically enhancing stone passage, as well as the effects of obstruction and indications for intervention of ureteral calculi.

OBSERVATION OF URETERAL CALCULI

It has long been recognized that many ureteral calculi pass spontaneously. The American Urological Association (AUA) clinical guidelines panel for the management of ureteral calculi recommends observation for stones less than 5 mm in size *(4)*. However, observation of ureteral calculi, although attractive because of its noninvasiveness, is associated with significant uncertainty. The time interval of spontaneous passage is important, as are the pain expectations, time off from work, and potential risk of renal injury (Fig. 1). Specifically, in order to select appropriate therapy, it is important to know which stones should be observed, how long a patient should expect to wait before stone passage, and which factors are predictive of spontaneous passage.

The likelihood of stone passage by size varies widely in the literature from 71–98% for stones under 5 mm in the distal ureter to 25–53% for stones 5–10 mm in the same location *(4)*. In a review of 75 patients with ureterolithiasis followed until spontaneous stone passage or intervention, Miller and Kane found that stone passage was dependent on a number of factors including stone size. Ninety-five percent of stones 2 mm and smaller passed spontaneously, whereas 83% of stones 2–4 mm and only 50% of stones over 4 mm passed spontaneously *(3)*. Miller and Kane also analyzed the impact of clinical factors including patient gender, age, stone size, location, pain medication requirements, and interval to stone passage. Multivariate analysis revealed that patient sex, age, and degree of pain were unrelated to interval to stone passage. Together, size, location, and side were statistically related to stone passage interval ($p = 0.012$). Stones that were smaller, more distal, and right sided were more likely to pass spontaneously and required fewer interventions. The time interval to stone passage was quite variable, however, and was highly related to location and size. The average interval to stone passage by size is summarized in Figure 1 and is typically 1–2 wk for stones less than 5 mm. For 95% of stones of a particular size to pass spontaneously, however, much longer intervals, up to 30–40 d, may be required. The likelihood of intervention in their cohort also went up with stone size from only 5% for 2 mm stones to 50% for over 4 mm stones.

Hubner et al evaluated a cohort of 100 patients managed with observation and found that no stone larger than 6 mm passed spontaneously *(5)*. They also found that complications increased significantly with time, with 20% complications after 4 wk compared

Table 1
Randomized Controlled Trials of Calcium Channel Blockers and Steroids for Stone Passage

Reference	N	Medication	Treatment arm		Control arm	
			Passage (%)	Days	Passage (%)	Days
Borchi (12)	86	Nifedipine + methylprednisolone	86	11.2	65	16.4
Porpiglia (13)	96	Nifedipine + deflazacort	79	7	35	20
Cooper (14)	70	Nifedipine	86		56	

to only 7% complications under 4 wk. Ibrahim analyzed prognostic factors in the conservative management of ureteral stones. Factors predictive of spontaneous stone passage for stones ≤10 mm included: duration of pain <30 d; pyuria <100 white blood cells/high powered field; lack of irregular stone surface and partial obstruction.

MEDICAL MANAGEMENT TO ENHANCE PASSAGE OF URETERAL CALCULI

Pain and Nausea Treatment

The cornerstone of medical management of ureteral stones has been pain control. The most common agents used are oral narcotics and nonsteroidal antiinflammatory medications. There is no evidence that oral narcotics either speed or diminish ureteral stone passage; however, patient comfort is necessary in order to tolerate observation. Oxycodone is a potent, well-tolerated oral narcotic that retains 50% of its effectiveness when taken orally and is used most commonly in combination with acetaminophen. Narcotics act primarily centrally. Because acute ureteral obstruction and oral narcotics can both lead to nausea, antiemetics are also beneficial to some patients. We most commonly use prochlorperazine in oral or suppository form, which has been shown to be superior to placebo in treating nausea and vomiting (7). Intravenous administration of intramuscular ketorolac is an effective treatment for acute renal colic. It blocks the synthesis of prostaglandin E2 from the renal medulla, thus decreasing glomerular filtration rate and urine output. It also acts centrally to decrease pain, acts locally to decrease ureteral spasm and may diminish ureteral edema (8–10). Ketorolac is a commonly used agent for control of acute colic but is used less commonly in the outpatient setting. A study of the prostaglandin synthesis inhibitor diclofenac sodium in 80 patients with ureterothiasis under 5 mm confirmed excellent analgesia in 84% of patients and suggested enhanced stone passage (57.5%) although there was no untreated control group (11).

Oral Steroids, Calcium Channel Blockers, and Beta Blockers

There has been growing evidence that the combination of oral steroids and long-acting calcium channel blockers enhances passage of ureteral calculi (Table 1). Borchi et al. performed a prospective randomized double blind study comparing 16-mg methylprednisolone and 40 mg of nifedipine daily to the same dose of steroid and placebo on 86 patients followed until stone passage or 45 d (12). The treatment group had a higher spontaneous passage rate (87 vs 65%, $p = 0.021$) and passed the stones more quickly (mean 11.2 vs 16.4 d, $p = 0.036$). The stones which successfully passed in this series were 6.4 and 5.3 mm in the different treatment groups, which is fairly large for spontaneous passage series.

In a similar prospective study, Porpiglia et al. studied 96 patients with distal ureteral stone under 1 cm (13). The patients were randomized between (1) oral 30-mg deflazacort and 30-mg slow-release nifedipine and (2) placebo. The passage rates were 79% in the treatment arm and 35% in the placebo arm ($p < 0.05$) and the treatment arm passed stones more quickly (mean 7 d vs 20 d, $p < 0.05$). Porpiglia et al. also examined the pain medication used by each patient and found that the steroid and nifedipine arm had significantly less pain medication usage, mean 15-mg sodium diclofenac vs 105 mg in the placebo arm. Transient hypotension and palpitations led to discontinuation in two patients of the treatment arm. Twenty-one percent of patients had side effects from treatment including headache and asthenia that did not require discontinuation. The treatment arm also experienced a mean decrease of systolic blood pressure of 15 mmHg.

Cooper et al. also performed a prospective randomized study comparing standard pain management and nausea medication to a group receiving the same regimen plus nifedipine, prednisone, and trimethoprim/sulfamethoxazole (14). They found the nifedipine/steroid/antibiotic group had higher spontaneous stone passage (86% vs 56%) and fewer lost work days (1.8 vs 4.9), emergency room visits, and surgical interventions. Because of the study design, it was impossible to determine which agent was responsible for the beneficial effects.

The mechanism by which calcium channel blockers enhance stone passage is not completely understood. Ureteral contractions are dependent on an active calcium pump. Calcium channel blockers appear to suppress the intensity of ureteral contractions (15) and, in an animal model (16), decrease the number of ureteral contractions per minute. For this reason, they are effective at relieving renal colic pain acutely (17). The improved passage is likely caused by diminished ureteral spasm in the region of the calculus and perhaps caused by direct ureteral relaxation. The mechanism of action of steroids is likely because of their antiinflammatory effects and presumably from effecting local inflammation and edema. A short course of oral steroids, as was used in the studies summarized, does not require a steroid taper after discontinuation.

β-blockers have been less extensively studied. In a prospective controlled trial involving 86 patients with distal ureteral stones, Bajor found that oxprenolol reduced the time to stone passage from 11 to 5.2 d without any significant side effects (18). The mechanism proposed for β-blockers is also ureteral smooth muscle relaxation.

Miscellaneous Agents Studied in Conservative Stone Management

Metoclopramide has been prospectively compared in 21 patients to opiates for relief of pain caused by ureteral colic (19). The pain relief at 10, 20, and 30 mins after treatment was thought to be comparable to opiates in this small group.

Glyceryl trinitrate (GTN) patches, 5 mg, identical to those used for patients with cardiac angina, have been studied in acute ureteral colic. In a preliminary study of various routes of administration of GTN in patients with ureteral colic, Hofstetter and Kriegmair found GTN to be beneficial (20). However, in a well designed, randomized, double-blinded study of 50 patients with under 10 mm stones, GTN did not demonstrate any advantage in stone-free rate, interval to stone passage, or number of episodes of pain over placebo (21).

Rowatinex, an oral medication of essential plant oils produced in Ireland, has been evaluated for its value in urolithiasis. In a prospective placebo controlled trial of 87 patients with ureteral stones, the overall stone expulsion rate was significantly higher in the Rowatinex group as compared to placebo: 81% and 59%, respectively *(22)*. The mechanism of action is unknown.

Because the ureteral dilation seen in pregnant women is likely caused by progesterone, it has been proposed as a treatment for ureterolithiasis *(23)*. Mikkelson et al. gave 24 patients with ureterolithiasis an IM injection of 250-mg hydroxyprogesterone and observed spontaneous stone passage in 75% of the new patients within 3 wk and claim this is superior to traditional control groups. Progesterone agents have not been studied in a well-designed, controlled study.

High Water Intake

Although increased fluid intake has been shown to be effective at diminishing stone recurrence rates, the utility of high fluid intake to improve stone passage is controversial. High fluid intake is commonly recommended in order to "flush" the stone out, but these instructions have little physiologic basis. The response to unilateral partial obstruction is an initial increase in renal blood flow and glomerular filtration rate and a subsequent decrease in both with continued obstruction. Ureteral pressure initially increases and stabilizes as ureteral coaptation is lost with progressive ureteral dilation. Initially, ureteral parastalsis increases but then decreases over time in the face of obstruction *(25)*. Therefore, after ureteral obstruction reaches a steady-state, increases in oral or intravenous fluids are not likely to affect the pressure in the obstructed kidney. Indeed, in cases of partial obstruction where ureteral peristalsis and coaptation is maintained, increasing fluid intake may drive the obstructed kidney to lose ureteral coaptation, thus worsening stone progression. It has been observed that when obstruction is relieved by percutaneous nephrostomy drainage, stone passage is enhanced, also arguing against the value of increased fluid intake during an acute stone episode. Additionally, in an animal model, percutaneous nephrostomy drainage was shown to be superior to stenting for spontaneous stone passage *(26)*.

Supporting increased fluid intake to enhance ureteral stone passage is a recent article by Kaid-Omar et al. *(27)*. In a nonrandomized observation study, 219 patients with ureteral stones under 6 mm were offered an intensive regimen of oral fluid intake. One hundred twenty-nine patients agreed to drink 3 L a day and 90 declined. The patients with high fluid intake had a greater stone passage rate (76% vs 14%, $p < 0.001$). They also had a significant increase in their urinary pH and a decreased stone recurrence rate. An obvious shortcoming of the study is the lack of randomization and the resulting potential for selection bias.

RENAL INJURY DURING PERIODS OF OBSERVATION

Limiting potential renal injury is an important goal in the management of ureterolithiasis. There is evidence that irreversible renal injury can occur with long periods of ureteral obstruction. The challenge is defining the degree of obstruction and deciding when to intervene. A historical method is to assign degree of obstruction based on the delay of the nephrogram and excretion of contrast on intravenous pyelography. Another method is to perform nuclear scintigraphy to assess degree of obstruction based on the excretion of radiopharmaceutical. Both methods are flawed because they represent a narrow observation of a phenomenon which is in flux. Many patients go from significant obstruction to minimal obstruction or stone passage within days. Degree of pain is also not a reliable indicator of degree of obstruction and we found that pain was not highly correlated to stone passage success or interval *(3)*.

The safe interval of observation is also not known. Holm-Nielsen et al found that a third of patients with unilateral ureteral obstruction lasting over 1 mo suffered irreversible renal injury that was difficult to predict based on clinical or radiographic data *(28)*. Irving et al. recently studied 54 patients with symptomatic unilateral ureterolithiasis with mercapto-acetyltriglycine radioisotope renography to monitor renal function *(29)*. They performed renal scans within 48 h of presentation, and again after stone treatment or 1 mo if treated conservatively. They intervened on any kidney whose differential function was under 45% (15 patients, 28%). When they compared the recovery of function of the 11 patients who had intervention in fewer than 7 d to the 4 patients whose intervention was after 7 d, the early intervention group had better recovery of function. A limitation of the study is that some of the patients who had intervention for diminished function likely underwent unnecessary intervention and would have passed the stones and had spontaneous recovery of function. These authors argue for nuclear renography and observation only for those patients with over 45% differential renal function.

OBSERVATION IN CHILDREN

There are few recent reports of the success of observation on ureteral calculi in children. Van Savage et al recently reviewed the outcome of 33 children with ureteral stones *(30)*. Twelve patients (36%) passed the stones spontaneously. The average size of the stones which passed was 2 mm whereas no stone over 4 mm passed spontaneously. This supports observation as a reasonable initial strategy for children with small distal stones and well controlled pain. The AUA clinical guidelines for ureteral stones are reasonable for children although the impact of stone size on particular treatments may need to be adjusted depending on the size of the child.

COST

The cost of conservative management of ureteral stones is multifactorial and complex. The obvious direct costs include the cost of outpatient visits, follow-up laboratory tests, radiographs, medications and emergency department visits. Indirect costs include lost wages from missed work and decreased work productivity caused by the effects of pain medication. The total cost of urolithiasis care is increased with the inappropriate attempt at observation for stones destined to require intervention. In a decision analysis model, Lotan et al found observation to be the least costly strategy of ureteral stone management if no costs, such as from emergency department visits, was incurred because of failed observation *(31)*.

INDICATIONS FOR INTERVENTION

Initial management of ureteral calculi should be based on patient history, comorbidities, symptoms, renal function, and stone size and location on imaging. Patients with solitary kidneys or bilateral ureteral stones require intervention and are poor candidates for observation. Similarly, patients with evidence of urinary infection in the face of a ureteral calculus are best managed with percutaneous nephrostomy or ureteral stenting and antibiotics before definitive management. Patients with normal renal function and ureteral stones under 6 mm should be considered for observation. Those with stones that are smaller and more distal are more likely to pass spontaneously. Miller and Kane found that 50% of patients with over 4 mm stones ultimately fail conservative management *(3)*. In our series, the most common reason for intervention was poor pain control followed by nonprogression after an adequate period of observation. Patients considering observation need to allow from 2 to 4 wk in order to give an adequate trial of intervention. Indications for intervention during that time include poor pain control, inability to tolerate oral pain medication, urinary infection, repeated emergency room visits, nonprogression on serial imaging, or a social situation which does not allow missed work or oral narcotics. Common professions that are poorly compatible with observation are physicians, pilots, and attorneys.

CONCLUSIONS

Conservative management is the preferred strategy for most patients with ureteral stones under 4 mm and should be considered for select patients with ureteral stones up to 8 mm in size. The likelihood of success diminishes as the size of the stone increases and for more proximal stones. Good pain control is critical for patient acceptance of observation. Serial monitoring should take place with clinical and radiographic assessment to ensure stone progression. There is strong evidence that oral calcium channel blockers and oral steroids may decrease patient pain and decrease the time interval of stone passage. Longstanding high-grade obstruction can contribute to irreversible renal injury; therefore vigilant follow-up of ureteral calculi is warranted with intervention for over 2 wk of high-grade obstruction or for nonprogression.

REFERENCES

1. Sierakowski R, Finlayson B, Landes RR, Finlayson CD, Sierakowski N. The frequency of urolithiasis in hospital discharge diagnoses in the United States. Invest Urol 1978; 15: 438.
2. Miller OF, Rineer SK, Reichard SR, et al. Prospective comparison of unenhanced spiral computed tomography and intravenous urogram in the evaluation of acute flank pain. Urology 1998; 52: 982–987.
3. Miller OF, Kane CJ. Time to Stone Passage for Observed Ureteral Calculi: A Guide for Patient Education. J Urol 1999; 162: 688–691.
4. Segura JW, Preminger GM, Assimos DG, et al. Ureteral stones clinical guidelines panel summary report on the management of ureteral calculi. J Urol 1997; 158: 1915.
5. Hubner WA, Irby P, Stoller ML. Natural history and current concepts for the treatment of small ureteral calculi. Eur Urol 1993; 24: 172.
6. Ibrahim AIA, Shetty SD, Awad RM, Patel KP. Prognostic factors in the conservative treatment of ureteric stones. Br J Urol 1991; 67: 358.
7. Medoff J. A double-blind evaluation of the antiemetic efficacy of benzquanamide, prochlorperazine and trimethobenzamide in office practice. Curr Ther Res 1970; 12: 706.
8. Gasparich JP, Mayo ME. Comparative effects of four prostoglandin synthesis inhibitors on the obstructed kidney in the dog. J Urol 1986; 135: 1088.
9. Larsen LS, Miller A, Allegra JR. The use of intravenous ketorolac for the treatment of renal colic in the Emergency Department. Am J Emerg Med 1993; 11: 197.
10. Lennon GM, Bourke J, Ryan PC, Fitzpatrick JM. Pharmacologic options for the treatment of acute ureteral colic. Br J Urol 1993; 71: 401.
11. Ahmad M, Chaughtai MN, Khan FA. Role of prostaglandin synthesis inhibitors in the passage of ureteric calculus. J Pak Med Assoc 1991; 41: 268.
12. Borchi L, Meschi T, Amato F, et al. Nifedipine and methylprednisolone in facilitating ureteral stone passage: a randomized, double-blind, placebo-controlled study. J Urol 1994; 152: 1095.
13. Porpiglia F, Destefanis P, Fiori C, Fontana D. Effectiveness of nifedipine and deflazacort in the management of distal ureteral stones. Urology 2000; 56: 579.

14. Cooper JT, Stack GM, Cooper TP. Intensive medical management of ureteral calculi. Urology 2000; 56: 575.

15. Andersson KE, Forman A, Effects of calcium channel blockers on urinary tract smooth muscle. Acta Pharmacol Toxicol 1986; 58: 193.

16. Salman S, Castilla C, Vela Navarette R, Action of calcium antagonists on ureteral dynamics. Acta Urol Esp 1989; 13: 150.

17. Capecchi S, Pignatelli R, Alegiani F, Emergency treatment of ureteral colic with nifedipine. Minerva Urol Nephrol 1991; 43: 287.

18. Bajor G. Beta-blocking agent facilitating the spontaneous passage of ureteral stones. Int Urol Nephrol 1990; 22: 33.

19. Muller TF, Naesh O, Svare E, Jensen A, Glyngdal P. Metoclopromide (Primperan) in the treatment of ureterolithiasis. A Prospective double-blind study of metoclopromide compared with morphatropin in ureteral colic. Urol Int 1990; 45: 112.

20. Hofstetter AG, Kriegmair M. Treatment of ureteral colic with glycerol trinitrate. Fortschritte Medizin 1993; 111: 286.

21. Hussain Z, Inman RD, Elves AWS, Shipstone DP, Ghiblawi S, Coppinger SWV. Use of glyceryl trinitrate patches in patients with ureteral stones: a randomized, double-blind, placebo-controlled study. Urology 2001; 58: 521.

22. Engelstein D, Kahan E, Servadio C. Rowatinex for the treatment of ureterolithiasis. J Urol (Paris) 1992; 98: 98.

23. Perlow DL. The use of progesterone for ureteral stones: a preliminary report. J Urol 1980; 124: 715.

24. Mikkelsen AL, Meyhoff HH, Lindahl F, Christensen J. The effect of hydroxyprogesterone on ureteral stones. Int Urol Nephrol 1988; 20: 257.

25. Weiss RM. Physiology and pharmacology of the renal pelvis and ureter. In: Campbell's Urology, 8th Ed., (Walsh PC, ed.). Saunders, Philadelphia, PA, 2002, pp. 377–409.

26. Lennon GM, Thornhill JA, Grainger R, McDermott TE, Butler MR. Double pigtail ureteric stent versus percutaneous nephrostomy: effects on stone transit and ureteric motility. Eur Urol 1997; 31: 24.

27. Kaid-Omar Z, Belouatek A, Driouch A, et al. Effects of diuretic therapy on spontaneous expulsion of urinary calculi, urinary pH, and crystalluria in lithiasic patients. Prog Urol 2001; 11: 450.

28. Holm-Nielsen A, Jorgensen T, Mogensen P, Fogh J. The prognostic value of probe renography in ureteric stone obstruction. Br J Urol 1981; 53: 504.

29. Irving SO, Calleja R, Lee F, Bullock KN, Wraight P, Doble A. Is the conservative management of ureteric calculi of >4 mm safe? B J Urol Int 2000; 85: 637–640.

30. Van Savage JG, Palanca LG, Andersen RD, Rao GS, Slaughenhoupt BL. Treatment of distal ureteral stones in children: similarities to the american urologic association guidelines in adults. J Urol 2000; 164: 1089.

31. Lotan Y, Gettman MT, Roehrborn CG, Cadeddu JA, Pearle MS. Management of ureteral calculi: a cost comparison and decision making analysis. J Urol 2002; 167: 1621.

25 Ureteral Stents

John S. Lam, MD and Mantu Gupta, MD

Key Words: Ureter; stent; obstruction; biomaterial.

INTRODUCTION

Ureteral stents have become an integral part of contemporary urologic practice over the past 20 yr. They are typically placed to prevent or relieve ureteral obstruction secondary to a variety of intrinsic or extrinsic etiologies that include obstructing ureteral calculi, ureteral strictures, congenital anomalies, retroperitoneal tumor or fibrosis, trauma, or iatrogenic injury. Ureteral stents are also commonly placed to provide urinary diversion or postoperative drainage, or to help identify and prevent inadvertent injury to the ureters before surgical procedures.

HISTORY OF STENTS

The concept of stenting the urinary system began as an adjunct to open surgery in order to facilitate upper tract drainage or align the ureter. Gustav Simon, in the 19th

From: Current Clinical Urology, *Urinary Stone Disease:*
A Practical Guide to Medical and Surgical Management
Edited by: M. L. Stoller and M. V. Meng © Humana Press Inc., Totowa, NJ

century, performed the first reported case by placing a tube in the ureter while performing an open cystostomy (1). In the early 1900s, Joaquin Albarrano created the first
catheter intended for use in the ureter (1). Although vulcanization of rubber was first
reported in 1839, early catheters were constructed from fabric coated with varnish (2).
The development of plastics, such as polyethylene and polyvinyl, allowed for stents to
become more rigid and easier to place; however, bladder irritation, infection, and problems with encrustation and migration still occurred (3,4). In 1952, Tulluch described the
use of polyethylene tubes to help repair ureters and fistulas in patients (5).

In 1967, the era of modern long-term indwelling ureteral stents began when Zimskind
and colleagues reported the use of open-ended silicone tubing as an indwelling stent
that was inserted endoscopically to bypass malignant ureteral obstruction or ureterovaginal fistulas (6). Straight silicone stents provided good internal drainage and
developed less encrustation than other compounds; however, they had no distal or
proximal features to prevent migration. Minor improvements followed with Marmar
closing the proximal end of the silicone stent to facilitate passage through severely
obstructed ureters (7) and Orikasa and associates utilizing a "pusher" to hold the stent
in place during wire removal (8).

Gibbons and colleagues made several modifications to prevent stent migration, including a distal flange to prevent proximal migration and sharply pointed barbs to prevent
downward migration and expulsion (9). This stent, however, was difficult to pass because the barbs increased the nominal 7 Fr stent to an actual 11 Fr. Proximal migration
remained a problem, and placement and removal of the stent was difficult. In 1974, the
Gibbons stent became the first commercially available "modern" internal ureteral stent.
Following the Gibbons stent, McCollough (10) and Hepperlen and associates (11)
designed single-pigtail stents that could be straightened and placed over a wire cystoscopically to prevent distal, but not proximal, migration. The migration issue was
resolved in 1978 when Finney reported the use of a "double-J" stent containing both
proximal and distal "J" hooks (12), and Hepperlen and Mardis described the use of a
pigtail arterial catheter (13).

Introduction of extracorporeal shockwave lithotripsy (SWL) and developments in
endourologic stone procedures dramatically increased the use of double-pigtail stents.
In the early 1980s, industry and research efforts started to focus on minimizing complications and identifying the "ideal" stent. Development of "firm" stents reduced
migration, but at the expense of a higher incidence of dysuria and loin or flank pain (14).
Surgical errors were also identified as a cause of stent migration (15). Among errors
reported were inadequate stent length, inadequate bladder or renal pelvis curl, proximal
curl remaining in the upper calyx, and inadequate fluoroscopic monitoring. Stents were
also reported to fail in specific types of cases. One series reported a 46% failure rate
at 30 d in patients with extrinsic ureteral obstruction (16). Other studies reported high
failure rates even in routine stent cases (17,18). The importance of properly testing new
materials became evident when polyethylene, a material with attractive biocompatibility, was discovered to become brittle and fractured easily with long-term exposure
to urine (19).

The word "stent" is commonly used in genitourinary reconstructive surgery. Two
related definitions of stent are given in most medical dictionaries. First, a stent is a
device used to maintain a bodily orifice, cavity, or contour; second, a stent is a catheter,
rod, or tube within a tubular structure to maintain lumenal patency or protect an
anastomosis or graft (20). Etymologically, the word stent is an eponym related to three

English dentists named Stent who contributed to improving a substance used for dental impressions at the end of the 19th century *(20)*. Transition of the dental impression compound into a urologic tool is attributed to J.F. Esser of Holland during World War I, as the name became associated with a support for oral skin grafts, which were later adopted in plastic surgery *(21)*. Urologic stenting first appeared in print beginning in the 1970s. Willard Goodwin, the originator of many commonly accepted urological procedures, wrote a brief commentary in 1972 titled, "Splint, Stent, Stint," concluding: "Urologists are always talking about putting a tube in a ureter or urethra. When they do this, it is not a splint. It may be a stent. It probably is never a stint. Perhaps the process is most properly described as leaving a tube or stent in an organ" *(22)*. The word "stent" became forged into the urologic literature when Montie, Stewart, and Levin explicitly defined the term: "When referring to an intraluminal device to maintain patency until healing has taken place, the stent is most appropriate" *(23)*.

PHYSIOLOGY OF THE STENTED URETER

In an unstented kidney, vesical pressures are only transmitted to the kidney in the state of diuresis; however, when the ureter is stented, bladder pressure can be transmitted back to the kidney *(24)*. Acute ureteral intubation causes an elevation of intrarenal pressure with a direct correlation to stent diameter, but the intrarenal pressure declines back to baseline after 3 wk *(24,25)*. This phenomenon is dependent on open tube flow, where a standing column of urine causes direct transmission of pressure from the bladder to the renal pelvis. Increased intrarenal reflux is noted in up to 90% of patients following stent placement for acute ureteral obstruction *(26,27)* that declines back to baseline after 3 wk *(25)*.

Urine flow is both extraluminal and intraluminal in the stented ureter, except in cases of ureteral obstruction, where flow may be entirely intraluminal *(12,28)*. As stent diameter increases, intraluminal flow increases *(29)*. Urine flow is multifactorial and depends on intrarenal pressure, internal stent diameter, stent length, intravesical pressure, and urine density *(25,26)*. Side holes have also been shown to play an important role. Stents without side holes drained 40–50% less efficiently than the identical stents with side holes *(30)*. Ureteral stents cause dilation of the ureter and urine flow becomes more extraluminal despite patency of the stent *(29,31)*. The dilation of the ureter may be caused by the cytotoxic effect of the foreign body; and/or infection may play a role *(32)*. Peristalsis is also diminished but usually returns in about 2 mo *(33)*. Stented ureters demonstrate thickened walls, increased mucus production, and histologic changes *(12)*.

PROPERTIES OF STENT MATERIALS

The modern day self-retained internal ureteral stent is a synthetic polymeric biomaterial device that can be placed by a variety of endourologic techniques, and is designed to retain its position within the ureter and drain urine between the renal pelvis and bladder. The urinary system is an unstable chemical environment and supersaturation of uromucoids and crystalloids at the interface between the material and urine creates a significant problem for long-term biocompatibility and biodurability of devices within this system. Mardis reviewed the basic properties of a ureteral stent, and optimization of these key features is needed to create the ideal stent *(34)*.

Elasticity and Memory

Elasticity and memory produces a stent's ability to maintain position within the ureter. The memory of polymeric elastomers produces an elastic stent that has coils on either end that can be straightened for passage over a guidewire. When the guidewire is removed, the coils reform to its preset configuration to maintain the device in position, thereby resisting stent migration. This property is a consequence of polymeric cross-linking, which results from physical or chemical bonding among macromolecular chains. The strength of this memory is the durometer, which can be varied within the same material and depends on the type of crosslinking used. As crosslinking increases, the durometer of the polymer changes from soft to hard.

Tensile Strength and Elongation Capacity

Variations in tensile strength reflect the mechanism of crystallization and crosslinking in biomaterials. Stents with a higher durometer, or more crosslinks, will have a greater tensile strength than stents made of the same material, but with a soft durometer. Higher tensile strength allows for creation of a higher internal to external diameter ratio and greater number of side-holes for improved drainage. Elongation capacity is the percent of elongation at stent breakage. Thermoplastic elastomeres, such as polyurethanes and a variety of other proprietary copolymers, generally have more elongation capacity than thermoset elastomeres, such as silicone (34).

Biodurability

Biodurability refers to a stent's ability to exist within the body without the adjacent system degrading stent structure and function. The urinary tract presents an unstable and hostile environment to stent function, replete with free radicals, oxidizers, enzymes, and a supersaturation of urinary mucoids and crystalloids. Stent degradation within the urinary tract has been reported for polyethylene, polyurethane, and silicone internal ureteral stents (34). Wide variations occur in the interface reactions between stent materials and the urinary system. This unpredictability requires that all stents be monitored at frequent intervals for maintenance of structure as well as function.

Biocompatibility

Biocompatibility is the utopian state where a material present within the ureter has no significant effect on the interface between itself and the urothelium adjacent to it, such as the ability to resist encrustation and infection. Currently available stents are well tolerated by the body for short periods; however, no stent is completely biocompatible. The biocompatibility of a stent may be enhanced with use of hydrophilic polymers that have low protein absorption and low bacterial adherence (35). In a study of a variety of stents, polyurethane has been shown to produce more epithelial effects than others (36,37).

Coefficient of Friction

Coefficient of friction describes how easily a stent is passed or exchanged. All commercial stent biomaterials present some surface friction generally dependent on the durometer of the biomaterial. A material with a higher durometer lowers the coefficient of friction, and consequently, soft durometer stents may be difficult to pass. Applying a hydrophilic coating reduces the surface coefficient of friction.

Radiopacity

Stents are best placed under fluoroscopic guidance, and radiopacity refers to the ease of stent visualization during fluoroscopy. All stents are radiopaque; however, some contain fillers that further enhance radiopacity, which is helpful when there is poor fluoroscopic equipment or the patient is large.

BIOMATERIALS

The use of biomaterials within the urinary tract dates back to ancient Egypt where lead and papyrus catheters were used for urinary drainage *(38)*. Ureteral replacement using glass, tantalum, or vitallium tubes were first described before World War II, but migration and obstruction limited their success *(39,40)*. In contemporary practice, devices constructed from synthetic polymeric compounds are the most useful materials implanted in the urinary tract. The advantages of these materials are that they are readily available, easily configurable, and have generally acceptable biocompatibility. Currently, self-retained internal ureteral stents are manufactured from "high polymers." Polymers are giant molecules of great variety and complexity. A typical polymeric chain has tens of thousands of chemical "monomers," which are linked by "polymerization." These chains are organized in various configurations resulting in complex and versatile macromolecules.

Polyethylene

Polyethylene consists of polyolefin polymers and was the first synthetic polymer employed to fashion ureteral stents. It is flexible, odorless, translucent, and nonreactive in the body. The stiffness of this material made it useful in the management of ureteral strictures *(30,36)*. On exposure to biological fluids, however, polyethylene was found to promote protein deposits, leading to an increased likelihood of crystalloid adherence, encrustation, and infection. Furthermore, long-term exposure of polyethylene to urine caused it to become brittle, risking fragmentation *(19,35)*.

Silicone

Silicone stents are composed of alternating silicone and oxygen atoms and remains the gold standard for tissue compatibility owing to its nontoxic, inert nature *(35)*. It is nonirritating and resistant to encrustation and thus ideal for long-term use. However, silicone stents migrate easily, have poor mechanical strength, and have a high coefficient of friction, making these stents difficult to use when negotiating strictures or tortuous ureters and difficult to pass or remove from the guidewire. Silicone stents have the lowest internal to external diameter ratio and the smallest side holes of all materials in order to prevent kinks or collapse.

Polyurethane

Polyurethane, a common generic class of condensation polymers derived from polyisocynate and a polyol, has been used in stent construction in an effort to combine the flexibility of silicone with the stiffness of polyethylene. Although polyurethane is highly versatile and inexpensive, it has been shown to induce significantly more epithelial ulceration and erosion than other materials *(37)*. Polyurethane also has limited durability and demonstrates slow in vivo biodegradation. These degradation products may be cytotoxic and as such, polyurethane stents are best employed as short-term implants *(37)*.

C-Flex

Proprietary modifications to silicone led to the development of C-Flex (Consolidated Polymer Technologies, Inc., Clearwater, FL), a silicone-modified styrene/ethylene/ butylene block thermoplastic copolymer. The partial silicone composition of C-Flex makes these stents softer than polyurethane and theoretically less likely to develop encrustation.

Silitek

Silitek (ACMI Corp., Southborough, MA) is a second-generation, polyester copolymer that followed silicone and polyurethane. Silitek is firm and resists extrinsic compression. It combines strength for placement control with flexibility for patient comfort. The UroPass, UroPass II, UroPass Obstruction, Single J Urinary Diversion, and pediatric 4.8-Fr stent (all from ACMI) are made of Silitek.

Percuflex

Percuflex (Boston Scientific Corp., Natick, MA) is a proprietary olefinic block copolymer developed by Boston Scientific/Microvasive, which becomes soft and flexible at body temperature. This material has excellent memory and strength, allowing these stents to be designed with a thinner wall and greater lumen diameter, while allowing for larger side holes without sacrificing tensile strength. The inert properties of Percuflex also offer excellent biocompatibility.

Tecoflex

Tecoflex (Thermedics, Inc., Woburn, MA) is a thermosensitive proprietary copolymer. Stents made with it have a smooth surface and a comparatively large inside diameter (4.5 Fr stent still has a 0.042″ internal diameter that accommodates a standard 0.038″ guidewire). This material allows for ink labeling instead of laser labeling, which may theoretically decrease the likelihood of encrustation from the rough surface created by the laser. The Quadra-Coil Multi-length, Classic Double PigTail, Lubri-Flex, and LithoStent, all from ACMI, are made of Tecoflex. Dual durometer Tecoflex stents, which include the Multi-Flex, Sof-Curl, and Double-J II, have a stiffer proximal segment to aid in accurate placement, while the softer distal segment improves patient comfort.

Other Proprietary Materials

Sof-Flex (Cook Urological Inc., Spencer, IN) is a proprietary compound from Cook Urological that is used in several of their stents. Other stent materials from Cook include Endo-Sof and Ultrathane. Pellethane (C.R. Bard, Inc., Covington, GA) is a proprietary copolymer from Bard, which allows for a variable durometer and is used in their Inlay stents. This material softens up to 50% when warmed to body temperature. Flexima is a newer proprietary material from Boston Scientific/Microvasive, designed to resist buckling during insertion. It is sold as a variable length stent called the Stretch VL from Boston Scientific/Microvasive. Vertex (Applied Medical Inc., Rancho Santa Margarita, CA) is a proprietary material from Applied Medical that is used in their ureteral stents.

Bioabsorbable Materials

Bioabsorbable polymeric materials are designed to retain their tissue-supporting properties for defined periods of time. After placement, they are gradually biode-graded into tissue-compatible compounds that are absorbed and replaced by healing tissue. Biodegradable devices were first developed for urological use in Finland in the late 1980's *(41)*. The main benefit of their use is the elimination of a second surgical intervention for removal. These stents will be most useful for clinical situations where temporary upper urinary tract drainage is desired, such as following endo-scopic or open ureteral surgery. Bioabsorbable materials used in urological stents are high molecular weight polymers of polylactic and polyglycolic acid *(41,42)*. Inves-tigators have designed short biodegradable stents that expand at body temperature to hold their position and degrade with time *(42,43)*. These stents do not communicate with the bladder or kidney and therefore would avoid vesicoureteral reflux and pos-sibly have a lower infection rate. An alternative strategy is a standard double-pigtail stent where degradation is controlled by modulating urinary pH to an alkaline level when the stent is no longer needed *(44)*. Currently, biodegradable stents require clinical trials in the United States to evaluate concerns of biocompatibility and ade-quate drainage of urine during stent degradation. Uniform stent degradation is diffi-cult to achieve and consequently, these stents tend to break off in chunks that are prone to obstruct the ureter.

Metals

Metallic superalloy titanium and nickel/titanium are materials currently used for permanently implanted stents, such as the Wallstent (Medinrent, Lausanne, Switzer-land) or the Memokath 051 (Engineers and Doctors of Copenhagen, Copenhagen, Den-mark), to relieve conditions such as malignant obstruction and ureteral strictures *(45–47)*. These stents gradually become covered with urothelium following implan-tation, thus preventing encrustation and infection. Problems associated with metal stents include collagenous ingrowth, hyperplastic epithelium, distal ureteral narrowing, intense fibrosis, and subsequent obstruction *(48,49)*. In an attempt to minimize the inflammatory process following stent placement and ensure ureteral patency, the use of stent-associated liposomal formulations of dexamethasone are currently under investi-gation *(50)*.

Hydrophilic Coatings

Hydophilic coatings consist of nondissolvable polymers that swell on contact with water and retain a large fraction of water within their polyanionic structure and that layers on its surface. The surface water of hydrophilic materials not only reduce their coefficient of friction, improving ease of stent insertion, but also contributes to bio-compatibility by reducing frictional irritation and cell adhesion at the biomaterial-urothelial interface *(51)*. This low interfacial tension may explain the ability of hydrogels to resist protein and crystalloid deposition on their surface *(52)*.

LSe is Cook Urological's ion implantation process, which attracts specific ions to the stent surface where they are implanted into the chemical structure. LSe is designed to reduce the coefficient of friction without presoaking in water and lower the surface energy of the stent; this is thought to help resist bacterial adhesion and development of encrustation *(53)*.

AQ is a hydrophillic coating made by Cook Urological that can be applied to any standard or specialty stent to lower the coefficient of friction. Other hydrophilic coatings include SL-6 by Applied Medical, and Hydro Plus by Boston Scientific/Microvasive.

Comparison of Biomaterials

Features of an ideal ureteral stent include: easy maneuverability, radiopacity, ability to relieve intraluminal and extraluminal obstruction, stability following placement, biological inertia, chemical stability in urine, resistance to encrustation and infection, excellent long-term flow, no causation of irritative voiding symptoms, and availability at an affordable price *(53)*. A comparison of properties among different stent materials is shown in Table 1. However, no contemporary stent incorporates all of these characteristics and there are too many different designs and biomaterials to attempt direct comparisons. In addition, the quality of study designs and conflicting results from many studies prevent supporting or contesting the use of any single design or biomaterial. The American Society for Testing and Materials (ASTM) has developed standards and test protocols for the evaluation of various materials that include polymeric biomaterials *(34)*. Most current methods of biocompatibility testing include cell culture techniques and animal models, controlled in vitro encrustation testing, and advanced microscopic and surface analytical techniques, such as X-ray photoelectron spectroscopy, atomic force microscopy, scanning electron microscopy, and energy-dispersive X-ray analysis.

STENT DESIGNS

Indwelling ureteral stents should be able to provide constant, unobstructed drainage and ensure stability of stent position. Stents with varying sizes, from 4.7 to 18 Fr in outer diameter, with side draining ports along their entire length have been developed for maximal urinary drainage. Maintenance of stent position is due to design of the distal ends as well as proper choice of stent length.

Double-J or Double-Pigtail Stents

These are the most popular ureteral stents. Double-J refers to an open hook configuration at either end of the ureteral stent, whereas a double-pigtail stent has a full retentive coil at either end. The Double-J stent is the original, silicone, closed-tipped stent to which ACMI/Surgitek holds the patent and has marketed since 1978 *(12)*. An open-tipped version is called the Uroguide. All stent manufacturers produce a basic double-pigtail stent, which have a variety of names, designs, and compositions. Standard double-pigtail stents must be sized correctly because those that are too long can cause bladder irritation, whereas those too short can migrate up the ureter. A 24-cm ureteral stent is well suited for most adults, but should be individualized based on the ureteral length of the patient.

Multiple-Coil Stents

Multiple-coil stents were designed to meet the "one size fits all" concept, which is advantageous for the urologist who does not have to worry about choosing the correct size, and the hospital which does not need to maintain an excessive inventory. Multiple-coil stents leave redundant length coiled in the bladder coiled so that the trigone is not irritated.

Table 1
Comparison of Properties Among Different Stent Materials

	Polyethylene	Polyurethane	C-Flex®	Silitek®	Percuflex®	Silicone
Biocompatibility	Low	Low	Intermediate–High	Intermediate	Intermediate–High	High
Biodurability	Low	Intermediate	Intermediate	Intermediate	Intermediate	Intermediate
Memory[a]	High	High	High	High	High	Low
Tensile strength[a]	High	High	Intermediate	High	Intermediate–High	Low
Elongation capacity	High	Intermediate	High	High	High	Low

[a] Dependent on durometer.

473

Specialty Stents

Open-ended ureteral catheters have no coils and thus are not suitable for long-term urinary drainage. However, they can be secured externally to a urethral catheter to provide temporary drainage. Open-ended stents are useful in helping to direct and advance the guidewire into the ureteral orifice. They can assist in the collection of upper urinary tract urine samples and permit retrograde pyelography. Furthermore, open-ended ureteral stents are commonly placed intraoperatively to identify the ureters in order to avoid inadvertent injury during abdominal or pelvic surgery.

Grooved stents have grooves spiraling down the exterior of the stent to improve extraluminal flow and are aimed at postlithotripsy or holmium laser cases, where passage of stone fragments is needed. The Towers peripheral stent is a grooved stent manufactured by Cook Urological. The outer diameter ranges from 6 to 8 Fr, and the length from 22 to 32 cm. The LithoStent by ACMI features 3 grooves spiraling down the exterior of the stent-like gutters designed to prevent ureteral strictures and urinomas; the lumen accommodates standard guidewires.

Tail stents are designed with a thinner, softer distal segment to increase patient comfort. They have a standard pigtail and a 6 or 7 Fr shaft at the proximal end, but the distal end tapers into an elongated 3-Fr closed-tip tail, which rests in the bladder. Drainage is achieved around the distal portion of tail stents, and consequently these stents are contraindicated when trauma to the distal ureter is suspected. Tail stents resist reflux because the distal third of the tail is occluded, and approx 3–5 cm of the tail's occluded portion lies within the intramural tunnel and the distal ureter. Upper tract symptoms in patients with tail stents could be attributed to either renal pelvic irritation or intermittent obstruction. Boston Scientific/Microvasive makes a tail stent called the Percuflex Tail Plus.

Injection stents are single-pigtail catheters that convert into an indwelling double-pigtail ureteral stent, obviating a second cystoscopy. It is ideal for patients undergoing SWL that need a double-pigtail stent postoperatively, but simultaneously require contrast instillation during the procedure for stone localization. Once the procedure is completed, the injection apparatus is removed leaving a double-pigtail stent.

Urinary diversion stents, made of various materials, have a single coil for the renal pelvis and a long straight end that is brought out for external drainage. Drainage holes are in the proximal end of the stent. They are commonly used to provide internal support to ureteral anastomoses created during various types of urinary diversion. This allows for accurate monitoring of urine output from each renal unit and facilitates removal of the stent after an adequate period of healing.

Endoureterotomy/endopyelotomy stents are used for temporary drainage from the ureteropelvic junction to the bladder following incision of a stricture. These internal stents have a tapering diameter with no sideports designed to prevent narrowing of the ureteral lumen while preventing ingrowth of the ureteral wall to the stent. The larger-caliber portion of the stent acts as a mold for the healing of the incised ureter. Applied Medical has a 7/10 Fr endopyelotomy stent for use with the Acucise endopyelotomy balloon catheter device. Cook Urological makes a 6/10 Fr and 7/14 Fr stent and Boston Scientific/Microvasive makes the RetroMax Plus in 7/14 Fr.

Subcutaneous urinary diversion (nephrovesical) stents are used as an alternative to percutaneous nephrostomy for urinary diversion in uremic cancer patients and in those with benign idiopathic ureteral obstruction, in which placement of ureteral stents have failed. The proximal end of the stent is inserted into the renal pelvis via a percutaneous nephrostomy puncture. A subcutaneous tunnel is created from the flank to the bladder, where the distal end of the stent is passed into the bladder via a suprapubic bladder puncture.

Fistula stent sets specifically assist in the internal management of ureteral fistulas. The stent has drainage ports solely in the pigtails, in order to reduce fluid pressure within the ureter. It is manufactured in several different diameters and lengths.

CLINICAL APPLICATIONS AND OUTCOMES

There are multiple indications for the placement of ureteral stents. They are often placed as part of therapy to relieve ureteral obstruction or promote healing of the ureter, or as prophylaxis against possible complications by assisting passage of a guidewire into a ureteral orifice or by passively dilating the ureter before interval ureteroscopy.

Urolithiasis

This is probably the most common indication for ureteral stenting. Contemporary management of renal calculi relies on endourologic techniques such as SWL, percutaneous nephrolithotomy (PCNL), and ureterorenoscopy (URS) *(54–57)*. Stenting can be performed as a therapeutic or prophylactic procedure. Indications for therapeutic stenting include: obstructive pyelonephritis secondary to an obstructing stone; renal failure secondary to bilateral obstructing stones or obstructing stone in a solitary kidney; refractory renal colic or pain; and relief of high grade and/or long-term obstruction. PCNL can be performed without need for postoperative ureteral stenting. Specific indications for postoperative stenting following PCNL include extensive perforation of the collecting system, need for subsequent SWL for large stone burden, ureteral obstruction secondary to edema or stone fragments, and persistent urinary leakage following nephrostomy tube removal.

The indications for ureteral stenting with SWL of renal calculi are less defined. Prophylactic stenting before SWL has been shown to prevent the development of 'steinstrasse' in patients with stones >20 mm *(58)*. However, opponents of stent use report an increased morbidity associated with stent placement with no differences in stone-free rates *(59,60)*. Furthermore, patients with ureteral stents placed before SWL were subjected to higher levels of total power during the procedure with no difference in stone-free rates among patients treated without a stent *(60)*. Urinary urgency (43 vs 25%), hematuria (40 vs 23%), duration of bladder discomfort (26 vs 13%), and duration of urinary frequency (31 vs 16%) was also significantly higher in patients with indwelling stents compared to those without *(60)*.

SWL of ureteral stones can be performed either by pushback of stone into the renal collecting system, bypass of stone with an externalized or internalized stent, or *in situ*. Data analyzed by the American Urological Association Ureteral Stones Clinical Guidelines panel did not support routine use of ureteral stents to improve efficiency and stone-free results of SWL, regardless of stone size *(61)*. Ureteral stenting before SWL of middle ureteral stones, however, may aid in the localization of stones overlying the bony pelvis, especially in the presence of significant ureteral obstruction, which diminishes the efficacy of intravenous contrast in aiding stone localization *(62)*. Advances in fiberoptics has allowed for the development of smaller ureteroscopes and advances in intracorporeal lithotripsy, such as the holmium:yttrium-aluminum-garnet (YAG) laser has allowed for uncomplicated ureteroscopy to be performed without routine stenting with minimal discomfort and a low incidence of postoperative complications *(63,64)*. However, ureteral stenting following ureteroscopy is recommended if complications occur, the stone is impacted, the ureteral orifice is formally dilated to 18 Fr, fragmentation is incomplete, or associated with a solitary kidney. In addition, stent placement after unsuccessful ureteroscopic stone extraction may facilitate spontaneous stone passage and dilates the ureter, making subsequent ureteroscopic procedures more successful *(65)*.

Pregnancy

Urolithiasis during pregnancy is relatively infrequent with the reported overall incidence of approx 0.07%, with 0.02% being symptomatic *(66)*. Although hypercalciuria, hyperuricosuria, and pregnancy-induced urinary stasis predispose to stone formation, the incidence of symptomatic urinary stones in this population is no greater than that for nonpregnant women of childbearing age *(66,67)*. These findings are likely a result of an increase in urinary lithogenic inhibitors (urinary magnesium, citrate, and glycoproteins) and urine volume during pregnancy *(67)*. Pain from renal colic is the most common nonobstetric reason for admission during pregnancy *(68)*. Approximately two-thirds of symptomatic stones presenting during pregnancy will pass spontaneously; therefore, a trial of conservative management with intravenous hydration, analgesics, antiemetics, and prophylactic antibiotics should be advocated initially *(69,70)*.

Azotemia, fever with obstruction, and urosepsis in the setting of urinary stone disease requires urgent percutaneous nephrostomy (PCN) or ureteral stent drainage, and the gravid state should not alter this approach. Indwelling ureteral stent or PCN drainage is recommended for interim treatment with definitive management delayed until postpartum for symptomatic urinary stones that do not pass or if obstruction persists for more than 3 or 4 wk *(71,72)*. Both can be placed with ultrasound guidance to avoid radiation exposure to the fetus. Encrustation is a concern during pregnancy because of gestational hyperuricosuria and hypercalciuria *(67)*. The authors recommend that ureteral stents be changed in gravid patients at 4–6-wk intervals. PCN offers a good alternative to stent drainage, especially early in pregnancy. The need for repeated stent changes is eliminated, and it can be converted to an indwelling stent for comfort as the patient nears term.

Definitive stone management during pregnancy has been performed with few complications. Both flexible and rigid ureteroscopy with holmium:YAG laser lithotripsy have allowed for successful and safe endoscopic removal of symptomatic stones during all stages of pregnancy, although this is not considered standard *(73–75)*. Other forms of intracorporeal lithotripsy that can be considered for treating stones during pregnancy are the pulsed-dye laser and pneumatic lithotriptor because these modalities deliver localized energy. In contrast, electrohydraulic lithotripsy (EHL) and ultrasonic lithotripsy may present theoretical risks to the fetus because electrical energy discharged from EHL could precipitate premature labor and the vibratory energy of ultrasonic lithotripsy may pose a risk to the developing ears of the fetus *(75)*. PCNL is rarely indicated during pregnancy; however, it has been safely performed in cases of repeated infection or obstruction despite percutaneous drainage *(72)*. Other options have included open stone surgery and early parturition. SWL is contraindicated in pregnancy because of a theoretical risk to the fetus and/or ovaries *(71)*.

Renal Transplantation

Urinary tract stones after renal transplantation can be a result of unsuspected donor calculus or caused by persistent hyperparathyroidism, recurrent urinary tract infections, foreign body such as suture or staple, obstruction, habitual decreased fluid intake, and type I renal tubular acidosis *(76)*. Because the renal transplant is denervated, the kidney transplant patient will not experience typical renal colic, and the diagnosis is suspected when renal function suddenly deteriorates or transplant pyelonephritis occurs. Upper tract stones are managed by the same techniques as stones in the normal urinary tract; however, negotiation of the transplanted ureter may be difficult or impossible because of tortuousity, thus favoring percutaneous techniques. SWL has been used successfully with the stone positioned in the shock wave path *(77)*.

Ureteral strictures and fistulas are the most frequent urologic complications in renal transplantation, occurring in 1–12% of patients *(78,79)*. Prospective studies have concluded that ureteral stenting is beneficial in reducing vesicoureteric leakage rates and obstruction in renal transplantation *(80)*. Furthermore, presence of a ureteral stent does not result in an increased incidence of urinary tract infection *(81)*.

Obstructive Urosepsis

Management of an obstructed urinary tract can be performed with ureteral stent or PCN drainage. The advantage of ureteral stenting is complete internalization of the stent without the need for an external drainage device; however, the advantage of PCN is a more definitive and reliable urinary drainage. Disadvantages of an indwelling stent include pain, encrustation, infection, and bladder irritability. Disadvantages of PCN include risk of renal and other organ injury during placement, their external nature, and the potential for dislodgment, erosion, bleeding, or infection. Both ureteral stents and PCN can be placed under intravenous sedation, although stenting usually occurs in the operating room with an anesthesiologist present. Both ureteral stenting and PCN have been demonstrated to effectively relieve obstruction and infection caused by ureteral stones and neither modality is superior in promoting more rapid recovery following drainage *(82)*. The decision on which mode of drainage to use should be based on surgeon preference and skill, presence of skilled interventional radiologists or urologists trained to perform PCN, operating room availability, and stone characteristics.

Extrinsic Ureteral Obstruction

Ureteral stenting has been widely used in the management of ureteral obstruction caused by pelvic malignancies or retroperitoneal fibrosis. Nevertheless, obstruction can still persist even after placement of large-caliber indwelling stents *(83)*. The combination of extrinsic compression against the stent and aperistaltic ureteral segments may impair urine drainage around well-placed stents. Stenting with single indwelling stents has been reported to fail in 50% of prostate cancer patients and 89% of patients with cervical cancer *(84,85)*. An option for patients failing previous stenting with a single 6-, 7-, or 8-Fr stent is to place two parallel ipsilateral ureteral stents, usually 8 Fr, which have been successfully used in the relief of obstruction (Fig. 1) *(86)*. Another option is the use of metal ureteral stents, which are intended for permanent implantation and have a radial force higher than the pressure exerted by the surrounding tissues. Varying success rates using these devices have been reported, ranging from 14 to 100% in patients with strictures of various etiologies and locations *(87,88)*. Multiple overlapping metal stents can be placed either alone or in combination with conventional indwelling ureteral stents in patients with long strictures. Not all patients with malignant strictures are candidates for metal stent implantation, especially those patients with distal ureteral

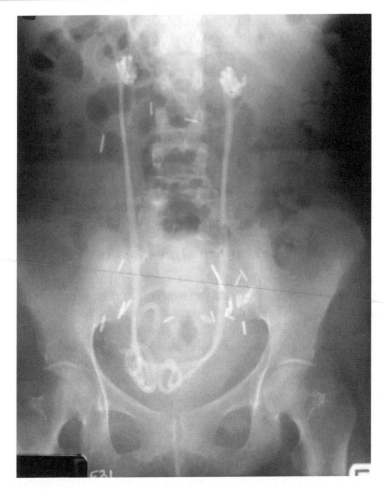

Fig. 1. KUB radiograph of bilateral parallel double-pigtail stents for malignant ureteral obstruction.

strictures because the stents may project into the bladder, prevent epithelization and result in early encrustation blockage and patient discomfort. Subcutaneous urinary diversion with nephrovesical ureteral stenting has also been reported to be successful in patients with ureteral obstruction secondary to malignancy or medical conditions, excluding them from more invasive procedures *(89,90)*.

Endoscopic and Open Surgery

Ureteral stenting has become complementary to ureteroscopic procedures to prevent either post-ureteroscopic ureteral edema or scarring of small mucosal lesions. Success rates for ureteral stenting following endoscopic balloon dilatation of ureteral strictures has been reported to be about 60% *(91)*. Primary insertion of ureteral stents has been shown to prevent or reduce the incidence of anastomotic stenosis and leakage following open ureteral repair *(92)*. Ureteral stents promote healing by providing a scaffold for epithelialization and by avoiding early flow urine through the defect. However, other studies have shown that ureteral healing is the same whether a stent is present or not *(93)*.

Endopyelotomy and endoureterotomy have become treatments of choice for uretero-pelvic junction obstruction and ureteral stricture, respectively, owing to a short conva-lescence period and absence of incision-related morbidity related to these procedures. Stenting is an integral part of the ureteral endoincision that prevents leakage of urine into the retroperitoneum and provides a mold for the ureteral epithelium to grow over. There remains debate over the size of the stent and optimal duration of postoperative stenting. A 6-wk duration of postoperative stenting is considered the gold standard based on experimental work by Davis, who showed that after a full-thickness incision through the narrowed segment of ureter, regeneration of the muscular layer was 90% complete by 6 wk *(94)*. However, others have demonstrated shorter duration of postoperative stenting in the successful outcome of endopyelotomy *(95)*. The size of ureteral stent to use following ureteral stricture incision remains just as controversial. A specialized endopyelotomy stent, one that measures 14 Fr at the ureteropelvic junction and tapers to 7 Fr, can be used *(96)*. These can be placed antegrade or retrograde, and can drain externally or internally. Placement of smaller 7 or 8 Fr internal ureteral stents have been reported to produce comparable results with that achieved by the standard 14/7 Fr endopyelotomy stent *(97)*. Smaller caliber stents, ranging in size from 4 to 10 Fr, have yielded satisfactory outcomes in 78–95% of patients *(97)*.

Preoperative ureteral stenting has been used to prevent ureteral injuries caused by gynecologic procedures, as well as general surgical procedures. However, some inves-tigators have reported that preoperative catheterization is not effective in preventing trauma and could even provoke it *(98,99)*. Transilluminating ureteral stents have been used for preventing ureteral injuries during gynecologic procedures *(100)*.

Trauma

Ureteral injuries can be secondary to external trauma, either blunt or penetrating, or more commonly are iatrogenic. In most cases, injury to the ureter diagnosed during the initial evaluation of the trauma is generally treated by open surgical repair. External ureteral trauma is almost exclusively associated with other injuries *(101)*. Principles of open surgical repair of ureteral injury include debridement and spatulation of the ureter, followed by a tension-free closure with absorbable suture over an indwelling ureteral stent. Delayed diagnosis of a missed or iatrogenic injury may be treated by percutaneous drainage of urinoma and retrograde or antegrade placement of a ureteral stent if the ureter is partially intact *(102)*. Following tangential injury to a portion of the ureteral wall by penetrating trauma or clamp or suture injury during surgery, passage of an indwelling ureteral stent may allow for complete healing with reasonable long-term results *(103)*. Ureteral stents may also be used safely and effectively to treat persistent or recurrent urinary extravasation resulting from major blunt renal trauma in appropriately selected patients *(104)*.

Fistulas

Ureteral fistulas can be classified based on location: ureterovaginal, ureterocutaneous, ureteroenteric, lymphaticoureteral, and ureteroretroperitoneal (urinoma) *(105)*. One of the earliest uses of ureteral stents was for treatment of ureterovaginal fistula in which polyethylene tubing was employed to affect closure *(5)*. The use of percutaneous ureteral stents to successfully treat urinary fistulas was first reported by Goldin *(106)*. Andriole and colleagues reported a 50% closure rate with use of an indwelling double-J stent in the management of upper urinary tract fistulas *(84)* and Chang and co-workers reported successful resolution in 10 of 12 ureteral fistulas treated with percutaneous antegrade ureteral stenting *(107)*.

STENT REMOVAL

There are no controlled studies or consensus on the ideal length of time to leave indwelling ureteral stents in place. In uncomplicated cases, stents can be removed in 2–3 d after ureteroscopy. In cases of ureteral perforation or concern regarding ureteral obstruction after instrumentation, an indwelling ureteral stent should remain in place for at least 1–2 wk. The majority of indwelling ureteral stents can be removed in the office with topical anesthesia using a flexible cystoscope and grasper. If the patient is unable to tolerate an office procedure, stent removal can be performed under anesthesia in the cystoscopy suite. In patients that are hospitalized, externalized ureteral stents can be used, and before stent removal, a ureterogram can be performed to document ureteral anatomy, passage or removal of stones, and lack of extravasation or obstruction.

Nonendourological techniques have been described for stent removal. Some stents are manufactured with a nylon suture attached to the distal end, which can be left at the urethral meatus allowing for removal after short-term drainage without the need for repeat cystoscopy. However, patients must be cautioned not to place tension on the string because this could potentially lead to unintentional dislodgment of the stent. The dangling suture may also be associated with a slight degree of incontinence. A wire introducer with a snail head coil at its distal end has also been described with some success for blindly grasping a stent within the bladder of women only *(108)*. Stent retrieval has been reported with indwelling stents incorporating a distal magnetic tip that can be retrieved by using a magnet *(109)*, and in stents with a stainless steel bead attached to its distal end, which can be removed by a urethral catheter that has a rare earth magnet attached to its proximal end *(110)*. The development of biodegradable stents will eliminate the need for invasive removal procedures *(42–44)*. All patients with indwelling ureteral stents should be told of the importance of appropriate follow-up and eventual stent removal. Extracting forgotten ureteral stents can be technically challenging and may require multiple cystoscopic and/or percutaneous procedures owing to potential stent friability and breakage.

COMPLICATIONS

Despite recent innovations and improvements in stent materials and designs, problems relating to indwelling ureteral stent use still occur, such as migration, occlusion, encrustation, breakage, and stone formation *(111)*.

Symptoms and Quality of Life

Patient discomfort associated with irritative voiding symptoms, flank and abdominal discomfort, and hematuria in the absence of urinary tract infection is the most common complication involving patients with indwelling ureteral stents *(112–114)*. It is presumed that the etiology for lower urinary tract symptoms is the distal portion of the stent traversing the intramural ureter and impinging on the bladder floor *(115,116)*. The cause of upper tract symptoms, which may occur in as many as 50% of patients, is thought to be secondary to vesicoureteral reflux. Many earlier studies comparing ureteral stents failed to report any significant differences between stents of different compositions and diameter *(113,114)*. However, more durable clinical studies have shown that "softer" stents composed of biomaterials with smaller durometer, likely result in a lower incidence of symptoms *(114)*. In another randomized, blinded study, smaller diameter stents were associated with less pain and improved patient tolerance *(117)*.

Migration

Migration of ureteral stents is a well-known complication *(118)*. Proximal or distal migration may occur despite the J shape of the stent and can be problematic. Stents with a full coil rarely migrate compared to those with the J configuration. Materials with good memory, such as polyurethane, have the least tendency for migration, whereas stents composed of softer materials, such as silicone, have the highest incidence of migration. Stent migration may occur if the stent is too short, resulting in proximal migration, or placed in massively dilated systems. One trick that can help prevent migration of the proximal coil into the ureter in a patient with a widely patent UPJ is to place the coil into a calyx with a relatively narrow infundibulum. Direct ureteroscopic removal and occasional use of percutaneous techniques may be needed to extract proximally migrated stents *(119)*. These stents can be tricky to retrieve ureteroscopically because they can be slippery and difficult to grasp, the distal coil displaces and distorts ureteral anatomy, and the tip to the stent can dig into the ureteral wall. One trick the authors have found useful in retrieving stents that have migrated into the distal ureter is the use of a stone basket to "catch" the distal tip instead of using a grasper. Another trick is to use rat tooth or 3-prong graspers and to place one of the prongs into a side-hole of the stent to prevent slippage when withdrawing.

Infection and Encrustation

Stent-related infection and encrustation are common complications, causing significant morbidity, and are the major limiting factors in long-term use of biomaterials within the urinary tract. The mechanism of encrustation in infected urine is identical to the formation of infected urinary stones, involving alkalization of urine owing to hydrolysis of urea by urease-producing organisms *(120)*. Magnesium and calcium precipitate in the alkaline environment produced by urea hydrolysis, forming magnesium ammonium phosphate ($NH_4MgPO_42H_2O$) and calcium hydroxyapatite ($Ca_{10}[PO_4]6H_2O$). It begins with the development of an organic biofilm, often consisting of albumin, Tamm-Horsfall protein, and alpha$_1$-microglobulin, covering the plastic surface, and can enhance crystal precipitation and aggregation events on the surface *(121)*. This biofilm also allows bacteria to be trapped and potentially be protected from antibiotics *(122)*. Stent encrustation in sterile urine is not completely understood, but it appears to be dependent on both the urinary constituents and properties of the biomaterial. Sterile encrustations are often composed of calcium oxalate *(123)*. Metabolic disorders, such as hypercalciuria, certain physiological states such as pregnancy, and even the intestinal microbial flora may contribute to accelerated encrustation of stents within a sterile urinary environment *(123–125)*. Presently, there are no biomaterials used in the urinary tract that are able to completely withstand the effects of the urinary environment.

Once established, stent-related encrustations and infections are often severe complications, necessitating stent removal if clinical cure is to be achieved. Stent colonization is frequent with rates ranging from 28 to 90% *(126)*. Use of urinary cultures to predict stent colonization has been reported to have a sensitivity of 31% and incidence of stent colonization does not correlate with indwelling time (127). In addition, administration of prophylactic antibiotic treatment does not prevent bacterial adherence to ureteral stents (127). Sterile pyuria is not infrequent and reflects foreign body reaction to the stent. In the absence of infection proven by culture, pyuria is generally inconsequential (30).

Encrustations may develop on ureteral stents intraluminally and extraluminally, reducing ureteral flow and causing obstruction of the renal unit, leading to impaired renal function. Encrustations may be multifactorial and risk factors include poor compliance, long indwelling times, sepsis, pyelonephritis, chronic renal failure, recurrent or residual stones, lithogenic history, metabolic abnormalities, congenital renal anomalies, and malignant ureteral obstruction (128). Interactions involved in the deposition of encrustation on stents also appear to be influenced by the chemical composition of the polymer, physical properties of its surface, presence of graft polymer coating conferring a hydrophilic/hydrophobic nature on the biomaterial, contact time with urine, solute content of urine, and intestinal microbial composition (123–125). The exact interval for changing or removing an indwelling ureteral stent to avoid significant encrustation is difficult to determine owing to multiple and unclear etiologies of stent encrustation. However, stent encrustation rates increase with the duration that the stent remains indwelling. At less than 6 wk, a 9.2% encrustation rate has been reported, which increases to 47.5% at 6–12 wk and 76.3% at more than 12 wk (128). The optimal indwelling period based on different series is 2–4 mo (111,128), however, it should be shorter in those patients with risk factors that predispose them for developing encrustations. Some recent developments in stent design, including the incorporation of antibiotic coatings covalently bound to the outer stent surface, are being used to decrease biofilm production and stent colonization, but are not yet proven to be clinically effective.

Retained/Fractured Stents

Retained stents, especially those encrusted, occur infrequently but can be a difficult and challenging problem that can lead to severe morbidity and sepsis if not managed carefully. Successful management of a retained ureteral stent requires careful planning and may require a combination of endourologic approaches that can be safely performed to remove the retained stent and any associated stone burden during a single anesthestic session (111). The authors feel the most important preliminary step is to obtain an excellent kidney-ureter-bladder (KUB) radiograph with tomographic views paying careful attention to the proximal coil and ureteral portions of the stent in order to determine whether it appears slightly "thicker" than it should (Fig. 2). These are subtle signs often missed by radiologists who are not familiar with the clinical situation. If no encrustations are present, cystoscopy is performed and gentle traction of the retained stent is attempted. If the patient complains of pain or the stent does not move easily, the authors do not proceed any further to avoid the risk of damaging the ureter. Occasionally, it is possible to remove enough of the stent beyond the urethral meatus and attempt to pass a guidewire through the stent to determine if the lumen of the stent is occluded and to possibly uncoil the proximal portion of the stent.

If encrustations are visualized on KUB radiograph or fluoroscopy, the authors do not advise attempted removal of the stent. Instead, ureteral access should be maintained with a wire placed adjacent to the encrusted stent. In some cases, this may be sufficient for facilitating removal of the retained stent. The authors recommend treatment of any bladder component of encrustation first. If bladder component encrustations are minor, a flexible or rigid alligator forceps or biopsy forceps can be used to separate the coils after

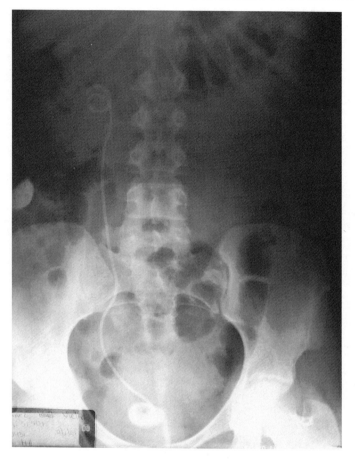

Fig. 2. KUB radiograph showing a retained ureteral stent with a calcified bladder stone encompassing the distal coil of the retained ureteral stent and a "thickened" proximal coil.

breaking off pieces of encrustation. A cystoscopic view of a large bladder stone encompassing the distal coil of the retained stent is shown (Fig. 3A). Otherwise, EHL can be used to break apart bladder encrustations and remove any stone-burden within the bladder (Fig. 3B). The least invasive and most efficacious way of managing encrustations on the proximal or ureteral portions of the retained stent is SWL, and subsequently gently tugging on the stent until it releases. If a lithotriptor is present in the room, this can be performed immediately and simultaneously. Otherwise, a small (4.7 Fr) ureteral stent can be placed adjacent to the existing stent. This will provide drainage if the renal unit is obstructed and passively dilate the ureter. The patient is then brought back for SWL at a later session. In no case should significant force be used to attempt stent extraction because this may result in severe ureteral injury, or the stent may break off, especially if it is brittle, making a terrible situation even worse. If a stent breaks off, ureteroscopy can be performed to retrieve the broken stent fragments within the ureter.

If the above fails, or if a ureteral component of encrustation is visible, retrograde ureteroscopy may be attempted after placing a safety wire. A small caliber (6 Fr) semi-rigid ureteroscope can be passed under direct vision along side the existing stent and encrustations can be fragmented using a holmium:YAG laser under low power (5 W).

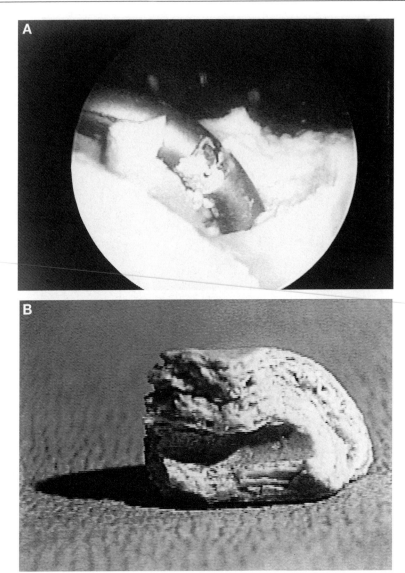

Fig. 3. Bladder component of stent encrustation. (**A**) Cystoscopic view of a retained indwelling ureteral stent with a large bladder stone encompassing the distal coil. (**B**) Fragment of encrustation.

If the ureter will not accommodate both ureteral stent and ureteroscope, a parallel 4.7 Fr ureteral stent can be placed and ureteroscopy can be reattempted after sufficient passive dilation has taken place. If this fails, or there is a large proximal stone burden, the patient can be placed in the prone position and a percutaneous approach may be attempted with removal of the stone burden and, if necessary, simultaneous antegrade ureteroscopy. Typically, a mid-posterior calyx is selected. If these approaches fail, laparoscopic or open surgery can be considered. An IVU demonstrates a malfunctioning stent with associated bladder and renal stones in a patient who failed to follow-up for over a year (Fig. 4 A,B). Following cystolitholapaxy, the retained stent was exchanged for a new stent and PCNL was performed at a later session to remove the remaining stone-burden.

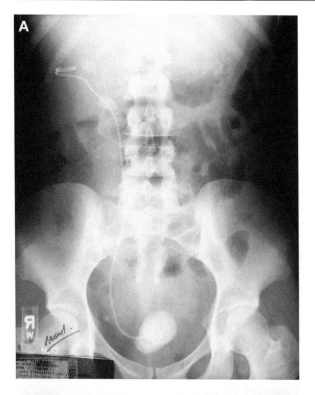

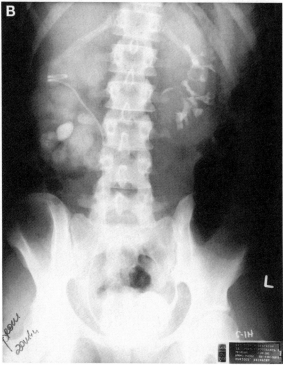

Fig. 4. IVU. (**A**) Scout film of a retained ureteral stent with renal and bladder stones. (**B**) Delay film showing a hydronephrotic and obstructed right renal unit with a persistent nephrogram and normal left renal unit.

It is important to monitor for a possible post-obstructive diuresis following exchange to a functional stent.

Prevention would be one way of avoiding the problem of retained stents, especially in poorly compliant patients. Some investigators have recommended a stent registry to keep track of indwelling stents placed in patients. Others have used a computerized tracking program, which significantly lowered the incidence of overdue indwelling ureteral stents from 12.5 to 1.2% over a 1-yr period *(129)*. Another option is to leave a distal traction suture attached and left at the urethral meatus after the stent is placed. This will remind the patient that a foreign body is in the urinary system and permit retrieval of the stent without cystoscopy. Straight ureteral stents connected to a urethral catheter have been used in poorly compliant patients. All straight-stent treated patients returned for follow-up, whereas only 45% of double-J stent treated returned for follow-up *(130)*. The development of biodegradable stents may also eliminate the need for stent removal.

A rare but described complication is the knotting of an indwelling ureteral stent. Most of these knots involve the proximal coiled end, necessitating difficult methods for extraction *(131)*. Previous reports have attributed knot formation to excessive length of the stent with one end abutting the wall of a dilated renal pelvis and then passing through the open loop *(132)*. Stent configuration, such as Double-J or multicoil, and flexibility may also be contributing factors *(131,132)*.

In vivo ureteral stent fracture has been reported to have an incidence of <1%; however, the consequences of fracture are severe *(133)*. Depending on the biomaterial, the elongation capacity of a stent decreases as a result of the urinary environment as well as the stresses and strains to which it is subjected in active patients. Stent fragmentation will have serious implications for the patient, as broken stent fragments may migrate either downward into the bladder or, more seriously, upwards toward the renal pelvis. Broken pieces from fractured stents have been removed by cystoscopy, ureteroscopy, percutaneous nephroscopy, or open surgery *(133,134)*.

False Passage/Erosion

Mucosal tears of the ureter are common, especially with ureteral dilation or on introduction of the beak of a scope. Submucosal passage and/or perforation with a ureteroscope, wire or stent can be dangerous, causing devascularization of the ureter. Subsequently this may cause stricture or, worse, necrosis of the ureter. Most injuries are minor and can be managed conservatively with a stent and postoperative antibiotics *(135)*. Microscopic hematuria is not uncommon with all ureteral stents *(9)*. Gross hematuria is rare and may indicate that the proximal or distal stent tip is eroding into the surrounding tissues *(6)*. Ureteral erosion can occur and lead to a periureteral collection or fistula formation *(136)*. These cases require surgical intervention. More frequent stent changes may minimize such complications.

PEARLS/TRICKS

Accurate and atraumatic stent placement is greatly enhanced by proper ureteral access using a guidewire under fluoroscopic guidance. Guidewires straighten the course to the ureter and secure the luminal path for low-friction passage of a stent, balloon dilator, or ureteroscope. Different types of guidewires have been developed, each designed with unique structural properties to help accomplish specific tasks. An appropriate guidewire

12. Finney RP. Experience with new double J ureteral catheter stent. J Urol 1978; 120: 678–681.

13. Hepperlen TK, Mardis HK. "Pig tail" stent termed means of lessening ureteral surgery. Clin Trends Urol 1978; 1: 405.

14. Lennon GM, Thornhill JA, Sweeney PA, et al. 'Firm' versus 'soft' double pigtail ureteric stents: A randomised blind comparative trial. Eur Urol 1995; 28: 1–5.

15. Slaton JW, Kropp KA. Proximal ureteral stent migration: An avoidable complication? J Urol 1996; 155: 58–61.

16. Docimo SG, Dewolf WC. High failure rate of indwelling ureteral stents in patients with extrinsic obstruction: Experience at 2 institutions. J Urol 1989; 142: 277–279.

17. Hubner WA, Plas EG, Trigo-Rocha F, et al. Drainage and reflux characteristics of antireflux ureteral double-J stents. J Endourol 1993; 7: 497–499.

18. Andriole GL, Bettmann MA, Garnick MB, et al. Indwelling double-J ureteral stents for temporary and permanent urinary drainage: Experience with 87 patients. J Urol 1984; 131: 239–241.

19. Papo J, Waizbard E, Merimsky E. Spontaneous breakage of a double-pigtail stent and bladder stone formation. J Urol 1986; 92: 617–619.

20. Bloom DA, Clayman RV, McDougal E. Stents and related terms: A brief history. Urology 1999; 54: 767–771.

21. Esser JF. Studies in plastic surgery of the face. Ann Surg 1917; 65: 297–315.

22. Goodwin WE. Splint, stent, stint. Urology Dig 1972; 11: 13–14.

23. Montie JE, Stewart BH, Levin HS. Intravasal stents for vasovasostomy in canine subjects. Fertil Steril 1973; 24: 877–883.

24. Payne SR, Ramsay JW. The effects of double J stents on renal pelvic dynamics in the pig. J Urol 1988; 140: 637–641.

25. Roos R, Lykoudis PS. The fluid mechanics of the ureter with an inserted catheter. J Fluid Mech 1971; 46: 265–271.

26. Hubner WA, Plas EG, Stoller ML. The double-J ureteral stent: in vivo and in vitro flow studies. J urol 1992; 148(2 Pt 1): 278–280.

27. Mosli HA, Farsi HM, al-Aimaity MF, et al. Vesicoureteral reflux in patients with double pigtail stents. J Urol 1991; 146: 966–969.

27. Ramsay JW, Payne SR, Gosling PT, et al. The effects of double J stenting on unobstructed ureters. An experimental and clinical study. Br J Urol 1985; 57: 630–634.

28. Brewer AV Elbahnasy AM, Bercowsky E, et al. Mechanism of ureteral stent flow: A comparative in vivo study. J Endourol 1999; 13: 269–271.

29. Mardis HK, Kroeger RM, Hepperlen TW, et al. Polyethylene double-pigtail ureteral stents. Urol Clin North Am 1982; 9: 95–101.

30. Lennon GM, Thornhill JA, Grainger R, et al. Double pigtail ureteric stent versus percutaneous nephrostomy: Effects on stone transit and ureteric motility. Eur Urol 1997; 31: 24–29.

32. Drake WM Jr, Carroll J, Bartone F, et al. Evaluation of materials used as ureteral splints. Surg Gynec Obstet 1962; 114: 47–51.

33. Patel U, Kellett MJ. Ureteric drainage and peristalsis after stenting studied using colour Doppler ultrasound. Br J Urol 1996; 77: 530–535.

34. Mardis HK, Kroeger RM, Morton JJ, et al. Comparative evaluation of materials used for internal ureteral stents. J Endourol 1993; 7: 105–115.

35. Denstedt JD, Wollin TA, Reid G. Biomaterials used in urology: Current issues of biocompatibility, infection, and encrustation. J Endourol 1998; 12: 493–500.

36. Mardis HK, Kroeger RM. Ureteral stents. Materials. Urol Clin North Am 1988; 15: 471–479.

37. Cormio L, Talja M, Koivusalo A, et al. Biocompatibility of various indwelling double-J stents. J Urol 1995; 153: 494–496.

38. Bitschay J, Brodny ML. A History of Urology in Egypt. Riverside Press, New York, NY, 1956, p. 76.

39. Lord JW, Eckel JH. The use of vitallium tubes in the urinary tract of dogs. J Urol 1942; 48: 412–420.

40. Lubash S. Experience with tantalum tubes in the reimplantation of the ureters into sigmoids in dogs and humans. J Urol 1947; 57: 1010–1027.

41. Kemppainene E, Talja M, Riihela E, et al. A bioresorbable urethral stent. Urol Res 1993; 21: 235–238.

42. Brauers A, Jung PK, Thissen H, et al. Biocompatibility, cell adhesion, and degradation of surface-modified biodegradable polymers designed for the upper urinary tract. Tech Urol 1998; 4: 214–220.

43. Lumiaho J, Heino A, Tunninen V, et al. New bioabsorbable polylactide ureteral stent in the treatment of ureteral lesions: An experimental study. J Endourol 1999; 13:107–112.

44. Schlick RW, Planz K. In vitro results with special plastics for biodegradable endoureteral stents. J Endourol 1998; 12: 151–155.

45. Pauer W, Eckerstorfer GM. Use of self-expanding permanent endoluminal stents for benign ureteral strictures: Mid-term results. J Urol 1999; 162: 319–322.

46. Kulkarni RP, Bellamy EA. A new thermo-expandable shape-memory nickel-titanium alloy stent for the management of ureteric strictures. BJU Int 1999; 83: 755–759.

47. Ahmed M, Bishop MC, Bates CP, et al. Metal mesh stents for ureteral obstruction caused by hormone-resistant carcinoma of the prostate. J Endourol 1999; 13: 221–224.

48. Thijssen AM, Millward F, Mai KT. Ureteral response to the placement of metallic stents: An animal model. J Urol 1994; 151: 268–270.

49. Desgrandchamps F, Tuhschmid Y, Cochand-Priollet B, et al. Experimental study of Wallstent self-expandable metal stent in ureteral implantation. J Endourol 1995; 9: 477–481.

50. Antimisiaris SG, Siablis D, Liatsikos E. et al. Liposome-coated metal stents: An in vitro evaluation of controlled-release modality in the ureter. J Endourol 1999; 14: 743–747.

51. Ratner BD, Hoffman AS. Synthetic hydrogels for biomedical applications. In: Hydrogels for Medical and Related Application, (Arrade JD, ed.). American Chemical Society, Symposium Series, No. 31, Washington, DC, 1976, p. 1.

52. Cox AJ. Effect of a hydrogel coating on the surface topography of latex-based urinary catheters: An SEM study. Biomaterials 1987; 8: 500–502.

53. Denstedt JD, Reid G, Sofer M. Advances in ureteral stent technology. World J Urol 2000; 18: 237–242.

54. Drach GW, Dretler S, Fair W, et al. Report of the United States Cooperative Study of Extracorporeal Shock Wave Lithotripsy. J Urol 1986; 135: 1127–1133.

55. Lingeman JE, Coury TA, Newman DM, et al. Comparison of results and morbidity of percutaneous nephrostolithotomy and extracorporeal shock wave lithotripsy. J Urol 1987; 138: 485–490.

56. Tawfiek ER, Bagley DH. Management of upper urinary tract calculi with ureteroscopic techniques. Urology 1999; 53: 25.

57 Grasso M, Ficazzola M. Retrograde ureteropyeloscopy for lower pole caliceal calculi. J Urol 1999; 162: 1904.

58. Sulaiman MN, Buchholz NP, Clark PB. The role ureteral stent placement in the prevention of Steinstrasse. J Endourol 1999; 13: 151–155.

59. Kirkali Z, Esen AA, Akan G. Place of double-J stent in an extracorporeal shock wave lithotripsy. Eur Urol 1993; 23: 460–462.

60. Preminger GM, Kettelhut MC, Elkins SL, et al. Ureteral stenting during extracorporeal shock wave lithotripsy: Help or hindrance? J Urol 1989; 142: 32–36.

61. Segura JW, Preminger GM, Assimos DG, et al. Ureteral stones clinical guidelines panel summary report on the management of ureteral calculi. J Urol 1997; 158: 1915–1921.

62. Nakada SY, Pearle MS, Soble JJ, et al. Extracorporeal shock-wave lithotripsy of middle ureteral stones: Are ureteral stents necessary? Urology 1995; 46: 649–652.

63. Denstedt JD, Wollin TA, Sofer M, et al. A prospective randomized controlled trial comparing nonstented versus stented ureteroscopic lithotripsy. J Urol 2001; 165: 1419–1422.

64. Hollenbeck BK, Schuster TG, Faerber GJ, et al. Routine placement of ureteral stents is unnecessary after ureteroscopy for urinary calculi. Urology 2001; 57: 639–643.

65. Jones BJ, Ryan PC, Lyons O, et al. Use of the double pigtail stent in stone retrieval following unsuccessful ureteroscopy. Br J Urol 1990; 66: 254–256.

66. Levine RJ, Hauth JC, Curet LB, et al. Trial of calcium to prevent preeclampsia. N Engl J Med 1997; 337: 69–76.

67. Swanson SK, Heilman RI, Eversman WG. Urinary tract stones in pregnancy. Surg Clin North Am 1995; 75: 123–142.

68. Rodriguez PN, Klein AS. Management of urolithiasis during pregnancy. Surg Gynecol Obstet 1978; 166: 604–608.

69. Strothers L, Lee LM. Renal colic in pregnancy. J Urol 1992; 148: 1383–1387.

70. Parulkar BG, Hopkins TB, Wollin MR, et al. Renal colic during pregnancy: A case for conservative treatment. J Urol 1998; 159: 365–368.

71. Denstedt JD, Razvi H. Management of urinary calculi during pregnancy. J Urol 1992; 148: 1072–1074.

72. Kavoussi LR, Albala DM, Basler JW, et al. Percutaneous management of urolithiasis during pregnancy. J Urol 1992; 148: 1069–1071.

73. Scarpa RM, DeLisa A, Usai E. Diagnosis and treatment of ureteral calculi during pregnancy with rigid ureteroscopes. J Urol 1996;155: 875–877.

74. Ulvik NM, Bakke A, Hoisaeter PA. Ureteroscopy in pregnancy. J Urol 1995; 154: 1660–1663.

75. Watterson JD, Girvan AR, Beiko DT, et al. Ureteroscopy and holmium:YAG laser lithotripsy: An emerging definitive management strategy for symptomatic ureteral calculi in pregnancy. Urology 2002; 60: 383–387.

76. Wheatley M, Ohld DA, Sonda LP III, et al. Treatment of renal transplant stones by extracorporeal shock-wave lithotripsy in the prone position. Urology 1991; 37: 57–60.

77. Pleass HCC, Clark KM, Rigg KS, et al. Urologic complications after renal transplantation: A prospective randomized trial comparing different techniques for ureteric anastomosis and the use of prophylactic stents. Transplant Proc 1995; 27: 1091–1092.

78. Loughlin KL, Tilney NL, Richie JP. Urological complications in 718 renal transplant patients. Surgery 1984; 95: 297–302.

79. Kinnaert P, Hall M, Janssen F, et al. Ureteral stenosis after kidney transplantation: True incidence and long-term follow-up after surgical correction. J Urol 1985; 133: 17–20.

80. Benoit G, Blanchet P, Eschwege P, et al. Insertion of a double pigtail ureteral stent for the prevention of urological complications in renal transplantation: A prospective randomized study. J Urol 1996; 156: 881–884.

81. Eschwege P, Blanchet P, Alexandre L, et al. Infectious complications after the use of double J ureteral stents. Transplant Proc 1996; 28: 2833.

82. Pearle MS, Pierce HL, Miller GL, et al. Optimal method of urgent decompression of the collecting system for obstruction and infection due to ureteral calculi. J Urol 1998; 160: 1260–1264.

83. Feng MI, Bellman GC, Shapiro CE. Management of ureteral obstruction secondary to pelvic malignancies. J Endourol 1999; 13: 521–524.

84. Andriole GL, Bettmann MA, Garnick MB, et al. Indwelling double-J ureteral stents for temporary and permanent urinary drainage: Experience with 87 patients. J Urol 1984; 131: 239–241.

85. Docimo SG, DeWolf WC. High failure rate of indwelling ureteral stents in patients with extrinsic obstruction: Experience at 2 institutions. J Urol 1989; 157: 277–279.

86. Fromer DL, Shabsigh A, Benson MC, et al. Simultaneous multiple double pigtail stents for malignant ureteral obstruction. Urology 2002; 59: 594–596.

87. Pauer W, Lugmayr H. Metallic wallstents: A new therapy for extrinsic ureteral obstruction. J Urol 1992; 148: 281.

88. Kulkarni R, Bellamy E. Nickel-titanium shape memory alloy Memokath 051 ureteral stent for managing long-term ureteral obstruction: 4-year experience. J Urol 2001; 166, 1750–1754.

89. Nakada SY, Gerber AJ, Wolf Jr JS, et al. Subcutaneous urinary diversion utilizing a nephrovesical stent: A superior alternative to long-term external drainage? Urology 1995; 45: 538–541.

90. Minhas S, Irving HC, Lloyd SN, et al. Extra-anatomic stents in ureteric obstruction: Experience and complications. BJU Int 1999; 84: 762–764.

91. Webber RJ, Pandian SS, McClinton S, et al. Retrograde balloon dilatation for pelviureteric junction obstruction. J Endourol 1997; 11: 239–242.

92. Finney RP. Double-J and diversion stents. Urol Clin North Am 1982; 9: 89–94.

93. Lee CK, Smith AD. Role of stents in open ureteral surgery. J Endourol 1993; 7: 141–144.

94. Davis DM. Intubated ureterotomy: A new operation for ureteral and ureteropelvic stricture. Surg Gynecol Obstet 1943; 76: 513.

96. Kumar R, Kapoor R, Mandhani A, et al. Optimum duration of splinting after endopyelotomy. J Endourol 1999; 13: 89–92.

96. Badlani GH, Smith AD. Stent for endopyelotomy. Urol Clin North Am 1988; 14: 445–448.

97. Pearle MS. Use of ureteral stents after endopyelotomy. J Endourol 1996; 10: 169–176.

98. Selvaggi FP, Battaglia M, Traficante A, et al. Obstetric and gynecological lesions of the ureter: Experience with 88 injuries. Int Urogynecol J 1991; 2: 81–84.

99. Sheikh FA, Kubchandani IT. Prophylactic ureteric catheters in colon surgery—how safe are they? Report of three cases. Dis Colon Rectum 1990; 33: 508–510.

100. Phipps JH, Tyrrell NJ. Transilluminating ureteric stents for preventing operative ureteric damage. Br J Obstet Gynaecol 1992; 99: 81.

101. Steers WD, Corriere JN Jr, Benson GS, et al.: The use of indwelling ureteral stents in managing ureteral injuries due to external violence. J Trauma 1985; 25: 1001–1003.

102. Watterson JD, Mahoney JE, Futter NG, et al. Iatrogenic ureteric injuries: Approaches to etiology and management. Can J Surg 1998; 41: 379–382.

103. Presti JC Jr, Carroll PR, McAninch JW. Ureteral and renal pelvic injuries from external trauma: Diagnosis and management. J Trauma 1989; 29: 370–374.

104. Haas CA, Reigle MD, Selzman AA, et al. Use of ureteral stents in the management of major renal trauma with urinary extravasation: Is there a role? J Endourol 1998; 12: 545–549.

105. Lang EK. Diagnosis and management of ureteral fistulas by percutaneous nephrostomy and antegrade stent catheter. Radiology 1981; 138: 311–317.

106. Goldin AR. Percutaneous ureteral splinting. Urology 1977; 10: 165–168.

107. Chang R, Marshall FF, Mitchell S. Percutaneous management of benign ureteral strictures and fistulas. J Urol 1987; 137: 1–26.

108. Yu DS, Yang, TH, Ma CP. Snail-headed catheter retriever: A simple way to remove catheters from female patients. J Urol 1995; 154: 167–168.

109. Macaluso JN Jr, Deutsch JS, Goodman JR, et al. The use of the Magnetip double-J ureteral stent in urological practice. J Urol 1989; 142: 701–703.

110. Taylor WN, McDougall IT. Minimally invasive ureteral stent retrieval. J Urol 2002; 168: 2020–2023.

111. Lam JS, Gupta M. Tips and tricks for the management of retained ureteral stents. J Endourol 2002; 16: 733–741.

112. Pollard SG, MacFarlane R. Symptoms arising from double-J ureteral stents. J Urol 1998; 139: 37–38.

113. Bregg, K., Rieble, R.A., Jr.: Morbidity associated with indwelling internal ureteral stents after shock wave lithotripsy. J Urol 1989; 141: 510–512.

114. Pryor JL, Langley MJ, Jenkins AD. Comparison of symptom characteristics of indwelling ureteral catheters. J Urol 1991; 145: 719–722.

115. Thomas R. Indwelling ureteral stents: Impact of material and shape on patient discomfort. J Endourol 1993; 7: 137–140.

116. McDougall EM, Denstedt JD, Clayman RV. Comparison of patient acceptance of polyurethane vs. silicone indwelling ureteral stents. J Endourol 1990; 4: 79–91.

117. Dushinski JW, Lingeman JE. Prospective randomized trial to evaluate patient comfort with regards to size of indwelling stent. J Urol 1997; 157 (Suppl): 43.

118. Oswalt GC Jr, Bueschen AJ, Lloyd LK. Upward migration of indwelling ureteral stents. J Urol 1979; 122: 249–250.

119. Bagley DH, Hoffman JL. Ureteroscopic retrieval of proximally located ureteral stents. Urology 1991; 37:446–448.

120. Tunney MM, Jones DS, Gorman PS. Biofilm and biofilm-related encrustation of urinary tract devices. Methods Enzymol 1999; 310: 558–566.

121. Santin M, Motta A, Denyer SP, et al. Effect of the urine conditioning film on ureteral stent encrustation and characterization of its protein composition. Biomaterials 1999; 20:1245–1251.

122. Wollin TA, Tieszer C, Riddell JV, et al. Bacterial biofilm formation, encrustation and antibiotic adsorption to ureteral stents indwelling in humans. J Endourol 1998; 12:101–111.

123. Keane PF, Bonner MC, Johnston SR, et al. Characterization of biofilm and encrustation on ureteric stents in vivo. Br J Urol 1994; 73:687–691.

124. Tieszer C, Reid G, Denstedt JD. Conditioning film deposition on ureteral stents after implantation. J Urol 1998; 160: 876–881.

125. Sidhu H, Holmes RP, Allison MJ, et al. Direct quantifications of the enteric bacterium *Oxalobacter formingens* in human fecal samples by quantitative competitive-template PCR. J Clin Microbiol 1999; 37:1503–1509.

126. Sofer M, Denstedt JD. Encrustation of biomaterials in the urinary tract. Curr Opin Urol 2000; 10: 563–559.
127. Lifshitz DA, Winkler HZ, Gross M, et al. Predictive value of urinary cultures in assessment of microbial colonization of ureteral stents. J Endourol 1999; 13: 735–738.
128. El-Faqih SR, Shamsuddin AB, Chakrabarti A, et al. Polyurethane internal stents in treatment of stone patients: Morbidity related to indwelling times. J. Urol 1991; 146:1817–1820.
129. Ather MH, Talati J, Biyabani R. Physician responsibility for removal of implants: The case for a computerized program for tracking overdue double-J stents. Tech Urol 2000; 6: 189–192.
130. Mydlo JH, Streater S. The applicability of using straight ureteral stents for the treatment of ureteral stones in presumably non-compliant patients. Urol Int 2001; 66: 201–204.
131. Kundargi P, Bansal M, Pattnaik PK. Knotted upper end: A new complication in the use of an indwelling ureteral stent. J Urol 1994; 151: 995–996.
132. Flam TA, Thiounn N, Gerbaud PF, et al. Knotting of a double pigtail stent within the ureter: An initial report. J Urol 1995; 154: 1858–1859.
133. El-Sheriff A. Fracture of polyurethane double pigtail stents: An in vivo retrospective and prospective fluoroscopic study. Br J Urol 1995; 76: 108–114.
134. Zisman A, Siegel YL, Siegmann A, et al. Spontaneous ureteral stent fragmentation. J Urol 1995; 153: 718–721.
135. Benjamin JC, Donaldson PJ, Hill JT. Ureteric perforation after ureteroscopy. Conservative management. Urology 1987; 29: 623–624.
136. Toolin E, Pollack H, McLean G, et al. Ureteroarterial fistula: A case report. J Urol 1994; 132: 553.

26 Anesthetic Considerations for Extracorporeal Shockwave Lithotripsy, Percutaneous Nephrolithotomy, and Laser Lithotripsy

Mark Ancheta, MD and Daniel Swangard, MD

Key Words: Anesthesia; sedation; pain; physiology.

INTRODUCTION

Extracorporeal shockwave lithotripsy (SWL) is the main outpatient treatment modality for urinary tract calculi. Anesthesia and analgesia are provided to treat the cutaneous, somatic, and visceral pain associated with SWL. Multiple anesthetic techniques have been used effectively. The decision to employ one technique over another depends on patient, as well as procedural, factors. Patient factors include intraoperative analgesia and sedation and minimizing adverse effects such as postoperative nausea and vomiting (PONV) and pruritis, which can prolong recovery and patient discharge. Procedural factors include providing satisfactory operating conditions for administration of shockwaves. This translates primarily into minimizing patient movement to allow for effective stone fragmentation. Cost effectiveness and optimal use of medical resources are attained with shorter

From: Current Clinical Urology, *Urinary Stone Disease:*
A Practical Guide to Medical and Surgical Management
Edited by: M. L. Stoller and M. V. Meng © Humana Press Inc., Totowa, NJ

treatment times and quicker postoperative recovery. To this end, anesthetic techniques may include intravenous (IV) anesthesia and analgesia, cutaneous local anesthesia, non-steroidal anti-inflammatory drugs (NSAIDs), patient-controlled analgesia/anesthesia (PCA), and neuraxial blockade with spinal or epidural anesthesia.

ANESTHETIC TECHNIQUE AND PERIOPERATIVE ANALGESIA

Monitored Anesthesia Care

Multiple regimens of IV anesthesia and analgesia for SWL have been studied. An advantage of IV analgesia and sedation or "monitored anesthesia care" (MAC) is quicker recovery profile compared to general anesthesia or epidural anesthesia (1). To determine the optimal opioid combination with propofol infusion, a study compared fentanyl and its analogs (including alfentanil, sufentanil, and remifentanil) with respect to their effects on recovery profile and adverse effects. Alfentanil had the worst recovery profile and the longest times to discharge, whereas remifentanil had the highest incidence of postoperative pain (2). Fentanyl provided excellent intraoperative and postoperative pain control. Another study found propofol infusion and fentanyl bolus to be superior to the combination of midazolam and alfentanil infusion with fewer episodes of desaturation (SpO_2 <90%), postoperative pain, and pruritis (3).

Remifentanil is a synthetic opioid with ultrashort duration of action owing to its plasma ester metabolism and is an attractive analgesic for use in SWL. During general anesthesia, remifentanil infusion in combination with desflurane and nitrous oxide (N_2O) compared to remifentanil and propofol produced shorter SWL procedure times, owing to less disruptive movements and episodes of respiratory depression, but a comparable recovery profile (4). When remifentanil infusion is compared to sufentanil boluses, there was less respiratory depression and PONV (5). But when remifentanil infusion is compared to the traditional combination of IV sedation with propofol and fentanyl bolus, it had a higher incidence of PONV resulting in slower recovery profile (6).

In an attempt to find an alternative analgesic that has favorable hemodynamic and respiratory profile, ketamine infusion was compared to alfentanil infusion. This study showed that although ketamine maintained higher mean arterial pressures and resulted in fewer episodes of bradypnea and desaturation (SpO_2 <90%), it was inferior to alfentanil because of ketamine's higher rate of intraoperative disruptive movements and postoperative confusion (7).

In summary, MAC using propofol infusion and fentanyl boluses for pain control seems to have the optimal balance of achieving a short recovery profile with the least amount of intraoperative, primarily patient movement, and postoperative adverse effects such as PONV and pruritis.

Cutaneous Anesthesia

Cutaneous local anesthesia has been studied as another method of reducing nocioceptive stimuli elicited from the shockwaves at the skin entry site. The eutectic mixture of local anesthetic (EMLA) with 2.5% prilocaine and 2.5% lidocaine can penetrate intact skin to provide cutaneous anesthesia. Studies have reported mixed results with EMLA's efficacy in decreasing the cutaneous pain associated with SWL. Most studies show that EMLA compared to placebo does not decrease analgesic requirements (8,9). But in another trial, EMLA decreased the analgesic requirements at 14 kV compared to placebo and was similar, in terms of pain scores, to IV fentanyl, intramuscular (IM) tramadol, and IM diclofenac (10,11). Compared to subcutaneous anesthesia with 2% lidocaine and 1:200,000 epinephrine, EMLA was equivalent with regard to supplemental opioid requirements (12). When EMLA was used as an adjunct to alfentanil continuous infusion or PCA, there was no opioid sparing effect and no improvement in recovery profile (13,14). The pain from SWL is from cutaneous and deep visceral origins and this may account for the apparent lack of decreased analgesic requirements effected by cutaneous anesthesia. Also, for optimal effect, EMLA must be applied topically at least 60–90 min before the painful stimulus. Based on these studies, there seems to be no added benefit in terms of improved recovery profile or patient comfort when EMLA is added to the anesthetic regimen for SWL.

Nonsteroidal Anti-Inflammatory Drugs

A local inflammatory response occurs within the urinary tract after fragmentation of the stone by high-energy shockwaves. NSAIDs have been studied for their anti-inflammatory effect and as adjuncts to opioid analgesics during SWL. IM diclofenac is similar to IV fentanyl and IM tramadol with respect to pain scores and opioid requirements; in addition, its use demonstrates less PONV and intraoperative episodes of desaturation (15). When diclofenac was included as part of an IV anesthetic with midazolam and fentanyl, there were reduced treatment times, better operating conditions with more shockwaves administered and a reduced requirement for opioids (16). Supplementing alfentanil PCA with diclofenac produced higher patient satisfaction as well (17). NSAIDs, as part of a balanced intravenous anesthetic, have an opioid-sparing effect and increase patient satisfaction owing to the reduction in side effects such as intraoperative hypoxia and PONV.

Patient-Controlled Analgesia

PCA for SWL allows the patient to rapidly control the level of sedation and comfort. In comparison to a continuous infusion, PCA with alfentantil produced equivalent pain control and study subjects used 31% less alfentanil (18). These patients were also able to tolerate higher discharge voltages and required fewer shocks to complete stone fragmentation leading to shorter treatment times (19). Combination of a sedative-hypnotic, such as propofol, and opioid PCA for SWL has been evaluated. PCA with propofol and alfentanil was superior to midazolam and alfentanil with less sedation and improved pulmonary status, including higher ventilatory rates, higher oxygen saturations, and less episodes of hypoxia (11% vs 30%) (20). Propofol's favorable recovery profile is attributed to its pharmacokinetics, having a short context-sensitive half time irregardless of the total cumulative dose administered. Cessation of propofol results in rapid awakening with minimal residual inhibition of the central nervous system. Remifentanil has also been used in PCA because of its ease of titration and rapid onset and short duration of action. When compared to PCA with remifentanil alone, PCA with remifentanil and propofol produced higher patient satisfaction, required less remifentanil, and had lower incidence of PONV (8% vs 27%) (21). However, in this study, the PCA was set at zero lockout and produced more adverse side effects, including higher incidence of apnea 52% vs 15% and oxygen desaturation 23% vs 7%. An appropriate lockout interval for PCA with remifentanil should improve the incidence of adverse effects while producing effective analgesia and sedation.

Neuraxial Anesthesia

Spinal anesthesia with the goal of producing a T6 level provides excellent operating conditions for SWL owing to its dense sensory and motor blockade. Intrathecal lidocaine is the prototypical agent used for this purpose. Unfortunately, the dense motor block with intrathecal lidocaine can prolong time to voiding and ambulation, leading to delayed discharge time. Alternatively, intrathecal opioids can provide similar sensory analgesia without the motor blockade associated with local anesthetics. A retrospective study has shown that intrathecal sufentanil compared to intrathecal lidocaine allowed for a higher number of shocks administered with a higher treatment success rate (22). Also, intrathecal sufentanil, when compared to 5% hyperbaric lidocaine, has a more favorable recovery profile (23,24). Intrathecal sufentanil 20 mcg reduced times to ambulation (79 ± 16 min vs 146 ± 57 min), tolerating oral intake (51 ± 21 min vs 81 ± 28 min), voiding spontaneously (80 ± 18 min vs 152 ± 54 min), and discharge (98 ± 17 min vs 166 ± 50 min) (23). The primary disadvantage of intrathecal opioids is the high incidence of pruritis. Despite having an incidence of 27–100% of pruritis with different doses of sufentanil, intrathecal opioid led to earlier discharge time vs intrathecal local anesthetic (23,24). The optimal dose of intrathecal sufentanil balances the benefits of superior analgesia without the adverse effects of pruritis and PONV. In a study comparing different doses of intrathecal sufentanil (12.5, 15, 17.5, and 20 mcg) for SWL, 20 mcg sufentanil had the lowest intraoperative and postoperative pain scores and required less supplemental sedation with propofol (25). Unfortunately, this dose of sufentanil also produced the highest rate of adverse effects (pruritis 100% and 13% PONV). The authors of this study recommended 15 mcg intrathecal sufentanil as the optimal dose for unilateral SWL because this dose, compared to 20 mcg intrathecal sufentanil, had a significant earlier time to discharge (84 ± 40 min vs 126 ± 48 min) (25). Another advantage to intrathecal opioid is the lack of a sympathetic blockade which typically results in more stable hemodynamics. Intrathecal sufentanil produced a smaller maximum decrease in mean arterial pressure (12.2 ± 12 mmHg vs 26.1 ± 12.4 mmHg) vs intrathecal lidocaine (24).

Continuous spinal anesthesia is also an option for SWL. A retrospective study of continuous spinal with 0.1% hyperbaric bupivacaine with a T4-T8 sensory level showed that it was safe to use such a technique. There was a 15% rate of sympathomimetic drug use, maximal systolic blood pressure decrease of 19.0% ± 9.8, maximal diastolic blood pressure decrease of 13.4% ± 13.3, maximal heart rate decrease of 7.2% ± 11.7, and a 6% incidence of post-dural puncture headache (26).

Spinal anesthesia with intrathecal opioids or local anesthetics can provide the necessary operating conditions for SWL. At this point, there are no randomized controlled studies evaluating the effectiveness of spinal anesthesia in comparison to general anesthesia or MAC.

General Anesthesia

SWL with cystoscopy for ureteral stent placement before lithotripsy requires general anesthesia or neuraxial anesthesia. A study compared epidural anesthesia with 1.5% lidocaine vs general anesthesia using propofol for maintenance of anesthesia without opioids. There was no difference in postoperative conditions or duration of SWL, but the general anesthesia group had a faster recovery time (127 ± 59 min vs 178 ± 49 min) (27).

COMPLICATIONS ASSOCIATED WITH ANESTHESIA FOR SWL

The main complications of anesthesia and SWL are related to the adverse effects of the anesthetic agents used. Opioids cause a dose dependent reduction in ventilatory rate leading to transient oxygen desaturation, as well as pruritis, nausea/vomiting, and sedation. Dolasetron reduces the incidence and severity of PONV in patients receiving opiods and may result in earlier discharge times (28). Intrathecal local anesthetics produce a motor block that can prolong recovery and also cause a decrease in sympathetic tone and consequently blood pressure. However, such hypotension is transient and most often easily treated with sympathomimetic drugs. However, to put these complications in perspective, a retrospective study of 600 SWL treatments with general anesthesia, epidural anesthesia, and local anesthesia showed the complication rate to be very low (29). In addition, the postoperative risk and outcomes associated with SWL are predictable. A retrospective study of 2203 patients undergoing general anesthesia, neuraxial anesthesia (spinal and epidural), and MAC showed that PONV and flank pain were the most common complaints. As with the previously mentioned study, this study also demonstrated that the peri-procedural complications with SWL were very low.

Owing to the nature of the shockwave energy, modifications to the technique of epidural placement should be made. A case has been reported in a patient who underwent epidural anesthesia during SWL. The patient suffered temporary neurological damage as a result of the air introduced into the epidural space during catheter placement (30). The use of air for the loss-of-resistance technique during epidural placement can introduce bubbles into the epidural and paravertebral spaces; this creates an air/tissue interface not usually present and thus a potential risk of damage to nearby tissue from the shockwaves. Therefore, saline should be used for loss-of-resistance to locate the epidural space.

REVIEW OF RELATIVE AND ABSOLUTE CONTRAINDICATIONS TO SWL

Most patients with urinary tract calculi will safely tolerate SWL without complications. But there is a select population of patients who may have an increased risk from shockwave therapy in which careful perioperative evaluation and planning can reduce risk. Traditionally, a number of clinical scenarios or conditions were considered absolute or relative contraindications to SWL, including calcified aortic or renal artery aneurysms, implanted cardiac pacemakers and defibrillators, coagulopathies, morbid obesity, cystine calculi, children, calculi in mid ureter and in anomalous kidneys, and calculi in distal ureter (31). In vitro and in vivo studies along with clinical experience have shown that with meticulous monitoring and treatment in the perioperative period, most, if not all, of these patients can undergo SWL safely.

Calcified aortic or renal artery aneurysms in close proximity to a stone are believed to have the risk of embolism or rupture of the vascular wall during SWL. Guidelines to decrease the risk of embolism or rupture of an ipsilateral calcified aneurysm suggest that the aneurysm should be asymptomatic, less than 2 cm for a renal artery aneurysm and less than 5 cm for an abdominal aortic aneurysm; also, a stone to aneurysm distance of ≥ 5 cm is recommended. The aneurysm should not lie along the parallel axis of the wave, and the energy setting should not exceed 18 kV in a Dornier HM3 unit (32–34).

Patients with an implantable pacemaker were considered to be at risk for electro-magnetic interference from the high-energy shockwaves. Clinical studies have shown that the risk is low, nonlethal, and the most serious complication was spontaneous deprogramming of the programmable pacemaker (35). Before undergoing SWL, it is reasonable to request that a patient undergo a pacemaker interrogation if none has been completed within 6 mo to document settings and proper functioning. A copy of the interrogation report should be made available to the anesthesiologist, in addition to a current 12-lead electrocardiogram. Most, if not all, pacemakers implanted in the last 10 yr are dual chamber devices that sense and pace in the right atrium, as well as the right ventricle. Biventricular pacemakers have recently come into practice and pace the right atrium as well as the left and right ventricles independently and are used in patients with end-stage congestive heart failure. Contemporary pacemakers require no reprogramming before SWL as it does not affect sensing or pacing functionality. In the unlikely event of interference/pacemaker malfunction, a magnet may be placed over the device during shockwave therapy; although important to confirm the magnet mode, magnet application usually converts the device to a fixed rate mode (nonsensing mode) such as DOO. Confirmation of the magnet mode requires the interrogation report mentioned previously. The method of returning the pacemaker to its original mode is simple, but different depending on manufacturer. The surgeon or anesthesiologist should consult with a cardiologist or the manufacturer if a magnet is applied during the procedure. Patients with piezoelectric rate responsive pacemakers should have this feature deactivated before SWL (31,36). Patients with implanted cardiac defibrillators may also safely undergo SWL without deactivation of such devices. Interrogation of all devices is indicated postoperatively by a cardiologist or electrophysiology nurse/technician to validate intact settings/functioning of the device before patient discharge (37).

In a study during nonsynchronized SWL with a spark plug lithotriptor (20–21 kV), there was an 18.4% incidence of unifocal, asymptomatic, premature ventricular contractions (PVC) without changes in hemodynamics or oxygenation (38). The PVCs were unpredictable in onset and without correlation to patient factors (age, history of coronary artery disease) or SWL factors (shockwaves or total energy delivered) and disappeared with resynchronization (38). There seems to be no known cardiac insult as a result of SWL. This is evidenced by the observed lack of angina, ischemic changes on electrocardiography, and rise in myocardial enzymes (CK-MB and troponin I) (39).

Patients with known coronary artery disease who are asymptomatic or have stable angina do not require additional preoperative stress testing. SWL is a low risk procedure with regard to perioperative cardiac morbidity. Delay of this procedure for cardiac reasons should be considered only in high-risk patients: those with current signs/symptoms of (1) unstable angina, (2) congestive heart failure, or (3) valvular heart disease. If preoperative history, physical exam, or ECG findings suggest a new or undiagnosed cardiac condition (angina, myocardial infarct, murmur, or carotid bruit), it is quite reasonable request a preoperative workup; in some cases, this may require postponement in the setting of this most often elective procedure. These guidelines apply also to low risk procedures such as percutaneous nephrolithostomy and laser lithotripsy to be mentioned later.

Patients with risk factors for coagulopathies have the potential for perirenal or intra-renal bleeding during SWL. Clinical studies have shown that patients with coagulopathies can safely undergo SWL when appropriate preoperative studies are done to evaluate for the presence of coagulopathy and treat the abnormalities *(31)*. Those patients with known inherited disorders of coagulation (hemophilia and von Willebrand disease) or acquired disorders of coagulation (cirrhosis, thrombocytopenia, and factor inhibitors) should be seen by a hematologist before procedure. A clear plan is required regarding the perioperative administration of clotting factors or other blood products. In addition, postoperative monitoring should be outlined by the hematologist. Communication among surgeon, anesthesiologist, and hematologist is essential. Many products, such as factor VIII, have short plasma half-lives and require an additional dose(s) in the postprocedure period. Coumadin should be stopped 5–7 d before the procedure and normal coagulation parameters confirmed just before the procedure. The clinical indications requiring coumadin therapy (i.e., heart valves, atrial fibrillation, and deep vein thrombosis etc.) are varied. In some cases, discontinuation of coumadin may require preoperative bridging therapy with lovenox or unfractionated heparin. It is recommended that one confer with a hematologist or internist regarding the appropriate perioperative plan for anticoagulation; this includes plans for both the preoperative and postoperative period.

If, by history and physical exam, there is no suspicion or history of bleeding dyscrasia, routine preoperative screening, such as PT/PTT or a platelet count, is not indicated. The approach to coagulation as outlined above also applies to percutaneous nephrolithotomy, and laser lithotripsy.

Morbid obesity poses a challenge for the successful treatment of renal calculi. The difficulties include a weight limitation on the Dornier HM3 gantry (not greater than 135 kg), the limited distance between the F1 and F2 focal points, and the damping effect of excess fat and muscle *(31)*. The distance limitation can be overcome by manipulating the proximal ureteral or renal pelvic stone to a more distal position that is closer to the skin level and use of second generation lithotriptors that have greater distance between the F1 and F2 focal points. The damping effect can be overcome by using higher energy shockwaves at increased frequency and abdominal compression *(31)*.

Cystine calculi do not have a strong acoustic interface and therefore do not fragment well. Limiting the size of the cystine calculi to <1.5 cm and undergoing previous chemolysis may improve the rate for successful fragmentation *(31)*.

There was concern for potential adverse effects of shockwave therapy on the immature kidney in the pediatric population, but none were found in animal studies *(40)*. To accommodate children, modifications to the Dornier HM3 gantry were made, including the addition of frame adaptations, slings, and hammocks. With shielding of the lungs and gonads, there seems to be no effect on linear body growth or renal function *(41)*. Children may safely undergo SWL, and reports suggest that children pass fragments more readily and have less pain *(31)*.

Calculi in the mid ureter and in anomalous kidneys may present a diagnostic and treatment challenge because they overly the pelvic bone making it difficult to locate the stones fluoroscopically and cause damping of shockwaves. To circumvent the nonoptimal location of these calculi, patients may be positioned prone in the gantry and a ureteral catheter placed to enhance localization *(42)*. Calculi in the distal ureter and below the pelvic brim may pose positioning problems and concerns for effects on fertility. Reports stating increased success rate used a horse riding position with intravenous or antegrade pyelography to enhance stone visualization, as well as a horizontal position *(43,44)*. SWL of the lower ureteral calculi is safe, without adverse effects on male or female fertility *(31)*.

The sole absolute contraindication to SWL is pregnancy, owing to adverse fetal effects from radiation exposure, anesthetic risks, and unknown potential effects from shockwaves *(31)*.

PERCUTANEOUS NEPHROLITHOTOMY

Introduction

Percutaneous nephrolithotomy (PCNL) is the preferred surgical technique for treatment of larger renal and ureteral calculi. The patient is anesthetized with general anesthesia and usually placed in the prone position to allow for instrumentation of the kidney. PCNL has a higher stone-free rate compared with SWL, especially for medium sized stones, but carries a higher risk of morbidity and mortality *(45,46)*.

Patient Positioning

Traditionally, PCNL is performed in the prone position and has some disadvantages owing to patient discomfort and adverse effects on the cardiopulmonary system. Great care must be taken during the transfer of the patient from the gurney (supine) to the operating table (prone), ensuring that the endotracheal tube does not become dislodged from excessive movement. Once prone, the anesthesiologist ensures a neutral cervical spine and appropriate positioning of the face pad around the eyes, nose, mouth and chin. The other members of the surgical team should take responsibility for proper patient positioning. This entails foam padding to avoid sustained pressure on the extremities (elbows/knees/heels), breasts, nipples, and gonads, as well as, avoidance of extreme range of motion of extremities to prevent dislocation, ligamentous injury and peripheral neuropathy. Cardiac preload can decrease from a compressed vena cava and restriction on ventilation can occur with a compressed abdomen from improper positioning. Bolsters should be used to free the abdomen from compression. Special consideration is required for morbidly obese patients who may require extra large bolsters or even a special table such as a Jackson. The supine position may be an alternative in certain clinical situations (morbid obesity) and has been shown to have comparable success and complication rate relative to the prone position, despite having a higher incidence of anteromedial renal displacement *(47)*.

Surgical Techniques

There are two technical approaches to PCNL. Subcostal access is preferred over supracostal access. Multiple studies have shown that subcostal access (below the 12th rib) compared to supracostal access has a lower incidence of respiratory pain (5% vs 37%) and lower systemic and intrathoracic complications (including pneumothorax, pleural effusions, bleeding requiring transfusion) *(48–50)*. With further analysis, the supra-11th rib puncture compared to the supra-12th rib puncture had higher pleural injuries and intrathoracic complications.

The technique of PCNL has evolved with different methods studied, including the mini-PCNL and tubeless PCNL. The mini-PCNL uses a smaller percutaneous tract dilator (22 Fr vs 30 Fr) and sheath whereas the tubeless-PCNL uses a double-J stent wire for drainage without a nephrostomy tube. In a study comparing the three different methods, the tubeless PCNL was the most cost efficient, with decreased total procedural cost and length of hospital stay, and least opioid requirements *(51)*. Other studies have confirmed the efficacy of tubeless PCNL, with reported stone free rates of 92–93% *(52,53)*.

Physiological Considerations and Complications of PCNL

There are potential physiological disturbances that may occur during PCNL. In a patient with compromised cardiopulmonary or renal function, fluid overload may become an issue with prolonged procedural time and excessive irrigation fluid. Fortunately, in patients with intact physiologic mechanisms to process the fluid load there seems to be no clinically significant electrolyte abnormalities associated with PCNL *(54)*. The absorbed fluid can also cause intraoperative hypothermia and female patients are more prone to a greater decline in temperature *(55)*. Therefore, accurate monitoring of core body temperature with an esophageal probe is indicated. Multiple studies have confirmed that renal puncture during PCNL does not result in a significant decline in renal function postoperatively as assessed by glomerular filtration rate and serum creatinine *(56)*.

Complications associated with PCNL are both minor and major *(57)*. The minor complications are postoperative fever, colic, and urinary tract infection. In a study comparing single dose vs short-term antibiotic prophylaxis in patients with sterile urine preoperatively, there was no difference in rates of bacteriuria, bacteremia, and postoperative fever *(58)*. This study suggests that a single intravenous dose of antibiotic at anesthetic induction is sufficient for infection prophylaxis. The major complications are septicemia, bleeding requiring blood transfusions, and intrathoracic injuries (pneumothorax and hemothorax) *(45)*.

Anesthetic Considerations

PCNL is usually accomplished with general anesthesia. Although there is limited data available that discuss different anesthetic techniques with reference to improving perioperative outcome, one study did examine the effect of single dose intrathecal morphine on pain and recovery after unilateral PCNL *(59)*. Supplementing general anesthesia with intrathecal morphine resulted in less analgesic requirement and improved mobility on postoperative day zero. Despite improved pain management and quicker return of bowel function, intrathecal morphine did not result in earlier discharge times. Owing to potential ventilatory difficulties associated with the prone positioning, patients are intubated with an endotracheal tube for the general anesthetic. Although general anesthesia is the common choice of anesthetic technique, epidural anesthesia is a safe alternative.

In summary, PCNL is indicated as a treatment option for renal and ureteric calculi of larger stones. Meticulous attention to patient positioning and improved surgical technique has decreased the risks associated with PCNL.

LASER LITHOTRIPSY

Intracorporeal lithotripsy is a direct approach to treating renal and ureteric calculi that are not amenable to treatment with SWL. Fragmentation of stones greater than 5 mm is necessary before extraction. There are different intracorporeal lithotriptors available and can be categorized as direct contact mechanical lithotriptors, devices that use shockwave effects, and laser systems *(60)*. Holmium:yttrium-aluminum-garnet (YAG) laser is the gold standard for laser lithotripsy, which unlike other laser modalities, can destroy all types of stones, including calcium oxalate monohydrate and cystine stones. Laser lithotripsy is advantageous because the devices are thin and flexible, can be used in all endoscopic instruments, and allow access to all parts of the urinary tract *(60)*.

Multiple studies have confirmed the safety and efficacy of laser lithotripsy, with overall stone-free rates ranging 89–97% (61–63). For treatment of proximal, middle, and lower ureteral stones, holmium:YAG laser lithotripsy was more effective than SWL with low risk of complications (64,65). High fragmentation rates of laser lithotripsy producing small fragments that easily pass the urinary tract may obviate the need for ureteral stenting (66). In studies comparing ureteral stenting to nonstenting after laser lithotripsy, the nonstented group had a significant reduction in severity of postoperative pain while not affecting the rate of postoperative sepsis, suggesting that ureteral stenting may not be necessary (67,68).

Laser lithotripsy is a low risk procedure. In a series of 598 patients treated with holmium:YAG laser lithotripsy, the overall complication rate was 4% and laser-related complications was <1% (62). The laser produces weak photoacoustic effects and has low risk of mechanical injury to organs. Nonlaser related complications are usually secondary to ureteroscopy. This risk may be reduced even further with the use of smaller caliber instruments (64).

Selected patient populations with relative or absolute contraindications to SWL may benefit from the treatment of laser lithotripsy. Patients with bleeding diathesis, including patients with liver dysfunction with a mean international normalized ratio of 2.3, thrombocytopenia, or on warfarin, can safely undergo laser lithotripsy without preoperative correction of the bleeding dyscrasia (61). Symptomatic stones during pregnancy can pose a treatment challenge, as pregnancy is the only remaining absolute contraindication to SWL. There are reports of a small number of pregnant patients with fetal gestational age ranges from 22 to 35 wk who have been successfully treated with laser lithotripsy with minimal or no use of fluoroscopy, resulting in no obstetric or urologic complications (53,69). Morbidly obese patients with symptomatic stones less than 1.5 cm can be effectively treated with laser lithotripsy (70). Children may also be safely treated with laser lithotripsy without risks of stricture or hydronephrosis (71). Patients with chronic renal insufficiency may also be treated with laser lithotripsy and avoid postoperative renal dysfunction (72).

In summary, intracorporeal laser lithotripsy is a safe, direct treatment of renal and ureteric calculi with low risk of complications, and may be safely used in patients with bleeding diathesis, pregnancy, morbid obesity, and patients with chronic renal insufficiency.

Anesthetic Options for Laser Lithotripsy

Patient immobility and comfort are goals for the anesthesiologist during laser lithotripsy. General anesthesia can provide a secure airway and avoidance of patient movement. Spinal anesthesia with a sensory level of T8-T10 is also an acceptable alternative owing to its rapid onset and relaxation of the pelvic floor and perineum. Adequate hydration will maintain hemodynamic parameters and will be useful for postoperative hematuria. Health care personnel in the operating room should wear protective eyewear to avoid the reflective laser beam.

SPECIAL CONSIDERATIONS FOR PATIENTS WITH SPINAL CORD INJURY

Patients with chronic spinal cord injury (SCI) are at an increased risk for urolithiasis. In addition, up to 85% of these patients with neurologic lesions above the major splanchnic sympathetic outflow (approx T6) are also at risk for autonomic hyperreflexia (AH) *(73)*. AH occurs when noxious stimuli below the neurologic lesion result in reflex sympathetic discharges without appropriate supraspinal control. The most common etiologies are bladder and bowel distention, but any noxious stimuli may induce the reflex. Signs and symptoms of AH include headache, diaphoresis, flushing, hypertension, and bradycardia or tachycardia. In a series of 20 patients with SCI undergoing SWL, one patient experienced AH, with a mean increase of systolic blood pressure by 44 mmHg, diastolic blood pressure by 24 mmHg, and bradycardia with a mean heart rate of 22 bpm *(74)*.

Several case reports have been published documenting the efficacy and safety of SWL and PCNL in patients with SCI *(74–80)*. Although the total number of patients is small, there appears to be a moderate success rate (53–100%) with low risk of AH (0–29%). Patients with SCI undergoing lithotripsy require general anesthesia or neuroaxial blockade (spinal/epidural) to attenuate/prevent AH. Preoperative consideration may include a bowel prep to maximize stone imaging and decrease bowel distention *(74)*. In a study of 69 patients with SCI undergoing urological surgery, laboratory evaluations revealed associated morbidities, including restrictive pulmonary dysfunction (69%), anemia (41%), hypoproteinemia (38%), and renal insufficiency (23%) *(81)*. Intraoperatively, management of AH includes removing the offending stimulus, treating the sympathetic response with antihypertensives and bradycardia with atropine or glycopyrolate *(82,83)*. Tachycardia may be treated with a short-acting beta blocker such as esmolol. Padding all pressure points will also decrease the risk of AH. Postoperatively, these patients continue to be at risk for AH and meticulous attention to pain control and avoidance of bowel/bladder distention are essential. The use of epidural anesthesia with local anesthetic to control AH in the postoperative period has been reported *(84)*.

In summary, patients with chronic spinal cord injury are at an increased risk for urolithiasis and require anesthesia for SWL, PCNL and laser lithotripsy to attenuate or prevent AH.

REFERENCES

1. Morgulis R, Yarmush J, Woglom J, Gelarden B. Alfentanil analgesia/sedation for extracorporeal shock wave lithotripsy: A comparison with general and epidural anesthesia. AANA J 1991; 59(6): 533–537.
2. Gesztesi Z, Sa Rego M, White P. The comparative effectiveness of fentanyl and its newer analogs during extracorporeal shock wave lithotripsy under monitored anesthesia care. Anesth Analg 2000; 90: 567–570.
3. Monk T, Boure B, White P, Meretyk S, Clayman R. Comparison of intravenous sedative-analgesic techniques for outpatient immersion lithotripsy. Anesth Analg 1991; 72: 616–621.
4. Coloma M, Chiu J, White P, Tongier W, Duffy L, Armbruster S. Fast-tracking after immersion lithotripsy: general anesthesia versus monitored anesthesia care. Anesth Analg 2000; 91: 92–96.
5. Beloeil H, Corsia G, Riou B. Remifentanil compared with sufentanil during extra-corporeal shock wave lithotripsy with spontaneous ventilation: a double-blind, randomized study. Br J Anaest 2002; 89(4): 567–570.
6. Burmeister M, Brauer P, Wintruff M, Graefen M, Blanc I, Standl T. A comparison of anaesthetic techniques for shock wave lithotripsy: the use of a remifentanil infusion alone compared to intermittent fentanyl boluses combined with a low dose propofol infusion. Anaesthesia 2002; 57: 877–881.
7. Monk T, Rater J, White P. Comparison of alfentanil and ketamine infusions in combination with midazolam for outpatient lithotripsy. Anesthesiology 1991; 74: 1023–1028.

8. Bierkens AF, Maes RM, Hendrikx JM, Erdos AF, de Vries JD, Debruyne FM. The use of local anesthesia in second generation extracorporeal shock wave lithotripsy: eutectic mixture of local anesthetics. J Urol 1991; 146(2): 287–289.

9. McDonald PF, Berry AM. Topical anaesthesia for extracorporeal shock wave lithotripsy. Br J Anaesth 1992; 69(4): 399, 400.

10. Tiselius H. Cutaneous anesthesia with lidocaine-prilocaine cream: a useful adjunct during shock wave lithotripsy with analgesic sedation. J. Urol 1993; 149: 8–11.

11. Basar H, Yilmaz E, Ozcan S, Buyukkocack U, Sari F, Apan A, Batislam E. Four analgesic techniques for shockwave lithotripsy: eutectic mixture local anesthetic is a good alternative. J Endourol 2003; 17(1): 3–6.

12. Honnens de Lichtenberg M, Miskowiak J, Mogensen P, Andersen JT. Local anesthesia for extracorporeal shock wave lithotripsy: a study comparing eutectic mixture of local anesthetics cream and lidocaine infiltration. J Urol 1992; 147(1): 96, 97.

13. Monk T, Ding Y, White P, Albala D, Clayman R. Effect of topical eutectic mixture of local anesthetics on pain response and analgesic requirement during lithotripsy procedures. Anesth Analg 1994; 79: 506–511.

14. Ganapathy S, Razvi H, Moote C, Parkin J, Yee I, Gverzdys S, Dain S, Denstedt, JD. Eutectic mixture of local anaesthetics is not effective for extracorporeal shock wave lithotripsy. Can J Anaesth 1996; 43(10): 1030–1034.

15. Ozcan S, Yilmaz E, Buyukkocak, Basar H, Apan A. Comparison of three analgesics for extracorporeal shock wave lithotripsy. ScanD J Urol Nephrol 2002; 36: 281–285.

16. Fredman B, Jedeikin R, Olsfanger D, Aronheim M. The opioid-sparing effect of diclofenac sodium in outpatient extracorporeal shock wave lithotripsy (SWL). J. Clin Anesth 1993; 5: 141–144.

17. Parkin J, Keeley FX, Timoney AG. Analgesia for shock wave lithotripsy. J Urol 2002; 167(4): 1613–1615.

18. Kortis HI, Amory DW, Wagner BK, Levin R, Wilson E, Levin A, Pitchford DE, Pollak P. Use of patient-controlled analgesia with alfentanil for extracorporeal shock wave lithotripsy. J Clin Anesth 1995; 7(3): 205–210.

19. Schelling G, Weber W, Mendl G, Braun H, Cullmann H. Patient-controlled analgesia for shock wave lithotripsy: the effect of self-administered alfentanil on pain intensity and drug requirement. J Urol 1996; 155(1): 43–47.

20. Uyar M, Uyar M, Ugur G, Bilge S, Ozyar B, Ozyurt C. Patient-controlled sedation and analgesia during SWL. J Endourol 1996; 10(5): 407–410.

21. Joo H, Perks W, Kataoka M, Errett L, Pace K, Honey R. A comparison of patient-controlled sedation using either remifentanil or remifentanil-propofol for shock wave lithotripsy. Anesth Analg 2001; 93: 1227–1232.

22. Nelson C, Francis T, Wolf S. Comparison of shockwave lithoripsy in patients receiving sufentanil or lidocaine spinal anesthesia. J Endo 2001; 15(5): 473–477.

23. Lau W, Green C, Faerber G, Tait A, Golembiewski J. Intrathecal sufentanil for extracorporeal shock wave lithotripsy provides earlier discharge of the outpatient than intrathecal lidocaine. Anesth Analg 1997; 84: 1227–1231.

24. Eaton M, Chhibber A, Green D. Subarachnoid sufentanil versus lidocaine spinal anesthesia for extracorporeal shock wave lithotripsy. Reg Anesth 1997; 22(6): 515–520.

25. Lau W, Green C, Faerber G, Tait A, Golembiewski J. Determination of the effective therapeutic dose of intrathecal sufentanil for extracorporeal shock wave lithotripsy. Anesth Analg 1999; 89: 889–892.

26. Shenkman Z, Eidelman L, Cotev S. Continuous spinal anaesthesia using a standard epidural set for extracorporeal shockwave lithotripsy. Can J Anaesth 1997; 44(10): 1042–1046.

27. Richardson M, Dooley J. The effects of general versus epidural anesthesia for outpatient extracorporeal shock wave lithotripsy. Anesth Analg 1998; 86: 1214–1218,.

28. Burmeister, M, Standl T, Wintruff M, Brauer P, Blanc I, Schulte am Esch J. Dolasetron prophylaxis reduces nausea and postanesthesia recovery time after remifentanil infusion during monitored anesthesia care for extracorporeal shock wave lithotripsy. Br J Anaesth 2003; 90(2): 194–198.

29. Knudsen F, Jorgensen S, Bonde J, Andersen J, Mogensen P. Anesthesia and complications of extracorporeal shock wave lithotripsy of urinary calculi. J Urol 1992; 148: 1030–1033.

30. Deam R, Scott D. Neurological damage resulting from extracorporeal shock wave lithotripsy when air is used to locate the epidural space. Anaesth Interns Care 1993; 21: 455–457.

31. Streem S. Contemporary clinical practice of shock wave lithotripsy: a reevaluation of contraindications. J Urol 1997; 157: 1197–1203.

32. Carey S, Streem. Extracorporeal shock wave lithotripsy for patients with calcified ipsilateral renal arterial or abdominal aortic aneurysms. J Urol 1992; 148(1): 18–20.

33. Hunter P, Finlayson B, Hirko R, Voreck W, Walker R, Walck S, Nasr M. Measurement of shockwave pressures used for lithotripsy. J Urol 1986; 136: 733–738.

34. Chaussy C. Extracorporeal Shock Wave Lithotripsy. New Aspects in the Treatment of Kidney Stone Disease. S. Karger, New York, NY, 1982.

35. Drach G, Weber C, Donovan J. Treatment of pacemaker patients with extracorporeal shock wave lithotripsy: experience from 2 continents. J Urol 1990; 143(5): 895, 896.

36. Cooper D, Wilkoff B, Masterson M, Castle L, Belco K, Simmons T, Morant V, Streem S, Maloney J. Effects of extracorporeal shock wave lithotripsy on cardiac pacemakers and its safety in patients with implanted cardiac pacemakers. PACE 1998; Pt. 1: 1607–1616.

37. Chung M, Streem S, Ching E, Mowrey K, Wilkoff B. Effects of extracorporeal shock wave lithotripsy on tiered therapy implantable cardioverter defibrillator. PACE 1999; 22(5): 738–742.

38. Greenstein A, Kaver I, Lechtman V, Braf Z. Cardiac arrhythmias during nonsynchronized extracorporeal shock wave lithotripsy. J. Urol 1995; 154: 1321, 1322.

39. Greenstein A, Sofer M, Lidawi G, Matzkin H. Does shock wave lithotripsy of renal stones cause cardiac muscle injury? A troponin I-based study. Urology 2003; 61(5): 902–905.

40. Kaji D, Xie H, Hardy B, Sherrod A, Huffman J. The effects of extracorporeal shock wave lithotripsy on renal growth, function, and arterial blood pressure in an animal model. J Urol 1991; 146: 544–547.

41. Newman D, Coury T, Lingeman J, Mertz J, Mosbaugh P, Steele R, Knapp P. Extracorporeal shock wave lithotripsy experience in children. J Urol 1986; 136: 238–240.

42. Jenkins A, Gillenwater J. Extracorporeal shock wave lithotripsy in the prone position: treatment of stones in the distal ureter or anomalous kidney. J Urol 1988; 139: 911–915.

43. Ackaert K, Dik P, Lock M, Kurth K, Schroder F. Treatment of distal ureteral stones in the horse riding position. J Urol 1989; 142: 955–957.

44. Becht E, Moll V, Neisius D, Ziegler M. Treatment of prevesical ureteral calculi by extracorporeal shock wave lithotriptsy. J Urol 1988; 139: 916–918.

45. Havel K, Saussine C, Fath C, Lang H, Faure F, Jacqmin D. Single tones of the lower pole of the kidney. Comparative results of extracorporeal shock wave lithotripsy and percutaneous nephrolithotomy. Eur Urol 1998; 33(4): 396–400.

46. Mays N, Petruckevitch A, Burney P. Results of one and two year follow-up in a clinical comparison of extracorporeal shock wave lithotripsy and percutaneous nephrolithotomy in the treatment of renal calculi. Scand J Urol Nephrol 1992; 26(1): 43–49.

47. Shoma A, Eraky I, El-Kenawy M, El-Kappany H. Percutaneous nephrolithotomy in the supine position: technical aspects and functional outcome compared with the prone technique. Urology 2002; 60(3): 388–392.

48. Radecka E, Brehmer M, Holmgren K, Magnusson A. Complications associated with percutaneous nephrolithotripsy: supra- versus subcostal access. A retrospective study. Acta Radiol 2003; 44(4): 447–451.

49. Munver R, Delvecchio F, Newman GE, Preminger GM. Critical analysis of supracostal access for percutaneous renal surgery. J Urol 2001; 166(4): 1242–1246.

50. Kekre N, Gopalakrishnan G, Gupta G, Abraham B, Sharma E. Supracostal approach in pecutaneous nephrolithotomy: experience with 102 cases. J Endourol 2001; 15(8): 789–791.

51. Feng M, Tamaddon K, Mikhail A, Kaptein J, Bellman G. Prospective randomized study of various techniques of percutaneous nephrolithotomy. Urology 2001; 58(3): 345–350.

52. Limb J, Bellman GC. Tubeless percutaneous renal surgery: review of first 122 patients. Urology 2002; 59: 527–531.

53. Lojanapiwat B, Soonthornphan S, Wudhikarn S. Tubeless percutaneous nephrolithotomy in selected patients. J Endourol 2001; 15: 711–713.

54. Kikreja R, Desai M, Sabnis R, Patel S. Fluid absorption during percutaneous nephrolithotomy: does it matter? J Endourol 2002; 16(4): 221–224.

55. Roberts S, Bolton DM, Stoller ML. Hypothermia associated with percutaneous nephrolithotomy. Urology 1994; 44(6): 832–835.

56. Kim S, Kuo R, Lingeman J. Percutaneous nephrolithotomy: an update. Curr Opin Urol 2003; 13: 25–241.

57. Gravenstein D. Extracorporeal shock wave lithotripsy and percutaneous nephrolithotomy. Anesthesiol Clin North Am 2000; 18(4): 953–971.

58. Dogan H, Sahin A, Cetinkaya Y, Akdogan B, Ozden E, Kendi S. Antibiotic prophylaxis in percutaneous nephrolithotomy: prospective study in 81 patients. J Endourol 2002; 16(9): 649–653.

59. Andreoni C, Olweny E, Portis A, Sundaram C, Monk T, Clayman R. Effect of single-dose subarachnoid spinal anesthesia on pain and recovery after unilateral percutaneous nephrolithotomy. J Endourol 2002; 16(10): 721–725.

60. Leveillee R, Lobik L. Intracorporeal lithotripsy: which modality is best? Curr Opin Urol 2003; 13: 249–253.

61. Watterson J, Girvan A, Cook A, Beiko D, Nott L, Auge B, Preminger G, Denstedt J. Safety and efficacy of holmium:YAG laser lithotripsy in patients with bleeding diatheses. J Urol 2002; 168(2): 442–445.

62. Sofer M, Watterson J, Wollin T, Nott L, Razvi H, Denstedt J. Holmium:YAG laser lithotripsy for upper urinary tract calculi in 598 patients. J Urol 2002; 167(1): 31–34.

63. Watterson J, Girvan A, Beiko D, Nott L, Wollin T, Razvi H, Denstedt J. Ureteroscopy and holmium:YAG laser lithotripsy: an emerging definitive management strategy for symptomatic ureteral calculi in pregnancy. Urology 2002; 60(3): 383–387.

64. Lam J, Greene T, Gupta M. Treatment of proximal ureteral calculi: holmium:YAG laser ureterolithotripsy versus extracorporeal shock wave lithotripsy. J Urol 2002; 167: 1972–1976.

65. Yip S, Lee F, Tam P, Leung S. Outpatient treatment of middle and lower ureteric stones: extracorporeal shock wave lithotripsy versus ureteroscopic laser lithotripsy. Ann Acad Med Singapore 1998; 27(4): 515–519.

66. Teichman J, Vassar G, Bishoff J, Bellman G. Holmium:YAG lithotripsy yields smaller fragments than lithoclast, pulsed dye laser or electrohydraulic lithotripsy. J Urol 1998; 159(1): 17–23.

67. Cheung M, Lee F, Leung Y, Wong B, Tam P. A prospective randomized controlled trial on ureteral stenting after ureteroscopic holmium laser lithotripsy. J Urol 2003; 169(4): 1257–1560.

68. Denstedt J, Wollin T, Sofer M, Nott L, Weir M, D'A Honey R. A prospective randomized controlled trial comparing nonstented versus stented ureteroscopic lithotripsy. J Urol 2001; 165(5): 1419–1422.

69. Carringer M, Swartz R, Johansson J. Management of ureteric calculi during pregnancy by ureteroscopy and laser lithotripsy. Br J Urol 1996; 77(1): 17–20.

70. Andreoni C, Afane J, Olweny E, Clayman R. Flexible ureteroscopic lithotripsy; first-line therapy for proximal ureteral and renal calculi in the morbidly obese and superobese patient. J Endourol 2001; 15:493–498.

71. Wollin T, Teichman J, Rogenes V, Razvi H, Denstedt J, Grasso M. Holmium:YAG lithotripsy in children. J Urol 1999; 162(5): 1717–1720.

72. Lee D, Bagley D. Long-term effects of ureteroscopic laser lithotripsy on glomerular filtration rate in the face of mild to moderate renal insufficiency. J Endourol 2001; 15: 715–717.

73. Colachis S. Autonomic hyperreflexia with spinal cord injury. J Am Paraplegia Soc 1992; 15(3): 171–186.

74. Kabalin J, Lennon S, Gill H, Wolfe V, Perkash I. Incidence and management of autonomic dysreflexia and other intraoperative problems encountered in spinal cord injury patients undergoing extracorporeal shock wave lithotripsy without anesthesia on a second generation lithotriptor. J Urol 1993; 149(5): 1064–1067.

75. Kilciler M, Sumer F, Bedir S, Ozgok Y, Erduran D. Extracorporeal shock wave lithotripsy treatment in paraplegic patients with bladder stones. Int J Urol 2002; 9(11): 632–634.

76. Kobayashi N, Yoshida K, Uchijima Y, Takeuchi S, Tosaka A, Saitoh H. Extracorporeal shock wave lithotripsy on patients with spinal cord injury with special reference to autonomic hyperreflexia. Hinyokika Kiyo 1995; 41(2): 107–111.

77. Robert M, Bennani A, Ohanna F, Guiter J, Averous M, Grasset D. The management of upper urinary tract calculi by piezoelectric extracorporeal shock wave lithotripsy in spinal cord injury patients. Paraplegia 1991; 33(3): 132–135.

78. Niedrach W, Davis R, Tonetti F, Cockett A. Extracorporeal shock-wave lithotripsy in patients with spinal cord dysfunction. Urology 1991; 38(2): 152–156.

79. Chang C, Chen M, Chang L. Autonomic hyperreflexia in spinal cord injury patient during percutaneous nephrolithotomy for renal stone: a case report. J Urol 1991; 146(6): 1601, 1602.

80. Culkin D, Wheeler J, Nemchausky B, Fruin R, Canning J. Percutaneous nephrolithotomy: spinal cord injury vs. ambulatory patients. J Am Paraplegia Soc 1990; 13(2): 4–6.

81. Okuyama A, Ueda M, Morimoto Y, Okuyama M, Kemmotsu O. Anesthetic management for urological surgery of patients with chronic spinal cord injury. Masui 1994; 43(7): 1033–1037.

82. Burnstein A, Richlin D, Sotolongo J. Nifedipine pretreatment for prevention of autonomic hyperreflexia during anesthesia-free extracorporeal shock wave lithotripsy. J Urol 1992; 147(3): 676, 677.

83. Dykstra D, Sidi A, Anderson L. The effect of nifedipine on cystoscopy-induced autonomic hyperreflexia in patients with high spinal cord injuries. J Urol 1987; 138(5):1155–1157.

84. Murphy D, McGuire G, Peng P. Treatment of autonomic hyperreflexia in a quadriplegic patient by epidural anesthesia in the postoperative period. Anesth Analg 1999; 89(1): 148, 149.

27 Complications of Urinary Stone Surgery

Ruben Urena, MD, Freddy Mendez-Torres, MD, and Raju Thomas, MD

Key Words: Infection; hemorrhage; complication; fistula.

INTRODUCTION

The surgical treatment of urinary tract calculi has changed enormously during the past two decades. With advances in fiberoptics, development of flexible instrumentation, and the widespread use of extracorporeal shockwave lithotripsy (SWL), open stone surgery (OSS) has mostly been replaced by minimally invasive procedures for managing both renal and ureteral calculi.

The trend of urologists involved in the management of patients with urinary tract stones is to choose the less invasive and more effective treatment modality, based on patient and stone characteristics. Among these minimally invasive techniques available are SWL, percutaneous nephrostolithotripsy (PCNL), retrograde ureteroscopic intrarenal surgery (RIRS), and laparoscopic stone surgery. Not infrequently, some of these techniques are used in combination in the treatment of complex stone disease, wherein SWL is combined with either PCNL (sandwich technique) or with RIRS.

As new and less invasive modalities and techniques have emerged, so has the awareness of identifying and treating associated complications.

From: Current Clinical Urology, *Urinary Stone Disease:*
A Practical Guide to Medical and Surgical Management
Edited by: M. L. Stoller and M. V. Meng © Humana Press Inc., Totowa, NJ

COMPLICATIONS OF EXTRACORPOREAL
SHOCKWAVE LITHOTRIPSY

The first clinical application of extracorporeal shockwave lithotripsy was reported by Chaussy et al. *(1)* in 1980. It received FDA approval in the United States in 1984 *(2)*. Since then, SWL indications have increased and gained widespread acceptance for the management of renal and ureteral lithiasis.

All lithotriptors rely on the coordination of their four basic components: (a) shockwave source, (b) shockwave focusing, (c) shockwave coupling, and (d) stone imaging. Knowing the basic functioning principles of a given lithotriptor is crucial for urologists to help select the one which will provide the best results while minimizing complications.

Shockwave generators are categorized according to their energy source. The three commercially available energy sources for lithotriptors are: (a) electrohydraulic, (b) piezoelectric, and (c) electromagnetic. Electrohydraulic energy is produced by applying electrical current between two electrodes; the spark-gap between the electrodes then produces a shockwave within a fluid medium that diverges from the point of origin to an ellipsoid or parabolic reflector, where it is reflected and redirected toward the second focal point where the stone is located. Varying the voltage applied to the electrode controls the intensity of shockwave energy. In piezoelectric generators, electrical current is applied to a dish containing an array of piezoelectric crystals. The vibration of the hemispherically arranged piezoelectric crystals generates a shockwave that converges at the target site. In electromagnetic generators, electric current is applied to a magnetic coil within a metallic membrane. The rapid movement of the metallic membrane generates a shockwave that is focused with an acoustic lens or parabolic reflector to the focal point where the lithiasis is located.

Clinical Expectations

With appropriate patient selection, 80 to 85% of simple renal calculi can be satisfactorily treated with SWL *(3–5)*. To get maximum stone fragmentation and to assure its elimination, patients' anatomic and stone characteristics should be considered. The stone-related factors include size, number, location, and composition; the patients' characteristics include the presence of a dependent or obstructed collecting system, body habitus, and weight *(6)*. Alternative treatment modalities, such as PCNL, have been recommended under such circumstances.

Although numerous reports have proven SWL to be safe, easy to use, and noninvasive *(7)*, it is often recognized as a form of trauma similar to renal contusions and occasionally resulting in adverse clinical sequelae *(8)*. Complications can present either from stone fragmentation or from the effects of the shockwaves as they penetrate tissue.

Stone Localization Technique

Either ultrasound (US) or fluoroscopy can be used for stone localization. Fluoroscopy allows for accurate "live" imaging of both renal and ureteral stones. The use of ultrasound avoids radiation exposure and allows for radiolucent stone localization. The use of lithotriptors which combines both fluoroscopic and US imaging modalities may improve stone localization while reducing or avoiding the risks of radiation exposure.

Shockwaves are directed and concentrated toward a defined focal point (F2), where the stone is located. The focal volume of the lithotriptors impacts the amount of tissue exposed to the shockwaves. Electrohydraulic lithotriptors are associated with a larger focal volume, thus delivering more shockwave energy and better stone fragmentation, but exposing surrounding body tissue to unnecessary shockwaves and producing more pain at the skin entry site. Piezoelectric lithotriptors have smaller focal volumes, and because of a low energy density at the skin entry site, are less painful.

First generation lithotriptors achieved shockwave coupling through a water bath. Thereafter, generations replaced the water bath for water cushions coated with acoustic gel, which allows for easier patient positioning.

Factors Affecting Fragmentation

The degree of stone fragmentation after lithotripsy depends on various factors. These include stone composition and fragility, stone burden (size and number), stone location, and the type of lithotriptor used. When adjusted for stone size, cystine and calcium oxalate monohydrate stones are the most resistant to SWL *(9–11)*. Next, in descending order, are hydroxyapatite, struvite, calcium oxalate dihydrate, and uric acid stones *(12,13)*. Stone composition can also affect the type of fragments produced. Struvite, uric acid, and calcium phosphate dihydrate fracture into smaller fragments that can be easily passed. On the other hand, cystine, brushite, and calcium oxalate monohydrate are difficult to fragment and are likely to produce relatively large fragments and, thus, are less likely to be eliminated *(12,14)*. Generally, brushite and calcium oxalate monohydrate stones less than 1.5 cm should be treated with SWL. For larger stones, PCNL or RIRS, if feasible, should be considered.

Complications Related To Stone Fragments

Much of the morbidity associated with SWL treatment results from the fate of the fragmented calculus. SWL can result in incomplete stone fragmentation, residual calculi, steinstrasse, and/or ureteral obstruction. Patients with lithiasis and an associated obstruction, such as ureteropelvic junction obstruction (UPJO), calyceal diverticulum, or distal ureteral obstructive calculus, have poor outcomes after SWL therapy unless their obstructive process is addressed first.

Stone Burden

Stone burden is perhaps the single most important factor in determining the appropriate treatment modality for the management of renal calculi *(15)* (Fig. 1). Initial studies reported stone-free rates of 91% for renal stones ≤ 2 cm *(16)*. More recently, the mean stone-free rates following SWL therapy for nonstaghorn renal calculi stratified by size have been reported as 79.9% for stones ≤ 1 cm (63–90% range), 64.1% for 1–2 cm stones (50–82.7% range), and 53.7% for stones >2 cm (33.3–81.4% range), and 27% at three mo for those >3 cm, with 77% of these patients requiring re-treatment *(17–22)*. For staghorn calculi, the overall stone-free rate with SWL monotherapy was found to be 51.2%, with 30.5% of patients requiring auxiliary procedures *(8)*. There exists an inverse relationship between SWL results and stone burden; the higher the stone burden, the lower the stone-free rates with a higher need for ancillary procedures and re-treatments. SWL should thus be considered as a first-line management for renal stones ≤ 2 cm, although stone composition and location have to be taken into consideration in the 1–2 cm group. For stones >2 cm, endoscopic treatment (i.e., PCNL, RIRS) should be considered as initial treatment, rather than SWL.

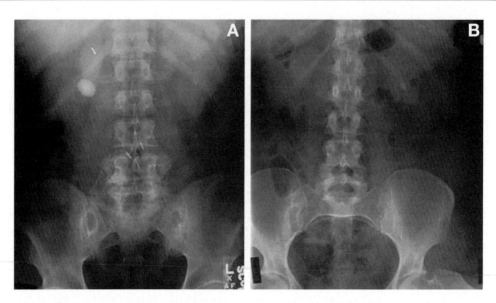

Fig. 1. (A) Right renal pelvic stone. **(B)** Adequate fragmentation and passage of <2-cm stone in the right renal pelvis.

Stone Location

Stone location has an impact on SWL outcome, with different stone-free results achieved depending on the location of the stones within the calyceal system. For upper and middle calyces, stone-free rates of 70–90% have been reported *(23)*. On the contrary, lower pole stones (LPS) have had limited success following SWL because of increased difficulty in passing fragments. In 1994, Lingeman et al. *(19)* reported an overall stone-free rate of 59% in a meta-analysis of patients with LPS treated with SWL. When stratified by stone size, the meta-analysis revealed stone-free rates of 74%, 56%, and 33% for stones ≤1 cm, 1.1–2 cm, and >2 cm, respectively. More recently, in 2001, the Lower Pole Study Group reported an overall stone-free rate of 37% for LPS after SWL, with only 21% of patients being rendered stone-free when the calculus was >1 cm. They concluded that PCNL should be considered the primary approach for LPS larger than 1 cm *(24)*.

Poor stone localization can lead to incomplete or poor stone fragmentation, which can result from stone migration, radiolucency, inadequate imaging equipment or technique, and the patient's body habitus. Constant fluoroscopic or ultrasonic imaging allows for realignment of the stone in case of stone movement or migration. In case of radiolucent stones, either intravenous urography or retrograde contrast injection through a ureteral catheter must be administered to identify the stone as a filling defect *(25)*. Sundaram et al. *(26)* described a technique in which a 4-Fr whistle tip ureteral catheter is passed alongside a previously inserted 6-Fr double-J stent and its tip positioned in the lower or mid third of the ureter for contrast material injection during lithotripsy. They found it to be successful in localizing radiolucent and poorly calcified renal stones during lithotripsy despite the presence of a double-J stent. Patient's body habitus, such as morbid obesity, skeletal anomalies (i.e., spinal deformity, limb contraction), and ectopic kidneys can make stone localization challenging. The increased distance from the skin surface to the stone in obese patients may not position the stone adequately within the lithotriptor's focal zone. US can be used to measure such distance pretreatment, so that a lithotriptor machine with a greater focal length and higher peak pressures (27,28) can be used to prevent ineffective SWL in these patients. The Medstone lithotriptor has been found to be advantageous to locate and treat lower third ureteral stones. This lithotriptor pinpoints the stone at the F2 point with remarkable ease as opposed to lithotriptors using fluoroscopy (29).

Although many patients have successful stone fragmentation after SWL, not all have complete passage of these stone fragments. Stone fragment passage varies over time according to several reported series. Drach et al. (30) described that up to 85% of patients have radiologic evidence of residual fragments in the kidney a few days after SWL. Others have reported spontaneous passage of most fragments during the first 3 mo after SWL (2,31,32), whereas others have reported continued fragment clearance up to 24 mo after treatment (33).

Residual Stone Fragments

The concept of clinically insignificant residual fragments (CIRF) after SWL was first introduced to describe stone fragments smaller than 5 mm, not composed of struvite, in asymptomatic patients with sterile urine (34). It is reported to be present in 12–30% of patients after SWL (33). However, concerns remain whether CIRF are really clinically insignificant. Streem et al. (33) and Zanetti et al. (35) at follow-up evaluations reported residual stones less than 4 mm in size after SWL to subsequently become symptomatic and/or required intervention in 43% and 22% of patients, respectively. Candau et al. (36) emphasized the importance of the size of the residual fragment, ≤2 mm vs 2–4 mm, as a risk factor for becoming symptomatic.

Besides the probability of small residual fragments becoming symptomatic or requiring intervention, they might act as a nidus for stone growth or increase the rate of regrowth. Stone recurrence rates have been much higher when stone fragments are present than when patients have been rendered completely stone free (17–80% vs 6–15%, respectively) (31,34,35,37–40). Similarly, Streem at al. (33) reported in a prospective study that residual fragments <4 mm after SWL were found to increase in size in 18%, decrease in 16%, and remain stable in 42%.

Residual stones from infectious stones can lead to postoperative bacteriuria, recurrent or antibiotic-resistant urinary tract infections, be a focus for septicemia, and lead to an increase in stone size (nidus). In case of metabolic stone disease, a stone-free status is encouraged, not just to prevent recurrences but to prolong the treatment intervals (17). Given the negative impact and long-term morbidity associated with residual fragments, the need of achieving a complete stone-free status in all patients cannot be overemphasized.

Steinstrasse and Management

Steinstrasse, or "stone street," is described as a long column of stone fragments within the ureter after SWL (41) (Fig. 2). It is a well-known complication after SWL treatment of larger renal and ureteral calculi. Different series have reported an incidence of 1–6%, with results varying using different types of lithotriptors (42–45). Its occurrence is related to the size and composition of the calculus being treated, the presence of a concomitant distal ureteral obstruction (i.e., calculus or stricture), and to the effectiveness of the lithotriptor in adequately fragmenting the stone.

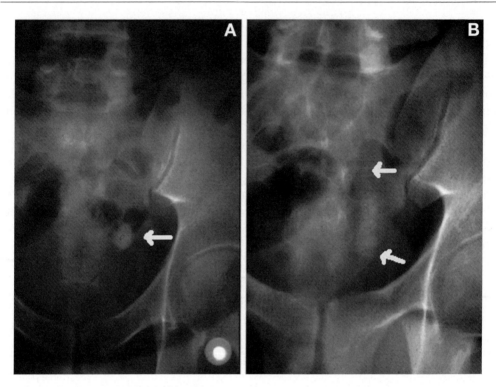

Fig. 2. (A) Large ureteral stone (arrow). **(B)** Same ureteral stone after SWL showing steinstrasse (between arrows) and renal obstruction.

Most steinstrasse are short, transient, and asymptomatic, or are passed causing just mild discomfort. However, larger steinstrasse can produce partial or complete ureteral obstruction and become symptomatic and/or cause sepsis. In this latter case, its early recognition and prompt management avoid escalation of symptoms and risk of urosepsis. Anuria may complicate steinstrasse in case of an obstructed solitary kidney or after bilateral SWL. In almost a third of patients, obstruction may be silent *(46)*, leading to ipsilateral renal function deterioration. In the absence of symptoms, silent obstruction can be ruled out with follow up renal US or intravenous pyelogram (IVP).

A decision to place a ureteral stent should be made after all the risk factors for steinstrasse development have been taken into consideration. Pre-SWL ureteral stents initially allow for the passage of urine and gravel through and around it, respectively. It is believed that the urine that refluxes from the bladder back to the kidney through the ureteral stent is responsible for contributing to ureteral peristalsis, which then aids to propel urine and gravel down to the bladder *(47)*. With time, the ureteral stent also produces passive ureteral dilation *(48,49)*, and this allows for passage of larger fragments.

Routine use of ureteral stents is not advocated because its use is not without associated potential morbidity. It has been found to produce discomfort and intolerance that may require its removal and even to have caused obstruction by itself *(50)*. Besides this, it increases the level of invasiveness and cost associated with delivery of SWL *(51)*.

Much debate has existed with regard to proper pre-SWL stenting based on stone size. Low et al. *(52)* found that placement of double J stents for improving stone-free rates, alleviating pain, or preventing ureteral obstruction in conjunction with SWL of solitary renal calculi <20 mm in diameter was unnecessary. In a study of 1087 patients, with stones ranging in size from 10 to 95 mm, Sulaiman et al. *(43)* reported that the use of ureteral stents had no effect on the incidence of steinstrasse for patients with lithiasis <2 cm, but they did find a much lower likelihood of steinstrasse and steinstrasse-associated symptoms in patients with lithiasis >2 cm in whom a stent was placed before SWL. Similarly, Al-Awadi et al. *(53)* found that the use of pre-SWL stents significantly lowered the incidence of steinstrasse in patients with a stone burden of 1.5–3.5 cm, and that the incidence of steinstrasse increased with the size of the calculi, whether a stent was placed before SWL or not. Despite the lack of evidence to support the use of stents in uncomplicated cases with smaller stones, a survey done by the American Urological Association revealed that one-fourth of the respondents use pre-SWL stent for renal pelvic stones up to 1 cm in size, and that more than half routinely stent patients with renal calculi of 1.5 cm *(54)*.

Patient selection is the key for steinstrasse prevention. The risks, benefits, and costs of pre-SWL ureteral stenting should be weighed. Although ureteral stents may not prevent steinstrasse nor improve stone-free rates in patients with larger stones, they prevent obstruction from steinstrasse and are recommended in patients with stone burden >2 cm *(43,44,51)*. Similarly, although associated with more irritative symptoms, pre-SWL ureteral stent placement is recommended when treating solitary kidneys with lithiasis 10–20 mm or solitary proximal ureteral stones <2 cm because they are associated with fewer hospital readmissions and emergency room visits *(55)*, besides assisting in stone localization.

The management of steinstrasse depends on the clinical situation. Asymptomatic or minimally symptomatic steinstrasse can often be managed conservatively as long as there is no risk of jeopardizing the renal function; in these cases, spontaneous stone clearance has been found to occur in 60–86% *(44,46,51,56)*. The treatment options for symptomatic steinstrasse vary according to its location in the ureter, size, grade of ureteral obstruction, and presence of urinary infection. They include percutaneous or endoscopic retrograde drainage and SWL. Steinstrasse should be treated in all cases when: conservative management fails, pain is refractory to medical treatment, there is distal unilateral or bilateral obstruction, obstruction in a solitary kidney, and/or urosepsis. Under any of these circumstances, prompt urinary tract decompression should be considered with either a retrograde stent placement or a percutaneous nephrostomy.

Most short steinstrasse clear without requiring any intervention, as reported by Kim et al. *(56)*, with 64% of their patients having steinstrasse of an average length of 2.6 cm, and being treated conservatively. The use of prophylactic antibiotics is recommended when conservative management is chosen, as well as are frequent radiologic and ultrasound examinations. Failure of steinstrasse to resolve with expectant management within 3–4 wk may necessitate intervention *(58)*. Whenever intervention is required, the least invasive and more effective procedure is advocated.

In situ SWL, in the absence of a distal obstruction and/or sepsis, can be used either for steinstrasse in the upper and lower ureter or for a leading ureteral calculus fragment. Success rates of up to 90% with minimal complications have been reported for repeated SWL *(43,56)*. *In situ* repeat SWL either disintegrates the lead fragment or mechanically loosens it *(44)*. Ureteroscopy with intracorporeal lithotripsy alone and/or with stone basket extraction are often used in uncomplicated cases of simple steinstrasse (column of gravel <5 cm and without urosepsis) *(59)* or in cases of a large ureteral leading fragment, whenever a guidewire can be passed beyond the obstruction. Even though success rates of almost 100% have been achieved with ureteroscopy *(43,58,60)*, caution is warranted because of a higher risk of ureteral perforation in these cases *(53)*. For steinstrasse in the distal ureter, either SWL or ureteroscopy could be attempted.

Complex steinstrasse with associated sepsis, or the inability to pass a guidewire through the site of obstruction, is an indication for percutaneous drainage. Percutaneous nephrostomy drainage alone, besides relieving obstruction and/or infection, decreases the intrapelvic pressure, which re-establishes ureteric peristalsis and thus permits the passage of stone fragments in up to 75% of cases *(44,58)*. PCNL can also be used for steinstrasse with or without ureterorenoscopy. In case of a combined approach, an antegrade guidewire can be passed through the nephrostomy tract and aid in the retrograde ureteroscopic approach. Ureteral meatomy *(61)* to facilitate fragment passage and retrograde steinstrasse irrigation *(62)* have been reported, but are rarely used today.

In summary, given the high likelihood of associated morbidity, if a patient has a high probability of steinstrasse formation, close follow-up with early intervention or prophylactic pre-SWL ureteral stenting should be considered *(45)*.

Infection

Many stones may harbor bacteria even though bacteriuria is only intermittently present, especially in patients who have been treated previously with antibiotics. It has been documented that in 5–16% of patients undergoing SWL, bacteriuria will develop despite a sterile urine culture before lithotripsy *(63)*. However, only 2–3% of these patients develop a symptomatic urinary tract infection (UTI) *(63)*. No significant correlation was found between the occurrence of bacteriuria and the number and size of the stones, nor was there any correlation between bacteriuria and the stone-free rate or the location of the calculi after SWL therapy *(64)*. There is evidence that urine cultures may not be a reliable indicator of bacteria within stones, making it difficult to predict all patients in whom infectious complications might develop after SWL.

Fragmentation of infectious stones, despite sterile urine, may release preformed bacterial endotoxins and viable bacteria into the surrounding medium that may be later absorbed systemically. The renal trauma and microvasculature disruption associated with SWL allow bacteria to enter the bloodstream. Although bacteremia has been reported in up to 14% after SWL *(65)*, the overall reported incidence of sepsis related to SWL therapy is less than 1% and 2.7% for nonstaghorn calculi and staghorn calculi, respectively *(66)*. The risk of sepsis increases if the urine culture is positive before SWL and especially in the presence of obstruction *(67)*. Therefore, bacteriologic evaluation of the urine is recommended in these patients and SWL should be performed only in cases in which there is no evidence of urinary tract infection and distal obstruction.

Controversy exists regarding the routine use of prophylactic antibiotics in SWL. Dincel et al. *(64)* found that there was a significantly higher risk of UTI in patients with struvite stones than in those with other types of stones (17.3% vs 2.1%). They concluded that although prophylactic antimicrobial therapy was justifiable among patients with a history of UTI or a suspected struvite stone, even in the absence of bacteriuria, it was of little value in patients with a calcium oxalate or calcium phosphate stone. Bierkens et al. *(68)*, in a prospective, placebo-controlled randomized study corroborated these findings. They noted that in a group of patients with documented sterile urine who received prophylactic antibiotics immediately before and after SWL, and a controlled group, the incidence of pyuria or bacteriuria did not change and that in both groups only 2–3% of the patients eventually had clinical and bacteriological signs of a UTI within 6 wk of SWL. Similarly, Clayman and colleagues *(63)* explained that their SWL treatment policy had changed and that only patients with a suspected struvite stone or those undergoing ureteral stent placements before lithotripsy received prophylactic antibiotics.

On the other hand, in a meta-analysis of multiple randomized studies, Pearle and Roehrborn *(69)* concluded that antibiotic prophylaxis before SWL in patients with sterile pretreatment urine cultures was efficacious in reducing the rate of post-SWL UTIs, and that it was both efficacious and cost-effective in all patients undergoing SWL when the need for inpatient treatment of urosepsis or pyelonephritis was taken into consideration. Preoperative antibiotics should thus be administered to patients who have radiographic or clinical features suggestive of infectious stones (i.e., struvite, staghorn calculus), in whom infection is highly suspected or with a positive urine culture, in patients with recurrent UTI, and in those undergoing any kind of endoscopic instrumentation associated with SWL.

Although less common, other infectious complications of SWL have been described. They include perinephric and psoas abscess, miliary tuberculosis, endocarditis, fungal and bacterial endophthalmitis, and death *(70–77)*. Knowledge of the potential existence of these infectious complications, coupled with early recognition and proper management, will minimize posttreatment morbidity.

Complications Secondary to Effects of SWL on Tissue: Renal Complications

BLEEDING

A variety of renal injuries can occur after SWL. Among these, the most common presenting sign is gross hematuria. Hematuria is commonly seen without clinical significance and usually resolves within the first 12 h *(2,78)*. It has been observed in patients receiving more than 2000 shocks *(2,78)*, and to occur regardless of the type of lithotriptor used. Although initially believed to be urothelial injury caused by stone fragments, it is now known to be the direct result from shockwave induced renal injury. Animal models without renal calculi produced parenchymal injury and hematuria following shockwave lithotripsy with either HM-3 or a piezoelectric lithotriptor *(79,80)*, as did patients who underwent biliary lithotripsy *(81)*. These studies confirm that hematuria resulted secondary to the renal injury from the shockwaves and not from the shock effect on the calculus.

Shockwave-induced renal trauma has been studied and identified radiographically, histopathologically, and by means of biochemical and isotope markers. In 63–85% of patients treated with SWL, renal injuries were noted with US, CT, MRI or quantitative radionuclide renography studies *(82–85)*. Radiographically, the renal lesions more frequently noted include perirenal hematoma, renal enlargement, renal fracture, loss of corticomedullary junction demarcation, and low signal intensity changes in perirenal fat *(86)*. Among these, hemorrhage and edema within or around the kidney are the most often seen. Diffuse or focal kidney enlargement and loss of corticomedullary junction are present in cases of intrarenal edema. MRI and CT scans have been proven to be more sensitive than ultrasound in detecting and monitoring these renal structural changes after SWL treatment *(84,87)*.

The urinary elevation of several enzymes and proteins has been used as biochemical markers to document shockwave injury to nephrons and the surrounding soft tissues. The elevated biochemical markers include proximal tubular enzymes, such as N-acetyl-β-D-glucosaminidase and β-galactosidase, renal brush border epithelial cells enzymes, γ-glutamyltransaminase and angiotensin converting enzyme and renal tubular enzymes β-microglobulin, as well as urothelial glycosaminoglycan and glucose, proteins, and immunoglobulin G alterations in cases of diffuse renal trauma *(88–101)*. Although most studies have found significant elevated levels of these biochemical markers, Krongrad et al. *(102)* did not find a statistically significant increase of these tubular enzymes, suggesting that their elevation was a result of a tubular defect in association with stone disease and not a response to SWL treatment. Other less specific markers have also been found to be transiently elevated after SWL, but are not just associated with shockwave-related injury to the kidney but also to adjacent organs and soft tissues. These include alkaline phosphatase, lactic dehydrogenase, glutamic-pyruvic transaminase, glutamic-oxaloacetic transaminase, C-reactive protein, S-100 protein, and creatinine kinase.

Histopathologic studies in animals and humans have also documented acute changes in the kidneys and surrounding tissues after SWL. Tubular, vascular, and interstitial changes have been localized to the plane of the pressure wave, in which disruption of the renal parenchymal cells have been found, as well as degenerative changes and accumulation of hemosiderin granules and cast material *(103)*. Dilation of veins with evidence of endothelial damage and thrombus formation was among the alterations found within the microvasculature *(103)*. The effect of increasing the number of shockwaves is translated into a higher rate of damage to the nephrons and especially to small- and medium-sized blood vessels within the F2 range. This explains why although electrohydraulic lithotriptors produce a larger lesion, electromagnetic lithotriptors, because of more cellular destruction at F2, are associated with a higher rate of subcapsular hemorrhage.

Retroperitoneal hematomas have been documented radiographically in intraparenchymal, subcapsular, and perirenal locations. These hematomas have been found to be produced primarily as a result of shockwave-induced vascular insult to thin-walled veins and walls of small arteries and glomerular and peritubular capillaries. Rupture of these interlobular and arcuate veins located in the corticomedullary junction makes this region of the kidney more vulnerable to SWL-related intrarenal hematoma and hemorrhage. Histopathology analysis after SWL has shown that although glomerular atrophy and sclerosis, as well as interstitial fibrosis and hyalinization of arcuate veins, are present, the rest of the renal parenchyma appears normal *(89,104)*, suggesting that SWL-related renal injury is focal and that this does not affect the majority of the renal parenchyma.

Perirenal and subcapsular fluid collections, either from bleeding or urine, occur in 24–32% of patients after SWL *(78,83,84)*. Their appearances vary from mild intraparenchymal contusions to large hematomas. Most hematomas are usually asymptomatic, with symptomatic hematomas being reported in less than 1% of patients *(105,106)*. These hematomas are more commonly found in hypertensive patients, especially those with poor blood pressure control at the time of treatment, and among patients on antiplatelet medication *(84,107,108)*. Other risk factors for increased hemorrhage and also related to vascular disorders, are advanced arteriosclerosis, primary coagulopathic disorders, diabetes mellitus, coronary artery disease, and obesity *(109,110)*. No correlation in the occurrence of hematomas was found when the voltage applied and number of shockwaves administered were evaluated *(109,110)*.

Although patients with uncorrected coagulopathies and thrombocytopenia have higher risk of hematoma formation, SWL has been successfully performed among both hemophiliac patients and patients with bleeding diathesis after adequate preoperative work up and corrective measures *(111,112)*. Most renal hematomas are managed conservatively. Perirenal fluid collection reabsorbs within a few days, whereas subcapsular hematomas may take from 6 wk to 6 mo to resolve radiographically *(88,113,114)*. Surgical management may be warranted in cases of persisting symptomatic renal hematomas or progressive renal function impairment *(106,115)*. Rarely, large hematomas may need blood transfusions or may produce a state of acute renal failure, which may result in death if the condition is not recognized and treated promptly.

RENAL FUNCTION POST-SHOCKWAVE LITHOTRIPSY

Ever since the early studies on the use of SWL were reported, efforts have been made to address its effects on renal function. To date, it has not been convincingly proven whether renal function is altered in all patients undergoing SWL, or if only in a subset of patients who are at risk. It is not clearly understood whether patients with two kidneys tolerate SWL therapy better than patients with just one kidney. Although acute renal failure has been described, the condition can be reversible *(116)* or associated with renal loss owing to either the presence of perirenal hematomas or silent obstruction *(117)*.

Extensive animal studies have been performed to evaluate the effects of SWL on glomerular filtration rate (GFR) and renal plasma flow (RPF). Willis et al. *(118)* first studied the effects of SWL on renal hemodynamics in anesthetized minipigs with and without pretreatment with verapamil. They found a significantly acute reduction in GFR and RPF of the shocked kidneys, as well as a significant reduction of the RPF of the contralateral unshocked kidney, but not of its GFR. Verapamil was found to blunt the SWL-induced reductions of urine flow, GFR, and RPF in the shocked kidneys and to eliminate the reduction of RPF in the unshocked kidneys. In another study using uninephrectomized and binephric minipigs, Willis et al. *(119)* found that although a reduction in GFR and RPF after SWL occurred in both groups, no differences were found in whole-animal GFR and RPF in either group before or after SWL. They attributed this to the compensatory renal hypertrophy and improved hemodynamics in solitary kidneys, which may acutely attenuate the renal vasoconstrictive effect of SWL *(119)*.

Similar results have been achieved after studying the effects of SWL on renal function in humans. Kaude et al. *(78)* and Thomas et al. *(85)* found an immediate decrease in effective renal plasma flow, measured by renal scans, in 30% of kidneys treated with SWL. The decrease in renal function has been related to the number of shocks received by the shocked nephron units at F2, where a transient reduction of intrarenal blood flow was observed *(120–122)*. These studies indicate that renal function is adversely affected acutely in some patients after SWL and that the primary change appears to be a vasoconstrictive response resulting in a decrease in both GFR and RPF.

BILATERAL SHOCKWAVE LITHOTRIPSY

Long-term studies of the role of SWL on renal function show variable results. Some studies have reported a reduction on GFR or an increase of serum creatinine whereas others found no difference. Five years after shockwave lithotripsy, Brito et al. *(123)* noted a 40% rise in serum creatinine and a 10% fall in the estimated RPF rate in seven patients. Cass *(20)* reported a significant decrease in GFR of >20% in 18% and 13% of patients after simultaneous bilateral SWL and after SWL to solitary kidneys, respectively. Thomas et al. *(85)* reported a statistically significant decrease in renal function RPF with synchronous bilateral SWL treatment. At 4.5 yr after shockwave lithotripsy in patients with a solitary kidney, Chandhoke et al. *(124)* also noted a decrease of 22% in the GFR, which was similar to the 29% long-term reduction in renal function recorded after percutaneous nephrolithotomy in solitary kidneys. SWL-induced renal trauma results in a potential focal scarring and a mild decrease in renal function, but this is less than that produced by PCNL.

Neal et al. confirmed that consecutive bilateral SWL treatments produced a significant overall loss of effective RPF among infant Rhesus monkeys treated with high dose 18 kilovolts (kV), 2000 shocks as opposed to the ones treated with low dose 15 kV, 1500 shocks *(125)*. Bilateral synchronous SWL has also been reported to be relatively safe and without risk of renal failure or deterioration of renal function in patients with bilateral urolithiasis. No clinical difference in the long-term effect on renal function, as measured by serum creatinine, was found in patients with bilateral renal calculi treated with SWL in a simultaneous vs a staged fashion *(126)*. Perry et al. *(127)* found bilateral synchronous SWL to be safe and effective monotherapy for bilateral urolithiasis. There was no renal function deterioration as per mean serum creatinine, which was found to be similar preoperatively and postoperatively (1.46 and 1.41 mg/dL, respectively, $p = 0.73$). Caution should be warranted as to proper patient selection to avoid bilateral obstruction and/or acute renal insufficiency. Serum creatinine is not the most accurate measure to evaluate follow up renal function status because one can lose up to 20% of renal function without significant change in the serum creatinine levels.

SOLITARY KIDNEY

Contrary to the previously cited studies, and despite the fact that there is a mild decrease in GFR in patients with solitary kidneys undergoing SWL, other studies have found SWL to be safe enough to be considered the treatment of choice *(128–130)*. Liou and Streem *(131)* also found no evidence that SWL, PCNL, or the combination of both techniques resulted in the deterioration of renal function in patients with a solitary kidney after a mean follow up of 53 mo. They concluded that any of these three treatment modalities are equally efficacious for preserving renal function. Because patients with solitary kidneys do not have a contralateral kidney that could compensate for the recovery of function of the treated kidney, long-term reduction in renal function is thought to occur secondary to the presence of multiple renal stones and repeat SWL.

RENAL INSUFFICIENCY

SWL in patients with stone-related renal insufficiency has also been addressed. The combination of ureteral stenting followed by phased SWL allowed these patients to achieve variable levels of improvement in the renal function *(132)*. Renal transplant patients can be safely managed with SWL. It is considered the treatment of choice for calyceal stones sized 5–15 mm in allograft kidneys *(133)*. As in cases of lithiasis in the mid ureter, SWL in allografted kidneys is performed in the prone position for better stone localization and treatment.

Nonrenal Complications

ADJACENT ORGANS

As the availability of SWL has increased, so have reports of shock-induced injuries to adjacent soft tissue and organs while the shockwaves travel toward the target organ. Although infrequent, unusual cases of gastric, splenic, pancreatic, colonic, cardiac, and vascular complications have been reported in the literature. Urinary fistulae and urinomas have also been reported.

Subcapsular splenic hematomas and even splenic rupture have occasionally been reported *(134–136)*. Subcapsular splenic hematomas can occur either immediately after SWL or months later. Conservative management has been advocated in selected cases of subcapsular splenic hematomas, although delayed splenectomy and even death from an infected hematoma and septic shock have been described *(137)*. These effects have occurred in patients with portal hypertension with severe coagulopathy and splenomegaly. Shockwave-induced injury to pancreatic tissue produces elevation of both serum and urinary amylase as well as of serum lipase *(138,139)*. Acute pancreatitis has been described after right side, left side, and bilateral renal or upper ureteral SWL. Although seldom clinically significant, cases of severe acute pancreatitis have occurred *(140)*.

FISTULAE

Infrequent cases of urinary fistulas, pyelocutaneous, ureterocolic, and ureterovaginal have been described to occur after SWL *(141–143)*. Both pyelocutaneous and ureterocolic fistulas were related to cases of xanthogranulomatous pyelonephritis *(141,142)*. Post-SWL urinoma secondary to rupture of the renal pelvis and renocutaneous fistula complete these groups of urinary collecting system injuries *(144,145)*.

Cardiac arrhythmias, primarily premature ventricular contractions (PVCs), occur in up to 60% after nonelectrocardiogram-gated SWL *(146–149)*. PVCs are usually not life threatening, and rapid resumption of the normal cardiac rhythm is achieved by synchronizing the SWL to the patient's electrocardiogram. SWL has safely been used in patients with aortic and renal aneurysms *(146–148)*. Although cases of dissection and rupture of calcified abdominal aortic aneurysms have been reported *(150–152)*, they are probably secondary to shockwave induced intimal injury. Using a tubless lithotriptor and with the patient in the supine position, Thomas et al have shown that real-time abdominal ultrasound can help to monitor the aneurysm during the shockwave lithotripsy procedure *(153)*. Caution should then be taken in patients with urolithiasis and calcified abdominal aortic aneurysms to properly focus the calculus at F2 and to not exceed the recommended number of shockwaves administered.

FERTILITY

Several studies have addressed, in both animals and humans, the effects of SWL regarding male and female reproductive function and fertility. Changes in DNA histograms resolved within 9 mo, but no statistically significant difference in the semen analysis, testosterone, or follicle-stimulating hormone was found after studying the effects of shockwaves on primate testicles *(154)*. In humans, microscopic hemospermia and a transient decrease in sperm density and motility have been found after SWL to distal ureteral lithiasis *(155)*. No histological differences were found in shockwave-treated rat ovaries when compared to control, nor were the pregnancy rates different among unilaterally oophorectomized rats subjected to direct, indirect, or no shockwaves *(156)*. Women of childbearing age, after receiving SWL to the distal ureter, were retrospectively found to have normal fertility and to have children without chromosomal anomalies *(157)*. No long-term sequelae or toxicity after SWL seems to exist in male or female gonads. SWL should not be used in pregnant women to avoid risks of miscarriage and to avoid shockwaves and/or radiation to the fetus.

Children

The short- and long-term effects of SWL on the pediatric population have also been studied. Thomas et al. *(158)* reported no statistically significant effect on linear body growth or renal function among children with urolithiasis treated with SWL. Although it has been found that SWL induces transient functional damage of tubular function in children, as per urinary enzymes activity that returns to baseline within 15 d *(159)*, it is considered an efficacious and safe treatment of upper tract urolithiasis in children without producing signs of damage to the growing kidney *(160,161)*. However, synchronous bilateral SWL may be inappropriate in the pediatric age group, because studies on infant primates showed the deleterious effects of synchronous bilateral SWL treatments *(125)*. The usual recommendation is to limit the amount of energy (such as kilovolts used) and the number of shockwaves used for treating pediatric urolithiasis.

Hypertension

Since its advent in 1980, the issue of SWL-induced changes in blood pressure has been controversial, and concern has surfaced as to the long-term risk of the development of hypertension. Abrupt onset of transient hypertension has been reported in association with a compressive perirenal hematoma. However, it is unclear whether the late occurrence of permanent hypertension is caused by SWL alone or the presence of nephrolithiasis, which by itself increases the relative risk of developing hypertension, or if it is related to aging of the patient, or multifactorial as a result of the combination of all of these factors.

In 1987, retrospective studies by Newman et al. *(162)* and Lingeman et al. *(163)* independently reported an excessive incidence of hypertension in 8% of patients following SWL after a 1-yr follow up. Similarly, Williams et al. *(164)* and Montgomery et al. *(165)* reported that 8% of treated patients developed severe hypertension within 21 mo after SWL and required treatment 12–44 mo after renal SWL on the Dornier HM-3. This study was of significant importance because it exceeded the annual incidence of new onset hypertension in men aged 30–60 yr, which was calculated to be 3–6% *(166)*.

Although this initial finding of an association between hypertension and SWL was alarming, other studies did not support this association. Yokoyama *(167)* found that in patients treated on the Dornier HM-3, after 18 mo an annualized increase in diastolic pressure and new onset of hypertension to be 0.78 mmHg and 0.65%, respectively. Significant elevation of diastolic pressure was noted in patients who received a larger number of shockwaves. Lingeman et al. *(168)*, in a study which included 731 patients who received SWL only, noted the annualized incidence of hypertension (2.4%) did not differ significantly from that in control patients (4%). Among patients who received SWL, no correlation was found between the incidence of hypertension and unilateral vs bilateral treatments, the number of shockwaves administered, the kilovoltage applied, or the power index (number of shockwaves times kilovoltage). However, as in Yokoyama and colleagues' study *(167)*, there was a significant rise in diastolic blood pressure

(DBP) after treatment with SWL (0.78 mmHg), which was not found in the control group (–0.88 mmHg). Later, an extended follow-up of this study after 4 yr reported an annualized incidence of new onset hypertension in SWL patients to be 2.1% compared to 1.6% in non-SWL patients. A statistically significant difference in the annualized DBP occurred in SWL-treated patients when compared to non-SWL patients. DBP decreased for both groups following treatment, but the decrease was significantly greater for those patients whose kidneys were not exposed to shockwaves *(169)*. Claro et al. *(170)* also found the incidence of hypertension after SWL to be similar to that of a normal population (3.92%), although the diastolic pressure was statistically higher after treatment.

More recently, Jewett et al. *(171)* reported the results of a prospective, randomized controlled trial of normotensive patients presenting with asymptomatic renal calculi. Patients were randomized to receive immediate SWL or be placed on an observation protocol, reserving SWL treatment for the onset of symptoms. At 24 mo follow-up, there was no observed difference in the incidence of new onset hypertension between the treatment and observation groups (2.7% in the SWL group and 2.5% in the observation group, for an overall incidence of 2.6%). In a similar study, Elves et al. *(172)*, studied the changes in BP over a mean of 2.2 yr in patients with small asymptomatic renal calculi randomized to observation or SWL and found no evidence that SWL causes changes in blood pressure. On the other hand, Strohmaier et al. *(173)* prospectively studied the BPs of stone patients undergoing different types of treatments (SWL, ureteroscopy, percutaneous nephrolithotomy/open surgery, spontaneous stone passage, and no treatment). At a 24 mo follow-up, in all groups, regardless of the stone location and type of treatment, SBP and DBP were significantly higher than the pretreatment levels, and they concluded that renal stone disease itself rather than the type of treatment was perhaps responsible for the increase in SBP and DBP.

Although renin-mediated hypertension (renovascular hypertension) has been associated with renal trauma, hypertension after SWL has not always been associated with an increase in renin production. To further investigate their association, studies have been done in animals and humans. Begun et al. *(174)* did not observe renin-mediated hypertension despite the excessive number of total shockwaves (20,000) delivered to the kidney of each minipig over a 4-mo period. On the contrary, Neal et al. *(175)* did find evidence of renin elevation after SWL on rhesus monkeys. Renin levels remained elevated over baseline in the infant monkeys but returned to normal values in the adult group of treated animals. In one of the few studies done in humans, Strohmaier et al. *(176)* studied endothelin production, which was thought to stimulate renin secretion and its effect on hypertension after SWL. They found only a slight and transient increase in active renin, whereas no correlation between endothelin and active renin was noted. They concluded that the increase in active renin was not mediated by endothelin and that the transient increase in active renin could not be attributed to the development of hypertension. Although an increase of renin levels after SWL could explain in part the early elevation in blood pressure after SWL, its long term occurrence cannot be explained solely based on renin production.

Assessment of the intrarenal resistive index (RI) by color Doppler ultrasonography at the level of the interlobar arteries is a noninvasive diagnostic modality for studying the renal vascular resistance and its associated changes in the arterial system. The intrarenal resistive index was originally found to be increased in 30% of patients immediately after SWL *(177)*. Later, statistically significant elevated resistive index levels were observed in 45% of patients older than 60 yr who had hypertension after SWL, whereas, in the normotensive patients, the resistive index was either stable or decreased *(179)*. Knapp et al. *(179)* also reported that post-SWL RI values surpassing 0.690 with 80% sensitivity and a 70% specificity may predict arterial hypertension. Intrarenal Doppler ultrasound is useful in patients older than 60 yr to find the high-risk group for arterial hypertension after SWL secondary to disturbances of renal perfusion as assessed by the RI.

SWL induced hypertension seems to be multifactorial, and none of its proposed etiology could by itself be responsible for its occurrence. Although DBP has been consistently found to be higher after SWL than in controls, no study has yet demonstrated its long-term clinical implications. In summary, high risk patients (i.e., altered renal function, older patients, preexisting hypertension) should be closely monitored before and after SWL.

COMPLICATIONS OF PERCUTANEOUS NEPHROSTOLITHOTOMY

The creation of a percutaneous tract specifically for stone removal was first reported by Fernstrom and Johannson *(180)* in 1976. Since then, numerous reports have established PCNL as a urologic procedure for managing select upper tract calculi. With subsequent advances in endoscopic equipment and energy sources, which safely and effectively fragment larger calculi, PCNL is now used as the procedure of choice for managing most complex renal calculi or even simple renal calculus associated with complex renal anatomy. Nevertheless, as the number and complexity of PCNL procedures increase, the potential for complications also increases. A high index of suspicion and prompt recognition and institution of appropriate treatment is fundamental to limit morbidity.

Factors Influencing Complications

Prevention of possible PCNL complications can be achieved through proper patient selection and a thorough knowledge of the topographic renal anatomy and its intrarenal vasculature for establishment of the percutaneous access. Knowledge of appropriate use and safety profile of the energy sources used for stone fragmentation is essential. Patient history and physical exam reveal associated co-morbidities, medications, previous surgeries, or body habitus that may contraindicate or delay the procedure. PCNL is absolutely contraindicated in cases of uncorrected bleeding diathesis or active urinary infection. Patients taking anticoagulation medications, (i.e., aspirin, clopidogrel bisulfate, and so on) should suspend taking them for 7–10 d before surgery and be screened for PT, PTT, platelets, and bleeding time before PCNL. Patients with urinary tract infection should receive bacteria-specific antibiotics and have a negative urine culture before PCNL. In the event of a UTI and obstruction, proper drainage (i.e., nephrostomy or ureteral stent) of the obstructed renal unit and broad-spectrum IV antibiotics should be initiated until the results of the urine culture are known. Once again, if UTI is suspected, PCNL should not be performed until a pretreatment urine culture rules out active infection. Relative contraindications include "corrected" bleeding abnormalities, anatomic abnormalities (i.e., horseshoe kidneys, pelvic kidneys), medical co-morbidities, and body habitus (i.e., morbid obesity, severe kyphoscoliosis).

Preoperative imaging studies are important to identify the number and locate the position of the stones, assess the intrarenal architecture and evaluate the relationship of the kidney and its surrounding organs for planning the preferred percutaneous access. Patients with simple renal pelvic or calyceal lithiasis, normal body habitus or absence of complex medical conditions most commonly only need an intravenous pyelogram (IVP) preoperatively to determine the renal calyx to be accessed. On the contrary, patients with staghorn calculus, calyceal diverticuli, abnormal body habitus, history of previous abdominal or renal surgery, and history of recurrent pyelonephritis should also have a CT scan study. CT scan allows better topographic evaluation of the planned renal access in relation to the pleura, diaphragm, liver, spleen, and of a retrorenal colon.

Patient Positioning

Proper patient position is achieved by placing the patient in the prone position and elevating the ipsilateral side 30°. This position helps to ventilate the patient and tends to bring the posterior calyces into a vertical position, which is helpful during the percutaneous renal access *(8)*. Foam padding of the chest, face, arms, and legs, as well as proper support of all extremities, should be emphasized. These safety measures are crucial to avoid pressure sores and temporary or permanent nerve injuries or limb paralysis.

Intraoperative Complications

Intraoperative complications can occur acutely during: (1) establishment of the percutaneous renal access; (2) during the percutaneous intrarenal surgery, or; (3) later during the postoperative period.

BLEEDING

During Percutaneous Access

Because of the extremely vascular nature of the kidney, bleeding from renal parenchyma always occurs to some degree during every percutaneous renal access. Significant blood loss is more likely to occur in patients with complex renal anatomy or when more than one percutaneous access site is needed, such as with treating staghorn calculi. Intrarenal anatomic consideration is of paramount importance in reducing the risk of tract bleeding. Therefore, determination of calyceal orientation and choice of the most favorable calyx for puncture are made before attempting percutaneous access and with the patient in the prone position mentioned above, using biplanar C-arm fluoroscopy or real-time ultrasound. The posterior calyx providing the most direct and shortest access to the targeted stone is preferred. A posterolateral puncture directed toward the papilla of a posterior calyx would be expected to traverse through the relatively avascular intersegmental renal zone *(181)*, and consequently be associated with less bleeding.

In a study done using polyester resin corrosion endocasts of the kidney collecting system and intrarenal vessels to identify the preferred anatomic point of puncture into a calyx, Sampaio and associates *(182)* reported that puncture through the infundibulum of the upper, middle, and lower poles was associated with vascular injury in 67.6%, 38.4%, and 68.2% of the kidneys, respectively. Puncture through the upper pole infundibulum should be avoided because the posterior segmental artery crosses the posterior surface of the infundibulum in 57% of cases *(183)*. Puncture through the fornix proved to be significantly safer and was associated with less than 8% venous injury and no arterial injuries. Consequently, the preferred point of entry into the collecting system is through the renal papilla, along the axis of the calyx. Proper alignment of the percutaneous access with the infundibulum's axis prevents excess torquing with the rigid nephroscope that otherwise would lead to renal trauma and subsequent bleeding. Direct puncture into the renal pelvis should be avoided because of the risk of injuring a large retropelvic vessel, which can be present in one third of cases *(157)*, or one of four segmental renal arteries, which traverses the anterior aspect of the renal pelvis and parenchyma.

During Tract Dilation

Beside the percutaneous access, tract dilation is another important step of percutaneous renal surgery that needs to be done carefully to minimize intraoperative bleeding. Several methods of tract dilation are available, including serial coaxial metal dilators (Alken set, Karl Storz, Culver City, CA), semirigid graded Amplatz dilators (Cook Urological, Spencer, IN), and balloon dilators. More recently, radially expanding single-step nephrostomy tract dilators have been described *(184)*. Irrespective of the tract dilation method used, caution should be taken to dilate the tract only up to the peripheral aspect of the collecting system under fluoroscopic guidance. The renal pelvis is at high risk for perforation and the hilar vessels may be injured if dilation is directed too far medially. Balloon dilators have been found to be associated with less bleeding than serial dilators *(185)*. Alken dilators, because of their metallic nature, are associated with an increased potential for tearing the renal pelvis medial wall and causing subsequent bleeding. Fluoroscopic monitoring under such circumstances is highly recommended. The Amplatz working sheath tamponades the renal parenchyma and should be kept within the collecting system after tract dilatation, and excessive angulation should also be avoided at all times to limit bleeding from parenchymal vascular trauma. Such working sheaths also allow for safe nephroscopic manipulations while maintaining a low pressure irrigation environment.

Renal hemorrhage is one of the most common and worrisome complications of percutaneous renal surgery. Although in experienced hands it has an incidence of 1% to 3%, a transfusion rate of up to 34% has been reported *(186–190)*. Differences in the transfusion rate have been noted to be influenced by different factors, such as operative technique (balloon dilators vs Amplatz dilators) *(185)*, patient's status (anemic vs nonanemic) *(190)*, stone complexity (i.e., nonstaghorn vs staghorn calculus), and number of access tracts needed *(191)*.

When bleeding occurs during the percutaneous access or during the tract dilation process, advancement of the nephrostomy sheath usually tamponades the bleeding allowing the procedure to continue. Removal or suctioning of blood clots within the collecting system is important for stone localization and for working in a clear field, thus avoiding injury to the urothelial lining. Dark-colored blood stream after stopping the fluid irrigation is usually of venous origin. If bleeding continues, obscuring endoscopic vision, placement of an appropriate nephrostomy tube and abandoning the planned procedure is recommended.

Intraoperative Bleeding

If heavy bleeding continues despite repositioning the access sheath and/or precludes adequate visibility, temporary interruption of the procedure is advised and tamponade maneuvers should be initiated.

A large-bore, 26-or 28-Fr Foley catheter should be inserted into the renal pelvis, clamped, and a diuretic administered intravenously. The nephrostomy should be left clamped for approx 30 min, while the bleeding and clots are tamponaded. Alternatively, a 30-Fr balloon dilator can be inflated over the working wire for approximately the same period of time or a council catheter can be inflated adjacent to a major injured vessel

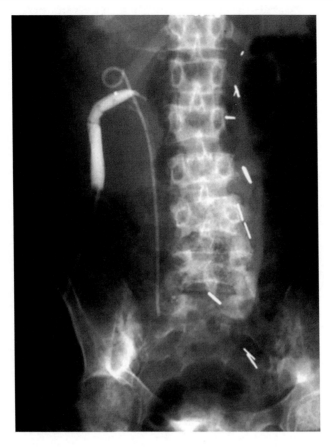

Fig. 3. A 24-mm, 10-cm high-pressure balloon in the nephrostomy tract to control renal hemorrhage. Note significant angulation of access tract, causing excessive angulation of Amplatz sheath during nephroscopy, likely the cause of bleeding.

(192) (Fig. 3). If the bleeding is controlled using these techniques and the patient is hemodynamically stable, the PCNL procedure can be restarted without angling the working sheath to avoid further bleeding. If unsure, it is highly recommended that further manipulations be abandoned and the procedure rescheduled.

When bleeding is not controlled with the aforementioned measures and the bleeding appears to be arterial in nature or when termination of the procedure is decided because of the hemodynamic condition of the patient, a specialized tamponade catheter (Kaye Catheter, Cook Urological, Spencer, IN) can be used in combination with serial hematocrit monitoring. The Kaye catheter is a large-diameter, occlusive balloon (36 Fr) with a built-in 14-Fr nephrostomy tube, which is passed over a 5-Fr ureteral stent. This catheter tamponades the nephrostomy tract and concurrently and effectively drains the renal pelvis while maintaining ureteral access. It is usually left inflated for 24 h, although it has previously been reported to be left inflated for as long as 2–4 d *(193,194)*. More recently, a new nephrostomy tube that combines the benefits of the re-entry Malecot design with those of the Kaye tamponade catheter has been developed *(195)*. It has been shown to be effective in high-risk patients in preventing and stopping bleeding from a percutaneous access site while maintaining ureteral access.

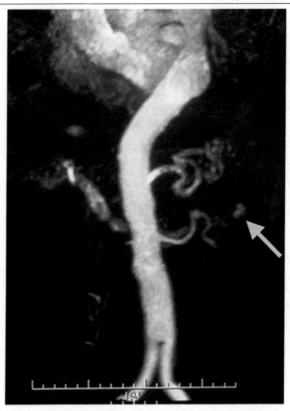

Fig. 4. Magnetic resonance angiography demonstrating a small pseudo-aneurysm and arterio-venous fistula in the left kidney following PCNL.

In cases in which, despite the expectant and supportive measures, there is evidence of continuous perioperative bleeding (arterial bleeding, dropping hematocrit, continued need for blood transfusion, hemodynamic deterioration and the presence of expanding perirenal hematoma), renal angiography and selective embolization of the injured vessels is indicated *(188,189,196–201)* (Fig. 4). However, most intraoperative bleeding precluding nephroscopic vision can be managed by placing a 26-Fr nephrostomy tube and returning at a later date for definitive percutaneous treatment.

Postoperative Bleeding

Delayed postoperative bleeding, either at the time of removal of the percutaneous nephrostomy drainage or several days to weeks thereafter, can occur secondary to an arterial laceration (i.e., segmental renal vessels), an arteriovenous fistula, or a pseudo-aneurysm. Bleeding at the time of removal of the nephrostomy tube from venous origin can be managed by reinserting the nephrostomy tube and leaving it for a few days until the urine clears. Bleeding from an arterial source usually does not respond well to this measure. In case of an arteriovenous fistula or a pseudoaneurysm, bleeding occurs days to weeks after the PCNL. Patient readmission to the hospital is advised, as is early stabilization with crystalloids and blood transfusion, if necessary. If the percutaneous tract is still patent, a balloon dilation catheter, a Kaye nephrostomy tamponade balloon catheter, or a Council catheter may be placed and inflated to limit the hemorrhage.

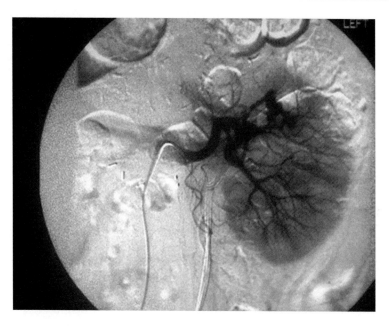

Fig. 5. A digital angiogram is performed to map the vascular supply to the pseudo aneurysm and arteriovenous fistula.

Immediate renal angiography should be performed to identify the bleeding site or the location of the arteriovenous fistula or pseudoaneurysm. Subsequently, selective or superselective embolization is attempted. In experienced hands, the blood transfusion rate is 2% and the need for renal embolization after PCNL is 1% *(202,206)* (Fig. 5). Hyperselective embolization is the least invasive and best treatment for massive hemorrhage after percutaneous nephrostolithotomy *(200,201)*. Patients whose bleeding is refractory to embolization should undergo open surgical exploration, with direct vascular repair, partial nephrectomy or nephrectomy.

Injury to the Collecting System and Fluid Extravasation

Although small perforations to the collecting system almost always occur to some extent, perforation of the renal pelvis rarely occurs. Because these can lead to some absorption of irrigation fluid, the use of physiologic irrigating solutions is emphasized. Major extraperitoneal perforations can be suspected if perirenal fat or other retroperitoneal structures are seen, or when a discrepancy of more than 500 mL between irrigant input and output is encountered. In case of intraperitoneal irrigant extravasation, abdominal distension can be observed. The amount of absorbed fluid also depends on the irrigant pressure and the length of procedure.

In case of minor perforations, premature termination of the procedure is usually not necessary if a low pressure irrigation system is being used. Smaller perforations usually seal within 24–48 h after termination of the procedure *(204)*. However, with more significant perforations, termination of the procedure and nephrostomy drainage are advisable. Intraperitoneal extravasation, though rare, may be treated by vigorous diuresis or with the use of peritoneal drainage *(205)*.

INJURY TO ADJACENT ORGANS

The retroperitoneal location of the kidney and its close relation to the diaphragm and pleura, liver, spleen, and right and left colon makes these organs vulnerable to possible injuries, especially while accessing the kidney percutaneously. Early injury recognition to any adjacent structure, as well as proper management of it, is vital to avoid further morbidity or death. Most of these complications can still be managed endourologically and/or in conjunction with interventional radiology, leaving open surgical exploration and repair for either major vascular complications or delayed unrecognized complications.

Lung and Pleural Cavity

Ideally, the renal percutaneous access should be done below the 12th rib and near the posterior axillary line to reduce the risk of pleural complications. Whenever the pleura is percutaneously crossed through an intercostal or supracostal approach, there is an increased risk of developing a pneumothorax, hemothorax, urothorax, or hydrothorax. Supracostal access tracts are associated with significantly higher intrathoracic and overall complication rates compared to subcostal access tracts, and consequently must be used with caution when no other alternatives are available *(206)*. Preoperative patient education and informed consents regarding the probability of pleural injury are highly recommended.

Intraoperatively, pleural violations are suspected by ventilatory difficulties and/or alterations in the respiratory parameters or with the presence of contrast within the pleural cavity during the nephrostogram at the end of the procedure. Postoperatively, ipsilateral chest pain or shortness of breath should also alert the surgeon to the possibility of a pleural injury. If diagnosed intraoperatively, either aspiration or placement of a chest tube should be decided at the end of the procedure. When diagnosed postoperatively, the decision of chest tube placement relies on the patient's respiratory status and grade of hemo/pneumothorax in the chest X-ray film. A renopleural fistula is suspected when there is continuous pleural effusion after chest tube drainage. This can be resolved by placing a ureteral double-J stent *(207)*. Postoperative pain management and incentive spirometry are essential after PCNL to allow the patient to breathe deeply and reduce the risk of atelectasis and associated febrile episodes.

Colon

The retroperitoneal colon is usually encountered anteriorly or anterolaterally to the lateral renal border. Therefore, the risk of colon injury is usually low. Colonic perforation may occur when the puncture site is placed lateral to the proposed posterior axillary line or in the rare event of a patient with a retrorenal colon. Displacement of the colon posterior to the kidney with increased risk of colon perforation is seen in elder patients with chronic constipation or patients with other causes of distended descending colon, patients with previous major abdominal surgery (i.e., jejunoileal bypass resulting in an enlarged colon), and in thin female patients with very little retroperitoneal fat *(208, 209)*. Other factors increasing the risk of colon injury include patients with left renal disease, mobile kidneys, anterior calyceal puncture, previous extensive renal surgery, horseshoe kidney, and kyphoscoliosis *(17,181,203,210,211)*. Ultrasound-guided renal percutaneous access can be performed in patients with increased risk of having a retrorenal colon *(212)*. A preoperative CT scan in the prone position is recommended if any possibility of colonic injury is suspected.

Colonic perforation should be suspected if the patient has intraoperative or immediate postoperative diarrhea or hematochezia, signs of peritonitis, or passage of gas or feces through the nephrostomy tract *(213)*. Otherwise, a postoperative nephrostogram before nephrostomy removal can reveal the presence of colonic contrast. In the absence of peritonitis or sepsis, most extraperitoneal colonic perforation can be successfully managed conservatively *(214)*. An indwelling Double J ureteral stent is inserted, the nephrostomy tube withdrawn under fluoroscopic guidance into the colon, and a Foley catheter is left in place in the bladder to maintain a low urinary pressure system. The patient should be given broad-spectrum antibiotics or triple antibiotic coverage and placed on a low-residue diet. This allows the renal collecting system to heal and the medial colonic wall to close. After 5 to 7 d, if the colostogram shows neither extravasation nor colonic communication with the collecting system, the Foley catheter is removed and the colostomy tube withdrawn, but still kept as a drain. Two to three days later, when the lateral colonic wall is expected to be closed, the tube is then completely removed. In case of intraperitoneal colonic perforation, peritonitis, sepsis, or failed conservative management, open surgical exploration should be performed.

Liver and Spleen

The liver and spleen may also be at risk of being injured during percutaneous access. In the absence of splenomegaly or hepatomegaly, injury to these organs is extremely rare with subcostal and lower pole punctures. The risk may be somewhat greater with upper pole punctures, especially if the puncture is performed during inspiration and/or if the puncture is above the 11th rib *(215–217)*. When performing upper pole punctures, a skin puncture site at the lateral border of the paraspinal muscles reduces the risk of liver or spleen injury.

Transhepatic percutaneous renal access is not without major risk, because it is similar to percutaneous procedures of the hepatobiliary system. Transhepatic tract dilation poses the risk of injuring the hepatic vasculature. However, in the absence of active bleeding, it can still be managed conservatively, leaving a transhepatic nephrostomy postoperatively, as well as an indwelling ureteral stent and bladder Foley catheter. The ureteral stent and bladder Foley catheter should be kept in place after the nephrostomy tube is removed to reduce the risk of renobiliary fistula. Active bleeding or injury to a major hepatic vessel requires open exploration and repair.

Splenic injuries are suspected in hemodynamically unstable patients with intra-abdominal bleeding undergoing left PCNL. The diagnosis is conducted with intraoperative abdominal ultrasound or with a postoperative abdominal CT scan. Although conservative management can be used in some patients with nonexpanding subcapsular hematomas, in most patients splenectomy is performed *(218)*.

INTRAOPERATIVE ENERGY SOURCE RELATED INJURIES

Independent of the type of lithotriptor used for PCNL, potential energy-related complications can be produced if improperly used. First, a thorough knowledge of the indications and safety profiles of the energy source being used is essential. Second, under no circumstance should the energy source be used unless there is proper visualization of the working field. If the working field is bloody or the presence of clots precludes adequate visualization, the case must be interrupted until proper hemostasis of any bleeding site is achieved and clots are removed.

Ultrasonic lithotriptors are rarely associated with energy-related intracorporeal complications. Nevertheless, caution is urged to not dig the probe against the urothelial lining to avoid perforation and bleeding. Similarly, overheating of the probe tip should be avoided. Periodic procedure interruption allows for crystals in the probe to cool, which prevents thermal injuries that can lead to strictures, especially at the UPJ. Overheating of the crystals can also cause the device to malfunction.

Electrohydraulic lithotripsy (EHL) is also relatively safe to use, although it can cause bleeding and renal pelvis perforation. Nephrostomy tube drainage, either alone or in conjunction with an indwelling ureteral stent, usually helps to heal the renal pelvis perforation adequately within a few days. EHL consequently has not been found to be associated with UPJ strictures.

Candela and Holmium laser lithotriptors have a high safety profile and a low complication rate, such as urothelial lining perforation (219). Holmium laser technology produces less urothelial penetration, thus posing some advantage over other laser modalities (i.e., tunable dye laser) in terms of causing less renal pelvis perforation when properly used. However, the Holmium laser, if directly in contact with transitional cell mucosa, can cause thermal injury. Also, direct contact of the Holmium laser can cut guidewires and stone baskets, and thus, direct contact with paraphernalia should be avoided.

A new lithotriptor composed of a Lithoclast Master and an ultrasonic device (EMS, Nyon, Switzerland) has been used for PCNL procedures. Clinical and laboratory assessment of this newly developed pneumatic lithotripsy device has validated its efficacy in fragmenting stones of all compositions and its overall safety associated with clinical application (218,220,221).

COMPLICATIONS OF URETEROSCOPY

Since its initial description by Young in 1912, ureteroscopy has come a long way and has gained widespread acceptance as an option for the treatment of multiple ureteric and renal conditions. Further advances in technology have led to the introduction of smaller caliber ureteroscopes with the capacity to accommodate accessory instruments necessary to perform diagnostic and therapeutic upper urinary tract procedures. Also, the advent of fiberoptic technology has provided the opportunity to create flexible scopes capable of reaching the renal pelvis and calyceal groups. Although ureteroscopy is being used for multiple purposes—including evaluation of filling defects in the upper urinary tract, evaluation of positive urine cytology, incision of strictures, uretero-pelvic junction obstruction, and ablation or resection of urothelial malignancies—the vast majority of ureteroscopic procedures are performed to fragment and extract ureteral stones.

Since its introduction into routine clinical practice in the early 1980s, the complications and adverse events associated with ureteroscopic procedures have decreased dramatically. Smaller caliber ureteroscopes, reliable and safer fragmentation devices and paraphernalia, and, above all, surgeons' experience in these procedures should be given credit.

Ureteroscopy, independent of its indications, should always be performed with the greatest margin of safety possible. To accomplish this, several steps should be performed during the procedure, including:

1. Complete cystoscopy and emptying of the bladder;
2. Retrograde pyelogram to evaluate ureteral anatomy and delineate plan of action, when indicated (Fig. 6). An adequate intravenous urogram may suffice;

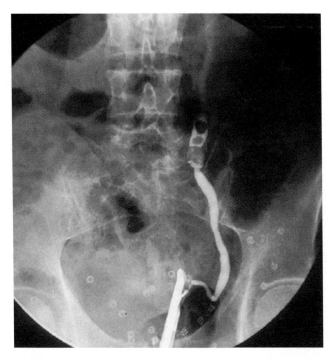

Fig. 6. Left retrograde pyelogram performed to delineate the course of a tourtous ureter associated with an impacted stone.

3. Placement of a safety wire under visual and fluoroscopic monitoring (we prefer to place an Amplatz Super Stiff™ guidewire because it straightens the ureter and facilitates access to the upper ureter);
4. Balloon dilation of the ureteral orifice and distal ureter only if necessary;
5. Careful passage of the rigid ureteroscope alongside the safety wire;
6. Careful passage of the flexible ureteroscope over a second guidewire under fluoroscopic imaging;
7. Judicious use of ureteral access sheath to facilitate recurrent and safe passage of rigid and flexible ureteroscopes.

The most critical step in ureteroscopic access is the placement of the safety wire. Fortunately, several different wires are available to facilitate access to the ureter. Size, tip design, surface coating, and shaft rigidity are the main characteristics that differentiate one guidewire from another.

After ureteroscopic access is obtained and the stone is directly visualized in the ureteroscopic field, the calculus is extracted intact or fragmented under direct vision for extraction. Several different devices are now available for stone fragmentation in the ureter:

1. Ultrasonic lithotriptor, which uses an electric current applied to a piezoceramic crystal creating vibrational energy that is transmitted to the stone via a rigid hollow probe for fragmentation and aspiration. This technology is very safe and activation of the probe in contact with the urothelium for short periods of time results in minimal tissue injury. The use of this technology in the ureter has decreased because of the advent of flexible laser fibers.

2. Pneumatic lithotriptor, which uses compressed nitrogen gas to launch a projectile against the handheld probe head, creating repeated impacts between the probe tip and the stone surface. Once the tensile forces of the stone are reached, stone breakage is obtained. There is an increased chance for proximal stone migration secondary to repeated impact. Although ureteral perforation can occur secondary to pneumatic lithotriptor use, the short burst of energy results only in superficial erosion or edema without subsequent complications (222).

3. EHL was the first modality of intracorporeal lithotripsy available. It relies on the effect of an electric discharge in a liquid medium, which creates a cavitation bubble that undergoes rapid expansion and contraction. This results in a shockwave that, when transmitted to the stone, fragments it. Severe damage to the ureteral mucosa can be caused by this lithotriptor, ranging from nonthermal perforation to extensive tissue damage secondary to the cavitation bubble (223).

4. Holmium: Yttrium-Aluminum-Garnet Laser is the most recent technology available for ureteral stone fragmentation. Laser devices rely on photothermal energy to fragment stones. The laser fibers are available in a range of sizes, from 200 to 1000 microns, and can be used through rigid and flexible endoscopes. To achieve optimal results and avoid tissue damage, the fiber should be in direct contact with the stone at the time of activation. Reported stone fragmentation rates range from 90 to 100% (224,225). The depth of tissue thermal injury with the Holmium: YAG ranges from 0.5 to 1 mm, and, because of this, it is extremely important to maintain the distance between the ureteral tissue and the probe tip greater than 1 mm (226). In practice, major soft tissue injuries with the Holmium: YAG lithotripsy are rare because the tip of the probe has to be in direct contact with the stone surface to be effective. Also, the low power settings required for lithotripsy are much lower than that used for tissue ablation. However, the Holmium: YAG laser can cut through guidewires and stone baskets and must be guarded against this occurrence.

Ureteral Injury

The rapid development of smaller and more efficient scopes has facilitated the use of ureteroscopy for the treatment of ureteral calculi. Although these advances have decreased the need for open ureteral surgery, iatrogenic injury can still occur with the endoscopic technique. Possible iatrogenic complications of ureteroscopy include ureteral perforation, stricture, false passage, ureteral avulsion, bleeding from the ureteral mucosa or adjacent structures, infection, and sepsis. Several studies have reported the overall complication rate associated with ureteroscopy to be between 1% and 15% (227–230). These complication rates have steadily decreased over the years.

Grasso et al. (231) reported on the complication rate for his series of 560 patients who underwent any type of ureteropyeloscopy. The reported incidence of pain, fever, false passage, and urinary tract infection were 5.5%, 1.4%, 0.4%, and 1.6%, respectively.

Ureteral perforation usually occurs during placement of a guidewire, especially in cases associated with long standing, impacted, obstructing ureteral stones. In cases in which the regular safety wire cannot be advanced with ease, a retrograde pyelogram should be performed to delineate the anatomy of the ureter and collecting system (Fig. 6). After the retrograde is performed, a wire covered with hydrophilic polymer (Glidewire™) can usually be advanced into the collecting system. If the ureter is tortuous, use of a 5-Fr open-ended ureteral catheter along with a Bentson tip guidewire is recommended (232). Despite these techniques, if advancing a wire is not possible, the renal unit should be drained proximally with a nephrostomy tube.

If the area associated with the ureteral stone is long and fibrotic, consideration for open or laparoscopic resection of the diseased segment should be made. Reconstruction after the resection can be made with an end-to-end anastomosis, Boari flap, Psoas hitch, transureteral–ureteral anastomosis, or ileal interposition, depending on the length and location of the defect. Ureteral stricture after ureteroscopy can also be secondary to ureteral perforation, submucosal false passage formation, or trauma of the ureteral wall while performing stone fragmentation or manipulation. Usually a small perforation or false passage, secondary to an incorrectly placed guidewire, will heal without serious complications with time and adequate stent drainage. However, balloon dilation over a perforating wire can convert a small perforation into a large laceration or avulsion. Major ureteral perforations can also be caused by excessive force applied to a rigid ureteroscope, especially over the iliac vessels. Another possible complication of ureteral tear could be the migration of the stone or fragment through the mucosal tear and the formation of a stone granuloma and subsequent ureteral stricture *(233)*.

Complications During Stone Manipulation

It is important to avoid basketing of large stones and subsequent extraction without fragmentation. It is obvious that a large stone that did not pass spontaneously would not necessarily pass while basketing without applying undue amount of tension to the ureter and the ureteropelvic junction. The most feared complication of this maneuver is the complete avulsion of the ureter with eversion into the bladder. Usually this complication will lead to a large ureteral defect and an even larger devascularized ureteral segment. In such patients, immediate exploration with attempted re-anastomosis of the ureteral ends is recommended. Failure to do so or failure in adequate healing because of devascularization will lead to ileal replacement of the ureter, renal auto-transplantation, or nephrectomy. Stone fragmentation and manipulation should be performed under direct vision.

Complications to Adjacent Structures

Another important consideration while performing ureteroscopic procedures should be avoiding trauma to adjacent vascular structures. This is especially important while performing ablative procedures in the area of the iliac vessels or with UPJ procedures in the presence of aberrant crossing vessels. Adequate preoperative imaging techniques should identify any potential problems.

It is extremely important to identify minor problems during ureteroscopy to avoid progression of the trauma. Adequate drainage of the kidney and aborting the procedure are always safe and acceptable options when a complication is encountered. Patients with postureteroscopy stent placement should be monitored and the stent removed promptly to prevent risk of stent calcification (Fig. 7).

Conclusion

The formula for a low rate of complication during ureteroscopic procedures is appropriate instrumentation, adequate fluoroscopic imaging, avoiding improper application of force to a rigid ureteroscope, placement of safety wire, avoiding advancement of instrument without direct visual imaging, safe application of fragmentation techniques, and knowing one's limitations at the time of the procedure.

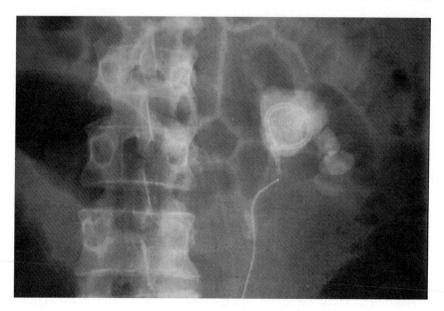

Fig. 7. Severely calcified and fragmented proximal curl of ureteral stent.

COMPLICATIONS RELATED TO OPEN SURGERY

In the era of minimally invasive surgery, the use of open surgery to treat urolithiasis has decreased dramatically. However, urologists should be proficient in these open surgical techniques in case they come across challenges such as a large staghorn calculus requiring intrarenal reconstruction of the collecting system or another stone not amenable to treatment with minimally invasive techniques (Fig. 8).

Before 1880, renal stone surgery was performed only in obstructed, grossly infected kidneys. At the time of perinephric abscess drainage, stones protruding from the kidney were removed or left to drain through the incision or fistulous tract. Severe intrarenal hemorrhage was the major complication associated with this procedure because of the lack of knowledge of the intrarenal vascular distribution. In 1880, Morris *(234)* described the first known nephrolithotomy in a nonabscessed kidney. Afterwards, he performed 34 consecutive renal surgeries for removal of stones, reporting a recovery rate of greater than 90%.

The later publication of *The Intrinsic Blood Vessels of the Kidney and Their Significance in Nephrotomy* by Max Brodel *(235)* in 1901 described the ramifications of the renal artery and the existence of an avascular plane between the anterior and posterior arterial segments. The further development of radiological techniques, including intra-operative X-rays and ultrasound, helped to further refine stone localization and make open renal surgery more accurate and easier *(236)*.

Open surgery today includes anatrophic nephrolithotomy, pyelolithotomy, radial serial nephrotomies, ureterolithotomy, cystolithotomy, and urethrolithotomy. Complications for these surgeries can be divided into: (a) those associated with renal exposure and (b) complications associated with surgical approach to the calculus. Herein, we review the complications associated with these surgical procedures.

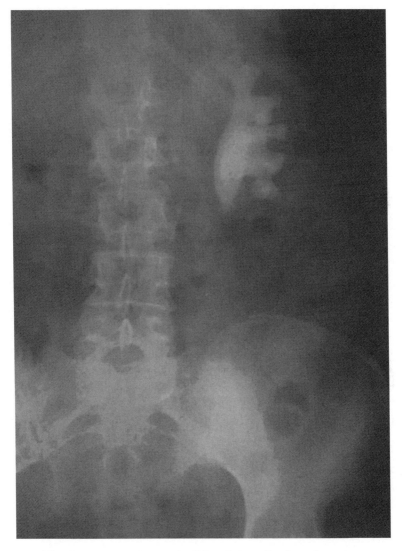

Fig. 8. Large staghorn calculi involving all calyceal groups.

Complications of Incisions and Renal Exposure

Several different skin incisions can be performed to approach the kidney. The decision of the surgical technique to be used depends on the surgeon's familiarity with different incisions available and the location of the urinary tract needing surgical intervention.

Standard Flank Incision

Standard flank incision, with or without rib resection, has been associated with increased postoperative pain and discomfort (because the muscles are incised), which can result in decreased ambulation and increased requirements of pain medication.

Inadvertent surgical division of the intercostal nerves results in denervation of the flank muscles, which can result in flank bulging after surgery not associated with true hernias. Honig et al. *(237)* reported that up to 15% of patients with flank incisions would develop flank bulges secondary to laxity of the flank muscles. Aside from denervation injuries, nerve trauma, and entrapment, flank pain is another complication that can occur after flank incisions. To avoid these complications, the intercostal nerve should be identified and preserved during dissection, if at all possible.

Another uncommon complication associated with the flank incision could be the formation of a flank hernia. Flank hernias are a rare problem and are more common in extremely obese, immunocompromised, or malnourished patients. Extreme caution should be taken during closure in these patients, and sometimes the use of internal retention sutures is necessary. Flank hernias should always be repaired in patients who are good surgical candidates, but, in severely debilitated patients with easily reducible hernias, a more conservative treatment should be considered.

Anterior Transperitoneal Approach

A transperitoneal approach can be difficult in obese patients because of the depth of the surgical field and because the panniculus and peritoneal contents can interfere with adequate visualization of the retroperitoneum. Also, violation of the peritoneum pre-disposes the patient to intestinal adhesion formation *(238)*. The potential spillage of infected urine into the peritoneal cavity with subsequent abscess and adhesion formation is another drawback for the transperitoneal approach.

Posterior Approaches

Posterior approaches can be used to gain access to the kidney and upper ureter in an extraperitoneal manner. This lumbotomy approach is usually well tolerated with mini-mal postoperative pain and early ambulation because few muscle groups are divided. The major drawback of this incision is the lack of exposure to the renal vessels during surgery. Thus, renal vein and artery control during iatrogenic vascular damage is extremely difficult to obtain. Another disadvantage of this approach is the fact that the renal unit moves anteriorly, away from the surgeon, during prone positioning of the patient.

Infection

There is a risk of wound infection in all skin incisions made for removal of urinary calculi. It is important to treat any urinary tract infection before performing any proce-dure for stone extraction, prompt identification of skin changes, and treatment with appropriate antibiotics. Local wound care is crucial in the treatment of this complication. One should identify high risk factors such as obesity and diabetes.

Pneumothorax

Pneumothorax is a complication associated not only with percutaneous renal access but also with open renal surgery. Pneumothorax occurs in fewer than 5% of patients undergoing open nephrolithotomy *(239)*. This complication is more common in patients with multiple previous renal surgeries and previous history of pyelonephritis or peri-renal abscess. After damage to the diaphragm and pleura is identified, primary closure with running absorbable suture can be performed after all the air is drained from the pleura with a 14-Fr red rubber catheter placed in a bowl of sterile water during complete expansion of the lungs by the anesthesiologist. Following this, a chest X-ray should be performed to assess whether any residual pneumothorax is present. If present and clinically significant, a chest tube should be inserted for at least 48 h and managed in a routine manner.

Complications Associated With Calculus Extraction

HEMORRHAGE

As with any surgical procedure, excessive bleeding is a possibility that has to be addressed. Although hemorrhage from the kidney during pyelolithotomy or nephrolithotomy is usually avoidable with good surgical techniques and gentle tissue handling, bleeding during an anatrophic or peripheral nephrolithotomy was seen in up to 10% of patients in Spirnak's reported series (240). To avoid this, control of the renal artery and vein should be obtained before incising the renal parenchyma. After vascular control is obtained, the renal incision should be obtained in the avascular plane of the kidney situated about 1 cm posterior to Brodel's white line. Intravenous injection of methylene blue can be used to demarcate the avascular plane. Any bleeding sites encountered during dissection should be closed using 3-0 absorbable sutures.

Postoperative bleeding usually results from inadequately controlled intrarenal vessels. Bed rest, IV fluids, and, if needed, blood transfusion will usually control the bleeding. If patients develop hemodynamic instability and cannot be managed medically, angiography and super-selective embolization should be performed. Re-exploration should be reserved for patients who fail embolization because of the higher incidence of renal loss.

ADJACENT ORGAN TRAUMA

Trauma to adjacent organs can occur, especially in infected or severely reactive renal units. While operating on the right kidney, attention should be paid on the duodenum, head of the pancreas, liver, short right adrenal vein, the inferior vena cava, and ascending colon. Inadvertent trauma to these structures can occur during blunt or sharp dissection or retractor placement.

On the left side, adjacent structures prone to damage include descending colon, the tail of the pancreas, and spleen. Conservative vs surgical management of trauma to adjacent organs is dependent on the degree of trauma, time elapsed before diagnosis, and clinical condition of the patient.

RETAINED STONE FRAGMENTS AND STONE MIGRATION

Intrarenal migration of calculi during open exploration and manipulation of the kidney is a common and serious problem. It is extremely important to obtain distal ureteral control with a vessel loop before making an incision in the renal pelvis. This maneuver will prevent distal migration of the stone while manipulating the kidney. The incision in the renal pelvis should be performed exactly over the stone after direct palpation. It is also important to make the incision away from the uretero-pelvic junction to avoid transection of this area and possible subsequent stricture formation.

If in doubt of the exact position of the renal stone, intraoperative X-ray should be taken to asses the exact position of the stone before performing the incision. When a large pelvis or ureteral incision is made or when some small fragments may have migrated, intraoperative placement of an indwelling ureteral stent is recommended to protect the closure and to avoid acute renal obstruction from distally migrated stone fragments.

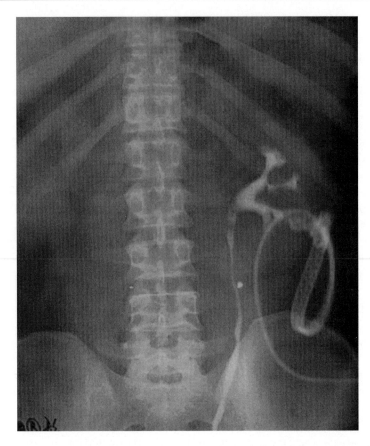

Fig. 9. Closed suction drain showing moderate extravasation of contrast material from the lower calyceal group after open renal surgery.

Inadvertent retention of stone fragments after open renal surgery is a common occurrence with reported incidence of up to 30% *(239)*. It is important to obtain intraoperative X-rays to compare them to preoperative studies and assess residual stones. For stones that are not reachable through the already-made pyelotomy, a flexible cystoscope/nephroscope can be used to gain access and remove these calculi. Fragmentation with Holmium: YAG laser or intact basketing are two possible ways of treating these hard-to-reach fragments. Postoperative SWL is another possible alternative to treat small-retained fragments in a nonoccluded system.

URINARY LEAKAGE

Persistent urinary leakage and urinary fistula formation, either pyelocutaneous, nephrocutaneus or ureterocutaneous, are problems that can be encountered after open surgery for renal stones. These complications are usually associated with distal obstruction, infection, and foreign bodies in the urinary system or devascularization of tissue secondary to surgical dissection. After these problems are diagnosed, adequate renal drainage with either indwelling ureteral stent or nephrostomy tube and indwelling bladder Foley catheter placement are usually enough to control the leakage. The majority of these extravasations resolves with adequate drainage (Fig. 9).

When the urinary leakage cannot drain to the exterior, a urinoma can form. To treat this, adequate drainage of the kidney is also necessary, and percutaneous drainage of the urinoma collection should be performed to avoid further complications such as abscess formation. To confirm the nature of the fluid collection, creatinine levels should be tested on the drained fluid and compared to serum levels.

Urinary leakage can be avoided with meticulous, watertight closure of the collecting system or ureter without tension. The use of 3-0 absorbable sutures in a continuous or interrupted manner is adequate for this purpose. Formation of large flaps of tissue should be avoided during dissection, and adequate drainage of the renal unit should be procured. In cases in which the leakage cannot be controlled with stents or nephrostomy tubes, re-exploration with resection of the diseased segment and reconstruction should be performed, following standard and time-tested urologic principles.

CONCLUSION

In conclusion, with a variety of options available for the treatment of symptomatic urolithiasis, a sound understanding of the principles of choosing a treatment option is essential. Potential complications should be known so that urologists can take every measure to prevent one.

REFERENCES

1. Chaussy C, Brendel W, Schmiedt E. Extracorporeally induced destruction of kidney stones by shockwaves. Lancet 1980; 13(2):1265–1268.
2. Chaussy C, Schmiedt E, Jocham D, Brendel W, Forssmann B, Walther V. First clinical experience with extracorporeally induced destruction of kidney stones by shockwaves. J Urol 1982; 127: 417–420.
3. Chaussy CG. ESWL: past, present and future. J Endourol 1988; 2: 97–105.
4. Krings F, Tuerk CH, Steinkogler I, Marberger M. Extracorporeal shock-wave lithotripsy treatment ("stir-up") promotes discharge of persistent calyceal stone fragments after primary extracorporeal shockwave lithotripsy. J Urol 1992; 148: 1040–1042.
5. Wickham JEA. Treatment of urinary tract stones. Br Med J 1993; 307: 1414–1417.
6. Grasso M, Loisides P, Beaghler M, Bagley D. The case for primary endoscopic management of upper urinary tract calculi: a critical review of 121 extracorporeal shock-wave lithotripsy failures. Urology 1995; 45: 363–371.
7. Chaussy C, Schmiedt E, Jocham D, Brendel W, Forssmann, Walther V. First clinical experience with extracorporeally induced destruction of kidney stones by shock waves. J Urol. 1982; 127(3): 417–420.
8. Lingeman JE, Lifshitz DA, Evan AP. Surgical management of urinary lithiasis. In: Campbell's Urology, 8th Ed., (Walsh PC, Retik AB, Vaughan ED, Wein AJ, eds.). Penn, Philadelphia, PA, 2002, pp. 3361–3451.
9. Zhong P, Preminger GM. Mechanisms of differing stone fragility in extracorporeal shockwave lithotripsy. J Endourol 1994; 8: 263–268.
10. Saw KC, McAteer JA, Fineberg NS, et al. Calcium stone fragility is predicted by helical CT attenuation values. J Endourol 2000; 14: 465–468.
11. Saw KC, McAteer JA, Monga AG, Chua GT, Lingeman JE, Williams JC Jr. Helical CT of urinary calculi: effect of stone composition, stone size, and scan collimation. AJR Am J Roentgenol 2000; 175: 329–332.
12. Pittomvils G, Vandeursen H, Wevers M, et al. The influence of internal stone structure upon the fracture behavior of urinary calculi. Ultrasound Med Biol 1994; 20: 803–810.
13. Saw KC, Lingeman JE. Lesson 20—management of calyceal stones. AUA Update Series 1999; 20: 154–159.
14. Dretler SP: Stone fragility. A new therapeutic distinction. J Urol 1988; 139: 1124–1127.

15. Motola JA, Smith AD. Therapeutic options for the management of upper tract calculi. Urol Clin North Am 1990; 17: 191–206.
16. Chaussy C, Schuller J, Schmiedt E, Brandl H, Jocham D, Liedl B. Extracorporeal shockwave lithotripsy (ESWL) for treatment of urolithiasis. Urology 1984; 23: 59–66.
17. Lingeman JE. Percutaneous procedures. In: Urinary Calculi, (Lingeman JE, Smith LH, Woods JR, Newman DM, eds.). Lea & Febiger, Philadelphia, PA, 1989, pp. 322–359.
18. Psihramis KE, Jewett MA, Bombardier C, Caron D, Ryan M. Lithostar extracorporeal shockwave lithotripsy: the first 1,000 patients. J Urol 1992; 147: 1006–1009.
19. Lingeman JE, Siegel YI, Steele B, Nyhuis AW, Woods JR. Management of lower pole nephrolithiasis: A critical analysis. J Urol 1994; 151: 663–667.
20. Cass AS. Comparison of first generation (Dornier HM-3) and second generation (Medstone STS) lithotriptors: Treatment results with 13,864 renal and ureteral calculi. J Urol 1995; 153: 588–592.
21. Murray MJ, Chandhoke PS, Berman CJ, Sankey NE. Outcome of extracorporeal shockwave lithotripsy monotherapy for large renal calculi. Effect of stone and collecting system surface areas and cost-effectiveness of treatment. J Endourol 1995; 9: 9–13.
22. Logarakis NF, Jewett MAS, Luymes J, Honey RJ. Variation in clinical outcome following shockwave lithotripsy. J Urol 2000; 163: 721–725.
23. Renner CH, Rassweiler J.: Treatment of renal stones by extracorporeal shockwave lithotripsy. Nephron 1999; 81: 71–81.
24. Albala DM, Assimos DG, Clayman RV, et al. Lower Pole I: a prospective randomized trial of extracorporeal shockwave lithotripsy and percutaneous nephrostolithotomy for lower pole nephrolithiasis-initial results. J Urol 2001; 166(6): 2072–2080.
25. Swanson SK. Excretory urography during extracorporeal shock-wave lithotripsy: a location alternative. Urology 1992; 39: 185–186.
26. Sundaram CP, Saltzman B. An effective technique to facilitate radiographic stone visualization with an internal stent during shockwave lithotripsy. J Urol 1998; 160(4): 1414, 1415.
27. Thomas R, Cass AS. Extracorporeal shockwave lithotripsy in morbidly obese patients. J Urol 1993; 150: 30–32.
28. Hoffmann R, Stoller ML. Endoscopic and open stone surgery in morbidly obese patients. J Urol 1992; 148: 1108–1111.
29. Thomas R, Macaluso JN, Vandenberg T, Salvatore F. An innovative approach to management of lower third ureteral calculi. J Urol 1993; 149: 1427–1430.
30. Drach GW, Dretler S, Fair W, et al. Report of the United States cooperative study of extracorporeal shockwave lithotripsy. J Urol 1986; 135: 1127–1133.
31. Graff J, Deidrichs W, Schultz H. Long-term follow-up in 1,003 extracorporeal shockwave lithotripsy patients. J Urol 1988; 140: 479.
32. Kohrmann KU, Rassweiler J, Alken P. The recurrence rate of stones following ESWL. World J Urol 1993; 11: 26–30.
33. Streem SB, Yost A, Mascha E. Clinical implications of clinically insignificant stone fragments after extracorporeal shockwave lithotripsy. J Urol 1996; 155: 1186–1190.
34. Newman DM, Scott JW, Lingeman JE. Two year follow up of patients treated with extracorporeal shockwave lithotripsy. J Endourol 1988; 2: 163–171.
35. Zanetti G, Seveso M, Montanari E, Guarneri A, Del Nero A, Nespoli R, Trinchieri A. Renal stone fragments following shockwave lithotripsy. J Urol 1997; 158: 352–355.
36. Candau C, Saussine C, Lang H, Roy C, Faure F, Jacqmin D. Natural history of residual renal stone fragments after ESWL. Eur Urol 2000; 37: 18–22.
37. Nijman RJ, Ackaert K, Scholtmeijer RJ, Lock TW, Schroder FH. Long-term results of extracorporeal shockwave lithotripsy in children. J Urol 1989; 142: 609–611.
38. Beck EM, Riehle RA. The fate of residual fragments after extracorporeal shockwave lithotripsy monotherapy of infection stones. J Urol 1991; 145: 6.
39. Fuchs AM, Wolfson BA, Fuchs GJ. Staghorn stone treatment with extracorporeal shockwave lithotripsy monotherapy: Long-term results. J Endourol 1991; 5: 45.
40. Nakamoto T, Sagami K, Yamasaki A, et al. Long-term results of endourologic treatment of urinary calculi: investigation of risk factors for recurrence or re-growth. J Endourol 1993; 7: 297–301.

41. Conlin MJ. Complications of extracorporeal shock-wave lithotripsy. In: Complications of Urologic Surgery, Prevention and Management, 3rd Ed., (Taneja SS, Smith RB, Ehrlich RM, eds.). WB Saunders, Philadelphia, PA, 2001, pp. 155–164.

42. McCullough, DL. Extracorporeal shock-wave lithotripsy. In: Campbell's Urology, vol. I, (Walsh PC, Retik AB, Stamey TA, et al., eds.). WB Saunders, Philadelphia, PA, 1992, pp. 2157–2182.

43. Sulaiman MN, Buchholz NP, Clark PB. The role of ureteral stent placement in the prevention of Steinstrasse. J Endourol 1999; 13(3): 151–155.

44. Sayed MA, el-Taher AM, Aboul-Ella HA, Shaker SE. Steinstrasse after extracorporeal shock-wave lithotripsy: aetiology, prevention and management. Br J Urol 2001; 88: 675–678.

45. Madbouly K, Sheir KZ, Elsobky E, Eraky I, Kenawy M. Risk factors for the formation of a steinstrasse after extracorporeal shock-wave lithotripsy: a statistical model. J Urol 2002; 167: 1239–1242.

46. Fedullo LM, Pollack HM, Banner MP, Amendola MA, Van Arsdalen KN. The development of steinstrassen after ESWL: frequency, natural history, and radiologic management. Am J Roentgenol 1988; 151: 1145–1147.

47. Fine H, Gordon RL, Lebensart PD. Extracorporeal shock-wave lithotripsy and stents: Fluoroscopic observations and a hypothesis on the mechanism of stent function. Urol Radiol 1989; 11: 37.

48. Ramsay JW, Crocker RP, Ball AJ, Jones S, Payne SR, Levison DA, Whitfield HN. Urothelial reaction to ureteric intubation: a clinical study. Br J Urol 1987; 60: 504, 505.

49. Saltzman, B. Ureteral stents indications, variations and complications. Urol Clin North Am 1988; 15: 481.

50. Bregg K, Riehle RA Jr. Morbidity associated with indwelling internal ureteral stents after shockwave lithotripsy. J Urol 1989; 141: 510–512.

51. Preminger GM, Kettelhut MC, Elkins SL, Seger J, Fetner CD. Ureteral stenting during extracorporeal shockwave lithotripsy: help or hindrance? J Urol 1989; 142: 32–36.

52. Low RK, Stoller ML, Irby P, Keeler L, Elhilali M. Outcome assessment of double-J stents during extracorporeal shockwave lithotripsy of small solitary renal calculi. J Endourol 1996; 10: 341–343.

53. Al-Awadi KA, Abdul Halim H, Kehinde EO, Al-Tawheed A. Steinstrasse: a comparison of incidence with and without J stenting and the effect of J stenting on subsequent management. Br J Urol 1999; 84: 618–621.

54. Hollowell CM, Patel RV, Bales GT, Gerber GS. Internet and postal survey of endourologic practice patterns among American urologists. J Urol 2000; 163: 1779–1782.

55. Chandhoke PS, Barqawi AZ, Wernecke C, Chee-Awai RA. A randomized outcomes trial of ureteral stents for extracorporeal shockwave lithotripsy of solitary kidney or proximal ureteral stones. J Urol 2002; 167: 1981–1983.

56. Kim SC, Oh CH, Moon YT, Kim KD. Treatment of steinstrasse with repeated extracorporeal shockwave lithotripsy: experience with piezoelectric lithotriptor. J Urol 1991; 145: 489–491.

57. Coptcoat MJ. The Steinstrasse: classification and management. In: Lithotripsy II. (Coptcoat MJ, Miller RA, Wickham JEA, eds.) BDI, London, 1987, pp. 133–137.

58. Coptcoat MJ, Webb DR, Kellet MJ, Whitfield HN, Wickham JE: The Steinstrasse: a legacy of extracorporeal lithotripsy. Eur Urol. 1988; 14(2): 93–95.

59. Newmark JR, Wong MYC, Lingeman JE. Complications. In: Smith's Textbook of Endourology, vol. I., (Smith AD, Bagley DH, Clayman RV, et al., eds.). Quality Medical, St. Louis, MO, 1996, pp. 680–693.

60. Weinerth JL, Flatt JA, Carson CC: Lessons learned in patients with large Steinstrasse. J Urol 1989; 142: 1425–1427.

61. Sigman M, Laudone V, Jenkins AD. Ureteral meatotomy as a treatment of Steinstrasse following extracorporeal shockwave lithotripsy. J Endourol 1988; 2: 41.

62. Rubenstein MA, Norris DM. Variation on water-pik technique for treatment of steinstrasse after ESWL. Urology 1988; 32: 429–430.

63. Clayman RV. Incidence of urinary tract infection in patients without bacteriuria undergoing SWL: comparison of stone types. J Urol 1999; 161: 727, 728.

64. Dincel C, Ozdiler E, Ozenci H, Tazici N, Kosar A. Incidence of urinary tract infection in patients without bacteriuria undergoing SWL: comparison of stone types. J Endourol 1998; 12: 1–3

65. Muller-Mattheis VG, Schmale D, Seewald M, Rosin H, Ackermann R. Bacteremia during extra-corporeal shockwave lithotripsy of renal calculi. J Urol 1991; 146: 733–736.

66. Lam HS, Lingeman JE, Barron M, et al. Staghorn calculi: analysis of treatment results between initial percutaneous nephrostolithotomy and extracorporeal shockwave lithotripsy monotherapy with reference to stone surface area. J Urol 1992; 147: 1219–1225.

67. Meretyk S, Bigg S, Clayman RV, Kavoussi LR, McClennan BL. Caveat emptor: calyceal stones and the missing calyx. J Urol 1992; 147: 1091–1095.

68. Bierkens AF, Hendrikx AJM, El Din K, de la Rosette JJMCH, Horrevorts A, Doesburg W, Debruyne FMJ: The value of antibiotic prophylaxis during extracorporeal shockwave lithotripsy in the prevention of urinary tract infections in patients with urine proven sterile prior to treatment. Eur Urol 1997; 31: 30.

69. Pearle MS and Roehrborn CE. Antimicrobial prophylaxis prior to shockwave lithotripsy in patients with sterile urine prior to treatment: a meta-analysis and cost-effectiveness analysis. Urology 1997; 49: 679.

70. Peiser J, Kaneti J, Lissmer L, Klain J, Blank C, Hertzanu Y. Perinephric inflammatory process following extracorporeal shockwave lithotripsy. Int Urol Nephrol 1991; 23: 107–111.

71. Davidson T, Tung K, Constant O, Edwards L. Kidney rupture and psoas abscess after ESWL. Br J Urol 1991; 68: 657, 658.

72. Kochakarn W, Ratana-Olarn K. Late perinephric abscess formation after extracorporeal shockwave lithotripsy. Br J Urol. 1991; 68(3): 323, 324

73. Greenwald BD, Tunkel AR, Morgan KM, Campochiaro PA, Donowitz GR. Candidal endophthal-mitis after lithotripsy of renal calculi. South Med J 1992; 85: 773, 774.

74. Kremer I, Gaton DD, Baniel J, Servadio C. Klebsiella metastatic endophthalmitis—a complication of shockwave lithotripsy. Ophthalmic Surg 1990; 21: 206–208.

75. Dogra PN, Jadeja NA. Urosepsis and ureteric strictures following extracorporeal shockwave lith-otripsy. Urol Int. 1994; 52: 109–112.

76. Silber N, Kremer I, Gaton DD, Servadio C. Severe sepsis following extracorporeal shockwave lithotripsy. J Urol 1991; 145: 1045, 1046.

77. Morano Amado LE, Amador Barciela L, Rodriguez Fernandez A, Martinez-Sapina Llamas I, Vazquez Alvarez O, Fernandez Martin J. Extracorporeal shockwave lithotripsy complicated with military tuberculosis. J Urol 1993; 149: 1532–1534.

78. Kaude JV, Williams CM, Millner MR, Scott KN, Finlayson B. Renal morphology and function immediately after extracorporeal shockwave lithotripsy. Am J Roentgenol 1985; 145: 305–313.

79. Jaeger P, Redha F, Uhlschmid G, Hauri D. Morphological changes in canine kidneys following extracorporeal shockwave treatment. Urol Res 1988; 16: 161–166.

80. Wilson WT, Morris JS, Husmann DA, Preminger GM. Extracorporeal shockwave lithotripsy: Comparison between stone and non-stone animal models of ESWL. J Endourol 1992; 6: 33.

81. Adwers JR. Gallstone lithotripsy: Early American results and the new reality. J Litho Stone Dis 1990; 2: 199.

82. Baumgartner BR, Dickey KW, Ambrose SS, Walton KN, Nelson RC, Bernardino ME. Kidney changes after extracorporeal shockwave lithotripsy: appearance on MR imaging. Radiology 1987; 163: 531–534.

83. Rubin JI, Arger PH, Pollack HM, et al. Kidney changes after extracorporeal shockwave lithotripsy: CT evaluation. Radiology 1987; 162: 21–24.

84. Knapp PM, Kulb TB, Lingeman JE, et al. Extracorporeal shockwave lithotripsy induced perirenal hematomas. J Urol 1988; 139: 700–703.

85. Thomas R, Roberts J, Sloane B, Kaack B. Effect of extracorporeal shockwave lithotripsy on renal function. J Endourol 1988; 2: 141.

86. Kaude JV, Williams JL, Wright PG, Bush D, Derau C, Newman RC. Sonographic evaluation of the kidney following extracorporeal shockwave lithotripsy. J Ultrasound Med 1987; 6: 299–306.

87. Dyer RB, Karstaedt N, McCullough DL, et al. Magnetic resonance imaging evaluation of imme-diate and intermediate changes in kidneys treated with extracorporeal shockwave lithotripsy. In: Shockwave Lithotripsy 2: Urinary and Biliary Lithotripsy, (Lingeman JE, Newman DM, eds.). Plenum, New York, NY, 1989, pp. 203–205.

88. Kishimoto T, Senju M, Sugimoto T, et al. Effects of high energy shockwave exposure on renal function during extracorporeal shockwave lithotripsy for kidney stones. Eur Urol 1990; 18: 290–298.

89. Recker F, Hofmann W, Bex A, Tscholl R. Quantitative determination of urinary marker proteins: a model to detect intrarenal bioeffects after extracorporeal lithotripsy. J Urol 1992; 148: 1000–1006.

90. Sakamoto W, Kishimoto T, Nakatani T, et al. Examination of aggravating factors of urinary excretion of N-acetyl-beta-D-glucosaminidase after extracorporeal shockwave lithotripsy. Nephron 1991; 58: 205–209.

91. Sen S, Erdem Y, Oymak O, et al. Effect of extracorporeal shockwave lithotripsy on glomerular and tubular function. Int Urol Nephrol 1996; 28: 309–313.

92. Karlin GS, Schulsinger D, Urivetsky M, Smith AD. Absence of persisting parenchymal damage after extracorporeal shock wave lithotripsy as judged by excretion of renal tubular enzymes. J Urol. 1990; 144(1): 13, 14.

93. Sakkas G, Becopoulos T, Karayannis A, Drossos G, Giannopoulou K. Enzymatic evaluation of renal damage caused by different therapeutic procedures for kidney stone disease. Int Urol Nephrol 1995; 27: 669–677.

94. Sarica K, Suzer O, Yaman O, Kupeli B, Baltaci S, Bilaloglu E, Tasman S. Leucine aminopeptidase enzymuria: quantification of renal tubular damage following extracorporeal shockwave lithotripsy. Int Urol Nephrol 1996; 28: 621–626.

95. Assimos DG, Boyce WH, Furr EG, Espeland MA, Holmes RP, Harrison LH, Kroovand RL, McCullough DL. Selective elevation of urinary enzyme levels after extracorporeal shockwave lithotripsy. J Urol 1989; 142: 687–690.

96. Morris JS, Husmann DA, Wilson WT, Preminger GM. Temporal effects of shockwave lithotripsy. J Urol 1991: 145: 881–883.

97. Jaeger P, Redha F, Marquardt K, Uhlschmid G, Hauri D. Morphological and functional changes in canine kidneys following extracorporeal shockwave treatment. Urol Int 1995; 54: 48–58.

98. Jung K, Kirschner P, Wille A, Brien G. Excretion of urinary enzymes after extracorporeal shockwave lithotripsy: a critical reevaluation. J Urol 1993; 149: 1409–1413.

99. Kishimoto T, Yamamoto K, Sugimoto T, Yoshihara H, Maekawa M. Side effects of extracorporeal shockwave exposure in patients treated by extracorporeal shockwave lithotripsy for upper urinary tract stone. Eur Urol 1986; 12: 308–313.

100. Wolff JM, Mattelaer P, Boeckmann W, Kraemer U, Jakse G. Evaulation of possible tissue damage in patients undergoing extracorporeal shockwave lithotripsy employing C-reactive protein. Scand J Urol Nephrol 1997; 31: 31–34.

101. Karlsen SJ, Berg KJ. Acute changes in kidney function following extracorporeal shockwave lithotripsy for renal stones. Br J Urol 1991; 67: 241–245.

102. Krongrad A, Saltzman B, Tannenbaum M. Enzymuria after extracorporeal shockwave lithotripsy. J Endourol 1991; 5: 209.

103. Rigatti P, Colombo R, Centemero A, et al. Histological and ultrastructural evaluation of extracorporeal shockwave lithotripsy-induced acute renal lesions: preliminary report. Eur Urol 1989; 16: 207–211.

104. Jaeger P, Redha F, Uhlschmid G, Hauri D. Morphological changes in canine kidneys following extracorporeal shockwave treatment. Urol Res 1988; 16: 161–166.

105. Maziak DE, Ralph-Edwards A, Deitel M, Wait J, Watt HJ, Marcuzzi A. Massive perirenal and intra-abdominal bleeding after shockwave lithotripsy: case report. Can J Surg 1994; 37: 329–332.

106. Dominguez Molinero JF, Arrabal Martin M, Mijan Ortiz JL, Lopez Carmona F, de la Fuente Serrano A, Zuluaga Gomez A. Renal hematomas secondary to extracorporeal shockwave lithotripsy. Arch Esp Urol 1997; 50: 767–771.

107. Ueda S, Matsuoka K, Yamashita T, Kunimi H, Noda S, Eto K. Perirenal hematomas caused by SWL with EDAP LT-01 lithotripter. J Endourol 1993; 7: 11–15.

108. Kostakopoulos A, Stavropoulos NJ, Macrychoritis C, Deliveliotis C, Antonopoulos KP, Picramenos D. Subcapsular hematoma due to ESWL: risk factors. A study of 4,247 patients. Urol Int 1995; 55: 21–24.

109. Newman LH, Saltzman B: Identification of risk factors in the development of clinically significant subcapsular hematomas following shockwave lithotripsy. In: Shock-wave Lithotripsy 2: Urinary and Biliary Lithotripsy, (Lingeman JE, Newman DM, eds.). Plenum, New York, NY, 1989, pp. 207–210.

110. Newman LH, Saltzman B: Identifying risk factors in development of clinically significant post-shock-wave lithotripsy subcapsular hematomas. Urology. 1991, 38: 35–38

111. Streem SB, Yost A. Extracorporeal shockwave lithotripsy in patients with bleeding diatheses. J Urol 1990; 144: 1347, 1348.

112. Donahue LA, Linke CA, Rowe JM. Renal loss following extracorporeal shockwave lithotripsy. J Urol 1989; 142: 809–811.

113. Umekawa T, Yamate T, Amasaki N, Ishikawa Y, Kohri K, Kurita T. Continuous evaluation for retroperitoneal hematoma following extracorporeal shockwave lithotripsy. Urol Int 1993; 51: 114–116.

114. Lemann J Jr, Taylor AJ, Collier BD, Lipchik EO. Kidney hematoma due to extracorporeal shockwave lithotripsy causing transient renin mediated hypertension. J Urol 1991; 145: 1238–1241.

115. Graham CW, Lynch SC, Muskat PC, Mokulis JA. Laparoscopic evacuation of a subcapsular renal hematoma causing symptomatic hypertension. J Endourol 1998; 12(6): 551–553.

116. Littleton RH, Melser M, Kupin W: Acute renal failure following bilateral extracorporeal shockwave lithotripsy without ureteral obstruction. In: Shockwave Lithotripsy 2: Urinary and Biliary Lithotripsy, (Lingeman JE, Newman DM, eds.). Plenum, New York, NY, 1989, pp. 197–201.

117. Hardy MR, McLeod DG. Silent renal obstruction with severe functional loss after extracorporeal shockwave lithotripsy: a report of 2 cases. J Urol 1987; 137: 91–92.

118. Willis LR, Evan AP, Connors BA, Reed G, Fineberg NS, Lingeman JA. Effects of extracorporeal shockwave lithotripsy to one kidney on bilateral glomerular filtration rate and PAH clearance in minipigs. J Urol 1996; 156: 1502–1506.

119. Willis LR, Evan AP, Connors BA, Fineberg NS, Lingeman JE. Effects of SWL on glomerular filtration rate and renal plasma flow in uninephrectomized minipigs. J Endourol 1997; 11: 27–32.

120. Kataoka T, Kasahara T, Kobashikawa K, Masuyama T, Watanabe K, Saito T, Ishida H, Yoshida H. Changes in renal blood flow after treatment with ESWL in patients with renal stones: studies using ultrasound color Doppler method. J Urol 1993; 84: 851–856.

121. Mostafavi MR, Chavez DR, Cannillo J, Saltzman B, Prasad PV. Redistribution of renal blood flow after SWL evaluated by Gd-DTPA-enhanced magnetic resonance imaging. J Endourol 1998; 12: 9–12.

122. Chan AJ, Prasad PV, Priatna A, Mostafavai MR, Sunduram C, Saltzman B. Protective effect of aminophylline on renal perfusion changes induced by high-energy shockwaves identified by Gd-DTPA-enhanced first-pass perfusion MRI. J Endourol 2000; 14: 117–121.

123. Brito CG, Lingeman JE, Newman DM, Kight JL, Heck LL. Long-term follow-up of renal function in ESWL-treated patients with solitary kidney. Abstract 299A. J Urol 1990; 143: 442.

124. Chandhoke PS, Albala DM, Clayman RV. Long-term comparison of renal function in patients with solitary kidneys and/or moderate renal insufficiency undergoing extracorporeal shockwave lithotripsy or percutaneous nephrolithotomy. J Urol 1992; 147: 1226.

125. Neal DE, Harmon EP, Hlavinka T, Kaack MB, Thomas R. Simultaneous bilateral extracorporeal shockwave treatment of the kidney in the primate model. J Endourol 1991; 1: 41–43.

126. Pienkny AJ, Streem SB. Simultaneous versus staged bilateral extracorporeal shockwaveshockwave lithotripsy: long-term effect on renal function. J Urol 1999; 162: 1591–1593

127. Perry KT, Smith ND, Weiser AC, User HM, Kundu SD, Nadler RB. The efficacy and safety of synchronous bilateral extracorporeal shockwave lithotripsy. J Urol 2000; 164: 644–647.

128. Kulb TB, Lingeman JE, Coury TA, et al. Extracorporeal shockwave lithotripsy in patients with a solitary kidney. J Urol 1986; 136: 786–788.

129. Karalezli G, Muftuoglu YZ, Sarica K, Yaman LS, Yurdakul T, Ozdiler E. Treatment of renal stones in a solitary functioning kidney with extracorporeal shockwave lithotripsy Urol Int 1993; 50: 86–89.

130. Zanetti GR, Montanari E, Guarneri A, Trinchieri A, Mandressi A, Ceresoli A. Long-term follow-up after extracorporeal shockwave lithotripsy treatment of kidney stones in solitary kidneys. J Urol 1992; 148: 1011–1014.

131. Liou LS, Streem SB. Long-term renal functional effects of shockwave lithotripsy, percutaneous nephrolithotomy and combination therapy: a comparative study of patients with solitary kidney. J Urol 2001; 166: 36; discussion 36–37.

132. Bhatia V, Biyani CS, al-Awadi K. Extracorporeal shockwave therapy for urolithiasis with renal insufficiency. Urol Int 1995; 55: 11–15.

133. Klingler HC, Kramer G, Lodde M, Marberger M. Urolithiasis in allograft kidneys. Urology 2002; 59: 344–348.

134. Chen CS, Lai MK, Hsieh ML, Chu SH, Huang MH, Chen SJ. Subcapsular hematoma of spleen—a complication following extracorporeal shockwave lithotripsy for ureteral calculus. Change Keng I Hsueh 1992; 15: 215–219.

135. Marcuzzi D, Gray R, Wesley-James T. Symptomatic splenic rupture following extracorporeal shockwave lithotripsy. J Urol 1991; 145: 547, 548.

136. Rashid P, Steele D, Hunt J. Splenic rupture after extracorporeal shockwave lithotripsy. J Urol 1996: 156: 1756, 1757.

137. Conde Redondo C, Estebanez Zarranz J, Amon Sesmero J, et al. Splenic hematoma after extracorporeal lithotripsy: apropos of a case. Arch Esp Urol 2002; 55: 943–946.

138. Kirkali Z, Kirkali G, Tanci S, Tahiri Y. The effect of extracorporeal shockwave lithotripsy on pancreatic enzymes. Int Urol Nephrol 1994; 26: 405–408.

139. Mullen KD, Hoofnagle JH, Jones EA. Shockwave-induced pancreatic trauma. Am J Gastroenterol 1991; 86: 630–632.

140. Hassan I, Zietlow SP. Acute pancreatitis after extracorporeal shockwave lithotripsy for a renal calculus. Urology 2002; 60: 1111.

141. Flood HD, Jones B, Grainger R. Ureterocolic fistula: a unique complication of extracorporeal shockwave lithotripsy. J Urol 1992; 147: 122–124

142. Srinivasan A, Mowad JJ. Pyelocutaneous fistula after SWL of xanthogranulomatous pyelonephritic kidney: case report. J Endourol 1998; 12: 13–14.

143. Kumar RV, Kumar A, Banerjee GK Ureterovaginal fistula: an unusual complication of stone fragments after extracorporeal shockwave lithotripsy in situ. J Urol 1994; 152: 2096,2097.

144. Alkibay T, Karaoglan U, Gundogdu S, Bozkirli I. An unusual complication of extracorporeal shockwave lithotripsy: urinoma due to rupture of the renal pelvis. Int Urol Neprhol 1992; 24: 11–14.

145. Collado A, Orsola A, Monreal F, Gausa-Gascon L, Rousaud A, Vicente J. Renocutaneous fistulae: a rare complication of extracorporeal shockwave lithotripsy. Int Urol Nephrol 1999; 31: 31–34.

146. Ector H, Janssens L, Baert L, De Geest H. Extracorporeal shockwave lithotripsy and cardiac arrhythmias. Pacing Clin Electrophysiol 1989; 12: 1910–1917.

147. Kataoka H. Cardiac dysrhythmias related to extracorporeal shockwave lithotripsy using a piezoelectric lithotriptors in patients with kidney stones. J Urol 1995; 153: 1390–1394.

148. Greenstein A, Kaver I, Lechtman V, Braf Z. Cardiac arrhythmias during nonsynchronized extracorporeal shockwave lithotripsy. J Urol 1995; 154: 1321, 1322.

149. Zanetti G, Ostini F, Montanari E, Russo R, Elena A, Trinchieri A, Pisani E. Cardiac dysrhythmias induced by extracorporeal shockwave lithotripsy. J Endourol 1999; 13: 409–412.

150. Lazarides MK, Drista H, Arvanitis DP, Dayantas JN. Aortic aneurysm rupture after extracorporeal shockwave lithotripsy. Surgery 1996: 122: 112, 113.

151. Taylor JD, McLoughlin GA, Parson KF. Extracorporeal shockwave lithotripsy induced rupture of abdominal aortic aneurysm. Br J Urol 1995; 76: 262, 263.

152. Neri E, Capannini G, Diciolla F, et al. Localized dissection and delayed rupture of the abdominal aorta after extracorporeal shockwave lithotripsy. J Vasc Surg 2000; 31: 1052–1055.

153. Thomas R, Cherry R, Neal DW. The use of extracorporeal shockwave lithotripsy in patients with aortic aneurysms. J Urol 1991; 146; 409, 410.

154. Hellstrom WJ, Kaack MB, Harrison RM, Neal DE Jr, Thomas R. Absence of a long-term gonadotoxicity in primates receiving extracorporeal shockwave application. J Endourol 1993; 7: 17–21.

155. Andreessen R, Fedel M, Sudhoff F, Friedrichs R, Loening SA. Quality of semen after extracorporeal shockwave lithotripsy for lower urethral stones. J Urol 1996; 155: 1281–1283.

156. McCullough DL, Yeaman LD, Bo WJ, et al. Effects of shockwaves on the rat ovary. J Urol 1989; 141: 666–669.

157. Vieweg J, Weber HM, Miller K, Hautmann R. Female fertility following extracorporeal shockwave lithotripsy of distal ureteral calculi. J Urol 1992; 148: 1007–1010.

158. Thomas R, Frentz JM, Harmon E, Frentz GD. Effect of extracorporeal shockwave lithotripsy on renal function and body height in pediatric patients. J Urol 1992; 148: 1064–1066.

159. Villanyi KK, Szekely JG, Farkas LM, Javor E, Pusztai C. Short-term changes in renal function after extracorporeal shockwave lithotripsy in children. J Urol 2001; 166: 222–224.

160. Shepherd P, Thomas R, Harmon EP. Urolithiasis in Children: Innovations in Management. J Urol 1988; 140: 790.

161. Brinkmann OA, Griehl A, Kuwertz-Broking E, Bulla M, Hertle L. Extracorporeal shockwave lithotripsy in children. Efficacy, complications and long-term follow-up. Eur Urol 2001; 39: 591–597.

162. Newman RC, Williams CM, Kaude J, Peterson J, Thomas WC. Hypertension following ESWL. Abstract 0/230, In Proceedings of the Fifth World Congress on Endourology and ESWL, 1987.

163. Lingeman JE, Kulb TB. Hypertension following ESWL. J Urol 1987; 137: 142A.

164. Williams CM, Kaude JV, Newman RC, Peterson JC, Thomas WC. Extracorporeal shock-wave lithotripsy: long-term complications. Am J Roentgenol 1988; 150: 311–315.

165. Montgomery BS, Cole RS, Palfrey EL, Shuttleworth KE. Does extracorporeal shockwave lithotripsy cause hypertension? Br J Urol 1989; 64: 567–571

166. Danneberg AL, Garrison RJ, Kannel WB. Incidence of hypertension in the Framingham Study. Am J Public Health. 1988; 78: 676–679.

167. Yokoyama M, Shoji F, Yanagizawa R, et al. Blood pressure changes following extracorporeal shockwave lithotripsy for urolithiasis. J Urol 1992; 147: 553–557; discussion 557, 558.

168. Lingeman JE, Woods JR, Toth PD. Blood pressure changes following extracorporeal shockwave lithotripsy and other forms of treatment for nephrolithiasis. JAMA. 1990; 263: 1789–1794.

169. Lingeman JE, Woods JR, Nelson DR. Commentary on ESWL and blood pressure. J Urol 1995; 154: 2–4

170. Claro JA, Lima ML, Ferreira U, Rodrigues NN Jr. Blood pressure changes after extracorporeal shock wave lithotripsy in normotensive patients. J Urol 1993; 150(6): 1765–1767

171. Jewett MA, Bombardier C, Logan AG, et al. A randomized controlled trial to assess the incidence of new onset hypertension in patients after shockwave lithotripsy for asymptomatic renal calculi. J Urol 1998; 160: 1241–1243.

172. Elves AW, Tilling K, Menezes P, Wills M, Rao PN, Feneley RC. Early observations of the effect of extracorporeal shockwave lithotripsy on blood pressure: a prospective randomized control clinical trial. BJU Int 2000; 85: 611–615.

173. Strohmaier WL, Schmidt J, Lahme S, Bichler KH. Arterial blood pressure following different types of urinary stone therapy. Presented at the 8th European Symposium on Urolithiasis, Parma, Italy, 1999. Eur Urol 2000; 38: 753–757.

174. Begun FP, Knoll CE, Gottlieb M, Lawson RK. Chronic effects of focused electrohydraulic shockwaves on renal function and hypertension. J Urol 1991; 145: 635–639.

175. Neal DE Jr, Kaack MB, Harmon EP, et al. Renin production after experimental extracorporeal shockwave lithotripsy: a primate model. J Urol 1991; 146: 548–550.

176. Strohmaier WL, Carl AM, Wilbert DM, Bichler KH. Effects of extracorporeal shockwave lithotripsy on plasma concentrations of endothelin and renin in humans. J Urol 1996; 155: 48–51.

177. Knapp R, Frauscher F, Helweg G, zur Nedden D, Strasser H, Janetschek G and Bartsch G. Age-related changes in resistive index following extracorporeal shockwave lithotripsy. J Urol 1995; 154: 955.

178. Janetschek G, Frauscher F, Knapp R, Hofle G, Peschel R, Bartsch G. New onset hypertension after extracorporeal shockwave lithotripsy: age related incidence and prediction by intrarenal resistive index. J Urol 1997; 158: 346–351.

179. Knapp R, Frauscher F, Helweg G, Judmaier W, Strasser H, Bartsch G, zur Nedden D. Blood pressure changes after extracorporeal shockwave nephrolithotripsy: prediction by intrarenal resistive index. Eur Radiol 1996; 6: 665–669.

180. Fernstrom I, Johannson B: Percutaneous pyelolithotomy: A new extraction technique. Scand J Urol Nephrol 1976; 10: 257.

181. Dyer RB, Assimos DG, Regan JD: Update on interventional uroradiology. Urol Clin North Am 1997; 24: 623.

182. Sampaio FJ, Zanier JF, Aragao AH, Favorito LA. Intrarenal access: 3-dimensional anatomical study. J Urol 1992; 148: 1769–1773.

183. Sampaio FJB, Aragao AHM: Anatomical relationship between the intrarenal arteries and the collecting system. J Urol 1990; 143: 679.

184. Goharderakhshan RZ, Schwartz BF, Rudnick DM, Irby PB, Stoller ML. Radially expanding single-step nephrostomy tract dilator. Urology 2001; 58(5): 693–696.

185. Davidoff R, Bellman GC. Influence of technique of percutaneous tract creation on incidence of renal hemorrhage. J Urol 1997; 157: 1229–1231.

186. Lang EK. Percutaneous nephrostolithotomy and lithotripsy: a multi-institutional survey of complications. Radiology 1987; 62: 25.

187. Roth RA, Beckmann CF. Complications of extracorporeal shockwave lithotripsy and percutaneous nephrolithotomy. Urol Clin North Am 1988; 15: 155.

188. Clayman RV, Surya V, Hunter D, et al. Renal vascular complications associated with percutaneous removal of renal calculi. J Urol 1984; 132: 228–230.

189. Carson CC, Brown MW, Weinerth JL. Vascular complications of percutaneous renal surgery. J Endourol 1987; 1: 181–187.

190. Stoller ML, Wolf JS Jr, St Lezin Ma. Estimated blood loss and transfusion rates associated with percutaneous nephrolithotomy. J Urol 1994; 152: 1977–1981.

191. Merhej S, Jabbour M, Samaha E, et al. Treatment of staghorn calculi by percutaneous nephrolithotomy and SWL: the Hotel Dieu de France experience. J Endourol 1998; 12: 5–8.

192. Gupta M, Bellman GC, Smith AD. Massive hemorrhage from renal vein injury during percutaneous renal surgery: endourological management. J Urol 1997; 157(3): 795–797.

193. Kaye KW, Clayman RV. Tamponade nephrostomy catheter for percutaneous nephrostolithotomy. Urology 1986; 27: 441.

194. Kerbl K, Picus DD, Clayman RV. Clinical experience with the Kaye nephrostomy tamponade catheter. Eur Urol 1994; 25: 94.

195. Goldfischer ER, Eiley DM, Smith AD. Novel hemostatic nephrostomy tube. J Endourol 1997; 11: 405–407.

196. Uflacker R, Paolini RM, Lima S. Management of traumatic hematuria by selective renal artery embolization. J Urol 1984; 132: 662–667.

197. Beaujeaux R, Saussine C, Al Fakir A, et al. Superselective endo-vascular treatment of renal vascular lesions. J Urol 1995; 153: 14.

198. Gallucci M, Fortunato P, Schettini M, Vincenzoni A. Management of hemorrhage after percutaneous renal surgery. J Endourol 1998; 12: 509–512.

199. Galek L, Darewicz B, Werel T, Darewicz J. Haemorrhagic complications of percutaneous lithotripsy: original methods of treatment. Int Urol Nephrol 2000; 32: 231–233.

200. Martin X, Murat FJ, Feitosa LC, et al. Severe bleeding after nephrolithotomy: results of hyperselective embolization. Eur Urol 2000; 37: 136–139.

201. Thomas R, Ruiz-Deya G, Mendez F, Shaw K, Lang E. Diagnosis and management of vascular complications from access procedures for percutaneous nephrostolithotripsy. Presented at Southeastern Section, Abstract #28. American Urological Association Meeting, Savannah, GA, 2003.

202. Kessaris DN, Bellman GC, Pardalidis NP, Smith AG. Management of hemorrhage after percutaneous renal surgery. J Urol 1995; 153: 604–608.

203. Fuchs GJ, Moody JA, Gutierrez-Aceves J, Barbaric JL. In: Complications of Percutaneous Renal Surgery. Prevention and Management, 3rd Ed. (Taneja SS, Smith RB, Ehrlich RM, eds.). WB Saunders, Philadelphia, PA, 2001: pp. 277–290.

204. Irby PB, Schwartz BF, Stoller ML. Percutaneous access techniques in renal surgery. Tech Urol 1999; 5: 29.

205. Carson CC, Nesbitt JA: Peritoneal extravasations during percutaneous lithotripsy. J Urol 1985; 134: 725.

206. Munver R, Delvecchio FC, Newman GE, Preminger GM. Critical analysis of supracostal access for percutaneous renal surgery. J Urol 2001; 166: 1242–1246.

207. Palou Redorta J, Banus Gassol JM, Prera Vilaseca A, Ramon Dalmau M, Morote Robles J, Ahmad Wahad A. Renopleural fistula after percutaneous nephrolithotomy. Urol Int 1988; 43: 104–106.

208. Hopper KD, Sherman JL, Williams MD, Ghaed N. The variable anteroposterior position of the retroperitoneal colon to the kidneys. Invest Radiol 1987; 22: 298–302.

209. Skoog SJ, Reed MD, Gaudier FA Jr, Dunn NP. The posterolateral and the retrorenal colon: Implications in percutaneous stone extraction. J Urol 1985; 134: 110–112.

210. LeRoy AJ, Williams HJ Jr, Bender CE, Segura JW, Patterson DE, Benson RC. Colon perforation following percutaneous nephrostomy and renal calculus removal. Radiology 1985; 155: 83–85.

211. Wolf JS. Management of intra-operatively diagnosed colonic injury during percutaneous nephrostolithotomy. Tech Urol 1998; 4: 160–164.

212. Thuroff J. Alken P. Ultrasound for renal puncture and fluoroscopy for tract dilation and catheter placement. Endourol Newslett 1987; 2(1).

213. Assimos DG. Complications of Stone Removal. In: Smith's Textbook of Endourology, vol. 21, (Smith AD, Bagley DH, Clayman RV, et al., eds.). Quality Medical, St Louis,, MO, 1996, pp. 298–308.

214. Gerspach JM, Bellman GC, Stoller ML, Fugelso P. Conservative management of colon injury following percutaneous renal surgery. Urology 1997; 49: 831–836.

215. Hopper KD, Yakes WF. The posterior intercostal approach for percutaneous renal procedures: Risk of puncturing the lung, spleen, and liver as determined by CT. Am J Roentgenol 1990; 154: 115–117.

216. Sampaio FJB. Surgical anatomy of the kidney. In: Smith's Textbook of Endourology. (Smith AD, Badlani GH, Bagley DH, et al, eds.). Quality Medical, St. Louis, MO, 1996, pp. 153–184.

217. Robert M, Maubon A, Roux JO, Rouanet JP, Navratil H. Direct percutaneous approach to the upper pole of the kidney: MRI anatomy with assessment of the visceral risk. J Endourol 1999; 13: 17–20.

218. Kondas J, Szentgyorgyi E, Vaczi L, Kiss A. Splenic injury: a rare complication of percutaneous nephrolithotomy. Int Urol Nephrol 1994; 26: 399–404.

219. Grasso M. Experience with the holmium laser as an endoscopic lithotrite. Urology 1996; 48: 199.

220. Teh CL, Zhong P, Preminger GM. Laboratory and clinical assessment of pneumatically driven intracorporeal lithotripsy. J Endouro. 1998; 12: 163–169.

221. Hofmann R, Olbert P, Weber J, Wille S, Varga Z. Clinical experience with a new ultrasonic and LithoClast combination for percutaneous litholapaxy. BJU Int 2002; 90: 16–19.

222. Denstedt JD, Razvi HA, Rowe E, Grignon DJ, Eberwein PM. Investigation of the tissue effect of a new device for intracorporeal lithotripsy: the Swiss lithoclast. J Urol. 1995; 153: 535–537.

223. Vorreuther R, Corleis R, Klotz T, Bernards P, Engelmann U. Impact of shock-wave pattern and cavitation bubble size on tissue damage during ureteroscopic electrohydraulic lithotripsy. J Urol 1995; 153: 849–853.

224. Denstedt JD, Razvi HA, Sales JL, Eberwein PM. Preliminary experience with Holmium: YAG laser lithotripsy. J Endourol 1995; 9: 255–258.

225. Gould DL. Holmium: YAG laser and its use in the treatment of urolithiasis: our first 160 cases. J Endourol 1998; 12: 23.

226. Johnson DE, Cromeens DM, Price RE. Use of the Holmium: YAG laser in urology. Lasers Surg Med 1992; 12: 353–363.

227. Thomas R. Rigid ureteroscopy: pitfalls and remedies. Urology 1988; 27: 328–334.

228. Blute ML, Segura JW, Patterson DE, Benson RC Jr, Zincke H. Impact of endourology on diagnosis and management of upper urinary tract urothelial cancer. J Urol 1989; 141: 1298–1301.

229. Low RK, Moran ME, Anderson KR. Ureteroscopic cytologic diagnosis of upper tract lesions. J Endourol 1993; 7(4): 311–314.

230. Fasihuddin Q, Hasan AT. Ureteroscopy: an effective interventional and diagnostic modality. J Pak Med Assoc 2002; 52: 510–512.

231. Grasso M, Bagley D. Small diameter, actively deflectable, flexible ureteroscopy. J Urol 1998; 160: 1648.

232. Thomas R: Catheterizing a Tortuous Ureter. J Urol 1998; 140: 778.

233. Abdel-Razzak OM, Bagley DH: Clinical experience with flexible ureteropyeloscopy. J Urol 1992; 148: 1788.

234. Morris H. A case of nephro-lithotomy or the extraction of a calculus from an undilated kidney. Trans Clin Soc Lond 1881; 14: 31.

235. Brodel M. The intrinsic blood vessels of the kidney and their significance in nephrotomy. Bull Johns Hopkins Hosp. 1901; 12: 10–13.

236. Robson AW. A method of exposing and operating on the kidney without division of muscles, vessels, or nerves. Lancet 1898; 1: 1315–1317.

237. Honig MP, Mason RA, Giron F. Wound complications of the retroperitoneal approach to the aorta and iliac vessels. J Vasc Surg 1992;15:25.

238. Moore RG, Partin AW, Adams JB, et al. Adhesion formation after retroperitoneal nephrectomy: laparoscopic versus open approach. J Endourol 1995; 9: 277.

239. Carlin BI, Paik M, Bodner DR, Resnick MI. Complications of urologic surgery prevention and management. In: Complications of Urologic Surgery, 3rd Ed. (Taneja SS, Smith RB, Ehrlich RM, eds.). WB Saunders Company, Philadelphia, PA, 2001, pp. 333–341.

240. Spirnak JP, Resnick MI. Anatrophic nephrolithotomy. Urol Clin North Am 1983; 10: 665–675.

28 Extracorporeal Shockwave Lithotripsy

Patient Selection and Outcomes

Christopher S. Ng, MD, Gerhard J. Fuchs, MD, and Stevan B. Streem, MD

CONTENTS

Key Words: Shockwave lithotripsy; nephrolithiasis; stone free; outcome.

INTRODUCTION

Since its first scientific and clinical descriptions by Chaussy more than 20 years ago, extracorporeal shockwave lithotripsy (SWL) has truly revolutionized the urologic management of stone disease and remains the sole noninvasive surgical treatment modality for urinary tract calculi (*1–3*). During the 1980s, the explosion of clinical experience with SWL was joined by that of other emerging "endo-urologic" modalities, such as percutaneous nephrolithotomy and ureteroscopy. As these technologies have continued to improve over the last decade, the relative roles of each endo-urologic approach have likewise continued to evolve. As is often the case, more controversies have been raised than have been settled as a result. This chapter details the contemporary role of SWL in the surgical management of urinary tract calculi and addresses areas of debate with its use.

PATIENT SELECTION

The indications for intervention with SWL for urinary tract stone disease remain unchanged. Thus, potential candidates for this treatment modality include patients with

From: Current Clinical Urology, *Urinary Stone Disease:*
A Practical Guide to Medical and Surgical Management
Edited by: M. L. Stoller and M. V. Meng © Humana Press Inc., Totowa, NJ

increasing stone size despite appropriate medical management or patients in whom the stones are associated with obstruction, refractory pain, urinary tract infection, or significant bleeding. In fact, the large majority of patients with urolithiasis who eventually present to the urologist will meet these criteria, and SWL will be the primary treatment of choice for almost all of such patients. Therefore, it becomes increasingly important not only to "rule out" certain absolute contraindications before proceeding with SWL, but also to identify correctly special patient conditions for which specific perioperative measures should be taken to allow for safe delivery of SWL. Furthermore, it is important to understand the technical limitations of SWL to allow for informed patient preference and improved patient selection.

Contraindications

Absolute contraindications to SWL include pregnancy, acute pyelonephritis or urinary sepsis, irreversible coagulopathy, implanted cardiac devices containing an abdominal crystalline component, and calcified vascular aneurysms located within 5 cm of the target stone, or measuring greater than 2 and 5 cm in absolute diameter for renal and aortic aneurysms, respectively. It is evident that these are very specific conditions that are presented by a minority of patients considered for SWL; nevertheless, they must be remembered, sought after, and ruled out.

Pregnancy remains an absolute contraindication to SWL, primarily owing to the potential risk to the fetus from radiation exposure, anesthesia, or the shockwaves (4). However, definitive clinical or scientific evidence to suggest either injury or safety is lacking, for obvious reasons. Interestingly, in a recent review of six women who were *post facto* determined to be 1–4 wk pregnant at the time of SWL, all women bore healthy children without chromosomal abnormalities (5). Furthermore, women of child-bearing age who undergo SWL do not appear to be at increased risk for infertility or fetal teratogenesis (6,7). Increased experience with piezoelectric lithotriptors with tiny focal points that enable radiation-free and anesthesia-free treatments may someday prove to be safe and effective during pregnancy.

Special Patient Conditions

Certain patient conditions, such as proximate calcified vascular aneurysms, implanted cardiac devices, and bleeding diatheses, were initially believed to be contraindications to SWL. However, clinical and scientific evidence accrued over the last two decades suggests that SWL can be performed safely in most of such patients, provided that certain guidelines are followed.

VASCULAR CALCIFICATIONS

Patients with calcified aortic or renal arterial aneurysms in close proximity to the target stone were once believed to be at risk for embolic events or aneurysm rupture from SWL. However, in vitro studies using calcified vascular tissue demonstrated no shockwave-induced injury (8,9). Furthermore, available clinical reports suggest that patients with ipsilateral calcified aneurysm could cautiously be selected as candidates for SWL if the aneurysm is asymptomatic and more than 5 cm away from the target stone, and if the diameter is less than 2 and 5 cm for renal artery and aortic aneurysms, respectively. In addition, the aneurysm should not be positioned in a path parallel to the shockwaves, and a lower level of energy should be used (10,11).

IMPLANTED CARDIAC DEVICES

The presence of implanted pacemakers or cardioverter defibrillators is no longer a contraindication to SWL, given that certain precautions are taken. An experienced cardiologist familiar with the device and a backup external device or corrective equipment should be readily available during the procedure. Devices must be thoroughly tested before and immediately after the procedure. Dual-chamber pacers should be set to a ventricular pacing mode only. Lastly, as mentioned above, patients with abdominally located devices containing piezoelectric crystals should not be treated with SWL owing to the risk of physical damage to the device (12–14).

COAGULOPATHY

Shockwave lithotripsy has been performed successfully in patients with significant *reversible* bleeding diatheses, such as hemophilia, hepatitis and cirrhosis, hypersplenism, and von Willebrand disease (15,16). The caveats in these or any such patient include the proper identification of the reversible coagulopathy and the appropriate normalization of bleeding and clotting studies before, during, and 24–48 h after SWL. Patients with irreversible coagulopathy should not be treated with SWL.

Technical Limitations

Based on the physics and the technical aspects of SWL, certain situations will limit the utility of SWL, including morbid obesity, unfavorable stone composition, and distal urinary tract obstruction. Although not contraindications *per se*, these limitations may reduce the overall efficacy of intervention, and reasonable expectations should be relayed to patients during counseling. With the incorporation of second and third generation lithotriptors, treating children is no longer a technical limitation, and in fact is associated with excellent results.

MORBID OBESITY

Several factors limit the utility of SWL in obese (greater than 300 pounds) patients. First, patients that exceed the weight limit of the machine, which currently can be as high as 400 lb, cannot be positioned at the focal point. Second, the focal length (maximum distance from stone to skin) of current machines ranges from 11 to 17 cm, which may still be too short for some obese patients (17). Third, the increased amount of intervening adipose and muscular tissue both dampen the peak shockwave focal pressure and hinder stone localization.

Various techniques have been used to overcome these limitations. Compression belts, similar to those used during intravenous pyelography, may decrease the focal length enough to reach the target stone. In addition, retrograde stone manipulation into the most posterior calyx may further decrease the focal length. Thomas and Cass described a technique of positioning the stone to within 4 cm beyond the focal point in the *z* (up and down) axis, along the so-called "extended shockwave pathway" (18). Their overall stone-free rate for SWL in obese patients was 68%, although these data were not stratified for the use of the extended shockwave pathway.

STONE IMPACTION AND COMPOSITION

Effective fragmentation of a given calculus by SWL requires a strong acoustic interface through a fluid medium. Impacted ureteral calculi lack such an interface between the surrounding ureteral walls and therefore respond poorly to SWL. In addition, certain stone compositions, particularly matrix and cystine, provide poor interfaces for fragmentation by SWL. Urinary matrix is composed primarily of proteins, water and sugars; most calcium stones are comprised of about 2–3% urinary matrix. However, matrix calculi contain about 65% urinary matrix, resulting in a gelatinous amorphous structure *(19)*. As such, there is no role for SWL in the management of matrix calculi *(20)*.

In contrast, pure cystine stones have a unique amino-acid crystalline structure containing repeated disulfide bonds, creating "hard" stones that are relatively resistant to SWL *(21)*. Because cystine calculi require larger numbers of shockwaves at higher energy levels to induce fragmentation, treatment with SWL should be limited to stones 1.5 cm or less in greatest diameter. Interestingly, cystine calculi with a calcium component, which are believed to be caused by the incorporation of calcium salts after partial chemical dissolution, tend to respond better to SWL than pure cystine calculi *(22)*. With careful patient selection, efficiency quotients *(see* "Comparing Apples to Apples" following) as high as 0.90 can be achieved with SWL monotherapy for small cystine stones that have failed medical therapy *(23)*.

DISTAL OBSTRUCTION

Stone-free results after SWL require adequate fragmentation and spontaneous passage through the urinary tract. Generally, SWL monotherapy in the setting of distal urinary tract obstruction is not recommended unless a simultaneous procedure to correct the obstruction is planned. This includes patients with obstruction caused by congenital renal anomalies, such as ureteropelvic junction obstruction. Of note, however, initial success rates for SWL in small series of horseshoe kidneys are unexpectedly high, ranging from 50 to 85%, although recurrence rates and auxiliary procedure rates approach 30% *(24)*.

Calyceal diverticular calculi have also been managed with success by SWL. In carefully selected patients with calculi measuring less than 1.5 cm associated with a radiographically patent calyceal diverticular neck, stone-free rates of 58% with symptomatic relief in 86% of patients can be achieved *(25)*.

OUTCOMES
Evaluating the Literature
DEFINITIONS OF SUCCESS AFTER SHOCKWAVE LITHOTRIPSY

As with any therapy for stone disease, the ultimate definition of success is "radiographically stone-free without symptoms." However, what is unique to SWL is that complete stone clearance relies on both adequate fragmentation and spontaneous passage. Therefore, the time to stone-free and symptom-free status may be prolonged after SWL compared to other urologic interventions. In turn, with the rapid increase in the world-wide experience with SWL, there exists a commensurate increase in the number of patients with small residual fragments after treatment. Such a finding is indeed inherent to the technique of SWL itself and has come to carry a much less ominous "prognosis" than it did before the advent of SWL. In fact, the presence of small asymptomatic residual fragments after SWL has been equated to successful treatment in some series, and as such, has been referred to as "clinically insignificant residual fragments." However, long-term follow-up studies evaluating the fate of these residual fragments after SWL suggest otherwise.

In a review of the long-term follow up of a very carefully selected group of 160 patients with anatomically normal upper tracts and 4 mm or less asymptomatic residual calcium oxalate or calcium phosphate calculi after SWL monotherapy for renal calculi, 18% of patients demonstrated growth of residual fragments (26). Furthermore, 43% developed a symptomatic episode, and 59% of these required intervention. By Kaplan-Meier estimations, the probability of developing a symptomatic episode within 5 yr after treatment was 71%. Fortunately, of patients that require urologic intervention for a symptomatic episode, the majority (79%) can be managed with repeat SWL alone, and 98% will require SWL and/or retrograde endoscopic procedures alone (26,27).

Candau and colleagues retrospectively reviewed 83 patients with residual fragments 4 mm or less at 3 mo after SWL. During a median of 40 mo follow up, 31 (37%) patients demonstrated an increase in stone burden, and 58% of these underwent a secondary procedure (28). Therefore, patients with residual stone fragments after SWL require continued surveillance and should be informed of the potential for recurrent symptomatic episodes and the possibility of secondary interventions. Furthermore, application of the term "clinically insignificant" to any residual stone after SWL may not be appropriate.

COMPARING APPLES TO APPLES

Owing to the wide variety of makes and models of lithotriptors, with different generators and energies, and subtle variations in overall patient care among investigators, it becomes difficult to make comparisons between series of reported data. For example, for a given stone-free rate, one machine may require multiple re-treatments or subsequent stent placements. Denstedt and colleagues (29) described the use of an "efficiency quotient" to take such factors into account as follows: efficiency quotient (EQ) = % stone-free divided by (100 + % re-treated + % auxiliary procedures). Therefore, a lithotriptor with an 85% stone-free rate, 10% re-treatment rate, and 15% rate of additional procedures would have an efficiency quotient of 0.68, whereas another machine which also has an 85% stone-free rate but with no re-treatments or ancillary procedures would have an EQ of 0.85. It is evident that despite the same stone-free rates, the two machines are not equally "efficient." This methodology is also useful in comparing results of SWL to other modalities, such as ureteroscopy or percutaneous nephrolithotomy. Unfortunately, only a small fraction of the current peer-reviewed literature reported EQs, and stone-free rates were the primary measure of success.

Renal Calculi

Overall results of SWL for solitary nonstaghorn renal calculi in any location vary from EQs of 0.45 to 0.82 for electrohydraulic lithotriptors and 0.42–0.67 for electromagnetic lithotriptors (24,30,31). However, two fundamental truths are well documented in the literature. First, stone-free rates are inversely proportional to the total stone burden. Second, stone-free rates are worse for calculi located in the lower pole of the kidney.

STONE BURDEN

Although there is no data defining the number of shockwaves that can safely be administered per kidney per session for any given lithotriptor and energy level, it is generally recommended that the safe maximum is approx 3000 to 3500 shockwaves. Therefore, one is inherently limited in the stone burden that can be treated per session.

Stone composition plays a key role in this determination. For example, it is generally recommended that calcium oxalate/phosphate stones larger than 2 cm and struvite stones larger than 3 cm be excluded from primary SWL monotherapy.

In contemporary series, overall stone-free rates for renal calculi measuring 10 mm or less range from 53.7 to 81%, regardless of location within the kidney. For 11–20 mm calculi, overall stone-free rates decrease to 38.4–66%. The widest range of success rates exist for calculi greater than 20 mm, from 28.1 to 83%, where stone location plays a greater role in the clearance of fragments. Lower pole stones >20 mm are associated with stone-free rates of 25–42% *(30,32,33)*. Interestingly, these contemporary data do not differ greatly from the first report by the US Cooperative Group in 1986, where 3-mo stone-free rates for stones <10 mm, 10–20 mm, and >20 mm were 81.9%, 78%, and 52.5%, respectively *(34)*.

STAGHORN CALCULI

The American Urological Association Nephrolithiasis Clinical Guidelines Panel evaluated the available literature before 1994 regarding the management of staghorn calculi *(35)*. The recommended guideline for a newly diagnosed staghorn calculus was primary percutaneous nephrolithotomy followed by SWL and/or repeat percutaneous procedures as needed. Furthermore, SWL monotherapy should not be used as first-line treatment.

Subsequent studies corroborated these recommendations. In a prospective randomized trial of percutaneous nephrolithotomy with or without SWL vs SWL monotherapy, the stone-free rates were 74% and 22%, respectively, and septic episodes occurred in 9% and 37% of patients, respectively *(36)*. Furthermore, we reviewed our experience with combination "sandwich" therapy, defined as primary percutaneous debulking followed by SWL and secondary percutaneous procedures, in 100 consecutive patients with staghorn calculi. Our stone-free rate was 63%, with 20% of patients developing fever or sepsis episodes during the course of treatment *(37)*. Interestingly, stone-free rates improved from 52% to 70% from the first 25 patients treated compared to the most recent 25 patients, implying a learning curve.

In summary, the current role for SWL in the management of staghorn calculi is merely as an adjunctive procedure to primary percutaneous intervention.

Lower Pole Renal Calculi

The optimal management of lower pole renal calculi continues to be an area of controversy and has recently received heightened attention within the endo-urologic community *(38)*. The anatomic disadvantage faced by lower pole calyceal stones becomes particularly important when considering SWL for definitive treatment, where spontaneous stone passage is just as crucial as adequate fragmentation. It was evident early in the world's experience with SWL that when stone-free rates were stratified by stone location, lower pole stones faired less well. In fact, in a large meta-analysis of the available data from 1986–1994, Lingeman and associates reported an overall stone-free rate of 62.2% for lower pole stones in 1931 patients. Interestingly, for stones less than 10 mm, stone-free rate was 74% compared to 33% for stones greater than 20 mm. Approximately half of all patients with stones 10–20 mm were stone free. In this retrospective comparison, the results of percutaneous nephrolithotomy (PCNL) were better than SWL for each size group, with an increasing advantage to PCNL as stone size increased.

Multiple retrospective studies have since reported similar findings. However, sufficient debate remained such that the Lower Pole Study Group was established to compare the efficacy of SWL and PCNL for the treatment of symptomatic lower pole renal calculi. In their initial report of a prospective, multicenter clinical trial of 128 patients with lower pole renal calculi less than 3 cm who were randomized to PCNL or SWL, overall stone-free rates at 3 mo were 95% and 37% respectively (38). When stratified by size, stone-free rates for SWL for stones <10 mm, 11–20 mm, and 21–30 mm were 63%, 23%, and 14%, respectively. EQ for SWL and PCNL for stones <10 mm were 0.51 and 0.91, respectively. For stones >10 mm, EQs were 0.16 and 0.82, respectively. However, SWL was associated with only an 11% rate of mostly minor complications. The conclusions from the Lower Pole Study Group were that SWL is recommended for lower pole stones 10 mm or less, whereas PCNL is recommended for lower pole stones >10 mm.

However, our own experience suggests that selected patients with stones 10–20 mm in size can be managed successfully with SWL. Such factors that must be considered in this regard are the same as those described above, and include but are not limited to presumed stone composition, concomitant medical problems, body habitus, and perhaps pyelocalyceal anatomy. The Lower Pole Study Group data, at the very least, provide the most objective information to date with which to counsel patients regarding the management of lower pole renal calculi.

ADJUNCTIVE PROCEDURES FOR LOWER POLE RENAL CALCULI

In attempts to improve on the stone-free rates of SWL for lower pole stones, a variety of adjunctive procedures have been used with varying results. Despite some encouraging reports, none have yet become routine to our clinical practice, but are nevertheless worthy of discussion. Brownlee and colleagues were first to report the use of "controlled inversion therapy," which involved placing the patient in a head-down position at a defined interval and duration after SWL (39,40). The goal of this procedure was to use gravity to their advantage to reposition stone fragments into more favorable calyces. Although this method indeed made theoretical sense, its practical utility was limited.

This idea was revisited with the addition of manual percussion (41,42). In a prospective randomized trial of inversion greater than 60°, forced diuresis and manual percussion for patients with lower pole residual fragments after SWL, an additional 37% were stone-free compared to 3% of those observed (41).

Other adjunctive procedures include lower pole irrigation using either antegrade or retrograde catheters (43,44), and repeat office treatment with a piezoelectric lithotriptor to merely "stir up" fragments (45). Again, despite isolated reports of favorable results with these measures, none have been employed with any regularity in our current practice.

THE ROLE OF LOWER POLE ANATOMY

In recognizing the marked variability of the anatomy of the renal collecting system, Sampaio and colleagues sought to categorize patients based of the anatomy of the lower pole calyx to predict who may have better outcomes after SWL (46,47). Others have subsequently contributed further to these analyses (48,49). In brief, from a representative pyelogram, measurements were obtained of the lower pole infundibular length and width as well as the angle of the infundibulum in relation to the renal pelvis and proximal ureter—the so-called "infundibulopelvic angle." Based on the retrospective review of stone-free status, cut-off values were determined to divide patients into "favorable" or "unfavorable" categories of lower pole renal anatomy.

However, using these methods, the Lower Pole Study Group found no significant correlation between lower pole anatomy and stone-free status (38). It is conceivable that the measurements of static images do not fully depict the dynamic system of lower pole drainage. In addition, there have been no reports on using these methods prospectively in clinical decision-making. Nevertheless, the role of evaluating lower pole anatomy is still being determined.

Ureteral Calculi

The indications for urologic intervention for ureteral calculi depend on many factors, including but not limited to stone size and location, stone shape and orientation, individual anatomy, and history of prior stone passage. Generally, stones 5 mm or less will pass spontaneously in up to 98% of cases, regardless of location within the ureter, whereas stones 5–10 mm have, at best, a 50% chance of passage (50). These probabilities are used to counsel patients regarding the options of watchful waiting vs intervention for ureteral calculi.

However, one cannot accurately predict how long it will take to spontaneously pass a given ureteral calculus. Thus, the duration and degree of renal colic as well as the development of other symptoms associated with stone passage may persuade the patient and surgeon to proceed with intervention, despite a high probability of passage. Certainly, any indication of infection or renal functional compromise associated with obstruction requires immediate temporary urinary diversion via ureteral stent or percutaneous nephrostomy tube and subsequent staged stone treatment.

In 1997, the Ureteral Stones Clinical Guidelines Panel reviewed the existing literature up through 1996 regarding the management of ureteral calculi (50). Owing to the marked inconsistency in the reporting of results, only broad categorizations could be made. Median stone-free rates after SWL for proximal ureteral calculi (above the iliac vessels) 10 mm or less vs greater than 10 mm were 84% and 72%, respectively, whereas those for distal stones (below the iliac vessels) were 85% and 74%, respectively. From the available data, there appeared to be no benefit to ureteral stenting or stone manipulation into the kidney (50,51).

However, more recent reports suggest less favorable results of SWL for larger ureteral calculi (>10 mm), with reported stone-free rates of 32–51% (33,52,53). In nonrandomized retrospective comparisons, ureteroscopic lithotripsy for ureteral calculi >10 mm was associated with 88–93% stone-free rates (52,53). From these data, primary SWL therapy for proximal or distal ureteral calculi should be limited to solitary stones 10 mm or less in size.

DISTAL URETERAL CALCULI

In recent series, stone-free rates after SWL for distal ureteral stones <20 mm were 73–100% (54–58). Although not stratified by size, the mean or median stone size was <10 mm in each series. The unmodified HM3 (Dornier Medical Systems, Inc., Marietta, Georgia) was associated with lower re-treatment and ancillary procedure rates compared to other lithotriptors. However, in select patients with small distal ureteral calculi, excellent results can be obtained using office-based electromagnetic or piezoelectric SWL under ultrasound guidance without anesthesia or heavy analgesia. In one study of 165 patients, 97% had stones <10 mm, and none were >15 mm. Stone-free rate at 3 mo was 99% with re-treatment in only 7% *(57)*.

Shockwave Lithotripsy Versus Ureteroscopy

With improved technology and expertise with ureteroscopy, the optimal management of distal, and even proximal, ureteral calculi less than 10 mm has come into debate. Peshcel and colleagues reported a randomized, prospective comparison between SWL and ureteroscopy for distal ureteral calculi of <10 mm *(55)*. Interestingly, repeat SWL was not part of the study, and all patients were to be "salvaged" on or before postoperative-day 43 by ureteroscopy only. There were no re-treatments in any patient in the ureteroscopy arm, and all patients were stone-free by 8 d. The re-treatment rates after SWL for stones <5 mm vs >5 mm were 15% and 5%, respectively. Although the results of both modalities in this series were excellent, it appears that ureteroscopy may have the greatest advantage over SWL in the setting of distal ureteral stones <5 mm. However, their level of expertise with ureteroscopy was indeed high given that their procedure times were much shorter for ureteroscopy than for SWL.

In a multicenter randomized prospective comparison of SWL and ureteroscopy for distal ureteral stones <15 mm, Pearle and associates emphasized the importance of secondary outcome parameters because stone-free rates were 100% in each group *(56)*. They favored SWL with the Dornier HM3 over ureteroscopy because of its higher efficiency, fewer complications, fewer postoperative symptoms and flank pain, and higher patient satisfaction.

It is evident that SWL and ureteroscopy are both excellent approaches for solitary distal ureteral calculi <10 mm in size, and the decision to proceed with either procedure still depends on the surgeon's expertise and informed patient preference.

Pediatric Urolithiasis

SWL has become an established and accepted treatment modality for urinary tract calculi in children. Long-term follow-up studies have found no adverse effects on renal function or morphology, blood pressure, or overall growth and development *(59–62)*. Furthermore, at 6 mo after SWL, no renal parenchymal scars were noted by di-mercapto-succinic acid (DMSA) renal scan, even after four sessions for staghorn calculi *(61, 63,64)*. Stone-free rates for solitary nonstaghorn renal calculi range from 80 to 100% *(61,62,65)*. In addition, a limited experience with SWL for renal calculi in premature infants has demonstrated excellent results, with all 8 patients stone-free by 8 wk after one session using a modified Dornier HM3 *(66)*.

SWL monotherapy is the treatment of choice for partial and complete staghorn calculi in children, affording far better results than those seen in the adult population. Stone-free rates of 73–83% have been reported *(63,64,67)*. Up to 5 SWL sessions per kidney have been administered, although most patients required one or two sessions. Despite multiple treatments with SWL, no renal parenchymal scars were noted by DMSA scan at 6 mo, and no changes in blood pressure were noted out to 9 yr *(63,64)*.

Excellent results from SWL for ureteral calculi in children have also been achieved. Initial stone free rates of 82% increase to 97% overall with additional SWL monotherapy for ureteral stones of any location. For calculi <10 mm, stone-free rates up to 100% have been reported *(68)*.

Pre-SWL ureteral stent placement in children, particularly for staghorn calculi, was shown to reduce the rate of obstructive complications and shorten hospital stay *(67)*.

Other technical considerations for children include lead shielding of the gonads, lungs, and thyroid when using fluoroscopy, and minimizing number of shockwaves and energy level. For infants, Styrofoam shielding of organs has also been used.

COMPLICATIONS

Steinstrasse

Post-SWL urinary obstruction owing to ureteral impaction of fragments is referred to as steinstrasse, or "street of stone," which connotes the classic radiographic findings. Steinstrasse occurs in up to 15% of radiography obtained within 48 h of SWL, and is found most commonly in the distal one-third of the ureter. Up to 50% of patients found to have steinstrasse require intervention, which most often involves either placement of a percutaneous nephrostomy tube or repeat SWL *(69,70)*.

Coptcoat and associates classified steinstrasse into three subtypes *(69)*. Type I consists of a column of dust or gravel, and is the most common type. Type II is caused by an impacted large "lead fragment" with dust or gravel stacked behind it. Type III refers to a column of large fragments.

The initial management of symptomatic steinstrasse consists of fluid hydration and analgesia. Persistent obstruction requires the placement of a percutaneous nephrostomy tube. Middle or upper pole access is preferred in case an antegrade approach is needed. Ureteral stent placement can be difficult and dangerous because the ureter is acutely inflamed and often tightly impacted with fragments. Subsequent intervention for failed conservative management is tailored to the type of steinstrasse. Most type I steinstrasse will pass with nephrostomy placement alone, which relieves the acute obstruction and, in turn, restores ureteral peristalsis. Type II steinstrasse may need repeat SWL or ureteroscopic lithotripsy to the lead fragment. Type III steinstrasse will need definitive management with SWL, ureteroscopy, or a percutaneous approach, depending on the location and stone burden. Open surgery has been required in 2–4% of patients with symptomatic steinstrasse *(69,70)*.

Preoperative placement of a ureteral stent may reduce the incidence of steinstrasse. In 400 patients randomized to stent or none before SWL for 1.5–3.5-cm renal calculi, the incidence of steinstrasse was 6% and 12%, respectively *(71)*. However, according to the authors, stenting did not seem to alter the presentation, treatment, or outcome of steinstrasse.

As an adjunct to endoscopic management of severe steinstrasse, ureteral meatotomy has been employed by the authors. Using a wide "cutting" incision of the ureteral orifice and judicious "spot" fulguration as needed, this technique provides improved ureteral drainage and easier ureteral access, and is particularly useful when multiple procedures for steinstrasse are anticipated. Resultant vesicoureteral reflux has not been found to be an issue in our experience.

Perirenal Hematoma

Perirenal hematomas, including intrarenal, subcapsular, and perinephric locations, can be detected in up to 30% by CT scan, however are clinically significant in less than 1% of patients. Risk factors for the development of post-SWL hematomas include hypertension (2.5% in controlled vs 3.8% in uncontrolled hypertension), coagulopathy, and acute urinary tract infection *(72,73)*.

Patients that present with severe ipsilateral flank pain despite oral analgesics within 48 h after SWL should be suspected to have a clinically significant perirenal hematoma. The initial evaluation should include a hematocrit level, abdominal X-ray, and renal ultrasound. If a hematoma is detected, the patient should be admitted to the hospital for intravenous hydration and analgesia and serial blood counts. Blood transfusions are given as warranted. Angiographic selective embolization or surgical intervention is rarely necessary.

In a recent yet unpublished review of 400 consecutive patients treated with SWL for renal calculi using the Storz Modulith SLX electromagnetic lithotriptor (Storz Medical, Kreuzlinsen, Switzerland) at our institution, fourteen (3.5%) developed perirenal hematomas. Thirteen were detected incidentally on routine follow-up ultrasound or CT scan. Only one patient (0.25%) developed symptoms and required hospitalization and blood transfusion. The development of a perirenal hematoma was not associated with higher energy levels or increased number of shockwaves administered.

The long-term outcome after development of a post-SWL hematoma is excellent. Up to 86% resolve in 2 yr. At 5 yr, there was no evidence of new onset hypertension or renal deterioration (73).

New-Onset Hypertension

Despite some debate regarding the development of new-onset hypertension after SWL, several long-term follow-up studies suggest that there is no significant increase in the incidence of new hypertension after SWL (74–76). Furthermore, a recent prospective randomized, albeit poorly powered, trial comparing SWL vs observation revealed no difference in the incidence of new-onset hypertension between groups at 12-mo follow-up (77). In addition, as mentioned above, even in a subset of patients who developed post-SWL hematoma in whom one might expect a Page kidney phenomenon, there was no evidence of new-onset hypertension or renal deterioration at 5 yr (73). Lastly, in a recent review of 228 patients with small asymptomatic calyceal calculi randomized to SWL or observation, 11% and 7% of patients, respectively, developed new-onset hypertension after a mean 2-yr follow-up, which was not statistically significant (78).

Renal Functional Effects

The risk of long-term renal deterioration after SWL is a legitimate concern, and has been yet another topic of debate. Several studies have suggested a decrease in glomerular filtration rate after SWL, particularly in those patients with pre-existing renal insufficiency, defined as serum creatinine >2 mg/dL or with solitary kidney (79,80).

However, more contemporary series demonstrated no deleterious effect of SWL on renal function. Pienkny and Streem compared 319 patients who underwent simultaneous bilateral SWL to 41 patients who underwent staged bilateral SWL (81). There was no clinically or statistically significant decrease in renal function in either group as measured by serum creatinine at a mean follow-up of 3.2 yr. Furthermore, there was no difference between groups. Perry and colleagues corroborated these findings in 120 patients who underwent simultaneous bilateral SWL, with a mean follow-up of 21 mo (82).

Further evidence toward the long-term safety of SWL regarding renal function was demonstrated by Liou and Streem in a recent series of 83 patients with a solitary kidney, who were treated with SWL, PCNL, or both and followed a mean of 4.4 yr with a maximum follow-up of 14 yr *(83)*. Renal function remained stable within treatment groups. As importantly, there was no difference in the effect on function among treatment groups. This finding implies that SWL, PCNL, and the two therapies combined are equally efficacious for preserving renal function in patients with a solitary kidney. Thus, the choice of therapeutic modality may be confidently based on stone size, configuration and presumed composition rather than on concerns regarding the long-term effects on renal function.

CONCLUSIONS

There is no doubt that SWL has revolutionized the urologic management of stone disease and remains the sole noninvasive surgical modality. However, there have been no significant advancements in its technology in the past decade. Conversely, ureteroscopic and percutaneous approaches have improved remarkably and continue to improve rapidly.

Therefore the relative role of SWL will indeed continue to evolve, perhaps into a more well-defined and limited capacity. It is interesting that current ureteroscopic procedures in skilled hands may be superior to SWL for small distal ureteral calculi. Thus it is not inconceivable that ureteroscopy may someday become superior to SWL for all upper tract calculi. So long as it proves to be better, we may be steering in the direction of more invasive rather than noninvasive interventions for stone disease. But for now, SWL continues to be the mainstay of endo-urologic management for most patients with urinary tract calculi.

REFERENCES

1. Eisenberger F, Chaussy C. Contact-free renal stone fragmentation with shock waves. Urol Res 1978; 6: 111.
2. Chaussy C, Brende, W, Schmiedt E. Extracorporeally induced destruction of kidney stones by shock waves. Lancet 1980; 2: 1265.
3. Chaussy C, Schmiedt E, Jocham D, et al. First clinical experience with extracorporeally induced destruction of kidney stones by shock waves. J Urol 1982; 127: 417.
4. Streem SB. Contemporary clinical practice of shock wave lithotripsy: a reevaluation of contraindications. J Urol 1997; 157: 1197.
5. Asgari MA, Safarinejad MR, Hosseini SY, et al. Extracorporeal shock wave lithotripsy of renal calculi during early pregnancy. BJU Int 1999; 84: 615.
6. Vieweg J, Weber HM, Miller K, et al. Female fertility following extracorporeal shock wave lithotripsy of distal ureteral calculi. J Urol 1992; 148: 1007.
7. Erturk E, Ptak AM, Monaghan J. Fertility measures in women after extracorporeal shockwave lithotripsy of distal ureteral stones. J Endourol 1997; 11: 315.
8. Vasavada SP, Streem SB, Kottke-Marchant K, et al. Pathological effects of extracorporeally generated shock waves on calcified aortic aneurysm tissue. J Urol 1994; 152: 45.
9. Abber JC, Langberg J, Mueller SC, et al. Cardiovascular pathology and extracorporeal shock wave lithotripsy. J Urol 1988; 140: 408.
10. Hunter PT, Finlayson B, Hirko RJ, et al. Measurement of shock wave pressures used for lithotripsy. J Urol 1986; 136: 733.
11. Carey SW, Streem SB. Extracorporeal shock wave lithotripsy for patients with calcified ipsilateral renal arterial or abdominal aortic aneurysms. J Urol 1992; 148: 18.
12. Cooper D, Wilkoff B, Masterson M, et al. Effects of extracorporeal shock wave lithotripsy on cardiac pacemakers and its safety in patients with implanted cardiac pacemakers. Pacing Clin Electrophysiol 1988; 11: 1607.
13. Drach GW, Weber C, Donovan JM. Treatment of pacemaker patients with extracorporeal shock wave lithotripsy: experience from 2 continents. J Urol 1990; 143: 895.

14. Chung MK, Streem SB, Ching E, et al. Effects of extracorporeal shock wave lithotripsy on tiered therapy implantable cardioverter defibrillators. Pacing Clin Electrophysiol 1999; 22: 738.

15. Partney KL, Hollingsworth RL, Jordan WR, et al. Hemophilia and extracorporeal shock wave lithotripsy: a case report. J Urol 1987; 138: 393.

16. Streem, S. B. and Yost, A. Extracorporeal shock wave lithotripsy in patients with bleeding diatheses. J Urol 1990; 144: 1347.

17. Hofmann R, Stoller ML. Endoscopic and open stone surgery in morbidly obese patients. J Urol 1992; 148: 1108.

18. Thomas R, Cass AS. Extracorporeal shock wave lithotripsy in morbidly obese patients. J Urol 1993; 150: 30.

19. Matthews LA, Spirnak JP. A matrix calculus causing bilateral ureteral obstruction and acute renal failure. J Urol 1995; 154: 1125.

20. Stoller ML, Gupta M, Bolton D, et al. Clinical correlates of the gross, radiographic, and histologic features of urinary matrix calculi. J Endourol 1994; 8: 335.

21. Ng CS, Streem SB. Medical and surgical therapy of the cystine stone patient. Curr Opin Urol 2001; 11: 353.

22. Kachel TA, Vijan SR, Dretler SP. Endourological experience with cystine calculi and a treatment algorithm. J Urol 1991; 145: 25.

23. Chow GK, Streem SB. Contemporary urological intervention for cystinuric patients: immediate and long-term impact and implications. J Urol 1998; 160: 341.

24. Renner C, Rassweiler J. Treatment of renal stones by extracorporeal shock wave lithotripsy. Nephron 1999; 81(Suppl 1): 71.

25. Streem SB, Yost A. Treatment of caliceal diverticular calculi with extracorporeal shock wave lithotripsy: patient selection and extended followup. J Urol 1992; 148: 1043.

26. Streem SB, Yost A, Mascha E. Clinical implications of clinically insignificant store fragments after extracorporeal shock wave lithotripsy. J Urol 1996; 155: 1186.

27. Chen RN, Streem SB. Extracorporeal shock wave lithotripsy for lower pole calculi: long-term radiographic and clinical outcome. J Urol 1996; 156: 1572.

28. Candau C, Saussine C, Lang H, et al. Natural history of residual renal stone fragments after ESWL. Eur Urol 2000; 37: 18.

29. Denstedt J, Clayman RV, Preminger GM. Efficiency quotient as a means of comparing lithotripters. J Endourol 1990; 4: 100.

30. Cass AS. Comparison of first generation (Dornier HM3) and second generation (Medstone STS) lithotriptors: treatment results with 13,864 renal and ureteral calculi. J Urol 1995; 153: 588.

31. Matin SF, Yost A, Streem SB. Extracorporeal shock-wave lithotripsy: a comparative study of electrohydraulic and electromagnetic units. J Urol 2001; 166: 2053.

32. Kosar A, Turkolmez K, Sarica K, et al. Calyceal stones: fate of shock wave therapy with respect to stone localization. Int Urol Nephrol 1998; 30: 433.

33. Logarakis NF, Jewett M A, Luymes J, et al. Variation in clinical outcome following shock wave lithotripsy. J Urol 2000; 163: 721.

34. Drach GW, Dretler S, Fair W, et al. Report of the United States cooperative study of extracorporeal shock wave lithotripsy. J Urol 1986; 135: 1127.

35. Segura JW, Preminger GM, Assimos DG, et al. Nephrolithiasis Clinical Guidelines Panel summary report on the management of staghorn calculi. The American Urological Association Nephrolithiasis Clinical Guidelines Panel. J Urol 1994; 151: 1648.

36. Meretyk S, Gofrit ON, Gafni O, et al. Complete staghorn calculi: random prospective comparison between extracorporeal shock wave lithotripsy monotherapy and combined with percutaneous nephrostolithotomy. J Urol 1997; 157: 780.

37. Streem SB, Yost A, Dolmatch B. Combination "sandwich" therapy for extensive renal calculi in 100 consecutive patients: immediate, long-term and stratified results from a 10-year experience. J Urol 1997; 158: 342.

38. Albala DM, Assimos DG, Clayman RV, et al. Lower pole I: a prospective randomized trial of extracorporeal shock wave lithotripsy and percutaneous nephrostolithotomy for lower pole nephrolithiasis-initial results. J Urol 2001; 166: 2072.

39. Rodrigues Netto N, Jr, Claro JF, Cortado PL, et al. Adjunct controlled inversion therapy following extracorporeal shock wave lithotripsy for lower pole caliceal stones. J Urol 1991; 146: 953.

40. Brownlee N, Foster M, Griffith DP, et al. Controlled inversion therapy: an adjunct to the elimination of gravity-dependent fragments following extracorporeal shock wave lithotripsy. J Urol 1990; 143: 1096.

41. Pace KT, Tariq N, Dyer SJ, et al. Mechanical percussion, inversion and diuresis for residual lower pole fragments after shock wave lithotripsy: a prospective, single blind, randomized controlled trial. J Urol 2001; 166: 2065.

42. D'A Honey RJ, Luymes J, Weir MJ, et al. Mechanical percussion inversion can result in relocation of lower pole stone fragments after shock wave lithotripsy. Urology 2000; 55: 204.

43. Nicely ER, Maggio MI, Kuhn EJ. The use of a cystoscopically placed cobra catheter for directed irrigation of lower pole caliceal stones during extracorporeal shock wave lithotripsy. J Urol 1992; 148: 1036.

44. Graham JB, Nelson JB. Percutaneous caliceal irrigation during extracorporeal shock wave lithotripsy for lower pole renal calculi. J Urol 1994; 152: 2227.

45. Krings F, Tuerk C, Steinkogler I, et al. Extracorporeal shock wave lithotripsy retreatment ("stir-up") promotes discharge of persistent caliceal stone fragments after primary extracorporeal shock wave lithotripsy. J Urol 1992; 148: 1040.

46. Sampaio FJ, Aragao AH. Limitations of extracorporeal shockwave lithotripsy for lower caliceal stones: anatomic insight. J Endourol 1994; 8: 241.

47. Sampaio FJ, D'Anunciacao AL, Silva EC. Comparative follow-up of patients with acute and obtuse infundibulum-pelvic angle submitted to extracorporeal shockwave lithotripsy for lower caliceal stones: preliminary report and proposed study design. J Endourol 1997; 11: 157.

48. Elbahnasy AM, Clayman RV, Shalhav AL, et al. Lower-pole caliceal stone clearance after shockwave lithotripsy, percutaneous nephrolithotomy, and flexible ureteroscopy: impact of radiographic spatial anatomy. J Endourol 1998; 12: 113.

49. Gupta NP, Singh DV, Hemal AK, et al. Infundibulopelvic anatomy and clearance of inferior caliceal calculi with shock wave lithotripsy. J Urol 2000; 163: 24.

50. Segura JW, Preminger GM, Assimos DG, et al. Ureteral Stones Clinical Guidelines Panel summary report on the management of ureteral calculi. The American Urological Association. J Urol 1997; 158: 1915.

51. Preminger GM, Kettelhut MC, Elkins SL, et al. Ureteral stenting during extracorporeal shock wave lithotripsy: help or hindrance? J Urol 1989; 142: 32.

52. Kupeli B, Alkibay T, Sinik Z, et al. What is the optimal treatment for lower ureteral stones larger than 1 cm? Int J Urol 2000; 7: 167.

53. Lam JS, Greene TD, Gupta M. Treatment of proximal ureteral calculi: holmium:YAG laser ureterolithotripsy versus extracorporeal shock wave lithotripsy. J Urol 2002; 167: 1972.

54. Turk TM, Jenkins AD. A comparison of ureteroscopy to in situ extracorporeal shock wave lithotripsy for the treatment of distal ureteral calculi. J Urol 1999; 161: 45.

55. Peschel R, Janetschek G, Bartsch G. Extracorporeal shock wave lithotripsy versus ureteroscopy for distal ureteral calculi: a prospective randomized study. J Urol 1999; 162: 1909.

56. Pearle MS, Nadler R, Bercowsky E, et al. Prospective randomized trial comparing shock wave lithotripsy and ureteroscopy for management of distal ureteral calculi. J Urol 2001; 166: 1255.

57. Jermini FR, Danuser H, Mattei A, et al. Noninvasive anesthesia, analgesia and radiation-free extracorporeal shock wave lithotripsy for stones in the most distal ureter: experience with 165 patients. J Urol 2002; 168: 446.

58. Hochreiter WW, Danuser H, Perrig M, et al. Extracorporeal shock wave lithotripsy for distal ureteral calculi: what a powerful machine can achieve. J Urol 2003; 169: 878.

59. Goel MC, Baserge NS, Babu RV, et al. Pediatric kidney: functional outcome after extracorporeal shock wave lithotripsy. J Urol 1996; 155: 2044.

60. Thomas R, Frentz JM, Harmon E, et al. Effect of extracorporeal shock wave lithotripsy on renal function and body height in pediatric patients. J Urol 1992; 148: 1064.

61. Lottmann HB, Archambaud F, Hellal B, et al. 99mTechnetium-dimercapto-succinic acid renal scan in the evaluation of potential long-term renal parenchymal damage associated with extracorporeal shock wave lithotripsy in children. J Urol 1998; 159: 521.

62. Brinkmann OA, Griehl A, Kuwertz-Broking E, et al. Extracorporeal shock wave lithotripsy in children. Efficacy, complications and long-term follow-up. Eur Urol 2001; 39: 591.

63. Orsola A, Diaz I, Caffaratti J, et al. Staghorn calculi in children: treatment with monotherapy extracorporeal shock wave lithotripsy. J Urol 1999; 162: 1229.

64. Lottmann HB, Traxer O, Archambaud F, et al. Monotherapy extracorporeal shock wave lithotripsy for the treatment of staghorn calculi in children. J Urol 2001; 165: 2324.

65. Villanyi KK, Szekely JG, Farkas LM, et al. Short-term changes in renal function after extracorporeal shock wave lithotripsy in children. J Urol 2001; 166: 222.

66. Shukla AR, Hoover DL, Homsy YL, et al. Urolithiasis in the low birth weight infant: the role and efficacy of extracorporeal shock wave lithotripsy. J Urol 2001; 165: 2320.

67. Al-Busaidy SS, Prem AR, Medhat M. Pediatric staghorn calculi: the role of extracorporeal shock wave lithotripsy monotherapy with special reference to ureteral stenting. J Urol 2003; 169: 629.

68. Landau EH, Gofrit ON, Shapiro A, et al. Extracorporeal shock wave lithotripsy is highly effective for ureteral calculi in children. J Urol 2001; 165: 2316.

69. Coptcoat MJ, Webb DR, Kellet MJ, et al. The steinstrasse: a legacy of extracorporeal lithotripsy? Eur Urol 1988; 14: 93.

70. Sayed MA, el-Taher AM, Aboul-Ella HA, et al. Steinstrasse after extracorporeal shockwave lithotripsy: aetiology, prevention and management. BJU Int 2001; 88: 675.

71. Al-Awadi KA, Abdul Halim H, Kehinde EO, et al. Steinstrasse: a comparison of incidence with and without J stenting and the effect of J stenting on subsequent management. BJU Int 1999; 84: 618.

72. Knapp PM, Kulb TB, Lingeman JE, et al. Extracorporeal shock wave lithotripsy-induced perirenal hematomas. J Urol 1988; 139: 700.

73. Krishnamurthi V, Streem SB. Long-term radiographic and functional outcome of extracorporeal shock wave lithotripsy induced perirenal hematomas. J Urol 1995; 154: 1673.

74. Yokoyama M, Shoji F, Yanagizawa R, et al. Blood pressure changes following extracorporeal shock wave lithotripsy for urolithiasis. J Urol 1992; 147: 553.

75. Claro Jde A, Lima ML, Ferreira U, et al. Blood pressure changes after extracorporeal shock wave lithotripsy in normotensive patients. J Urol 1993; 150: 1765.

76. Bataille P, Cardon G, Bouzernidj M, et al. Renal and hypertensive complications of extracorporeal shock wave lithotripsy: who is at risk? Urol Int 1999; 62: 195.

77. Jewett MA, Bombardier C, Logan AG, et al. A randomized controlled trial to assess the incidence of new onset hypertension in patients after shock wave lithotripsy for asymptomatic renal calculi. J Urol 1998; 160: 1241.

78. Elves AW, Tilling K, Menezes P, et al. Early observations of the effect of extracorporeal shockwave lithotripsy on blood pressure: a prospective randomized control clinical trial. BJU Int 2000; 85: 611.

79. Chandhoke PS, Albala DM, Clayman RV. Long-term comparison of renal function in patients with solitary kidneys and/or moderate renal insufficiency undergoing extracorporeal shock wave lithotripsy or percutaneous nephrolithotomy. J Urol 1992; 147: 1226.

80. Cass AS. Renal function after extracorporeal shock wave lithotripsy to a solitary kidney. J Endourol 1988; 8: 15.

81. Pienkny AJ, Streem SB. Simultaneous versus staged bilateral extracorporeal shock wave lithotripsy: long-term effect on renal function. J Urol 1999; 162: 1591.

82. Perry KT, Smith ND, Weiser AC, et al. The efficacy and safety of synchronous bilateral extracorporeal shock wave lithotripsy. J Urol 2000; 164: 644.

83. Liou LS, Streem SB. Long-term renal functional effects of shock wave lithotripsy, percutaneous nephrolithotomy and combination therapy: a comparative study of patients with solitary kidney. J Urol 2001; 166: 36; discussion 36, 37.

29   Indications and Outcomes of Ureteroscopy for Urinary Stones

Matthew T. Gettman, MD and Joseph W. Segura, MD

Key Words: Ureteroscopy; surgical treatment; renal calculus; staghorn calculus; ureteral calculus.

INTRODUCTION

Since the earliest reports on ureteroscopic techniques by Marshall, Goodman, and Lyon et al., technologic advances and physician innovation have dramatically expanded the diagnostic and therapeutic applications for ureteroscopy *(1–3)*. Although ureteroscopic techniques were initially limited to diagnostic evaluation of the distal ureter, the development and ongoing refinement of semi-rigid and flexible ureteroscopes now make nearly all areas of the urinary tract accessible *(4,5)*. In addition, the introduction of new technology has broadened the therapeutic implications for ureteroscopy beyond the realm of urinary stones to include definitive management of ureteropelvic junction obstruction, ureteral strictures, and select patients with transitional cell carcinoma (TCC) involving the upper urinary tract *(6–9)*. Furthermore, the diagnostic applications of ureteroscopy are increasingly realized for surveillance of select patients with upper-tract TCC and for the evaluation of patients with essential hematuria *(9,10)*.

Despite the versatility of modern ureteroscopy, definitive treatment of urinary stones remains the most common indication for performing ureteroscopic techniques *(11–13)*. Indeed, ongoing technologic advances have made ureteroscopic stone interventions

From: Current Clinical Urology, *Urinary Stone Disease:*
A Practical Guide to Medical and Surgical Management
Edited by: M. L. Stoller and M. V. Meng © Humana Press Inc., Totowa, NJ

more effective and less complicated than ever before *(14)*. This chapter summarizes the current indications and outcomes for ureteroscopic treatment of urinary stones in adults with renal or ureteral stones above (i.e., proximal ureteral stones) or below (i.e., distal ureteral stones) the pelvic brim.

URETEROSCOPIC MANAGEMENT OF URETERAL CALCULI

Both ureteroscopy and shockwave lithotripsy are widely used treatments for ureteral stones; therefore the optimal choice of therapy remains controversial. In most cases, either treatment modality can provide a successful therapeutic outcome. Accordingly, more invasive therapies for management of ureteral stones are rarely required. Conversely advances in minimally invasive stone treatment, excellent success rates, and low complication rates have diminished enthusiasm for conservative approaches to ureteral stones.

The fact remains that the majority of symptomatic patients spontaneously pass their ureteral stones *(15–18)*. Immediate intervention for ureteral calculi is absolutely warranted in the presence of urinary infection, complete ureteral obstruction, significant symptoms prompting multiple office visits, or for patients with occupational requirements precluding conservative treatment (e.g., pilot). For all other patients, stone size and location influence the likelihood of spontaneous stone passage and the recommendations for intervention. In a meta-analysis of 327 articles, Segura and colleagues reported that spontaneous passage occurred in 29–98% of stones <5 mm in diameter above the iliac vessels, and in 71–98% of stones <5 mm in diameter below the iliac vessels *(15)*. For stones with a diameter 5–10 mm, spontaneous passage occurred in 10–53% of proximal calculi and 25–53% of distal calculi. Similarly, Ueno and associates evaluated the frequency of spontaneous stone passage among 520 patients and noted a 55% overall spontaneous stone passage rate *(16)*. For stones measuring <4 mm, 4–6 mm, and >6 mm in diameter, spontaneous stone passage was observed in 80%, 59%, and 21% of patients, respectively. In a multivariate analysis of factors associated with spontaneous passage of ureteral calculi, Miller and Kane similarly found that smaller, more distal stones on the right side were more likely to spass pontaneously and required fewer surgical interventions *(17)*. In a recent report by Coll et al., spontaneous ureteral stone passage rates, regardless of size, were 48%, 60%, 75%, and 79% for stones located in the proximal ureter, middle ureter, distal ureter, or at the ureterovesical junction, respectively *(18)*.

When a conservative approach to ureteral stones is contraindicated or fails, the choice to proceed with ureteroscopic stone treatment is influenced not only by stone size and location but also by stone composition, body habitus, patient and surgeon preference, and previous surgical treatments. To streamline treatment selection, recommendations based on clinical outcomes data have been devised for ureteral stones located above or below the pelvic brim *(15)*.

Distal Ureteral Calculi

For stones located below the pelvic brim, ureteroscopy represents a major accomplishment in endo-urology. Among early reports published before the advent of smaller ureteroscopes and improved intracorporeal lithotripsy, a success rate of 73–94% was reported for distal stones *(15,19–21)*. These early success rates quickly made ureteroscopy a favored treatment for distal calculi. However, the risk of intraoperative complications, related primarily to the use of larger ureteroscopes, remained a concern early in the era of ureteroscopy. For instance, Blute et al. reported a 95% distal stone extraction rate in 1988, but they also noted a 20% overall complication rate and a 6.6% incidence of severe complications such as ureteral perforations, ureteral avulsions, or ureteral strictures *(19)*. Among other initial ureteroscopy series, the incidence of perioperative ureteroscopic complications ranged from 29 to 42% *(20,21)*. Using modern ureteroscopic techniques and instrumentation, the success rates for distal stones have remained favorable. In 26 reports published between 1996 and 2002 (representing 2733 patients), the cumulative stone-free rate was 96% (Table 1). Furthermore, modern ureteroscopy is associated with a low perioperative complication rate. Among contemporary series published between 1996 and 2002, the incidence of ureteral stricture is <2% and the incidence of ureteral perforation is <4% *(23,24,27,28,38)*. In addition, based on technical characteristics and safety of the Holmium: yttrium-aluminum-garnet (Ho:YAG) laser, ureteroscopic lithotripsy of ureteral and renal stones in patients with uncorrected bleeding diatheses has been successfully performed *(47,48)*. Based on these excellent success rates and low complication rates, the authors favor ureteroscopic management for most patients with distal ureteral stones.

Technical and practical issues make ureteroscopy favorable for distal stones. On a practical basis, access in the lower ureter can be achieved nearly all of the time with a semi-rigid or flexible instrument. In addition, most patients have a successful outcome following a single surgical procedure. In contemporary series, the retreatment rate for distal calculi following ureteroscopy is 4% (range 0–7%) (Table 1). The effectiveness of intracorporeal lithotripsy using the Ho:YAG laser makes treatment of all distal ureter stones a reality, regardless of composition. In nine series using Ho:YAG laser lithotripsy, ureteroscopic success rates for distal stones were 93–100% (3,30,31,34,39-41,43). Furthermore, stone burden is less of a limiting factor and consideration when choosing ureteroscopic management of distal ureteral stones given the efficacy of modern laser lithotripsy. Among 69 patients with distal ureteral stones treated by Cheung et al. with the Ho:YAG laser, differences in treatment success rates for stones <1.0 cm ($n = 56$ stones, success rate = 100%) and >1.0 cm ($n = 13$, success rate = 92%) were not statistically significant *(45)*. Even troublesome calcium oxalate monohydrate and cystine stones can effectively be treated using Ho:YAG laser lithotripsy. In addition, the majority of patients undergoing ureteroscopy are treated as outpatients and the overall cost of intervention is less than that reported for shock-wave lithotripsy or more invasive stone therapies *(49)*.

Despite these advantages of ureteroscopy, the optimal choice of distal stone treatment remains controversial. Although open surgery is essentially obsolete for distal stones, the choice of minimally invasive therapy remains highly debated. In an attempt to clarify treatment recommendations, the American Urological Association (AUA) formed the Ureteral Stones Clinical Guidelines Panel *(15)*. For distal stones ≤5 mm in diameter, the guidelines panel recommended an initial conservative approach with periodic evaluation. For stones requiring intervention, the use of blind stone basketing techniques was strongly opposed. Ureteroscopy or shockwave lithotripsy was recommended as the first-line treatment for distal stones. The recommendation to proceed with more invasive treatments, such as open ureterolithotomy, was reserved for salvage procedures or unusual clinical circumstances *(15)*.

Given the controversy associated with distal stone treatment, retrospective studies comparing minimally invasive treatment modalities have been reported *(25–28,34,50)*.

Table 1
Treatment of Distal Ureteral Stones With Ureteroscopy

First author	Year	Patients	Size of ureteroscope (Fr)	Modality of stone removal	LOS (days)	Stone-free rate	Complications	Second procedure
Hosking (22)	1996	68	6.0	Intact	NR	97% (66/68)	0% (0/68)	0% (0/68)
Jung (23)	1996	156	6.5	Alexandrite laser	NR	94.5% (148/156)	0% (0/156)	5% (8/156)
Netto (24)	1997	322	11.5	Intact	0.15	98.1% (316/322)	4.3% (14/322)	0% (0/322)
Kupeli (25)	1998	430	9.5–12.0	EHL, USL, PL	NR	91.9% (395/430)	12.6% (54/430)	NR
Bierkens (26)	1998	80	7.2	Pulsed dye	3.2	99% (79/80)	0% (0/80)	7% (6/80)
Eden (27)	1998	134	7.0–11.5	PL	1.1	89.5% (120/134)	2.2% (3/134)	6.0% (8/134)
Park (28)	1998	66	7.9–11.5	Intact, PL	NR	86.4% (57/66)	NR	NR
Pearle (29)	1998	48	6.9–8.5	Alexandrite laser	NR	94% (45/48)	NR	NR
Devarajan (30)	1998	102	7.5	Ho:YAG	NR	93% (95/102)	NR	5% (5/102)
Yip (31)	1998	34	8.5–9.5	Intact, Ho:YAG	NR	94% (32/34)	NR	6% (2/34)
Peschel (32)	1999	40	6.5–9.5	Intact, PL	NR	100% (40/40)	0% (0/40)	0% (0/40)
Tawfiek (33)	1999	34	6.0–9.8	Intact, EHL, PL, Ho:YAG	Outpt	100% (34/34)	0% (0/34)	0% (0/34)
Turk (34)	1999	96	7.5–9.5	Intact, Pulsed dye laser	NR	95% (92/96)	5.2% (5/96)	3.1% (3/96)
Puppo (35)	1999	220	7.0–8.0	EHL, PL	NR	99.6% (219/220)	NR	6.3% (14/220)
Strohmaier (36)	1999	40	7.5–9.5	Intact, EHL	NR	97% (39/40)	NR	NR
Hendrik (37)	1999	52	6.0–9.5	EHL, Pulsed dye laser	4.4	96% (50/52)	25% (22/87)	NR
Pardalidis (38)	1999	228	11.5	USL, EHL	1.3	92% (219/238)	2.5% (6/238)	4.2% (10/238)
Scarpa (39)	1999	81	4.8–14.0	Ho:YAG	NR	100% (81/81)	1% (2/150)	7% (10/150)
Matsuoka (40)	1999	30	NR	Ho:YAG	NR	93% (28/30)	3% (1/30)	0% (0/30)
Pearle (41)	2000	32	6.9–11.5	Alexandrite, Ho:YAG, EHL	75% Outpt	100% (29/29)	25% (8/32)	0% (0/32)
Delvecchio (42)	2000	15	8.5	PL	NR	100% (15/15)	0% (0/15)	0% (0/15)
Hollenbeck (43)	2001	103	6.9	Intact, Ho:YAG	NR	96% (99/103)	14% (14/103)	4% (4/103)
Yagisawa (44)	2001	5	8.0	PL	NR	100% (5/5)	NR	0% (0/5)
Cheung (45)	2001	69	6.5–7.0	Intact, Ho:YAG	NR	99% (68/69)	13% (60/69)	1% (1/69)
Sofer (3)	2002	237	6.9, 9.5, 11.5	Ho:YAG, EHL	NR	98% (232/237)	4% (24/598)	6% (38/598)
Desai (46)	2002	11	7.0, 8.0	PL	NR	100% (11/11)	0% (0/11)	0% (0/11)
TOTAL	1996–2002	2733	4.8–14.0	—	—	96% (2615/2733)	8% (213/2693)	4% (109/2526)

USL, ultrasonic lithotripsy; EHL, electrohydraulic lithotripsy; PL, pneumatic lithotripsy; Ho:YAG, holmium laser; NR, not reported; Outpt, outpatient.

574

Turk and Jenkins recommended ureteroscopy for distal stones after reviewing patients treated with a Dornier HM3 lithotripter (44 patients) or Dornier MFL5000 lithotripter (47 patients) versus ureteroscopy (96 patients). Stone-free rates favored ureteroscopy (95%) over shock-wave lithotripsy (83% for the HM3, 77% for the MFL5000). Complications, however, only occurred in the ureteroscopy cohort (34). Eden et al. similarly reported a 90% stone-free rate for 134 ureteroscopy patients and found that ureteroscopic stone-free rates were not size dependent (27). In a study comparing shock-wave lithotripsy and ureteroscopy, Anderson et al. reported stone-free rates of 96% for the Dornier HM3 lithotripter, 84% for Lithostar lithotripter, and 100% for ureteroscopy (50). Despite the higher success rates for ureteroscopy, the researchers recommended first-line therapy with shockwave lithotripsy and salvage therapy with ureteroscopy. Similarly, Park et al. favored shockwave lithotripsy as first-line therapy for distal stones <1.0 cm and reserved ureteroscopy for salvage therapy (28). The researchers did however recommend ureteroscopy as first-line therapy for stones >1.0 cm. In their 2-yr experience, stone-free rates after a single session were 86% for ureteroscopy and 80% for shockwave lithotripsy. For stones <1.0 cm, Park et al. noted shockwave lithotripsy stone-free rate of 83%, but this decreased to 44% for stones >1.0 cm in diameter. The combined ureteroscopy stone-free rate was 88% for all stones regardless of size (28). Bierkens et al. reported that ureteroscopy patients required less time to become stone free than patients treated with shock-wave lithotripsy (26). Comparing 44 patients treated with a Siemens Lithostar lithotripter to 80 patients treated with pulsed-dye ureteroscopic lithotripsy, success rates of 99% and 81% were recorded for ureteroscopy and shock-wave lithotripsy, respectively. Nonetheless, the researchers recommended shockwave lithotripsy for smaller stones and ureteroscopy only for larger distal stones. Kupeli et al. compared results of ureteroscopic lithotripsy in 430 patients with shock-wave lithotripsy performed using a Siemens Lithostar lithotripter in 726 patients (25). The stone-free rate for ureteroscopy was 92%, whereas the stone-free rate for shockwave lithotripsy was only 42%. Based on these findings, the group recommended ureteroscopy as the favored treatment for stones in the distal ureter.

Prospective randomized trials have compared shockwave lithotripsy and ureteroscopy for management of distal stones. Peschel et al. noted 100% ureteroscopic stone-free rates (n = 40) and 90% shockwave lithotripsy stone-free rates using a Dornier MFL5000 lithotripter (n = 40). For stones <5 mm and >5 mm in diameter, the shockwave lithotripsy stone-free rates were 95% and 85%, respectively (32). No complications were noted in either group, but operative time favored the ureteroscopy treatment arm. In addition, patient satisfaction was 100% for the ureteroscopy treatment arm and 85% for the shockwave lithotripsy treatment arm. Based on these results, ureteroscopic stone extraction was recommended as first-line therapy for distal stones (32). On the other hand, Pearle and colleagues prospectively randomized 32 patients with distal stones (diameter <1.5 cm) to ureteroscopy or shockwave lithotripsy using a Dornier HM3 lithotripter (41). A 100% stone-free rate was noted in both groups, but patients treated with shockwave lithotripsy had significantly shorter operative times. In addition, shockwave lithotripsy was associated with fewer perioperative complications, less postoperative discomfort, and greater overall patient satisfaction. Based on these results, the researchers recommended shockwave lithotripsy with a Dornier HM3 lithotripter as first-line treatment for distal stones (41).

In summary, the optimal choice of therapy for distal ureteral stones remains controversial and is influenced by many clinical factors as well as patient and physician preference. Given the excellent success rates, the authors favor ureteroscopy for management of most patients with distal stones. At the same time, however, shockwave lithotripsy is also associated with excellent success rates. Although comparative studies have been performed, universally accepted conclusions can not be formulated. Given the conflicting outcomes data, both ureteroscopy and shockwave lithotripsy are acceptable first-line treatment for most patients with distal stones. Nonetheless, ureteroscopy does appear preferable to shockwave lithotripsy for salvage therapy and for patients with stones located in multiple regions of the ureter. Furthermore, in the rare case of a very large (>1.5 cm) stone in the distal ureter, more invasive laparoscopic or open treatments may also have a role in providing efficacious single-session therapy.

Proximal Ureteral Calculi

Building on the success of ureteroscopy for distal calculi, attention has focused on the ureteroscopic management of stones located in the proximal ureter. In this role, analogous to the use of shockwave lithotripsy for distal ureteral stones, ureteroscopy has remained less widely accepted and more controversial than shockwave lithotripsy. The decreased enthusiasm for ureteroscopic treatment of proximal ureteral stones is in part attributable to the increased technical demands required for successful treatment and to the higher risk of complications. Moreover, the historical success rates associated with ureteroscopic treatment of proximal ureteral stones were suboptimal compared to the results of other treatment modalities (15). In general, the low success rates were attributable to inability to reach the stone, inability to fragment the stone, or cephalad stone migration during treatment. Technological advances such as introduction and downsizing of the flexible ureteroscopes and the development of Ho:YAG laser have greatly improved interest and efficiency of ureteroscopy for proximal ureteral stone treatment (14,23,28,30,31,33,35,40,51). In addition, ureteroscopy has also been reported as more cost effective than other therapeutic modalities (5,49,52).

A number of other factors suggest that ureteroscopy may be advantageous for treatment of proximal ureteral stones. In treating proximal stones with shockwave lithotripsy, success rates have been inversely proportional to stone size and less efficacious for patients with impacted stones (53,54). In the era of Ho:YAG lithotripsy, ureteroscopy is less dependent on stone volume and has been effectively used to treat patients with impacted stones. Similar to ureteroscopic treatment of stones in the distal ureter, advanced intracorporeal lithotripsy also makes safe fragmentation of all stone compositions in the proximal ureter. On the other hand, the type of lithotripsy device is an important factor to consider when treating proximal ureteral stones with shockwave lithotripsy. Lithotripsy using the Dornier HM3 lithotripter can be associated with significantly higher success rates than the newer less powerful machines that are more commonly used today (52). Also, retreatment is a common problem when using shockwave lithotripsy to treat patients with proximal ureteral stones. For the Dornier HM3 lithotripter and newer generation lithotripsy machines, retreatment rates are in the range 9–33% and 24–68%, respectively (52). In addition, as the number of shockwave lithotripsy retreatments increases, Pace et al. reported that the efficacy of additional intervention is decreased and that auxiliary procedures may be required to achieve a stone-free status (55). Conversely, ureteroscopy for proximal ureteral stones can provide many patients with the possibility of successful treatment in a single session.

In an attempt to streamline the decision making process, the Ureteral Stones Clinical Guidelines Panel of the AUA has also devised treatment guidelines for proximal ureteral stones *(15)*. In similar fashion as distal ureteral calculi, stones likely to spontaneously pass can be approached conservatively with periodic evaluation. For all other stones, definitive treatment was recommended. The recommended first-line therapy for stones with a diameter <1.0 cm in the proximal ureter was shockwave lithotripsy. Ureteroscopy or more invasive percutaneous nephrolithotomy was recommended for salvage treatment or if shockwave lithotripsy was contraindicated. For stones >1.0 cm in the proximal ureter, the guidelines panel recommended either shockwave lithotripsy, ureteroscopy, or percutaneous nephrolithotomy as first-line treatment *(15)*.

Since the formulation of the AUA treatment guidelines, treatment outcomes have improved for ureteroscopic treatment of proximal ureteral stones. In 24 series (representing 1130 patients) published since 1995 that have used smaller-caliber ureteroscopes and improved intracorporeal lithotrites, the overall stone-free rate was 86% and the retreatment rate was 11% (Table 2). The contemporary results are much higher than the median stone-free rates of 44–56% reported by the Ureteral Stones Clinical Guidelines Committee for ureteroscopic treatment of proximal ureteral stones *(15)*. In recent series the incidence and severity of ureteroscopic complications have also decreased when treating proximal ureteral stones *(3,5,12,14,33,51)*. With ureteroscope downsizing and the introduction of other modern ureteroscopic tools, the incidence of significant complications such as ureteral perforation and ureteral stricture was 2% and <1%, respectively, in five Ho:YAG lithotripsy series with abstractable data *(31,33,40,51,53)*. In addition, the stone-free ranges for Ho:YAG lithotripsy in the proximal ureter are 73–100% *(3,30,31,39,40,45,51)*. Besides Ho:YAG lithotripsy, favorable fragmentation and stone-free rates for proximal stones have been reported using other forms of intracorporeal lithotripsy including electrohydraulic lithotripsy, pneumatic lithotripsy, and the pulsed dye laser *(42,46,52,55,56)*. Proximal stone migration, observed in 40–48% of stones treated with pneumatic lithotripsy, has been a treatment concern with this form of intracorporeal lithotripsy especially in the proximal ureter; however a number of innovative devices have recently been introduced to prevent this complication *(42,46,56)*.

Recent series have better defined the contemporary role for ureteroscopic treatment of patients with proximal ureteral stones. In a report by Elashry et al., the introduction of the 7.5-Fr flexible ureteroscopes was reported to significantly decrease the need for dilation of the ureteral orifice, postoperative analgesia requirements, and need for postoperative hospitalization *(13)*. In multiple reports from New York University and Thomas Jefferson University, success has been reported using the smaller flexible ureteroscopes to effectively manage upper tract stones in a single treatment session *(4, 11,12,33,51)*. Furthermore, the role of ureteroscopy for salvage therapy in patients with proximal ureteral stones has been documented. Erhard et al. reported a stone-free rate of 97% for proximal ureteral calculi in a cohort of patients in which 55% had failed a previous stone treatment *(51)*. As with distal ureteral stones, ureteroscopy also appears reasonable for patients with stones located in the proximal ureter and other places in the urinary tract. Among 327 proximal ureteral or renal stones approached using small-caliber flexible ureteroscopes and intracorporeal lithotripsy, Grasso and Bagley noted that rigid ureteroscopy had been performed to treat distal ureteral stones in 23% of cases *(12)*. In the proximal ureter, ureteroscopic treatment appears to decrease the time interval required to become stone-free after treatment. Grasso retrospectively evaluated 112 patients with upper stones treated with shockwave lithotripsy or ureteroscopy. In the first month, a 45% stone-free rate was observed for shockwave lithotripsy whereas a 95% stone-free rate was noted for ureteroscopy *(5)*.

Table 2
Treatment of Proximal Ureteral Stones With Ureteroscopy

First author	Year	Patients	Size of ureteroscope (Fr)	Modality of stone removal	Stone-free rate	LOS (days)	Complications	Second procedure
Grasso (5)	1995	27	6.9, 7.5	Pulsed dye, EHL	96% (26/27)	NR	NR	4% (1/27)
Jung (23)	1996	40	6.5	Alexandrite laser	68% (27/40)	NR	5% (1/40)	28% (11/40)
Yang (52)	1996	43	6.9	EHL	84% (36/43)	2.5	9% (4/43)	14% (6/43)
Erhard (51)	1996	39	6.9–13	EHL, Ho:YAG, Pulsed dye	99% (38/39)	NR	NR	3% (1/39)
Harmon (14)	1997	17	6–11.5	Intact, EHL, USL,	77% (13/17)	NR	NR	NR
Yip (31)	1998	18	8.5, 9.5	Ho:YAG	78% (14/18)	NR	NR	6% (1/18)
Park (28)	1998	12	7.9–11.5	Intact, PL	75% (9/12)	NR	NR	NR
Pearle (29)	1998	51	6.9–8.5	Alexandrite laser	69% (35/51)	NR	NR	NR
Kupeli (25)	1998	15	9.5, 12.0	EHL, USL, PL	66% (10/15)	NR	40% (6/15)	NR
Grasso (12)	1998	84	>8.0	Pulsed dye, EHL, Ho: YAG	97% (82/84)	NR	NR	NR
Devarajan (30)	1998	114	7.5	Ho: YAG	88% (77/114)	NR	NR	11% (12/114)
Puppo (35)	1999	62	7.0–8.0	EHL, PL	99% (61/62)	NR	NR	26% (16/62)
Matsuoka (40)	1999	40	NR	Ho: YAG	80% (32/40)	NR	5% (2/40)	15% (6/40)
Scarpa (39)	1999	22	4.8–9.5	Ho:YAG	100% (22/22)	NR	1% (2/150)	7% (10/150)
Maheshwari (54)	1999	20	8.5	USL, PL	85% (17/20)	1-2	10% (2/20)	45% (9/20)
Hendrikx (37)	1999	32	6.0–9.5	EHL, Pulsed dye	81% (26/32)	4.4	25% (22/87)	NR
Tawfiek (33)	1999	29	6.0–9.8	Intact, EHL, PL, Ho:YAG	97% (28/29)	NR	0% (0/29)	3% (1/29)
Dretler (56)	2000	29	6.9–7.5	Ho:YAG, EHL	90% (26/29)	NR	0% (0/29)	10% (3/29)
Hollenbeck (43)	2001	81	6.9, 7.5	Intact, Ho:YAG	78% (63/81)	NR	17% (14/81)	9% (7/81)
Cheung (45)	2001	42	6.5, 7.0	Intact, Ho:YAG	73% (32/44)	NR	5% (2/44)	24% (10/42)
Yagisawa (44)	2001	14	8.0	PL	86% (12/14)	NR	NR	14% (2/14)
Sofer (3)	2002	194	7.5–10.5	Ho:YAG, EHL	97% (188/194)	99% Outpt.	4% (7/194)	6% (12/194)
Lam (53)	2002	81	7.5	Ho:YAG, Intact	97% (30/31)	0	0% (0/81)	3% (1/31)
Desai (46)	2002	24	7.0, 8.0	PL	100% (24/24)	NR	0% (0/24)	0% (0/24)
TOTAL	1995–2002	1130	4.8–13.0	—	86% (928/1082)	—	7% (62/877)	11% (109/997)

USL, ultrasonic lithotripsy; EHL, electrohydraulic lithotripsy; PL, pneumatic lithotripsy; Outpt., outpatient.

Studies comparing ureteroscopy to other treatment modalities have also attempted to define optimal stone therapy in the proximal ureter; however the small numbers of patients in many of the ureteroscopy treatment arms remain a limitation. Park et al. retrospectively compared ureteroscopic stone extraction to shockwave lithotripsy with a Dornier MPL9000 lithotripter *(28)*. In their 2-yr experience, 301 patients were treated with shockwave lithotripsy, but only 12 patients were treated with ureteroscopy. Stone-free rates after a single session were 75% and 72% for ureteroscopy and shockwave lithotripsy, respectively. Despite these results, the group recommended ureteroscopy predominantly as salvage therapy for shockwave lithotripsy failures. Strohmaier and associates also compared ureteroscopy to shockwave lithotripsy for treating patients with proximal ureteral calculi *(36)*. The stone-free rate for primary shockwave lithotripsy was 76%, whereas primary ureteroscopy was successful for the single patient undergoing this treatment. Stones successfully treated with shockwave lithotripsy had a mean diameter of 6.8 mm, whereas shockwave lithotripsy failures had a mean diameter of 9.4 mm. All patients failing shockwave lithotripsy selected secondary treatment with ureteroscopy and this secondary procedure was associated with an overall 97% stone-free rate. These results again confirm the efficacy of ureteroscopy for salvage therapy after failed shockwave lithotripsy. Grasso et al. compared the efficacy of ureteroscopy (27 patients) to shockwave lithotripsy on a Siemens Lithostar lithotripter (27 patients) for large proximal stones *(5)*. Stone-free rates of 62% and 97% were achieved for shockwave lithotripsy and ureteroscopy, respectively. Importantly, combined retreatment and auxiliary treatment rates were significantly higher for the shockwave lithotripsy cohort when compared to the ureteroscopy cohort (37% vs 3.7%). In addition, treatment costs were higher and postoperative visits were more common in the shockwave lithotripsy group *(5)*. Likewise, Lam et al. recently compared shockwave lithotripsy to Ho:YAG lithotripsy in 67 patients with proximal ureteral stones. Among stones >1.0 cm in diameter, the initial stone-free rate was 93% for ureteroscopy and 50% with shockwave lithotripsy performed with a DoLi 50 lithotripter *(53)*. For stones <1.0 cm in diameter, the initial stone-free rates were 100% and 80% for ureteroscopy and shockwave lithotripsy, respectively. The researchers recommended shockwave lithotripsy as first-line therapy for stones <1.0 cm because the procedure was less invasive. For stones >1.0 cm, ureteroscopy was recommended as first-line treatment *(53)*.

Based on the results of contemporary ureteroscopy series, the indications for ureteroscopic treatment of proximal ureteral stones appear to be evolving. Similar to the AUA guidelines published in 1997, we favor shockwave lithotripsy as first-line therapy for most proximal ureteral stones <1.0 cm in diameter. Ureteroscopy appears indicated as salvage therapy after failed shockwave lithotripsy for calculi <1 cm in diameter. Based on series published since 1996, the authors tend to favor ureteroscopy as an alternative to shockwave lithotripsy for proximal ureteral calculi >1 cm in diameter, especially if a Dornier HM3 lithotripter is not available. In addition, ureteroscopy appears advantageous for impacted proximal ureteral stones and as a treatment alternative for obese patients that are not candidates for shockwave lithotripsy. Furthermore, ureteroscopy appears more effective than shockwave lithotripsy for patients that present with stones in more than one area of the collecting system.

URETEROSCOPIC MANAGEMENT OF RENAL CALCULI

Although technologic advances make all areas of the kidney accessible, indications for ureteroscopic treatment of renal calculi remain debated. The current mainstays of therapy are shockwave lithotripsy and percutaneous nephrolithotomy; however ureteroscopy has been evaluated as an alternative to these treatment modalities. Because shockwave lithotripsy is the least invasive treatment option for small renal stones, this treatment modality has been preferable and effective, particularly when performed with the Dornier HM3 lithotripter. For stone burdens >2.0 cm in diameter, a percutaneous approach is classically selected. For larger diameter renal stones, a combination of minimally invasive therapies is often required to achieve a stone-free state. In similar fashion for ureteral stones, the AUA has also devised treatment guidelines for management of staghorn calculi (57). Given the dramatic advances in minimally invasive techniques, open surgery is rarely required for treating renal stones. The indications for treatment of renal calculi, regardless of treatment approach, include urinary tract obstruction, an attempt to prevent the loss of renal function, renal colic, and an attempt to prevent recurrent urinary tract infections. Selection of specific therapy traditionally has been influenced by stone burden, stone configuration (i.e., staghorn vs nonstaghorn calculus), individual patient characteristics (i.e., anatomy, underlying medical conditions), stone composition, and to some degree patient preference. The relatively new ureteroscopic treatment of renal calculi is increasingly reported and indications and outcomes can be considered in relationship to stone configuration (staghorn vs nonstaghorn).

Nonstaghorn Renal Stones

Before the advent of small-caliber flexible ureteroscopes, the role of ureteroscopy in the management of renal calculi was extremely limited. For the most part, ureteroscopic removal of a renal stone was typically reserved for the incidental stone encountered during diagnostic ureteroscopy. Although early reports described approx 50% success rate for ureteroscopic treatment of renal calculi, the cumulative success rate for 13 series (comprising 681 patients) published since 1996 was 84% (33) (Table 3). Among the same series, the cumulative incidence of complications was 4.4% and the cumulative incidence of secondary interventions was 17% (Table 3). To date, ureteroscopic treatment of renal calculi has been most favored for patients with contraindications to other minimally invasive treatments, but ureteroscopy is also increasingly used at some centers for standard patients and as an alternative to other treatments for lower-pole stones.

Recent series have effectively demonstrated the role of ureteroscopy in management of renal stones. Using 1.9-Fr electrohydraulic lithotripsy probes and flexible ureteroscopes, Elashry et al. reported a success rate of 92% when treating renal stones (58). In another report published early in the era of Ho:YAG laser lithotripsy, Grasso reported an 88.5% success rate among 26 patients following one treatment (59). In an expanded series reported by Fabrizio et al., an overall success rate of 89% was noted among 100 patients undergoing Ho:YAG laser lithotripsy (4). In 68% of patients, laser lithotripsy was selected because stones were located concurrently in multiple regions of the collecting system. In addition, a stone burden of >6 mm in diameter was noted in 67% of patients. Other indications for ureteroscopic treatment of renal calculi included patients previously failing shockwave lithotripsy, obese patients, and patients with anatomic abnormalities (4). In a recent report by Sofer et al, a similar success rate of 84% was reported among 56 patients with renal calculi that were treated exclusively with the Ho:YAG laser (3). In the era of Ho:YAG lithotripsy, ureteroscopy can also be used to treat renal stones regardless of stone composition. In two small series, cystine stones with diameter less than 3 cm have been effectively treated using ureteroscopic techniques (61,63). In this manner, ureteroscopy appears to be indicated for patients that are

Table 3
Treatment of Renal Stones With Ureteroscopy

First author	Year	Patients	Scope size	Stone removal modality	Location (n)				Stone type (n)		Stone free rate	LOS (d)	Complication rate	Second proc.
					Upper	Mid	Lower	Pelvis	Staghorn	Nonstaghorn				
Elashry (58)	1996	17	7.5–9.4	EHL			17			37	88% (15/17)	NR	NR	12% (2/17)
Grasso (59)	1996	29	7.5	Ho:YAG	7	2	20		3	26	88% (23/26)	NR	NR	12% (3/26)
Grasso (60)	1998	45	7.5	Ho:YAG; EHL	5	6	11	23		NR	76% (34/45)	NR	6% (3/51)	35% (18/51)
Grasso (12)	1998	193	<8.0	Pulsed dye, EHL, Ho:YAG	43	25	80	45		NR	79% (152/193)	NR	NR	NR
Fabrizio (4)	1998	100	7.5–9.8	EHL, Ho:YAG, Intact	Renal (other locations)=37		63			NR	98% (98/100)	0.5	6% (6/100)	0% (0/100)
Rudnick (61)	1999	5	NR	EHL		1	5	2		5	50% (4/8)	1	80% (4/6)	50% (3/6)
Tawfiek (33)	1999	59	7.5–9.8	Intact, EHL, PL, Ho:YAG	11	7	23	18		NR	88% (64/73)	NR	NR	NR
Grasso (62)	1999	79 (90)	7.5	Ho:YAG			90		22	68	76% (53/70)	NR	13% (9/70)	31% (22/70)
Kourambas (63)	2000	3	7.5	Ho:YAG	1		2	2		3	66% (2/3)	0	0% (0/3)	0
Hollenbeck (64)	2001	72	6.9–7.5	Intact, Ho:YAG, EHL			72			72	88% (38/43)	83% outpt.	19% (14/72)	13% (9/72)
Lee (65)	2001	9	NR	Ho:YAG		1	1	7	2	7	100% (9/9)	NR	NR	NR
Kourambas (7)	2001	14	7.5	Ho:YAG			NR			NR	79% (11/14)	NR	0% (0/14)	NR
Sofer (3)	2002	56	7.5–10.5	Ho:YAG, EHL			NR			NR	84% (47/56)	99% Outpt	NR	NR
TOTAL	1996–2002	681 (698)	7.5–10.5	—			—		—	—	84% (550/657)	—	4.4% (14/316)	17% (57/342)

Proc., procedure; outpt., outpatient.

581

not candidates for repeat percutaneous nephrolithotomy or for cystine stone patients that fail shockwave lithotripsy.

Among the renal stones treated with ureteroscopic techniques, management of stones located in the lower pole has generated significant interest. The mainstays of treatment for lower-pole stones have been percutaneous removal and shockwave lithotripsy. Percutaneous treatment of lower-pole stones assures the patient an almost certain treatment success, yet the procedure is more invasive and can be associated with significant complications. A percutaneous approach is also contraindicated in some patients with multiple medical problems or severe anatomic deformities. Although shockwave lithotripsy is appealing, the overall success rates using this treatment modality for lower-pole stones are only 50–80% (66). When stratified by stone size, shockwave lithotripsy is associated with a stone free rate of 63–76% for stones <1.0 cm in diameter and 45–59% for stones 1.0–2.0 cm in diameter (64). The introduction of the flexible steerable ureteroscope provides the chance to merge the higher success rates of percutaneous surgery with the minimally invasiveness of shockwave lithotripsy. Nonetheless, ureteroscopic treatment of lower-pole stones can be much more challenging than the other treatment options despite the technologic advances in ureteroscopy.

Ureteroscopic treatment of lower-pole stones has been performed by directly treating the stone in the lower pole or by displacing the stone to a more favorable location before intracorporeal lithotripsy (67). Using either approach, initial success rates for ureteroscopic treatment of lower-pole stones have been 76–88% (33, 58,62,64,67). In a recent report comparing in situ treatment of lower-pole stones to treatment after displacement, Schuster et al. found nonsignificant differences in success rates for stones <1.0 cm in diameter (77% vs 89%). For stones >1.0 cm in diameter, however, the 29% success rate associated with in situ stone treatment was significantly less than the 100% success rate associated with treatment after stone displacement (68). In an early report using in situ stone treatment, Elashry et al. used 1.9 Fr. EHL probes to achieve an 87% success rate among 17 patients with 37 lower-pole stones at a mean follow-up of 8.7 mo (58). The researchers suggested EHL was the only lithotrite with adequate flexibility to routinely access the lower pole and was also the most cost-effective mode of intracorporeal lithotripsy. In other studies, however, efficacy of Ho:YAG lithotripsy has now also been reported for lower-pole stones. Hollenbeck et al. evaluated ureteroscopic treatment for 60 patients undergoing 66 interventions for lower-pole stones <2.0 cm in diameter (mean 8.7 mm) (64). Using flexible ureteroscopy and intracorporeal lithotripsy when required, the researchers noted a 79% stone-free rate after a single procedure and an 88% success rate after a second procedure in four patients (64). Nonetheless, the researchers recommended shockwave lithotripsy as first-line therapy for lower-pole stones <1.0 cm. For patients failing initial shockwave lithotripsy, ureteroscopy was recommended as salvage therapy. For stone diameters between 1.0 and 2.0 cm, ureteroscopy was favored as first-line therapy because better results were achieved than historical results with shockwave lithotripsy, and ureteroscopy was less invasive than percutaneous nephrolithotomy. Grasso and Ficazzola also investigated the results of ureteroscopic treatment of 90 lower-pole stones based on stone burden (62). They stratified results based on stone diameter with groupings of <1.0 cm, 1.1–2.0 cm, and >2.0 cm in diameter and noted fragmentation rates of 94%, 95%, and 45%, respectively. After a second treatment for stones >2.0 cm in diameter, the success rate increased to 82% (62). A similar success rate of 87% was also reported at 3 mo follow-up in a report by Tawfiek and Bagley for 23 lower-pole stone patients with a mean diameter of 7 mm (33).

In addition to type of intracorporeal lithotripsy, patient anatomy has been another factor considered in the treatment of lower-pole stones. For patients undergoing shock-wave lithotripsy of lower-pole stones, Elbahnasy et al. previously evaluated the impact of patient anatomy on successful stone clearance *(69)*. Among the anatomic factors considered, they noted an acute infundibulopelvic angle, a narrow infundibular width, and a long lower-pole infundibular length as negative predictors of successful shockwave lithotripsy treatment. Grasso and Ficazzola similarly studied the impact of anatomic factors on ureteroscopic lithotripsy of lower-pole stones and noted an infundibular length >3.0 cm and the presence of infundibular strictures as adverse predictors of outcome *(62)*. In their series, they reported a 21% failure rate secondary to inability to access the lower-pole stone or inability to render the patient stone-free after fragmentation. As such, when either of these anatomic factors were encountered preoperatively, the researchers recommended percutaneous treatment of lower-pole stones rather than ureteroscopic treatment *(62)*.

Inability to ureteroscopically access the lower-pole stone with the intracorporeal lithotrite or stone basket is a particularly vexing problem. Not uncommonly, the stone can be accessed with the ureteroscope alone but decreased deflection of the ureteroscope with the addition of the stone basket or lithotrite through the working channel precludes adequate stone access. To overcome this limitation, Landman et al. recently recommended the use of unsheathed nitinol baskets within the standard working channel of commonly available flexible ureteroscopes to additionally improve active deflection by approx 15–20° and to improve irrigant flow approx 2- to 30-fold when compared to similar studies performed with sheathed nitinol baskets *(70)*.

Whereas the results of prospective studies comparing ureteroscopic treatment of lower-pole stones to other treatment modalities are currently unavailable, Albala et al. have previously published the results of treating lower-pole stones with shockwave lithotripsy and percutaneous nephrolithotomy *(71)*. They noted that percutaneous nephrolithotomy provided superior results, regardless of stone burden. Specifically, the success rates for stones <1.0 cm was 63% with shockwave lithotripsy compared to 100% with percutaneous nephrolithotomy. For shockwave lithotripsy, the success rates were 23% for stones between 1.0 and 2.0 cm and 14% for stones >2.0 cm in diameter *(71)*. Based on retrospective data now available for lower-pole stones, outcomes data for ureteroscopy appears more comparable to percutaneous nephrolithotomy and the treatment modality also appears more beneficial because it is less invasive.

In summary, the role of ureteroscopy in the management of nonstaghorn renal calculi appears to be expanding. In 2006, ureteroscopic treatment of renal stones appears indicated as a salvage therapy following failed shockwave lithotripsy and as first-line therapy when the other commonly employed first-line treatment modalities are contraindicated. Ureteroscopy also compares favorably to percutaneous nephrolithotomy from a standpoint of treatment morbidity when considering treatment of obese patients in which shockwave lithotripsy is contraindicated. Similar to recommendations for patients with multiple ureteral stones, ureteroscopy is favored for patients with stones located concurrently in the kidney and ureter and for patients with anatomic abnormalities precluding treatment with shockwave lithotripsy or percutaneous lithotripsy. Finally, ureteroscopic treatment has emerged as a very effective intervention for select patients with lower-pole stones. Although ureteroscopy is increasingly used for management of the standard renal stone patient, additional outcomes data comparing ureteroscopy and the other treatment options are warranted before ureteroscopic treatment of all renal stones becomes commonplace. Likewise, the results of ongoing comparative studies will further clarify the role of ureteroscopy in the management of lower-pole stones.

Staghorn Renal Calculi

Widespread enthusiasm is lacking for the primary management of staghorn calculi with ureteroscopic techniques. Although ureteroscopic management of select patients with staghorn calculi has been reported, the technique is challenging, often labor intensive, and can be associated with a high incidence of ancillary treatments. When the AUA treatment guidelines were published for staghorn stones in 1994, ureteroscopic management was not considered in the treatment armamentarium for staghorn stones *(57)*. In general, first-line therapy for staghorn calculi remains percutaneous nephrolithotomy followed by shockwave lithotripsy and/or repeat percutaneous nephrolithotomy. Based on the AUA guidelines, neither open surgery nor shockwave lithotripsy alone should be considered as first-line treatments for staghorn stones in the standard patient. For smaller volume branched stones, the AUA guidelines recommended percutaneous nephrolithotomy and shockwave lithotripsy as equally effective treatment options when the anatomy was normal or near normal. Also, as an option, open surgery was considered appropriate therapy when the stone could not be treated effectively by percutaneous nephrolithotomy or shockwave lithotripsy. In addition, nephrectomy was considered a reasonable option for a poorly functioning kidney bearing a staghorn stone. The recommended AUA guidelines were also reported as the most cost-effective methods for treatment of staghorn stones in a previous investigation *(57)*.

Advances of ureteroscopy have made ureteroscopic treatment of select patients with large-volume branched calculi a technical possibility. In a limited clinical experience published since 1994, successful ureteroscopic treatment of staghorn calculi has been reported *(59,60,72,73)*. Feasibility of ureteroscopically treating staghorn calculi also appears to be increasing in the era of Ho:YAG lithotripsy. Grasso et al. treated a group of 45 patients with minor staghorn calculi of noninfectious etiology and found a stone-free rate of 76% after a single treatment *(60)*. Following a second procedure in eight patients with residual fragments, the investigators achieved a 91% stone-free rate. With the ureteroscopic approach, second procedures were commonly performed for patients with large branched calculi or stone burdens in excess of 3.0 cm to exclude the presence of large residual fragments. In the series by Grasso et al. a second procedure was performed in 15 patients and identified fragments in 53% ($n = 8$) *(60)*. Among 25 patients with a minimum follow-up of 6 mo, 15 patients (60%) were stone-free, 6 patients had small fragments (24%), and 4 patients had stone regrowth (16%) The researchers recommended ureteroscopic stone treatment only for patients with noninfectious stones. When matrix stones were encountered, the group recommended a conversion to percutaneous nephrolithotomy *(60)*. In addition to ureteroscopic monotherapy of staghorn stones, combination therapies incorporating ureteroscopy have also been reported *(73)*. In one of the earliest reports on ureteroscopic treatment of staghorn calculi, Dretler et al. used staged therapy with primary pulsed dye laser lithotripsy and secondary shockwave lithotripsy to treat eight patients with staghorn stone burdens *(72)*. Although a mean of 2.8 procedures was performed for each patient and the mean length of hospitalization was 3.5 d, eventually 88% of the patients became stone-free *(72)*. Likewise, in the era of Ho:YAG laser lithotripsy, Mugiya et al. noted the combination of ureteroscopy and shockwave lithotripsy resulted in a 61% stone-free rate for complete staghorn calculi and an 80% stone-free rate for partial staghorn calculi *(73)*.

Although feasibility of ureteroscopic treatment of staghorn calculi represents a true technical milestone in the management of renal stones, additional experience is required to delineate the role of ureteroscopic stone treatment for staghorn calculi. At the present time, ureteroscopic treatment of staghorn calculi appears warranted only for patients that are not candidates for the traditional treatment modalities. Furthermore, ureteroscopic treatment of minor staghorn calculi should not be performed for patients with matrix stones or infectious stones. In reality, given the advances in anesthesia and the advances in percutaneous treatment of renal calculi, treatment of staghorn calculi with ureteroscopic techniques appears limited. Nonetheless, as additional experience and technologic advances are incorporated into the ureteroscopic treatment of staghorn calculi, indications for primary treatment of staghorn calculi in the standard patient may ultimately increase. The authors still favor the staghorn calculi treatment guidelines as previously published by the AUA *(57)*.

CONCLUSIONS

The indications and outcomes for ureteroscopic management of ureteral and select renal stones continue to increase and improve. Given the technologic advances, essentially all areas of the collecting system can be accessed with the ureteroscope. In our opinion, the strongest indication for ureteroscopic management of ureteral stones is for patients with calculi located below the pelvic brim. For stones located above the pelvic brim, ureteroscopy is an increasingly successful treatment, but may still remain less advantageous to shockwave lithotripsy in many cases, especially when performed with a Dornier HM3 lithotripter. In the kidney, the ureteroscopic indications for stone treatment are even less established, but encouraging results have recently been reported for stones especially located in the lower pole of the kidney.

The coexistence of multiple effective treatment modalities for management of ureteral calculi and renal calculi has created controversy. The battle for optimal treatment of ureteral and renal calculi has been amplified with the increased use of ureteroscopy secondary to improvements in ureteroscope design and instrumentation. Patient preference, physician familiarity, and instrument availability are factors that may influence the selection of stone treatment. Only prospective, randomized trials employing state of the art technology and equivalent physician expertise will determine the optimal treatment algorithms for ureteral and renal calculi and help resolve management controversies. In reality, optimal treatment of ureteral and renal stones will likely continue to require one of a number of minimally invasive therapeutic modalities that are tailored specifically to the characteristics of the patient.

REFERENCES

1. Marshall VF. (1964) Fiberoptics in urology. J Urol 1964; 91: 110.
2. Goodman TM. Ureteroscopy with a pediatric cystoscope in adults. Urology 1977; 9: 394.
3. Lyon ES, Kyker JS, Schoenberg HW. Transurethral ureteroscopy in women: a ready addition to the urological armamentarium. J Urol 1978; 119: 35–36.
4. Sofer M, Watterson JD, Wollin TA, Nott L, Razvi H, Denstedt JD. Holmium:YAG laser lithotripsy for upper urinary tract calculi in 598 patients. J Urol 2002; 167: 31–34.
5. Fabrizio MD, Behari A, Bagley DH Ureteroscopic management of intrarenal calculi. J Urol 1998; 159: 1139–1143.
6. Grasso M, Beaghler M, Loisides P. The case for primary endoscopic management of upper urinary tract calculi: II. Cost and outcome assessment of 112 primary ureteral calculi. Urology 1995; 45: 372–376.

7. Biyani CS, Cornford PA, Powell CS. Ureteroscopic endopyelotomy with the holmium: YAG laser. Eur Urol 2000; 38: 139–143.

8. Kourambas J, Delvecchio FC, Preminger GM. Low-power holmium laser for the management of urinary tract calculi, strictures, and tumors. J Endourol 2001; 15: 529–532.

9. Elliott DS, Segura JW, Lightner D, Patterson DE, Blute ML. Is nephroureterectomy necessary in all cases of upper tract transitional cell carcinoma? Long-term results of conservative endourologic management of upper tract transitional cell carcinoma in individuals with a normal contralateral kidney. Urology 2001; 58: 174–178.

10. Nakada SY, Elashry OM, Picus D, Clayman RV. Long-term outcome of flexible ureterorenoscopy in the diagnosis and treatment of lateralizing essential hematuria. J Urol 1997; 157: 776–779.

11. Grasso M. Ureteropyeloscopic treatment of ureteral and intrarenal calculi. Urol Clin North Am 2000; 27: 623–631.

12. Grasso M, Bagley D. Small diameter, actively deflectable, flexible ureteropyeloscopy. J Urol 1998; 160: 1648–1654.

13. Elashry OM, Elbahnasy AM, Rao GS, Nakada SY, Clayman RV. Flexible ureteroscopy: washington university experience with the 9.3F and 7.5F flexible ureteroscopes. J Urol 1997; 157: 2074–2080.

14. Harmon WJ, Sershon PD, Blute ML, Patterson DE, Segura JW. Ureteroscopy: current practice and long-term complications J Urol 1997; 157:28–32.

15. Segura JW, Preminger GM, Assimos DG, Dretler SP, Lingeman JE, Macaluso JN, Jr. Ureteral stones clinical guidelines panel summary report on the management of ureteral calculi. J Urol 1997; 158:1915–1921.

16. Ueno A, Kawamura T, Ogawa A, Takayasu H. Relation of spontaneous passage of calculi to size. Urology 1977; 10: 544–546.

17. Miller OF, Kane CJ. Time to stone passage for observed ureteral calculi: a guide for patient education. J Urol 1999; 162: 688–690.

18. Coll DM, Varanelli MJ, Smith RC. Relationship of spontaneous passage of ureteral calculi to stone size and location as revealed by unenhanced helical CT. AJR 2002; 178: 101–103.

19. Blute ML, Segura JW, Patterson DE. Ureteroscopy. J Urol 1988; 139:510–512.

20. Keating MA, Heney NM, Young HH 2nd, Kerr WS Jr, O'Leary MP, Dretler SP. Ureteroscopy: the initial experience. J Urol 1986; 135: 689–693.

21. Daniels GF Jr, Garnett JE, Carter MF. Ureteroscopic results and complications: experience with 130 cases. J Urol 1988; 139: 710–713.

22. Hosking DH, Bard RJ. Ureteroscopy with intravenous sedation for treatment of distal ureteral calculi: a safe and effective alternative to shock wave lithotripsy. J Urol 1996; 156: 899–901.

23. Jung P, Wolff JM, Mattelaer P, Jakse G. Role of lasertripsy in the management of ureteral calculi: experience with alexandrite laser system in 232 patients. J Endourol 1996; 10: 345–348.

24. Netto NR Jr., De Almeida Claro J, Esteves SC, Andrade EFM. Ureteroscopic stone removal in the distal ureter. Why change? J Urol 1997; 157: 2081–2083.

25. Kupeli B, Biri H, Isen K, et al. Treatment of ureteral stones: comparison of extracorporeal shock wave lithotripsy and endourologic alternatives. Eur Urol 1998; 34: 474–479.

26. Bierkens AF, Hendrikx AJM, De La Rosette JJ, et al. Treatment of mid and lower ureteric calculi: extracorporeal shock–wave lithotrispy vs laser ureteroscopy. A comparison of costs, morbidity, and effectiveness. Br J Urol 1998; 81: 31–35.

27. Eden CG, Mark IR, Gupta RR, Eastman J, Shrotri NC, Tiptaft RC. Intracorporeal or extracorporeal lithotripsy for distal ureteral calculi? Effect of stone size and multiplicity on success rate. J Endourol 1998; 12: 307–312.

28. Park H, Park M, Park T. Two-year experience with ureteral stones: extracorporeal shockwave lithotripsy v ureteroscopic manipulation. J Endourol 1998; 12: 501–504.

29. Pearle MS, Sech SM, Cobb CG, et al. Safety and efficacy of the Alexandrite laser for the treatment of renal and ureteral calculi. Urology 1998; 51:33–38.

30. Devarajan R, Ashraf M, Beck RO, Lemberger RJ, Taylor MC. Holmium:YAG lasertripsy for ureteric calculi: an experience of 300 procedures. Br J Urol 1998; 82: 342–347.

31. Yip KH, Lee CW, Tam PC. Holium laser lithotripsy for ureteral calculi: an outpatient procedure. J Endourol 1998; 12: 241–246.

32. Peschel R, Janetschek G, Bartsch G. Extracorporeal shock wave lithotripsy versus ureteroscopy for distal ureteral calculi: a prospective randomized study. J Urol 1999; 162: 1909–1912.

33. Tawfiek ER, Bagley DH. Management of upper urinary tract calculi with ureteroscopic techniques. Urology 1999; 53: 25–31.

34. Turk TM, Jenkins AD. A comparison of ureteroscopy to in situ extracorporeal shock wave lithotripsy for the treatment of distal ureteral calculi. J Urol 1999; 161:45–46.

35. Puppo P, Ricciotti G, Bozzo W, Introini C. Primary endoscopic treatment of ureteric calculi. Eur Urol 1999; 36: 48–52.

36. Strohmaier WL, Schubert G, Rosenkranz T, Weigl A. Comparison of extracorporeal shock wave lithotripsy and ureteroscopy in the treatment of ureteral calculi: a prospective study. Eur Urol 1999; 36: 376–379.

37. Hendrikx AJ, Strijbos WE, deKnijff DW, Kums JJ, Doesburg WH, Lemmens WA. Treatment for extended-mid and distal ureteral stones: SWL or ureteroscopy? Results of a multicenter study. J Endourol 1999; 13: 727–733.

38. Pardalidis NP, Kosmaoglou EV, Kapotis CG. Endoscopy vs. extracorporeal shockwave lithotripsy in the treatment of distal ureteral stones: ten years' experience. J Endourol 1999; 13: 161–164.

39. Scarpa RM, De Lisa A, Porru D, Usai E. Holmium:YAG laser lithotripsy. Eur Urol 1999; 35: 233–238.

40. Matsuoka K, Iida S, Inoue M, et al. Endoscopic lithotrispy with the holmium:YAG laser. Lasers Surg Med 1999; 25: 389–395.

41. Pearle MS, Nadler R, Bercowsky E, et al. Prospective randomized trial comparing shock wave lithotripsy and ureteroscopy for management of distal ureteral calculi. J Urol 2001; 166: 1255–1260.

42. Delvecchio FC, Kuo RL, Preminger GM. Clinical efficacy of combined lithoclast and lithovac stone removal during ureteroscopy. J Urol 2000; 164: 40–42.

43. Hollenbeck BK, Schuster TG, Faerber GJ, Wolf JS Jr. Comparison of outcomes of ureteroscopy for ureteral calculi located above and below the pelvic brim. Urology 2001; 58: 351–356.

44. Yagisawa T, Kobayashi C, Ishikawa N, Kobayashi H, Toma H. Benefits of ureteroscopic pneumatic lithotripsy for the treatment of impacted ureteral stones. J Endourol 2001; 15: 697–699.

45. Cheung MC, Lee F, Yip SKH, Tam PC. Outpatient holmium laser lithitripsy using semirigid ureteroscope: is the treatment outcome affected by stone load? Eur Urol 2001; 39: 702–708.

46. Desai MR, Patel SB, Desai MM, et al. The Dretler stone cone: a device to prevent ureteral stone migration-the initial clinical experience. J Urol 2002; 167: 1985–1988.

47. Kuo RL, Aslan P, Fitzgerald KB, Preminger GM. Use of ureteroscopy and holmium:YAG laser in patients with bleeding diatheses. Urology 1998; 52: 609–613.

48. Watterson JD, Girvan AR, Cook AJ, et al. Safety and efficacy of holmium:YAG laser lithotripsy in patients with bleeding diathesis. J Urol 2002; 168: 442–445.

49. Lotan Y, Gettman MT, Roehrborn CG, Cadeddu JA, Pearle MS. Management of ureteral calculi: a cost comparison and decision making analysis. J Urol 2002; 167: 1621–1629.

50. Anderson KR, Keetch DW, Albala DM, Chandhoke PS, McClennan BL, Clayman RV. Optimal therapy for the distal ureteral stone: extracorporeal shock wave lithotropsy versus ureteroscopy. J Urol 1994; 152: 62–65.

51. Erhard M, Salwen J, Bagley DH. Ureteroscopic removal of mid and proximal ureteral calculi. J Urol 1996; 155: 38–42.

52. Yang SSD, Hong JS. Electrohydraulic lithotripsy of upper ureteral calculi with semirigid ureteroscope. J Endourol 1996; 10: 27–29.

53. Lam JS, Greene TD, Gupta M. Treatment of proximal ureteral calculi: holmium:YAG laser lithotripsy versus extracorporeal shock wave lithotripsy. J Urol 2002; 167: 1972–1976.

54. Maheshwari PN, Oswal AT, Andankar M, Nanjappa KM, Bansal M. Is antegrade ureteroscopy better than retrograde ureteroscopy for impacted large upper ureteral calculi? J Endourol 1999; 13: 441–444.

55. Pace KT, Weir MJ, Tariq N, Honey RJ. Low success rate of repeat shock wave lithotripsy for ureteral stones after failed initial treatment. J Urol 2000; 164: 1905–1907.

56. Dretler SP. Ureteroscopy for proximal ureteral calculi: prevention of stone migration. J Endourol 2000; 14: 565–567.

57. Segura JW, Preminger GM, Assimos DG, et al. Nephrolithiasis clinical guidelines panel summary report on the management of staghorn calculi. J Urol 1994; 151: 1648–1651.
58. Elashry OM, DiMeglio RB, Nakada SY, McDougall EM, Clayman RV. Intracorporeal electrohy-draulic lithotripsy of ureteral and renal calculi using small caliber (1.9F) electrohydraulic litho-tripsy probes. J Urol 1996; 156:1581–1585.
59. Grasso M. Experience with the holmium laser as an endoscopic lithotrite. Urology 1996; 48: 199–206.
60. Grasso M, Conlin M, Bagley D. Retrograde ureteropyeloscopic treatment of 2 cm. or greater upper urinary tract and minor staghorn calculi. J Urol 1998; 160: 346–351.
61. Rudnick DM, Bennett PM, Dretler SP. Retrograde renoscopic fragmentation of moderate-size (1.5–3.0-cm) renal cystine stones. J Endourol 1999; 13: 483–485.
62. Grasso M, Ficazzola M. Retrograde ureteropyeloscopy for lower pole caliceal calculi. J Urol 1999; 162: 1904–1908.
63. Kourambas J, Munver R, Preminger GM. Ureteroscopic management of recurrent renal cystine calculi. J Endourol 2000; 14: 489–492.
64. Hollenbeck BK, Schuster TG, Faerber GJ, Wolf JS Jr. Flexible ureteroscopy in conjunction with in situ lithotripsy for lower pole calculi. Urology 2001; 58: 859–863.
65. Lee DI, Bagley DH. Long-term effects of ureteroscopic laser lithotripsy on glomerular filtration rate in the face of mild to moderate renal insufficiency. J Endourol 2001; 15: 715–717.
66. Lingeman JE, Siegel YI, Steele B, Nyhuis AW, Woods JR. Management of lower pole nephroli-thiasis: a critical analysis. J Urol 1994; 151: 663–667.
67. Kourambas J, Delvecchio FC, Munver R, Preminger GM. Nitinol stone retrieval-assisted ureter-oscopic management of lower pole renal calculi. Urology 2000; 56: 935–939.
68. Schuster TG, Hollenbeck BK, Faerber GJ, Wolf JS. Ureteroscopic treatment of lower pole calculi: comparison of lithotripsy in situ and after displacement. J Urol 2002; 168: 43–45.
69. Elbahnasy AM, Clayman RV, Shalhav AL, et al. Lower-pole caliceal stone clearance after shock-wave lithotripsy, percutaneous nephrolithotomy, and flexible ureteroscopy: impact of radiologic spatial anatomy. J Endourol 1998; 12: 113–119.
70. Landman J, Monga M, El-Gabry EA, et al. Bare naked baskets: ureteroscope deflection and flow characteristics with intact and disassembled ureteroscopic nitinol stone baskets. J Urol 2002; 167: 2377–2379.
71. Albala DM, Assimos DG, Clayman RV, et al. Lower pole I: a prospective randomizd trial of extrcorporeal shock wave lithotripsy and percutaneous nephrostolithotomy for lower pole neph-rolithiasis-initial results. J Urol 2001; 166: 2072–2080.
72. Dretler SP. Ureteroscopic fragmentation followed by extracorporeal shock wave lithotripsy: a treatment alternative for selected large or staghorn calculi. J Urol 1994; 151: 842–846.
73. Mugiya S, Ohhira T, Un-No T, Takayama T, Suzuki K, Fujita K. Endoscopic management of upper urinary tract disease using a 200-μm holmium laser fiber: initial experience in Japan. Urology 1999; 53: 60–64.

30 Ureteroscopy

Technical Aspects

Assaad El-Hakim, MD, Beng Jit Tan, MD,
and Arthur D. Smith, MD

CONTENTS

Key Words: Ureter; nephrolithiasis; instrumentation; ureteroscope.

INTRODUCTION

Ureteroscopy has gained widespread use for diagnosis and treatment of diseases of the upper urinary tract. Ureteroscopy came as an extension of cystoscopy and was based to a large extent on technologic advances in instrumentation. In 1912, Young and McKay passed a rigid cystoscope into the dilated ureter of a boy with posterior urethral valves *(1)*. Since then, vast alterations in the concept and design of endoscopes occurred. Miniaturization of both rigid and flexible ureteroscopes was made possible mainly by fiberoptic imaging technology. Ancillary instruments for ureteral access, stone fragmentation and retrieval, and other diagnostic and therapeutic applications have also been developed. In this chapter, we review the technical aspects of ureteroscopy, including ureteral access and instrumentation available for endoscopic stone management.

ACCESS

A complete patient history, physical examination, laboratory tests, and upper tract imaging should be obtained in preparation for either diagnostic or therapeutic uretero-

From: Current Clinical Urology, *Urinary Stone Disease:*
A Practical Guide to Medical and Surgical Management
Edited by: M. L. Stoller and M. V. Meng © Humana Press Inc., Totowa, NJ

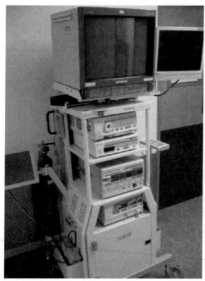
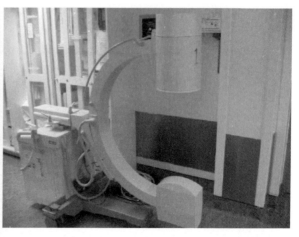

Fig. 1. Video/Camera equipment and portable C-arm fluoroscopy unit.

scopy. The procedure must be planned appropriately depending on the collecting system anatomy and the pathology in question. Previous pelvic surgery, radiation therapy, or trauma may lead to anatomical abnormalities of the upper tracts. Likewise, a urethral stricture or significant prostatic enlargement may make access difficult. An in-depth discussion of how to overcome a difficult access is presented in the *Pearls and Tricks* section at the end of this chapter. We routinely administer preoperative prophylactic antibiotics and use pneumatic compressive sleeves on the lower extremities to prevent deep venous thrombosis. Basic requirements to obtain ureteral access include a cystoscopy table, camera/video equipment, and a fluoroscopy unit (Fig. 1). The operating table must be radiolucent, equipped with stirrups, and allow for a drainage system. Occasionally, the position of the table must be altered to achieve better access to the ureter. A camera/video system allows the surgeon to operate in a comfortable position with the advantage of a magnified view. The assistant surgeon can follow the procedure simultaneously, and mentoring is likewise facilitated. Fluoroscopy is mandatory to obtain access and perform adequate tasks. All of the following maneuvers require fluoroscopic guidance, including retrograde pyelography, insertion of guidewires, stents, and balloon dilation. We do not recommend carrying out the procedure in a cystoscopy suite with overhead fluoroscopy, as this results in exposure of the urologist to excessive radiation. The use of an appropriately positioned C-arm allows the majority of the radiation to be absorbed by the patient.

The patient is positioned in dorsal lithotomy. All pressure points must be padded carefully. The leg ipsilateral to the ureter to be explored is slightly extended, lowered, and abducted. This position enhances maneuverability by straightening the distal ureter. General or regional anesthesia is preferred for therapeutic ureteroscopy, although deep sedation may be an option in selected cases. Access to the ureter begins by identifying the ureteral orifice. A rigid cystoscope with a 30° lens, or alternatively a flexible cystoscope, is introduced into the bladder. Once the ureteral orifice has been located, a guidewire is introduced gently (Fig. 2A). An open-ended ureteral stent is used to stabilize the wire and guide its entrance into the orifice. At this point, a retrograde pyelogram can be performed if necessary, using open ended or olive tip ureteral catheter.

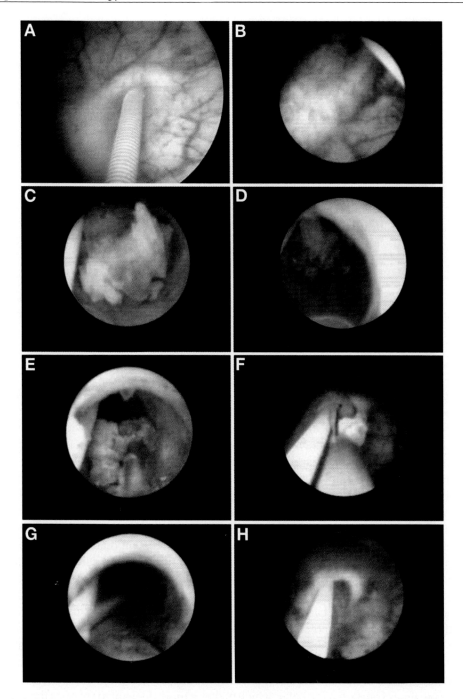

Fig. 2. (A) The ureteral orifice is located cystoscopically and a regular guidewire is introduced. **(B)** The ureter is engaged with the rigid ureteroscope with the wire at 12-o'clock position tenting up the ureteral orifice. Note that the ureteral orifice was not dilated in this case. **(C)** The distal ureteral stone is visualized. **(D)** The holmium-laser fiber is placed on the stone surface before activating the laser. **(E)** The stone is vaporized and fragmented in small pieces. **(F)** Fragments that are less likely to pass spontaneously are removed using a stone basket. **(G,H)** The distal ureter and the ureteral orifice at the end of the procedure; notice that minimal trauma to the urothelium was sustained.

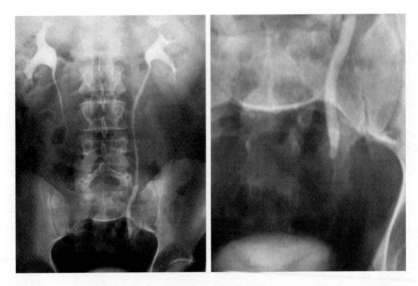

Fig. 3. Intravenous pyelogram (15 min) of a 45-year-old man with left distal ureteral stone. This patient underwent left rigid ureteroscopy and holmium-laser lithotripsy as shown in Fig. 2.

Ureteral Dilation

Today, technologic breakthroughs allow us to use very small ureteroscopes that permit easy access to the ureter without prior dilation (Fig. 2B). However, this is not always possible, and in many cases ureteral dilation is required. In general, dilation up to 15 or 18 Fr is more than sufficient *(2)*. Before proceeding with dilatation, a retrograde pyelogram must be obtained to clearly outline the anatomy of the ureter (Fig. 3).

Dilation should be simple, efficient, fast, and cause minimal or no iatrogenic trauma. General indications include dilation of the ureteral orifice and intramural ureter before ureteroscopy, and dilation of a ureteral stricture or narrowing.

Balloon dilators are the most preferred and probably the most used dilating devices. They are available in different sizes, raging from 3 to 30 Fr in diameter and from 1 to 20 cm in length. The shaft length ranges from 30 cm for urethral dilation up to 150 cm for ureteral dilation. Quality balloons allow for even distribution of pressure along the entire length of the balloon, while keeping the external diameter constant. Each balloon dilator has a recommended safe inflation pressure that ranges from 8 to 17 atm.

Balloon dilators accept a regular (0.035- or 0.038-in.) guidewire over which they can be advanced. In the deflated state, the balloon collapses to essentially the size of the catheter shaft to allow for smooth advancement and withdrawal from the urinary tract. After multiple inflations and deflations the balloon will not collapse to its initial deflated size and its surface becomes somewhat irregular, which makes it more difficult to advance the balloon forward. For this reason, it is easier to start dilating at the most proximal point of the ureter and after deflation, pulling the balloon backward. If multiple dilations are required this maneuver is repeated as necessary to the ureteral orifice. Two radiopaque markers are located at each end of the balloon and thus indicate its proper position. In addition, balloon dilators have various tip designs. Longer-tip dilators have a more tapered balloon shape once inflated, whereas shorter tip dilators allow for a more complete expansion of the distal end of the balloon, flush with the tip of the dilator.

Various types of inflation devices are available. The LeVeen device (Boston Scientific, Microvasive) is a 10-mL syringe with a spiral piston that allows gradual and controlled inflation, and avoids pressure fluctuations. The addition of a pressure manometer gauge permits constant monitoring of the balloon pressure, which must remain within manufacturer's range.

After retrograde pyelogram, the radiopaque markers of the balloon are positioned using fluoroscopy around the desired location. The balloon dilator must be held tightly in position to prevent it from migrating during inflation. Diluted contrast material is used to fill the balloon and inflation is monitored fluoroscopically. We use a 6-Fr/65-cm long shaft with an 18-Fr/4-cm long balloon. The maximum pressure of this balloon is 16 atm. Inflation is maintained for approx 1–2 min. At the point of narrowing, a circumferential constriction of the balloon, called a waist, can occur under low pressure, and then disappears. If the waist persists then further dilation is required and it is preferable to deflate the balloon and repeat the procedure after moving the balloon 0.5–1 cm either proximally or distally. Inflation pressures of less than 15 atm are usually sufficient in more than 90% of cases (3). Balloon dilation should never be performed at the level of a ureteral stone. This may result in ureteral perforation and stone extrusion.

Early in ureteroscopic experience, the distal ureter was routinely dilated to 24 Fr to facilitate passage of larger rigid ureteroscopes. Although such dilation is considered excessive nowadays, Garvin and Clayman demonstrated that no distal ureteral strictures occurred on excretory urogram obtained in 86 out of 131 patients who underwent aggressive ureteral dilation (24 Fr) and ureteral stent insertion after ureteroscopic stone extraction. A follow-up cystogram in 30 patients showed low-grade vesicoureteral reflux in 20% of the patients and none of these individuals was symptomatic. However, mucosal tears and extravasation of contrast were seen in 52% and 19% of patients, respectively (4).

If balloon dilation is not successful, a backup form of dilation should be available. The following are alternative mechanical dilating devices, but none are equivalent to balloon dilators: Teflon or polyethylene dilators, telescoping metal ureteral dilators, metal bougies, and multibeaded, acorn metal dilators. Finally, another system of ureteral dilation is hydraulic pump dilation. We will discuss briefly each of these options.

Teflon or polyethylene dilators are graduated individual dilators from 6 to 18 Fr that are passed over a regular guidewire through the cystoscope sheath (by increments of 2 Fr). Also available is a single 14-Fr Teflon dilator with the tip tapering down to 6 Fr over the distal 4 cm. Dilation is accomplished in one passage with the latter. Lesions of the ureteral wall secondary to linear shearing can occur with both types of dilators, and their use is not recommended in the presence of distal stones or steinstrasse (5).

Telescoping metal dilators are coaxial hollow tubes that follow the same principle as percutaneous renal access dilation. This technique has been abandoned owing to the high associated rate of iatrogenic injuries. Metal bougies are flexible olive- or acorn-shaped 9–15-Fr dilators. They are passed over a guidewire through a cystoscope sheath. A modification of this system consists of five individual olive-shaped dilators ranging from 8.5 Fr to 15 Fr, strung together on a spring wire. The advantage of this method is single passage of the dilator (6).

In contrast to mechanical-type dilators, the hydraulic Ureteromat (Karl Storz, Culver City, CA) system involves a pressure irrigation pump connected to the ureteroscope that provides a controlled pulsatile flow of irrigant at the tip of the instrument. It has a maximum flow of 400 mL/min and a maximum pressure of 200 mmHg. The irrigant

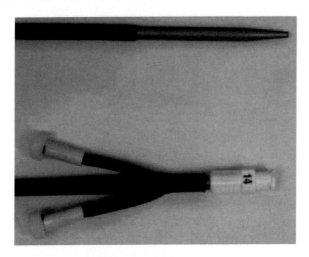

Fig. 4. Ureteral access sheath.

is directed at the center of the ureteral orifice, stretching its edges and dynamically dilates it. The system is activated throughout the procedure for enhanced visibility. The underlying rationale is to achieve temporary inversion of the ureteral peristaltic waves *(7)*.

Access Sheaths

Ureteral access sheaths and peel-away introducers are coaxial systems composed of an external Teflon sheath over a polyurethane introducer that are passed over a guidewire. Internal sheath diameter varies from 9.5 Fr to 14Fr and length from 20 cm to 60 cm. The dilator tip tapers to 6 Fr to provide one-step gradual dilation (Fig. 4). The access sheath provides a continuous working channel for the introduction of ureteroscopes and instruments. The main advantage is to facilitate repeated instrument exchanges while protecting the ureter from potential trauma. The sheath may minimize damage to the flexible ureteroscope. Potential drawbacks include ureteral wall injury during initial introduction and access sheath kinking in the prostatic urethra of male patients. In addition, the sheath may not be very useful for distal ureteral stones.

There has been a recent resurgence in the use ureteral of access sheaths. Preminger's group randomized 62 ureteroscopic procedures to 12/14 Fr ureteral access sheath vs no access sheath. The access sheath appeared to facilitate semirigid and flexible ureteroscopy by decreasing operative time and costs. There was no significant difference in postoperative symptoms, early complication rate or stone-free status in the access sheath and nonaccess sheath groups in patients not requiring additional balloon dilatation *(8)*. In another report of 71 ureteroscopic procedures using the access sheath the ureteral stricture rate was 1.4% at 3 mo follow-up or greater *(9)*.

Using an in vitro cadaveric model, application of the ureteral access sheath during flexible ureteroscopy or percutaneous nephrolithotomy resulted in decreased intrarenal pressures and increased irrigant flow *(10,11)*. Another potential advantage of the access sheath is that it facilitates retrograde balloon hot wire incision of ureteropelvic junction obstruction, and allows direct vision assessment of the incision depth with a ureteroscope afterwards *(12)*.

We have found ureteral access sheaths particularly useful in flexible ureteroscopy for upper ureteral and intrarenal stones. Repeated access is greatly facilitated and stone fragments can be easily extracted while the ureter is constantly protected.

Safety Wires

Use of safety guidewires is imperative to obtain access to the ureter. The 0.035-in. or 0.038-in. guidewires are standard for most ureteroscopic procedures. Other wires such as the hydrophilic Teflon wire should also be available. During ureteroscopy the guidewire plays a very important role. It is needed to gain and secure access, to pass instruments and scopes, and to insert a ureteral stent. It also serves for reorientation during surgery, either under direct vision or with fluoroscopy. The guidewire helps to straighten ureteral kinks and tortuosities, and to align the ureteral orifice with the bladder neck. Basically, a guidewire is for ureterorenoscopy what a retractor is for open surgery. It is always preferable to have a safety wire in place during the whole procedure, regardless of whether flexible or rigid scopes are being used. For a more detailed description of the composition and various designs of guidewires please refer to the Instrumentation section.

Incision

To obtain access to the upper tract beyond the ureteral meatus an endoscopic incision of the ureter may be required. In the case of an impacted stone at the level of the ureteral orifice, a direct vision incision of the ureteral orifice can be performed at the 12-o'clock position. This is achieved using a cold knife urethrotome or the Holmium:yttrium-aluminum-garnet (YAG) laser. A guidewire can then be inserted past the stone to secure access.

Other indications for endoureterotomy include ureteral strictures, ureteropelvic junction obstruction, ureterovesical junction obstruction, and ureteral anastomotic strictures (uretero-intestinal stricture, ureteral reimplantation stricture, and renal transplant anastomotic stricture). Cold knife, Holmium:YAG laser, and controlled cutting balloon catheter (Acucise catheter) have all been used for the various indications of endoureterotomy, in either a retrograde or antegrade manner *(13)*. It is, however, beyond the scope of this chapter to discuss the outcomes of all these techniques.

INSTRUMENTATION

Ureteroscopes

Rigid Ureteroscope

Initial exploration of the ureter was performed using rigid pediatric cystoscopes *(1,14)*. Modern rigid ureteroscopes are miniaturized instruments, which have either fiberoptic light bundles or rod-lens optical system. The rod-lens system provides excellent optical quality but does not allow torquing of the scope as that may result in a dark crescent area appearing on the side of the image. The fiberoptic imaging bundles take up less space than the rod lens system and have no image artifacts. Most modern rigid ureteroscopes use this optical technology. Along with the advent of smaller working instruments, newer ureteroscope diameters range from 6.9 to 9.4 Fr and are equipped with one or two separate working channels ranging from 2.1 to 5.4 Fr in size. The angle of view is usually 0–5°. These ureteroscopes thus have a larger working channel than instruments of a

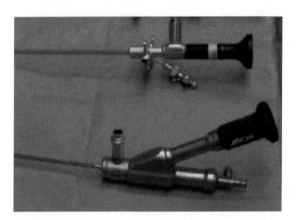

Fig. 5. Straight, working–channel, rigid ureteroscope with an offset eyepiece as compared to a standard rigid ureteroscope.

similar outer diameter with rod lens imaging systems. Their smaller size allows for easier access to the upper urinary tract, less trauma to the urothelium (Fig. 2G, H), and possibly less postoperative pain *(15)*. The standard eyepiece design is in line with the shaft of the scope; however, most companies have developed ureteroscopes with an offset eyepiece when rigid ultrasound probes were first introduced for ureteroscopic lithotripsy (Fig. 5). The offset eyepiece can be fixed or movable. The tip of the ureteroscope is usually beveled for smoother excursion. As mentioned previously, ureteroscopes with one or two working channels are available. The advantage of having two separate working channels is the minimal impact on irrigant flow during insertion of instruments. However single channels usually have a larger diameter. With the introduction of laser lithotripsy, large working channels are probably less needed and a 3.4 Fr channel is probably adequate for most procedures. These small-caliber instruments can be inserted without dilatation of the ureteral orifice in the majority of cases, and are useful for most diagnostic and therapeutic procedures.

During rigid ureteroscopy, the ureteroscope is passed in the urethra alongside the safety guidewire up to the bladder. The ureter is carefully engaged with the wire at 12-o'clock position tenting up the ureteral orifice (Fig. 2B). Alternatively, the ureter can be accessed with the wire at 6 o'clock position and the scope inverted 180° so that the tip elevates the ureteral orifice initially. Under both direct and fluoroscopic guidance, the ureteroscope is advanced up the ureter keeping the wire in view at all times. If difficulty is encountered, a second guidewire can be passed through the working channel of the ureteroscope up to the level of the kidney. This facilitates directing the tip of the scope and controlled progression over the wire. The initial safety wire will serve to gently open the ureteral lumen. Other correctable causes should be thought out when encountering difficulty advancing the ureteroscope, such as an over-distended bladder, inadequate dilation of the distal ureter, or anatomic abnormalities such as the presence of a large prostatic median lobe or intrinsic or extrinsic narrowing of the ureter.

Continuous irrigation is very important to ensure adequate visibility during either rigid or flexible ureteroscopy. Gravity irrigation is often insufficient owing to the narrow and long working channels of ureteroscopes. Several irrigation devices are available that generate higher flow at the tip of the instrument. We prefer pressurized irrigation using a pneumatic sleeve applied around the normal saline bag. The hydraulic Ureteromat system used for ureteral dilation also provides effective irrigation throughout the procedure. Two 60-mL syringes attached to a Y connector can be used in alternation to manually inject irrigation solution by the operator assistant.

FLEXIBLE URETEROSCOPE

Marshall described the first clinical use of a flexible ureteroscope in 1964 *(16)*. By the 1980s, the flexible fiberoptic ureteroscope had evolved from a passive diagnostic tool to an active therapeutic instrument *(17)*. With continued improvement of endoscopic instrumentation and development of new energy sources, modern flexible ureteroscopes now have the ability to access the entire collecting system and have become indispensable in the treatment of upper tract calculi, strictures, and tumors. The newest generation of flexible ureteroscopes have even greater active tip deflection and narrower shaft diameters; both factors facilitate passage of scopes into the upper tract and access to lower calyceal pathologies *(18)*.

Image and light transmission in flexible ureteroscopes uses fiberoptic technology. The light cord can either be separate and plug onto the ureteroscope, or be incorporated into the scope as an integral cord. Both types of light connection transmit more than enough light to the internal ureteroscopic fiberoptic system. The depth of image (or field of view) is limited in most flexible ureteroscopes; thus, flexible ureteroscopes are equipped with focusing mechanisms and image magnification to compensate for that loss. In addition to the active tip deflection, flexible ureteroscopes possess secondary passive deflection. Secondary passive deflection is possible by an additional flexible segment of the ureteroscope shaft located just proximal to the active deflection level. This allows access to most parts of the collecting system *(19)*. The principal advantage of this segment is to allow advancement of the tip of the endoscope in the lower infundibulum. The point of deflection can be effectively moved more proximally along the shaft of the ureteroscope to give equivalent lengthening of the tip.

Currently available flexible ureteroscopes have a tip diameter from 6 to 8.4 Fr and a shaft diameter from 7.2 to 9.9 Fr in size. Most ureteroscope working channels are 3.6 Fr in diameter, although larger channels, up to 4.5 Fr, exist. Many instruments, including stone baskets, graspers, and biopsy forceps are now available in sizes 3 Fr or less.

Active tip deflection is possible in two directions (down/up), and ranges from 160 to 185° for the downward direction and from 120 to 180° for the upward direction. Recently, two manufacturers (ACMI, Santa Barbara, CA and Storz, Culver City, CA) introduced a newer generation of flexible ureteroscopes (DUR-8 Elite and 11278 AU, respectively) with enhanced active tip deflection (down/up: 310/170° and 270/270°, respectively). The DUR-8 Elite has a second lever to control an additional point of deflection (130°) located more proximally on the shaft (Fig. 6), and the Storz 11278AU has a single lever that provides maximal deflection. Active tip deflection and irrigant flow rate are invariably decreased by the introduction of instruments in the working channel of flexible ureteroscopes. In a comparison of the newer models with their predecessors Chiu et al. found that although the tip deflections of all ureteroscopes were compromised by the insertion of endoscopic tools, new ureteroscopes were less affected. However, the irrigant flow rate of these new scopes was decreased compared to their respective older models *(20)*.

Flexible and rigid ureteroscopes are used in a complementary fashion to access the entire upper urinary tract. A flexible ureteroscope is introduced into the ureter over a

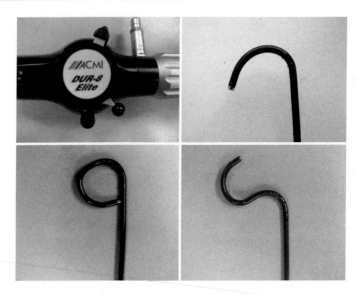

Fig. 6. The DUR-8 Elite flexible ureteroscope from ACMI has a second lever to control an additional point of deflection located more proximally on the shaft.

guidewire and under fluoroscopic guidance. During either flexible or rigid uretero-scopy, the bladder should not be overdistended and pressure in the upper tract should be kept to a minimum. A retrograde pyelogram is performed to outline the upper-tract collecting system anatomy, and the flexible ureteroscope is advanced under both direct vision and fluoroscopic guidance into all minor and major calices to map the entire system. When instruments are introduced, the tip of the scope must be straightened to avoid damage to its internal sheath. Access to the lower calyx can be challenging if the infundibulopelvic angle is acute, the lower calyx infundibulum is long and the intrarenal collecting system is dilated. Once positioned in the renal pelvis, the combination of maximal active deflection and advancement of the flexible endoscope causes buckling of the secondary-deflecting segment. This maneuver directs the tip of the instrument near the lower pole infundibulum, and by reversing the active deflection and continuing to advance the endoscope, the lower pole calyceal system can be entered. Secondary deflection is required in approx 60% of lower calyceal access. In the remaining cases active deflection alone is sufficient and the tip is deflected toward the lower pole infun-dibulum as soon as the ureteroscope passes the ureteropelvic junction. Alternatively, the ureteroscope is deflected in the renal pelvis and then withdrawn into the lower calyx. A guidewire can be directed and coiled in the lower calyx and then the scope advanced over the wire. Prone positioning of the patient with the head down 20° has been shown to provide the broadest angle of entry to the lower pole infundibulum *(21)*. Lower pole stones can be treated *in situ* or moved, with flexible 2.5 Fr graspers or a basket, into a position that allows better visualization. Use of a head-down position with the ipsilateral flank elevated may help the stone or fragments to migrate cephalad and become more accessible.

Great care must be taken in handling and sterilizing these delicate instruments. One study showed that flexible ureteroscopes were used for an average of 3–13 h before they needed repair. The most fragile part of these instruments was the deflection unit *(22)*.

RESECTOSCOPE

Ureteroresectoscopes incorporate working elements much like standard resectoscopes. The tip of these resectoscopes can be insulated to permit use of electrocautery. Working elements include resecting loops, cold and hot knife blades, and fulgurating electrodes. A ureteral resectoscope is used in a similar fashion to a standard resectoscope. However, the former carries the disadvantage of having a smaller diameter. The working space is also limited within the ureter lumen. It can be used to obtain tissue for pathologic evaluation of a suspicious upper urinary tract lesion as well as to treat known upper tract transitional cell carcinoma. Deep resection of the ureter is avoided to prevent deep thermal injury to the ureteral wall and ureteral perforation. The base of the lesion and the surrounding areas can be fulgurated with electrocautery using the resectoscope loop. Placement of a ureteral stent is recommended after completion of the resection.

Wires

Guidewires secure the ureteral lumen and serve as guidance to introduce various instruments and working tools. Different types of guidewires are available, each designed with particular properties to help accomplish specific tasks. In most ureteroscopies, a standard 145 to 150 cm long, 0.035 or 0.038 in., polytetrafluoroethylene (PTFE)–coated guidewire can be used to secure ureteral access.

Guidewire diameter range from 0.018 in. (0.46 mm) to 0.045 in. (1.15 mm). Available lengths vary from 80 to 260 cm. The distal 3–8 cm of most guidewires are designed to be soft and flexible to minimize trauma. Bentson and Newton wires have longer flexible tips up to 15 cm. Guidewire tips are either straight, angled, or have a "J" configuration. Some wires have floppy tips at both end, which facilitates flexible ureteroscope back loading and also minimizes damage to the internal endoscopic channel.

The basic design of a guidewire consists of a solid stainless steel core around which is wrapped a coiled spring wire. The outer surface of the spring wire can be coated with various materials to decrease friction between the wire and the instruments passed over it. These coatings include PTFE, Teflon, and different types of hydrophilic polymers. Several guidewire manufacturers have developed hydrophilic polymer coatings with minimal friction and very slippery and flexible qualities. These properties are helpful to negotiate a ureteral kink or bypass an impacted stone. It is essential that the hydrophilic guidewire be wet with water or saline to activate the surface polymer. The core part provides rigidity to the guidewire and can be either fixed or moveable. If moveable, the core part can be withdrawn longitudinally from the outer spring wire, thus varying the flexibility and rigidity of the guidewire tip. By increasing the diameter of the solid core, the guidewire stiffness can be increased as well. Amplatz Super Stiff wires (Boston Scientific, Microvasive) are constructed with a larger flat core component, which provides resistance to buckling or kinking owing to greater intrinsic rigidity.

Baskets

Baskets are available in different sizes and designs. The main components are the handle, the control wire, the sheath and the basket itself. The basket is opened by advancing the control wire out of the sheath and closed by pulling it back into the sheath. Baskets differ in their design (shape, number of wires, tip configuration), material, handle type, sheath diameter (2.0–7.0 Fr), and working length. Helical and nonhelical designs (spherical and elliptical and so on) are available, with three or more wires. Double-wire designs can add strength and may ease opening of the ureteral lumen. The tip is a small extension at the distal end of the basket where wires reassemble. Tipless or 0-tip baskets are now available; their main advantage is to reduce the likelihood of mucosal damage and perforation. Filiform tips (up to 15 cm) projecting beyond the basket are available in some designs. Filiform-tipped baskets can be helpful for passing the basket beyond the stone ureteroscopically and to re-advance it easily if the stone is not engaged in the open basket.

The material used to build a basket influences its strength, malleability and memory. Nitinol alloy (nickel-titanium) provides for some of these characteristics. The nitinol wire memory allows the basket to retain its shape after extreme torsion. The wire shape alters characteristics of the basket. Most baskets possess cylindrical wires, but flat-wire and delta wire designs are also available. Flat-wire baskets can be used for ureteroscopic biopsy and excision of papillary tumors on a stalk. The Segura basket, which is a flat wire basket, cannot be rotated because it can damage the ureteral mucosa. Delta-wire design offer a larger surface section of each wire within the cylindrical sheath; thus, the overall strength can be increased for the same sheath size, or alternatively, a smaller sheath diameter becomes possible for the same basket strength. Basket modification with a central channel is also available for laser fiber lithotripsy, in case of stone entrapment.

Lithotrites

Small ureteral stones can be extracted intact during ureteroscopy; however, larger stones require fragmentation. Intracorporeal ureteral lithotripsy presents different challenges from lithotripsy during percutaneous nephrolithotomy owing to anatomical and technical considerations. Four ureteral lithotrites are available, namely, electrohydraulic (EHL), pneumatic (ballistic), ultrasonic, and laser lithotripsy. Laser and EHL are flexible lithotrites, whereas pneumatic and ultrasonic are rigid lithotrites.

ELECTROHYDRAULIC LITHOTRITES

The first report of ureteral lithotripsy with EHL using a rigid ureteroscope was in 1985 *(23)*. The use of smaller EHL probes through flexible ureteroscopes started in 1988 *(24)*. EHL produces an electrical spark, which generates a shock wave within a liquid environment that fragments the stone *(25)*. Flexible probes range in diameter from 1.6 to 5 Fr. There is little difference in fragmentation ability among the different probes, but use of smaller probes is beneficial because irrigation is improved. However, larger probes have enhanced durability *(26)*. EHL works efficiently in normal saline, eliminating the risk of hyponatremia with sterile water *(27)*.

Unfortunately, EHL has a narrow margin of safety owing to the risk of damage to the ureteral mucosa, and ureteral perforation. Despite technological advancement, ureteral perforation remains an issue of concern with reported rates of 0 *(28)* to 39% *(29)*. Perforation may occur even when the probe is not in direct contact with the ureteral wall, and the risk is proportional to the energy used *(25)*. The risk of perforation may be higher for impacted stones especially when vision is impaired by minor bleeding commonly encountered during EHL *(30)*. Compared to Holmium:YAG lithotripsy, retropulsion of calculi occurs more frequently with EHL, and stone fragments are larger requiring repeated basketing *(31)*.

EHL successfully fragments 90–98% of stones but the 3-mo stone-free rate is lower because some large fragments may be retained *(28,29)*. Stone-free rates decrease with ureteral stones larger than 15 mm (67%) and are significantly lower than those seen with Holmium:YAG lithotripsy (100%) *(31)*.

The flexible nature of EHL probes is the major advantage of this lithotrite. It allows intracorporeal lithotripsy throughout the entire upper urinary tract with both rigid and flexible ureteroscopes. In addition, EHL is the least expensive intracorporeal device. On average 1–1.3 probes are used for each procedure, except with harder stones *(28)*.

The small 1.6 and 1.9 Fr probes must be used for ureteral lithotripsy. The probe is positioned about 1 mm from the stone surface and should be extended at least 2 mm distal to the tip of the ureteroscope to prevent damage to the lens. It is recommended to limit the energy used when treating ureteral stones to minimize the risk of perforation. The goal of the treatment is to create fragments that can be removed or fragments that are likely to pass spontaneously. Attempts to reduce the stone to fragments smaller than 2 mm are not recommended, because damage to the mucosa may occur *(27)*.

PNEUMATIC

The Swiss lithoclast was the first pneumatic lithotrite, introduced in the early nineties. It uses a "jackhammer" effect by which a small metal projectile in the hand piece of the instrument is propelled by controlled bursts of compressed air against the head of the metal probe at a frequency of 12 cycles per second. The probe tip is placed against the stone, which fragments on impact. The discharged probe is brought back into its former position by a piece of rubber bushing placed around the base of the probe. Pneumatic devices are still the most popular forms of ureteral lithotripsy in Europe.

Probes for the pneumatic lithotrites are rigid and range from 2.4 Fr (0.8 mm) to 7.5 Fr (2.5 mm) in diameter. A flexible Nitinol probe has been developed recently that is able to fragment calculi through semirigid and actively deflectable, flexible ureteroscopes with no reported complications *(32)*. However, use of flexible probes through deflected ureteroscopes significantly decreases fragmentation power *(33)*. Another improvement of this technology has been the introduction of a suction device connecting to the lithoclast probe that allows evacuation of small stone fragments *(34)*.

Successful fragmentation of ureteral stones of various compositions has been reported in 73–96% of cases *(35,36)*. This is similar to reported success rates of EHL.

Pneumatic lithotripsy may be more advantageous for large and hard stones encountered during percutaneous nephrolithotomy or cystolitholapaxy. Although less practical for ureteral lithotripsy, pneumatic devices have a significantly lower risk of ureteral perforation compared to EHL, ultrasonic, and laser lithotripsy *(37)*. On average, the risk of ureteral perforation is less than 1% *(35,36,38)*. Furthermore, because no heat is produced during lithotripsy, the risk of thermal injury to the urothelium is eliminated.

Another advantage of pneumatic lithotrites is their relatively low cost and low maintenance. Although they are more expensive than EHL, there are no disposable costs and the probes have a long life span. Disadvantages include the rigid nature of the probe, which requires straight working channel rigid ureteroscopes with an offset eyepiece. Also, pneumatic ureteral lithotripsy is accompanied by a relatively high rate of stone propulsion up to 17% *(38)*. Technical difficulty may be encountered if the stone can not be stabilized in a dilated ureter. Fixation of ureteral stones with a basket or proximal placement of a ureteral occlusion balloon is sometimes necessary. Fixation of the stone is rarely difficult in the kidney or the bladder.

ULTRASONIC

Ultrasonic lithotripsy is a major modality for the treatment of kidney stones during percutaneous nephrolithotomy, however, its use is limited in ureteroscopy owing to the nonflexible probe design and relatively large diameter. The ultrasound probe works by exciting a piezoceramic plate located in the ultrasound transducer. The plate then resonates and generates ultrasonic waves at a frequency of approx 23–25,000 Hz. Ultrasound energy is transformed into longitudinal and transverse vibrations of the hollow steel probe, which transmit the energy to the calculus. The ultrasonic lithotriptor system is connected to a suction pump so that debris from the stone are removed continuously with irrigating fluid during lithotripsy. In addition, the flow of fluid through the hollow probe serves to cool the instrument. Heat may develop at the end of the probe because irrigation is limited during ureteroscopy and because the small probe lumen is more prone to clogging. Ultrasonic probes are available at sizes ranging from 2.5 to 12 Fr. The 2.5-Fr probe is solid and has no hollow center for suction. Therefore, when it is used in the ureter, heat dissipation is slow. Bending of the probe results in energy loss at the convexity of the kink (39).

The advantage of ultrasonic lithotripsy is simultaneous fragment removal. However, the rigid nature of ultrasonic probes and their large diameter limits its use in ureteroscopic lithotripsy. An ureteroscope with an offset eyepiece and a large working channel is required. Excellent results have also been reported for distal ureteral stones easily accessible to the rigid ureteroscope (33).

LASER

The special features of laser light allow considerable energy to be transmitted in a highly concentrated manner. Lasers are named after the laser medium generating a specific wavelength. Initial lithotrites used continuous-wave lasers that heated the stone until vaporization occurs. Excessive temperature was needed to melt the stone making continuous-wave lasers clinically unusable (40). The development of pulsed lasers solved this dilemma. Pulsed energy generates very high power density at the stone surface with concomitant heat dissipation.

Pulsed lasers create a "plasma" bubble that generates a shock wave responsible for stone fragmentation, except for holmium laser (41). The holmium:YAG laser produces an elongated cavitation bubble that generates a weak shock wave compared with the strong shock wave produced by other pulse lasers. In fact, Holmium laser lithotripsy occurs primarily through a photothermal mechanism that causes stone vaporization (42). The first commercially available laser lithotrite was the pulsed-dye laser, which employed a coumarin green dye as a liquid laser medium. The 200-μm flexible fiber allowed the use of flexible ureteroscopes. Overall success rates were 80–95% (42). However, calcium oxalate monohydrate stones were more difficult to treat and yielded larger fragments (43), and cystine stones did not absorb the laser wave length and were not fragmented (44). Other limitations of the coumarin pulsed-dye laser included the initial high cost, and the cost of toxic disposable dye and maintenance. The flashlamp pumped Q-switched alexandrite laser was proposed as an alternative to the pulsed-dye laser. It operated at a wavelength of 750 nm as opposed to the coumarin laser wavelength of 504. This solid-state laser was equally efficacious, compact, and with no toxic chemicals.

Recent developments in laser lithotripsy led to the Holmium:YAG laser (Fig. 7). The properties of this laser make it a great clinical tool: monochromatic, directional and

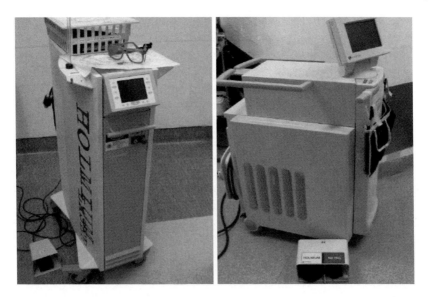

Fig. 7. Two holmium:YAG laser generators from different manufacturers.

coherent. The holmium laser operates at a wavelength of 2140 nm in the pulsed mode, which is highly absorbed by water and results in superficial cutting or coagulation. The zone of thermal injury associated with laser ablation ranges from 0.5 to 1.0 mm in depth *(45)*. The Holmium:YAG laser, similar to the EHL, allows the use of flexible instruments throughout the entire collecting system. However, when compared with EHL, holmium laser is safer and more efficient. Whereas EHL may cause injury to the ureter even when the probe is activated several millimeters away from the ureteral wall, the holmium laser can be safely activated at a distance of 0.5–1 mm from the ureteral wall *(46)*. The ability of the holmium laser to fragment all stones regardless of composition is a clear advantage over the pulsed-dye laser. Successful fragmentation of ureteral stones of all compositions is reported to be up to 100% of cases, with a stone-free rate as high as 95%. Perforation and stricture rates are 1.1% and 1.2%, respectively *(47,48)*.

Currently, the holmium laser is the most effective and versatile intracorporeal lithotriptor with a good margin of safety. Further advantages include significantly smaller stone fragments compared with other lithotrites, resulting in small stone debris, which are easily irrigated and reduce the need for stone retrieval. Retropulsion is less likely owing to the weak shock wave. In addition, the holmium laser is more compact than the coumarin laser, requires minimal maintenance, and is ready for use 1 min after it is turned on. The major disadvantage of the holmium laser is the initial high cost of the device and the cost of the laser fibers. However, the holmium laser has multiple soft tissue applications and can be used for treating benign prostatic hyperplasia, strictures, and urothelial tumors.

During lithotripsy, the laser fiber should be placed on the stone surface before activating the laser (Fig. 2D). Caution must be exercised when operating the holmium laser near a guidewire or a basket because it is capable of cutting through metal. Furthermore, the laser fiber should extend at least 2 mm beyond the tip of the endoscope to avoid damage to the lens or the working channel of the endoscope. Holmium laser fibers are available in 200-, 365-, 550-, and 1000-μm diameters, as well as end- or side-firing fibers. However, only the 200- and 365-µm diameter fibers are used for flexible intracorporeal lithotripsy. Treatment should be started with low energy. Usually 0.6–1.2 Joules at a rate of 5–15 Hz provides adequate lithotripsy. High-pulse energy narrows the safety margin and may increase stone retropulsion and mucosal damage. Stone fragmentation with the holmium laser occurs by small perforations at the surface of the stone. The surgeon should move the laser fiber over the stone surface, vaporizing the stone rather than fragmenting it until fragments are small enough to pass spontaneously (Fig. 2E) or are able to be safely retrieved (Fig. 2F). Fragments larger than 4 mm are produced by all types of endoscopic lithotrites, with the exception of the Holmium:YAG laser *(49)*.

Other laser lithotriptors are currently being developed. The erbium:YAG (Er:YAG) laser operates at a wavelength of 2940 nm and fragments stones through a photothermal mechanism like the Ho:YAG laser. Experimental studies demonstrated that Er:YAG lithotripsy is more efficient than Ho:YAG lithotripsy because optical energy is better absorbed by urinary calculi at 2940 nm wavelength compared with 2140 nm. However, a major limitation of Er:YAG lithotripsy to date has been the lack of clinically useful optical fibers to transport the laser energy through endoscopes *(50)*.

LASER SAFETY

The cornea will absorb laser energy. Under prolonged exposure, aqueous flare, cataracts, or corneal burn may occur. The holmium laser beam is invisible. All procedure room personnel, including the patient, should wear appropriate laser safety eyewear while the laser is in operation. Access to the operation room must be restricted and laser-warning signs should be posted at all entrances. Ocular hazards can result from direct, reflected, or scattered laser exposure. In fact, the holmium laser properties are such that when using energy levels applied for stone disease (i.e., less than 15 W), the operator's retina might be damaged only if it were positioned at a distance of 10 cm or less from the fiber *(26)*. The required eye protection for coumarin green laser causes pronounced blue-yellow color confusion, whereas alexandrite laser causes mild red-green color confusion. The eyewear for holmium laser does not compromise color vision *(51)*.

Laser exposure on unprotected skin may cause skin injuries. Pigment darkening, photosensitive reactions, and severe skin burns may occur. Moreover, the laser lithotriptor should not be used in the presence of flammable anesthetics. All room personnel should be trained in laser safety.

A potential side effect of holmium laser lithotripsy is the production of cyanide gas when uric acid stones are treated; this has been reported in vitro. However, review of clinical experience suggests no significant cyanide toxicity from holmium laser lithotripsy *(52)*.

PEARLS AND TRICKS

On many occasions, an urologist is challenged in obtaining ureteral access in patients with abnormal ureteral anatomy. Patients may present with a ureteral orifice that is difficult to find or an orifice that is stenotic and strictured from previous surgery. Carefully evaluate for ureteral anomalies related to number (duplication), position (ectopy), or morphology (ureterocele); watch for urine efflux. Severe inflammation within the bladder and mucosal edema may hide the ureteral orifices. This is commonly seen in patients with cystitis, or a chronic indwelling catheter. Locating the ureteral orifice is also difficult in a patient with prior ureteral reimplantation. In Politano-Leadbetter or Anderson ureteral reimplantation, laterality of the ureters is maintained, and the orifice is located either in the orthotopic position or slightly closer to the bladder neck. In patients who have undergone a Cohen cross-trigonal reimplantation, the ureteral orifice is found exiting the contralateral side of the bladder. In the extavesical seromuscular Lich-Gregoire technique, commonly used in kidney transplants, the ureter enters near the posterior wall or the dome of the bladder. In patients who have undergone ileal interposition, the ileal segment is usually anastomosed to the posterolateral wall of the bladder. The anastomosis is often patulous and is easily visualized by endoscopy. Regardless of the situation, caution must be taken when attempting ureteral access in patients whose distal ureteral anatomy is abnormal. The use of a flexible cystoscope is of great help in these difficult cases to reach and access the ureteral orifice in the most optimal direction. Straight or angled tipped hydrophilic wires offer the best chance to secure access. They can later be exchanged for a regular guidewire over an open ended ureteral catheter. In cases where the orifice is obscured by inflammation, edema, or scarring, intravenous indigo carmine or methylene blue helps to locate a hidden orifice.

Benign Prostatic Hyperplasia Median Lobe

One of the more common, and often difficult, tasks is locating the ureteral orifices in a patient with benign prostatic hyperplasia and a large median lobe. The transmural ureter often assumes a J-hook configuration as it enters the bladder.

If the ureteral orifice is not readily identified, first make sure the irrigation fluid is clear. Rotate the cystoscope 180° to use the rounded beak of the scope to gently retract the middle lobe off the interureteric ridge and expose the orifice. This configuration also provides a more direct angle into the distal bend of the ureter, allowing for easier passage of the wire. A 70° lens can aid viewing around a large median lobe or finding an ectopic orifice. A flexible cystoscope can also be helpful as mentioned before. Occasionally, using an angled tipped guidewire that is directed gently back and forth on the interureteric ridge can sometimes reveal the ureteral orifice opening and find its way into the distal ureter. A rigid ureteroscope may also be used to introduce a guidewire into a ureter. If all these maneuvers fail, percutaneous renal access with antegrade passage of a guidewire down the ureter and into the bladder may become necessary.

Ureteral Kinks

Ureteral kinks sometimes pose a difficult problem in securing access and progressing proximally during ureteroscopy. These kinks are secondary to multiple causes including abdominal masses, prior retroperitoneal or endoscopic surgery, distal obstruction and elongation of the ureter, and vascular abnormalities.

First, an attempt is made to pass a hydrophilic guidewire past the area of concern. An angled tipped wire over an open-ended ureteral catheter offers a good chance to steer past the kink. Alternatively, different angiocatheters with various tip configurations can be used to support the glide wire and orient its tip in the desired direction. We find the Cobra angiocatheter very useful in these situations. Placing the patient in a steep Trendelenberg position slightly displaces the kidneys cephalad and may help straighten the ureter. If these maneuvers fail, inflating a balloon dilator distal to the ureteral kink and exerting gentle traction under fluoroscopic guidance can align the ureter and facilitate passage of the guidewire. Once a glide wire is passed beyond the kink, it should be exchanged to a regular wire, or preferably to a superstiff wire, to straighten the ureter.

SUMMARY

Ureteroscopy and intracorporeal lithotripsy is highly successful thanks to multiple modern instruments and tools. However, always remember that the ureter is fragile and if there are significant technical difficulties in achieving the goal, place a stent and come back at a later date. Passive ureteral dilation usually ensues within 48 h.

REFERENCES

1. Young HH, McKay RW. Congenital valvular obstruction of the prostatic urethra. Surg Gynecol Obstet 1929; 48: 509.
2. Ford TF, Parkinson MC, Wickham JE. Clinical and experimental evaluation of ureteric dilatation. Br J Urol. 1984; 56(5): 460–463.
3. Huffman JL, Bagley DH. Balloon dilation of the ureter for ureteroscopy. J Urol. 1988; 140(5): 954–956.
4. Garvin TJ, Clayman RV. Balloon dilation of the distal ureter to 24F. an effective method for ureteroscopic stone retrieval. J Urol 1991; 146(3): 742–745.
5. Eshghi M. Dilatation of ureteral orifice for ureterorenoscopy. Urol Clin North Am 1988; 15(3): 301–314.
6. Smith AD. Rapid dilatation of ureteral orifice for ureteroscopy. Urology 1985; 26(4): 407.
7. Pérez-Castro E. Ureteromat; Method to facilitate ureterorenoscopy and avoid dilatation. Urol Clin North Am 1988; 15(3): 315–321.
8. Kourambas J, Byrne RR, Preminger GM. Does a ureteral access sheath facilitate ureteroscopy? J Urol 2001; 165(3): 789–793.
9. Delvecchio FC, Auge BK, Brizuela RM, et al. Assessment of stricture formation with the ureteral access sheath. Urology 2003; 61(3): 518–522.
10. Rehman J, Monga M, Landman J, et al. Characterization of intrapelvic pressure during ureteropyeloscopy with ureteral access sheaths. Urology 2003; 61(4): 713–718.
11. Landman J, Venkatesh R, Ragab M, et al. Comparison of intrarenal pressure and irrigant flow during percutaneous nephroscopy with an indwelling ureteral catheter, ureteral occlusion balloon, and ureteral access sheath. Urology 2002; 60(4): 584–587.
12. Auge BK, Wu NZ, Pietrow PK, Delvecchio FC, Preminger GM. Ureteral access sheath facilitates inspection of incision of ureteropelvic junction. J Urol 2003; 169(3): 1070–1073.
13. Hafez KS, Wolf JS Jr. Update on minimally invasive management of ureteral strictures. J Endourol 2003; 17(7): 453–464.
14. Goodman TM. Ureteroscopy with pediatric cystoscope in adults. Urology 1977; 9(4): 394.
15. Abdel Razzak OM, Bagley DH. Rigid ureteroscopes with fiberoptic imaging bundles: features and irrigating capacity. J Endourol 1994; 8(6): 411–414.
16. Marshall VF. Fiber optics in urology. J Urol 1964; 91: 110–114.
17. Aso Y. Takayasu H, Ohta N, Tajima A. Flexible ureterorenoscopy Urol Clin North Am 1988; 15: 329–338.
18. Parkin J, Keeley FX, Jr, Timoney AG, Flexible ureteroscopes: a user's guide. BJU Int 2002; 90: 640–643.
19. Grasso M, Bagley D. Small diameter, actively deflectable, flexible ureteropyeloscopy. J Urol 1998; 160(5): 1648–1653.
20. Chiu KY, Cai Y, Marcovich R, El-Hakim A, Smith AD, Lee BR. Comparison of the mechanical, flow, and optical properties of contemporary flexible ureteroscopes. Urology 2003; 62(5): 800–804.
21. Bercowsky E, Shalhav AL, Elbahnasy AM, Owens E, Clayman RV. The effect of patient position on intrarenal anatomy. J Endourol 1999; 13(4): 257–260.
22. Afane JS, Olweny EO, Bercowsky E, et al. Flexible ureteroscopes: a single center evaluation of the durability and function of the new endoscopes smaller than 9Fr. J Urol 2000; 164(4): 1164–1168.
23. Green DF, Lytton B. Early experience with direct vision electrohydraulic lithotripsy of ureteral calculi. J Urol 1985; 133(5): 767–770.
24. Begun FP, Jacobs SC, Lawson RK. Use of prototype 3F electrohydraulic electrode with ureteroscopy for treatment of ureteral calculus disease. J Urol 1988; 139(6):1188–1191.

25. Vorreuther R, Corleis R, Klotz T, Bernards P, Engelmann U. Impact of shock wave pattern and cavitation bubble size on tissue damage during ureteroscopic electrohydraulic lithotripsy. J Urol 1995; 153: 849–853.

26. Segura JW. Intracorporeal lithotripsy. AUA Update Series 1999; 18: 66–71.

27. Denstedt JD, Clayman RV. Electrohydraulic lithotripsy of renal and ureteral calculi. J Urol 1990; 143: 13–17.

28. Elashry OM, DiMeglio RB, Nakada SY, McDougall EM, Clayman RV. Intracorporeal lithotripsy of ureteral and renal calculi using small caliber (1.9 Fr) electrohydraulic lithotripsy probes. J Urol 1996; 156: 1581–1585.

29. Basar H, Ohta N, Kageyama S, Suzuki K, Kawabi K. Treatment of ureteral and renal stones by electrohydraulic lithotripsy. Int Urol Nephrol 1997; 29: 275–280.

30. Hofbauer J, Hobarth K, Marberger M. Electrohydraulic versus pneumatic disintegration in the treatment of ureteral stones: A randomized, prospective trial. J Urol 1995; 153: 623–625.

31. Teichman JMH, Rao RD, Rogenes VJ, Harris JM. Ureteroscopic management of ureteral calculi. Electrohydraulic versus holmium:YAG lithotripsy. J Urol 1997; 158: 1357–1361.

32. Tawfiek ER, Grasso M, Bagley DH. The initial use of the Browne Pneumatic Impactor. J Endourol 1997; 11: 121–124.

33. Grocela JA, Dretler SP. Intracorporeal lithotripsy. Urol Clin North Am 1997; 24: 13–23.

34. Delvecchio FC, Kuo RL, Preminger GM. Clinical efficacy of combined lithoclast and Lithovac stone removal during ureteroscopy. J Urol 2000; 164: 40–42.

35. Knispel HH, Klan R, Heicappell R, Miller K. Pneumatic lithotripsy applied through deflected working channel of mini-ureteroscope: Results in 143 patients. J Endourol 1998; 12: 513–515.

36. Keeley FX, Pillai M, Smith G, Krisofos M, Tolley DA. Electrokinetic lithotripsy: Safety, efficacy and limitations of a new form of ballistic lithotripsy. Br J Urol 1999; 84: 261–263.

37. Piergiovanni M, Desgrandchamps F, Cochand-Priollet B, et al. Ureteral and bladder lesions after ballistic, ultrasonic, electrohydraulic or laser lithotripsy. J Endourol 1994; 8: 293–299.

38. Murthy PV, Rao HS, Meherwade S, Rao PV, Srivastava A, Sasidharan K. Ureteroscopic lithotripsy using mini-endoscope and Swiss lithoclast: Experience in 147 cases. J Endourol 1997; 11: 327–330.

39. Marberger M. Disintegration of renal and ureteral calculi with ultrasound. Urol Clin North Am 1983; 10: 729–742.

40. Mulvaney WP, Beck CW. The laser beam in urology. J Urol 1968; 99: 112–115.

41. Floratos DL, Rosette JJM. Lasers in urology. Br J Urol 1999; 84: 204–211.

42. Vassar GJ, Teichman JMH, Glickman RD. Holmium:YAG lithotripsy efficiency varies with energy density. J Urol 1998; 160: 471–476.

43. Coptcoat MJ, Ison KT, Watson G, Wickham JEA. Lasertripsy for ureteric stones in 120 cases: Lessons learned. Br J Urol 1988; 61: 487–489.

44. Bhatta KM, Prien EL, Dretler SP. Cystine calculi-rough and smooth: A new clinical distinction. J Urol 1989; 142: 937–940.

45. Wollin TA, Denstedt JD. The holmium laser in urology. J Clin Laser Med Surg 1998; 16: 13–20.

46. Santa-Cruz RW, Leveille RJ, Krongard A. Ex vivo comparison of four lithotriptors commonly used in the ureter: What does it take to perforate? J Endourol 1998; 12: 417–422.

47. Grasso M, Chalik Y. Principles and applications of laser lithotripsy: Experience with the holmium laser lithotrite. J Clin Lasers Surg Med 1998; 16: 3–7.

48. Devarajan R, Ashraf M, Beck RO, Lemberger RJ, Taylor MC. Holmium:YAG lasertripsy for ureteric calculi: An experience of 300 procedures. Br J Urol 1998; 82: 342–347.

49. Teichman JM, Vassar GJ, Bishoff JT, Bellman GC. Holmium:YAG lithotripsy yields smaller fragments than lithoclast, pulsed dye laser or electrohydraulic lithotripsy. J Urol 1998; 159: 17–23.

50. Chan KF, Lee H, Teichman JM, et al. Erbium: YAG laser lithotripsy mechanism. J Urol 2002; 168(2): 436–441.

51. Teichman JM, Johnson AJ, Yates JT, et al. Color vision deficits during laser lithotripsy using safety goggles for coumarin green or alexandrite but not with holmium:YAG laser safety goggles. J Urol 1998; 159(3): 683–689.

52. Teichman JMH, Champion PC, Wollin TA, Denstedt JD. Holmium:YAG lithotripsy of uric acid calculi. J Urol 1998; 160: 2130–2132.

31 Percutaneous Nephrolithotomy

Indications and Outcomes

Paul K. Pietrow, MD

CONTENTS

HISTORY
INDICATIONS
CONTRAINDICATIONS
OUTCOMES
COMPLICATIONS
REFERENCES

Key Words: Nephrolithiasis; kidney; percutaneous access; nephrolithotomy.

HISTORY

The management of renal calculus disease underwent drastic changes in the early 1980s with the arrival of percutaneous surgery and shockwave lithotripsy within several years of each other. Previously, patients were managed with an array of open procedures, including pyelolithomy, ureterolithotomy and anatrophic nephrolithotomy. The opportunity to effectively manage renal calculi in a percutaneous manner has drastically reduced patient morbidity when compared to an open, flank approach. Fernstrom and Johansson were the first to describe a percutaneous approach to the renal collecting system for the management of calculi *(1)*. Much of the early pioneering efforts were performed at the University of Minnesota and were made possible by the arrival of improved equipment and of an effective ultrasonic device that could be used to destroy and remove stones of varying compositions *(2)*. Although the availability of improved access devices, nephroscopes and lithotrites have made this procedure more facile and safe, the basic principles and techniques have not changed dramatically over the past 20 yr.

From: Current Clinical Urology, *Urinary Stone Disease:*
A Practical Guide to Medical and Surgical Management
Edited by: M. L. Stoller and M. V. Meng © Humana Press Inc., Totowa, NJ

Table 1
Indications for Percutaneous Nephrolithotomy

Strong
- Calculi >2–3cm
- Staghorn calculi
- Complex calculi (multiple calyces)

Possible
- >1 cm calcium oxalate monohydrate calculi
- >1 cm cystine calculi
- Calyceal diverticular calculi
- >1 cm lower pole calculi
- >1 cm renal calculi in patients with urinary diversions
- >1 cm renal transplant calculi
- Calculi associated with UPJ obstruction
- Large proximal ureteral calculi

INDICATIONS

Although significantly less morbid than open surgery, percutaneous nephrolithotomy (PCNL) is still the most invasive approach to urinary lithiasis when compared to ureteroscopy or extracorporeal shockwave lithotripsy (SWL). Consequently, this technique is generally reserved for specific needs (Table 1). Bulky stones greater than 2 cm are frequently best treated with a percutaneous approach to minimize repeat treatments and trauma to the kidney. Complete stone clearance can also avoid the risk of steinstrasse if the ureter is unable to accommodate a large bolus of stone debris. These concerns are especially true of staghorn calculi or complex stones that occupy multiple calyces. Some stones are simply too dense or organic in nature to respond well to SWL and may be best served with an initial percutaneous approach. Calcium oxalate monohydrate calculi are noted to be the densest stones and often experience incomplete fragmentation *(3,4)*.

Cystine stones are also resistant to shockwave energy, likely owing to their organic origin and their tight crystalline formation. Additionally, residual cystine fragments can easily act as "seed calculi" leaving the patient with multiple smaller stones rather than their initial large calculus. In light of these difficulties, many authors advocate a percutaneous approach for cystine stones even less than 2 cm in order to achieve complete stone clearance *(5,6)*.

Some stones smaller than 2 cm may be best treated with a percutaneous approach if they reside within difficult anatomic locations. Calyceal divertula have a tight neck that will not allow the easy passage of stone debris. If the diverticulum is inaccessible from a retrograde ureteroscopic approach, then percutaneous access can clear any stone material and allow either destruction of the urothelial lining or creation of a wider infundibular orifice (or both) *(7,8)*. Owing to obvious anatomic constraints, this technique is best reserved for posterior calyces.

Stones within a lower pole calyx may have a difficult time clearing out of this region into the pelvis and down the ureter following SWL. A well-controlled large randomized trial has demonstrated that percutaneous nephrolithotomy is superior to SWL for lower pole calculi *(9)*. The difference was particularly dramatic for stones larger than 1 cm.

Table 2
Contraindications for Percutaneous Nephrolithotomy

Absolute	*Relative*
• Uncontrolled coagulopathy	• Ectopic kidney
• Active urinary tract infection	• Fusion anomalies
	• Severe dysmorphism
	• Morbid obesity

Several authors have identified anatomic features of the lower pole collecting system that might allow for the easy clearance of fragments after SWL. These include the presence of an obtuse infundibular/renal pelvis angle (>70°), a short infundibular length (<3 cm) and a wide infundibular neck (>5 mm) *(10)*.

Patients with urinary diversions and moderate-to-large calculi may be best served with PCNL if retrograde access is too difficult or if the presence of infected stones and colonized urine preclude the use of shockwave lithotripsy. These patients fare well if they are covered with broad spectrum antibiotics and pre-placement of the percutaneous access 1–2 d before their procedure *(11)*.

Urinary lithiasis within a kidney transplant may require a percutaneous antegrade approach if the stone or the patient are not amenable to SWL. In addition, transplant ureters can be difficult to access in a retrograde fashion owing to angulation and narrowing at the uretero-vesical anastomosis.

The presence of co-existing pathology may also require a percutaneous approach. Patients with large calculi and a ureteroplevic junction obstruction (UPJO) may be best served by performing a PCNL and an antegrade endopyelotomy in the same sitting. Care must be taken to discern the difference between a primary UPJO causing stone or a stone causing a secondary UPJO.

CONTRAINDICATIONS

Several conditions can preclude the use of a percutaneous route to remove renal calculi (Table 2). An uncontrolled coagulopathy (either pathophysiologic or pharmacologic) puts the patient at too great of a risk for severe hemorrhage. Because each kidney receives 5–10% of the total cardiac output with each beat of the heart, uncontrolled hemorrhage can be rapid and require transfusion, selective arterial embolization or even nephrectomy. Significant amounts of irrigating fluids are absorbed during a PCNL owing to extravasation into the retroperitoneal space and the opening of venous sinuses within the renal parenchyma. The presence of an active urinary tract infection, therefore, places the patient at a greater risk of bacteremia of even septicemia with vascular collapse.

Renal anatomic abnormalities may make it difficult to adequately and safely access the collecting system. This includes renal ectopia (e.g., pelvic kidney) or fusion anomalies (e.g., horseshoe kidney). Although these anomalies are not absolute contraindications for the performance of a PCNL, good spatial orientation, excellent preoperative imaging and a very healthy respect for surrounding viscera and vasculature are crucial *(12)*. Patients with a solitary kidney should be approached with care. Any surgical intervention runs the risk of permanent injury to the sole functioning renal unit.

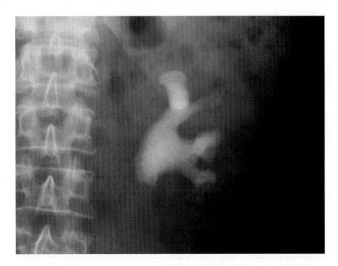

Fig. 1. Large, branched staghorn calculus completely filling the collecting system of a left kidney.

OUTCOMES

The technical success of percutaneous nephrolithotomy has made this technique the standard of care for many calculi and scenarios as outlined in the Indications section. A careful assessment of results, however, reveals that the expected outcomes and risks vary with the specific application.

Staghorn Calculi

Staghorn calculi (either partial or complete) represent a unique challenge for the endourologist (Fig. 1). The sheer bulk of the stone burden and the complex branched anatomy of the collecting system require careful planning regarding access and plurality of access tracts. Additionally, these calculi are typically associated with an infectious etiology. Antibiotics are never able to completely penetrate the interstices of a complex stone, running the risk of a release of bacteria and endotoxin during stone ablation *(13)*. Despite these warnings, however, PCNL remains the standard of care for staghorn calculi, replacing anatrophic nephrolithotomy and other open approaches.

Results from many authors have demonstrated the superiority of PCNL over SWL alone. In 1994, the evidence was compelling enough to prompt the AUA Guidelines Committee to recommend PCNL as first line therapy, often combined with SWL to ablate calculi in difficult to reach calyces *(14)*.

Second-look PCNL may also be added to the end of this regimen to "clean-up" any residual fragments left after the shockwave lithotripsy. This technique has been dubbed "sandwich therapy." Stone-free rates tend to range from 70 to 100% with this approach, with acceptable complication rates. Randomized trials have been performed comparing a combination of PCNL with SWL vs SWL alone. One particularly noteworthy analysis from Meretyk et al. demonstrated a stone-free rate of 74% with combination therapy vs 22% with SWL alone *(15)*. Nearly half of all shockwave lithotripsy patients had septic episodes whereas the combination patients had an 8% rate. Finally, 26% of the monotherapy patients required ancillary procedures over 6 mo vs 4% of the combination patients over one additional month.

Chandhoke has demonstrated that initial combination therapy is more cost effective than shockwave monotherapy *(16)*. This is especially notable when the stone surface area exceeds 500 mm^2 when measured in its greatest dimensions. This implies a calculus at least as large as 2.2 × 2.2 cm, clearly within the parameters of a typical staghorn calculus.

More recently, some centers have moved away from a sandwich technique, relying on aggressive PCNL at the first sitting. This may require the use of a supracostal access or a multi-tract access at the first procedure *(17–19)*. These same approaches may remove so much stone burden that there is no longer a need for the "meat" portion of the sandwich (SWL) or the second-look PCNL.

Others have moved away from the removal of all residual fragments, electing to treat small remnants with aggressive medical therapy *(20)*. This therapy should be directed by the information gained from a complete metabolic evaluation and/or stone analysis. Anatomic abnormalities (UPJ obstruction, caliceal diverticulum) or genetic predisposition (cystinuria) that played a role in the formation of the original calculus should be addressed if possible. Residual fragments should be small and expected to have a reasonable chance of spontaneous passage. The presence of infected fragments is generally frowned on as these can easily act as "seed" calculi and reinfect the patient's urinary tract.

Simultaneous Bilateral Percutaneous Nephrolithotomy

Several authors from various institutions and nations have described the performance of bilateral PCNL in one operative setting to avoid the costs and risks of multiple anesthetics *(21–24)*. All authors provide the caveat that the decision to proceed on to the second side is determined by the clinical result and the relative ease of performance of the first side. Significant hemorrhage, prolonged stone extraction time, multiple access tracts and instability of vital signs all warrant the cessation of surgery after completion of the initial side. The most symptomatic side is usually approached first. Alternatively, the renal unit most at risk of injury owing to obstruction or bulky stone burden may be treated initially. Two of the series compared bilateral PCNL patients to either unilateral PCNL or staged PCNL *(22,23)*. Both demonstrated increased transfusion requirements for the bilateral patients but noted that this was more closely related to number of nephrostomy tracts employed and the relative stone burden addressed. That is, smaller stone burdens addressed with one nephrostomy tract on each side appeared to lose as much blood as an equal stone burden on a unilateral patient treated via two nephrostomy tracts.

These same authors report that they are able to proceed on to bilateral PCNL in the majority of patients selected. Both Dushinski and Maheshwari reported that 94–96% of patients were able to be treated with a bilateral approach when surgically planned *(21, 24)*. However, none of the authors are able to identify how many patients were screened for a bilateral approach and deemed too risky for consideration of such an undertaking. Judicious patient screening, careful technique on the initial side, and sound intraoperative judgment are all crucial for the safe performance of a bilateral, synchronous nephrolithotomy.

Supracostal Access

As the kidney lies within the retroperitoneum, the lower pole is displaced ventrally and laterally by the body of the psoas muscle. As a result, the upper pole of the kidney

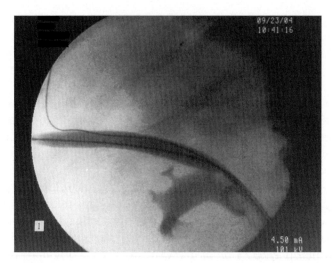

Fig. 2. Dilating balloon traversing percutaneous tract via puncture above the 12th rib. Calculi are visible as filling defects within the renal pelvis.

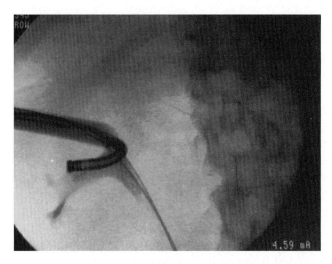

Fig. 3. A flexible cystoscope is introduced through the upper pole access and directed into an upper, lateral calyx to confirm complete stone clearance.

represents the most superficial access point during a posterior percutaneous approach. Entry into the lower pole can be hampered by the presence of adipose tissue and/or large buttocks. In addition, entry into the collection system sometimes requires unimpeded endoscopic access to the ureteropelvic junction or proximal ureter. For these reasons, some authors have advocated the use of an upper pole access during PCNL. Depending on the height of the kidney in the retroperitoneum, this may require that the tract gains entry above the 12th or even the 11th rib. This approach has been termed "supracostal" (Fig. 2). Although not without risk, this approach offers excellent visualization of the upper pole, the lower pole and the UPJ. The use of flexible nephroscopy also allows reasonable access into many (if not all) of the lateral calyces (Fig. 3).

Indeed, Wong and Leveillee have demonstrated that a primary upper pole access is effective for a series of staghorn and complex calculi that were all at least >5 cm in size *(17)*. By employing flexible endoscopes, a Holmium laser, nitinol baskets and second-look PCNL, the authors were able to able to render 95% of the patients stone-free. This did require an average of 1.6 procedures per patient. Complications were reasonable. They report a 2% transfusion rate, a 3% incidence of pneumothorax and 12% of the patients experiencing a postoperative febrile episode.

Gupta et al. reported a series of 62 patients who underwent supracostal access for PCNL. All tracts were above the 12th but below the 11th ribs *(25)*. With this approach, 90% of the patients were either stone-free or reduced to clinically insignificant fragments. The staghorn patients fared well with an 84% stone-free rate. Chest complications developed in 5% of the patients, all of which were managed with chest tube decompression. The authors conclude that fear of chest complications should not preclude the use of supracostal access if it is needed for adequate access. As expected, they also advocate the acquisition of an upright chest radiograph at the end of every supracostal PCNL.

Munver et al. have also outlined an extensive series of patients, reporting on the complication rates of 98 supracostal access tracts *(26)*. Seventy-two of these tracts were above the 12th rib, whereas 26 were above the 11th. Not surprisingly, the higher the access tract the greater the rate of complications. Seven patients (7%) had intra-thoracic problems, all managed with chest tube drainage. Of note, the authors also compared the supracostal patients to a contemporary series of subcostal PCNL patients and noted only one intrathoracic event out of 202 subcostal tracts (0.5%).

Multiple Access Percutaneous Nephrolithotomy

Clustered or staghorn calculi may be too complex to completely reach with the rigid nephroscope through one single access tract. As noted previously, some remnant stones can be reached with a flexible nephroscope through one access (especially if it is through the upper pole). Alternately, some have advocated the placement of additional nephrostomy tracts to reach isolated calyces and bulky remnants *(27)*. Indeed, this tactic has been employed since the early development of the percutaneous technique *(28)*. Most authors report increases in transfusion rates as the number of tracts increase.

Tubeless PCNL/Reduced Drainage PCNL

Although percutaneous nephrolithotomy is clearly effective, there is no doubt that it creates significant discomfort. Many endourologists have tried various measures to reduce postoperative pain without sacrificing efficacy or safety. One approach involves the placement of a small drainage catheter at the end of the procedure. It is presumed that the reduced diameter of the nephrostomy tube can reduce pain after the operative procedure. Pietrow and colleagues randomized patients to standard 22 Fr catheter drainage vs 10 Fr drainage utilizing a small locking loop catheter *(29)*. Patients demonstrated significantly less pain in the immediate perioperative period if they had the smaller tube, although this advantage waned quickly and was no different at the 14 d postoperative follow-up. Importantly, there was no difference in complications or in hematocrit change between the two groups. Moreover, many of these patients were treated through a supracostal approach, which is generally considered more painful.

Others have also studied this modification. A recent investigation by Liatkos et al. randomized patients to receive either a standard 24 Fr Malecot re-entry catheter or an

18 Fr catheter with a tail-less stent following PCNL *(30)*. This study found that those patients with the smaller tube and the tail-less stent had less pain than the standard cohort. Of note, these authors did not assess the patients' perception of pain until their 2-wk postoperative visit. Although the patients appeared more comfortable, it is hard to distinguish whether this difference is caused by the smaller drainage catheter or to the presence of a tailless stent.

Bellman has promoted a tubeless technique in selected patients. In this approach, the full PCNL is performed in the usual fashion *(31,32)*. If the patient meets strict criteria, an internal ureteral stent is placed, the nephrostomy access tract is removed and the skin is closed. Patients must not require a second-look procedure and must therefore be rendered stone-free during their operation. Significant intraoperative hemorrhage, large stone volume, prolonged procedure times and a risk of infection have all been used as exclusion criteria for a tubeless procedure. Using these parameters, Bellman and colleagues have demonstrated decreased postoperative pain and decreased analgesic requirements from those treated in a standard fashion. They do not report any increase in complications nor in transfusion requirement. This technique has been duplicated by others with similar results, confirming its safety and efficacy.

The ability to apply this technique beyond these strict guidelines has been proposed and several have explored methods to close the tract to limit postprocedural hemorrhage. Noller and colleagues have employed fibrin glue to seal the access tract at the end of the procedure and have reported satisfactory results with small changes in hematocrit and no need for transfusion *(33)*.

Clayman and colleagues have used a novel hemostatic agent (Flo-Seal Matrix, Baxter Healthcare Corp., Deerfield, IL) to fill the access tract before removal of the final safety wire *(34)*. A ureteral occlusion balloon is placed at the edge of the calyx to keep the material next to the parenchyma and out of the collecting system. Both of these approaches may allow a wider application of the tubeless technique. All authors repeat the caveat that the procedure must be uncomplicated and that there must be no need for re-entry into the collecting system.

In an interesting prospective, randomized study, Desai et al. compared standard large bore drainage to small catheter drainage and a tubeless technique *(35)*. The patients met reasonable, but strict exclusion criteria that prevented an increased risk of complication from any of the methods. The authors found that patients in the tubeless group had the least postoperative analgesic requirement, followed by the small-bore catheter group. Additionally, these patients had the shortest duration of urine leak through the nephrostomy tract. As in earlier studies, there was no difference in transfusion requirements among the three groups.

Intracorporeal Lithotriptors

The performance of a successful percutaneous nephrolithotomy is dependent on the ability to gain safe access into the collecting system and on the ability to fragment and remove calculi once the stone has been encountered. The development of an effective handheld ultrasonic device has been crucial to the efficacy of this procedure. After its introduction in the early 1980s, it quickly became the instrument of choice owing to its ability to fragment calculi of all compositions. The hollow channel and continuous suction allow debris to be removed at the same time, thereby keeping the operative field free of fragments and clot. Although the ultrasonic device can address all stones, it can be slow and tedious when applied to very hard calculi such as calcium oxalate monohydrate.

Pneumatic devices have also been employed. These instruments use compressed nitrogen gas to drive a piston in the instrument, which subsequently fragments the calculi into increasingly smaller pieces. These pieces must be extracted with a grasper or with an ultrasonic device once the stone has been ablated. Although quite effective for stones of all densities, the time required to remove all the fragments can also be significant and tedious.

More recently, a combination device has been introduced that places a thin pneumatic probe within the central channel of an ultrasonic probe. Early studies from several investigators are promising and demonstrate faster operative times with no increase in complications. Pietrow et al. compared two cohorts of patients, one treated with the combination device and the second with an ultrasonic device alone *(36)*.

The combination instrument was able to treat all stones regardless of composition. Operations were quicker with the new instrument, with all gains coming from reduced fragmentation time. Hofman et al. have reported similar results, noting a decrease in disintegration time of 30–50% when applied to an in vitro model. The device was equally effective in a clinical setting, reducing operative times through the rapid disintegration of the target calculus *(37)*.

COMPLICATIONS

The list of potential complications from PCNL is long and varied. The percutaneous access must traverse multiple tissue layers and planes, including skin, subcutaneous fat, muscle, fascia, perirenal fat, and parenchyma. In addition, difficulties can arise from the location of the access tract, trauma to the renal parenchyma, injury to the collecting system, hemorrhage, fluid shifts or even the physiologic stress of surgery. Rarely, other structures may be abnormally displaced and are at risk of inadvertent damage. An incomplete list includes: colon, small bowel, spleen, liver, gallbladder, and the great vessels.

Transfusion rates generally run in the low single digits, but have been reported as high as 50% in some older series. Hemorrhage can arise from the parenchyma of the kidney, from branches of the renal vasculature or from the torn edges of the urothelium. As mentioned in previous sections, increasing the number of access tracts will increase the need for transfusion. A rare but impressive source of postoperative hemorrhage is from the formation of an arteriovenous fistula along the percutaneous tract (Fig. 4). These patients can present with massive hematuria and usually require embolization (Fig. 5) or even nephrectomy.

Urinary tract infection and sepsis are always a risk during this procedure owing to colonization of the urine and sequestration of bacteria within the calculi. Careful attention to preoperative urine cultures and the liberal use of perioperative antibiotics can minimize the risk of overwhelming infections. Patients with known or suspected struvite calculi should be treated with extra care. Rubenstein et al. have demonstrated that even patients with neurogenic bladders and known urine colonization can be safely treated with this technique *(11)*. These authors have advocated the placement of the nephrostomy access one day before the scheduled procedure to allow time for observation and the early treatment of signs of systemic infection.

Colonic perforation has been reported from multiple authors and sites *(38–40)*. This particular complication is thought to be caused by the presence of a retrorenal colon or caused by the placement of the access tract in too lateral a location. Very thin patients may be at higher risk, as are females and left-sided procedures. Surgeons may not notice the problem until after the case has been completed, because the nephrostomy access

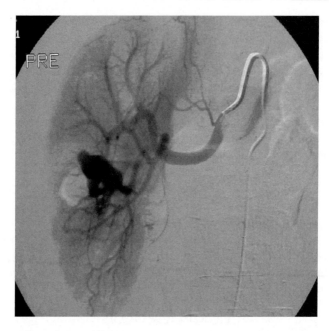

Fig. 4. Angiogram demonstrating a large pseudoaneurysm in the right kidney. This patient presented 2 wk after uneventful PCNL with massive gross hematuria.

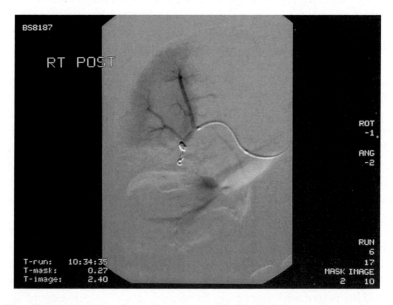

Fig. 5. Same patient after selective embolization of the pseudoaneurysm.

sheath will likely tamponade the defect and "bypass" the injury. Patients may develop significant fevers or abdominal pain in the postoperative period. Feculent material may be visible in the urine, the urine leak may cause watery diarrhea or stool may exude from the nephrostomy tract. Most authors recommend the placement of a ureteral catheter or stent to attempt to divert the urine down towards the bladder and away from the nephrocolonic fistula. In addition, the nephrostomy should be pulled back into the colon to allow the fistula to heal spontaneously. Colon resection is always a distinct possibility but is usually avoided.

Intrathoracic complications can arise from upper pole or supracostal access tracts when the pleura are violated. Pneumothorax, hydrothorax, or hemothorax have been reported. Intraoperative manifestations may include difficulty with mechanical ventilation, poor oxygenation, hypotension or cardiovascular collapse. The fact that the patient is usually in a prone position for this procedure can make recognition and management of a severe intrathoracic complication quite challenging for the anesthesiologist. Most of these patients can be managed with the placement of a draining chest tube, which may be placed intraoperatively if the complication is recognized during the procedure *(41)*. Intraoperative fluoroscopy can be used to diagnose the condition with poor penetration of the ipsilateral lung field or for the correct interpretation of a collapsed lobe.

REFERENCES

1. Fernstrom I, Johansson B. Percutaneous pyelolithotomy. Scand J Urol Nephrol 1976; 10: 257.
2. Castaneda-Zuniga WR, Clayman R, Smith A, Rusnak B, Herrera M, Amplatz K. Nephrostolithotomy: percutaneous techniques for urinary calculus removal. 1982. J Urol 2002; 167(2 Pt 2): 849–853.
3. Dretler SP. Stone fragility—a new therapeutic distinction. J Urol 1988; 139(5): 1124–1127.
4. Zhong P, Preminger GM. Mechanisms of differing stone fragility in extracorporeal shockwave lithotripsy. J Endourol 1994; 8(4): 263–268.
5. Cranidis AI, Karayannis AA, Delakas DS, Livadas CE, Anezinis PE. Cystine stones: the efficacy of percutaneous and shock wave lithotripsy. Urol Int 1996; 56(3): 180–183.
6. Katz G, Lencovsky Z, Pode D, Shapiro A, Caine M. Place of extracorporeal shock-wave lithotripsy (ESWL) in management of cystine calculi. Urology 1990; 36(2): 124–128.
7. Canales B, Monga M. Surgical management of the calyceal diverticulum. Curr Opin Urol 2003; 13(3): 255–260.
8. Schwartz BF, Stoller ML. Percutaneous management of caliceal diverticula. Urol Clin North Am 2000; 27(4): 635–645.
9. Albala DM, Assimos DG, Clayman RV, et al. Lower pole I: a prospective randomized trial of extracorporeal shock wave lithotripsy and percutaneous nephrostolithotomy for lower pole nephrolithiasis-initial results. J Urol 2001; 166(6): 2072–2080.
10. Elbahnasy AM, Clayman RV, Shalhav AL, et al. Lower-pole caliceal stone clearance after shockwave lithotripsy, percutaneous nephrolithotomy, and flexible ureteroscopy: impact of radiographic spatial anatomy. J Endourol 1998; 12(2): 113–119.
11. Rubenstein JN, Gonzalez CM, Blunt LW, Clemens JQ, Nadler RB. Safety and efficacy of percutaneous nephrolithotomy in patients with neurogenic bladder dysfunction. Urology 2004; 63(4): 636–640.
12. Raj GV, Auge BK, Weizer AZ, et al. GM. Percutaneous management of calculi within horseshoe kidneys. J Urol 2003; 170(1): 48–51.
13. McAleer IM, Kaplan GW, Bradley JS, Carroll SF, Griffith DP. Endotoxin content in renal calculi. J Urol 2003; 169(5): 1813, 1814.
14. Segura JW, Preminger GM, Assimos DG, et al. Nephrolithiasis Clinical Guidelines Panel summary report on the management of staghorn calculi. The American Urological Association Nephrolithiasis Clinical Guidelines Panel. 1994; J Urol 151(6): 1648–1651.
15. Meretyk S, Gofrit ON, Gafni O, Pode D, Shapiro A, Verstandig A, Sasson T, Katz G, Landau EH. Complete staghorn calculi: random prospective comparison between extracorporeal shock wave lithotripsy monotherapy and combined with percutaneous nephrostolithotomy. J Urol 1997; 157(3): 780–786.
16. Chandhoke PS. Cost-effectiveness of different treatment options for staghorn calculi. J Urol 1996; 156(5): 1567–1571.
17. Wong C, Leveillee RJ. Single upper-pole percutaneous access for treatment of > or = 5-cm complex branched staghorn calculi: is shockwave lithotripsy necessary? J Endourol 2002; 16(7): 477–481.

18. Lam HS, Lingeman JE, Mosbaugh PG, et al. Evolution of the technique of combination therapy for staghorn calculi: a decreasing role for extracorporeal shock wave lithotripsy. J Urol 1992; 148 (3 Pt 2): 1058–1062.

19. Martin X, Tajra LC, Gelet A, Dawahra M, Konan PG, Dubernard JM. Complete staghorn stones: percutaneous approach using one or multiple percutaneous accesses. J Endourol 1999; 13(5): 367, 368.

20. Delvecchio FC, Preminger GM. Management of residual stones. Urol Clin North Am 2000; 27(2): 347–354.

21. Maheshwari PN, Andankar M, Hegde S, Bansal M. Bilateral single-session percutaneous nephrolithotomy: a feasible and safe treatment. J Endourol 2000; 14(3): 285–287.

22. Silverstein AD, Terranova SA, Auge BK, et al. Bilateral renal calculi: assessment of staged v synchronous percutaneous nephrolithotomy. J Endourol 2004; 18(2): 145–151.

23. Holman E, Salah MA, Toth C. Comparison of 150 simultaneous bilateral and 300 unilateral percutaneous nephrolithotomies. J Endourol 2002; 16(1): 33–36.

24. Dushinski JW, Lingeman JE. Simultaneous bilateral percutaneous nephrolithotomy. J Urol 1997; 158(6): 2065–2068.

25. Gupta R, Kumar A, Kapoor R, Srivastava A, Mandhani A. Prospective evaluation of safety and efficacy of the supracostal approach for percutaneous nephrolithotomy. BJU Int 2002; 90(9): 809–813.

26. Munver R, Delvecchio FC, Newman GE, Preminger GM. Critical analysis of supracostal access for percutaneous renal surgery. J Urol 2001; 166(4): 1242–1246.

27. Martin X, Tajra LC, Gelet A, Dawahra M, Konan PG, Dubernard JM. Complete staghorn stones: percutaneous approach using one or multiple percutaneous accesses. J Endourol 1999; 13(5): 367, 368.

28. Young AT, Hulbert JC, Cardella JF, et al. Percutaneous nephrostolithotomy: application to staghorn calculi. AJR Am J Roentgenol 1985; 145(6): 1265–1269.

29. Pietrow PK, Auge BK, Lallas CD, et al. Pain after percutaneous nephrolithotomy: impact of nephrostomy tube size. J Endourol 2003; 17(6): 411–414.

30. Liatsikos EN, Hom D, Dinlenc CZ, et al. Tail stent versus re-entry tube: a randomized comparison after percutaneous stone extraction. Urology 2002; 59(1): 15–19.

31. Bellman GC, Davidoff R, Candela J, Gerspach J, Kurtz S, Stout L. Tubeless percutaneous renal surgery. J Urol 1997; 157(5): 1578–1582.

32. Limb J, Bellman GC. Tubeless percutaneous renal surgery: review of first 112 patients. Urology 2002; 59(4): 527–531.

33. Noller MW, Baughman SM, Morey AF, Auge BK. Fibrin sealant enables tubeless percutaneous stone surgery. J Urol 2004; 172(1): 166–169.

34. Lee DI, Uribe C, Eichel L, et al. Sealing percutaneous nephrolithotomy tracts with gelatin matrix hemostatic sealant: initial clinical use. J Urol 2004; 171(2 Pt 1): 575–578.

35. Desai MR, Kukreja RA, Desai MM, et al. A prospective randomized comparison of type of nephrostomy drainage following percutaneous nephrostolithotomy: large bore versus small bore versus tubeless. J Urol 2004; 172(2): 565–567.

36. Pietrow PK, Auge BK, Zhong P, Preminger GM. Clinical efficacy of a combination pneumatic and ultrasonic lithotrite. J Urol 2003; 169(4): 1247–1249.

37. Hofmann R, Weber J, Heidenreich A, Varga Z, Olbert P. Experimental studies and first clinical experience with a new Lithoclast and ultrasound combination for lithotripsy. Eur Urol 2002; 42(4): 376–381.

38. LeRoy AJ, Williams HJ Jr, Bender CE, Segura JW, Patterson DE, Benson RC. Colon perforation following percutaneous nephrostomy and renal calculus removal. Radiology 1985; 155(1): 83–85.

39. Wolf JS Jr. Management of intraoperatively diagnosed colonic injury during percutaneous nephrostolithotomy. Tech Urol 1998; 4(3): 160–164.

40. Gerspach JM, Bellman GC, Stoller ML, Fugelso P. Conservative management of colon injury following percutaneous renal surgery. Urology 1997; 49(6): 831–836.

41. Ogan K, Pearle MS. Oops we got in the chest: fluoroscopic chest tube insertion for hydrothorax after percutaneous nephrostolithotomy. Urology 2002; 60(6): 1098, 1099.

32 Percutaneous Nephrolithotomy

Technical Aspects

Sangtae Park, MD, MPH, Maxwell V. Meng, MD, and Marshall L. Stoller, MD

CONTENTS

Key Words: Percutaneous; nephrolithotomy; renal; tract dilation; urological.

INTRODUCTION

In 1976, Fernstrom and Johansson reported the first successful percutaneous nephrolithotomy (PNL) in three patients *(1)*. Since then, advances in the design of nephroscopes and new methods to fragment large calculi have increased the safety and efficacy of this operation. PNL is an integral part of modern urological training *(2)* and is widely performed in both academic and community settings *(3)*. Recently, the American Urology Association (AUA) published its guidelines *(4)* regarding management

From: Current Clinical Urology, *Urinary Stone Disease:*
A Practical Guide to Medical and Surgical Management
Edited by: M. L. Stoller and M. V. Meng © Humana Press Inc., Totowa, NJ

of staghorn stones, and PNL holds a central position in the surgical approach for these cases.

In general, PNL can be considered a four-step operation: percutaneous renal access, tract dilation, stone fragmentation and extraction, and postextraction drainage. Each of the above steps requires meticulous attention to detail, and in cases where one method fails, an alternative maneuver may be required. PNL can thus be technically challenging, with potential for severe complications. In this chapter, we review the technical considerations for successful PNL.

PREOPERATIVE PREPARATION

The patient should be counseled of the potential risks and benefits of PNL, including the risks of injury to adjacent organs (5–7), transfusion (8), renal loss, and sepsis (9). Minor complications have been reported in 11–25% of cases, whereas major complications occur in 1–7% of cases (10). The only absolute contraindication to PNL is uncorrected coagulopathy. Patients should discontinue aspirin and nonsteroidal anti-inflammatory drugs 7–10 d before surgery.

Standard preparation includes a type and screen of the blood and culture-specific antibiotics in those with severe urinary tract infection. Although objective data are scant, prophylactic antibiotics in the form of first generation cephalosporin are given before percutaneous access and continued for 24 h following surgery. Bowel preparation is not routinely performed. Before surgery, the surgical team should ensure equipment availability that is in good working order. Although deep sedation has been used, general endotracheal anesthesia is preferred by most because this allows optimal airway control in the prone patient. Furthermore, in upper pole punctures, breath holds can be performed more precisely, allowing for increased safety.

POSITIONING

Following endotracheal intubation, the patient is placed on the operating table in a prone position. Ipsilateral ureteral catheterization can be performed before or after prone positioning. Most surgeons routinely place an angiographic exchange catheter and only rarely use an ureteral occlusion balloon. Prevention of neuromuscular injury associated with positioning is important and thus the surgeon should take an active role in patient positioning. The endotracheal tube, face, and cervical spine are protected. The shoulder and elbow joints are flexed to angles less than 90° and well-padded. The knees are flexed. Bolsters are placed longitudinally from the shoulder to the iliac crest, preventing undue pressure on the medially positioned breasts and male genitalia. The shoulders, hips, and legs are secured with heavy tape and any hindrance to movement of the fluoroscopy unit should be addressed. The back is prepped and draped. A commonly used drape is the neurosurgical craniotomy set with a fluid collection pouch and clear plastic adhesive at the surgical site. This protects the operating staff and room from the high volume of irrigant required during these procedures. It also helps maintain body temperature as patients frequently lose 2°C while positioning and preparing the patient before the incision.

There have been some reports of performing PNL in the supine (11) or lateral positions. Certainly, the supine position is preferable in the transplant kidney (12) and possibly the lateral position in a morbidly obese patient (13). However, in the overwhelming majority of cases, the prone position is preferred.

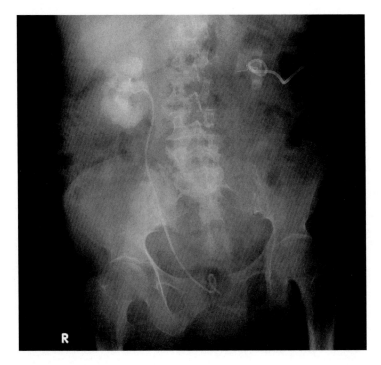

Fig. 1. Severe bilateral nephrolithiasis. This patient required three separate punctures of the right kidney to clear the stone burden.

RENAL ACCESS

The importance of appropriate preoperative imaging cannot be understated when PNL is being considered in a patient with urolithiasis. CT has emerged as the preoperative study of choice owing to its high sensitivity and specificity *(14–16)* (Fig. 1). Although unenhanced CT is traditionally used for urolithiasis, contrast-enhanced CT's can be reformatted to demonstrate the stone and surrounding calyceal anatomy in a fashion similar to intravenous urography (IVU) *(17)*. Renal fusion defects or heterotopia (e.g., horseshoe kidney) *(18)*, perirenal anatomy (e.g., retrorenal colon, severe vertebral deformities) *(19)*, and extrarenal pathology can also be detected, and these may significantly impact the percutaneous surgical approach.

Although many urologists personally obtain renal access in the operating room ("single session" renal access and tract dilation), some prefer to obtain access preoperatively by the radiologist. The advantages of single session access are that it is more convenient for the patient as he or she is asleep during the entire procedure. Also, the urologist can pick the specific calyx and perform multiple punctures at his or her discretion. Furthermore, the urologist is not dependent on another specialty or the availability of the radiologist in scheduling the procedure. Potential disadvantages are that it may require additional training, longer operating room times, increased radiation exposure to the urologist, and technically difficult punctures may be easier to perform using the more versatile, advanced equipment typically found in the radiology suite *(20)*. The ability to choose the specific calyx to puncture is overwhelmingly the most important issue, and therefore, the single session PNL is preferred by the authors.

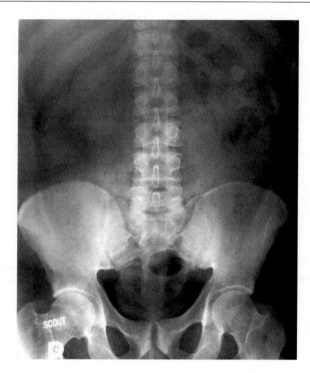

Fig. 2. Left calyceal diverticulum. Direct puncture into the diverticulum, with stone extraction and infundibulotomy performed.

After reviewing the preoperative studies, the surgeon decides on the optimal approach for stone extraction, while keeping in mind the potential limitations and complications of each approach. In general, lower and middle pole punctures are associated with fewer complications and preferred if complete stone eradication is possible via this approach *(21,22)*. Puncture into the fornix or papilla of a posterior calyx is ideally suited to minimize vascular injury and to assure direct access to the renal pelvis and indirect access to an anterior calyx. Infundibular and direct renal pelvis punctures are not recommended because vascular injury is more likely and can occur in up to 70% of cases.

Unless an anterior calyceal diverticular stone is being targeted (Fig. 2), anterior calyces should not be punctured because the majority of stone may be inaccessible using this approach. Furthermore, there is an increased risk of colonic injury and a tendency for severe torquing of the kidney using the rigid nephroscope that can crack the renal parenchyma and lead to increased hemorrhage.

Upper pole puncture is suitable if the majority of stone burden is located superiorly, if lower pole access could not clear all the stones, or if antegrade endopyelotomy is being considered as part of the procedure *(21,23,24)*. Pleural and pulmonary injuries are the main risks of upper pole puncture, but hepatic and splenic complications have been reported, and the surgeon should be cognizant of these potential issues *(10)*. Overall, hydropneumothorax has been reported to range between 9 and 37%, but in only 2–8% were they significant enough to require intervention *(25)*. Although needle aspiration of the hydropneumothorax is sufficient in most cases, larger collections may require tube thoracostomy drainage for 1 or 2 d *(26)*.

Multiple access is a technique to be considered when there is a large stone burden or if there are narrow, angulated infundibuli that cannot be addressed completely using a single access (Fig. 1). In such cases, maximal stone clearance is achieved using the first tract, then subsequent punctures are made targeting residual calcifications. If significant hemorrhage is encountered after the first puncture, the procedure should be concluded with a plan to return for a second stage.

Fluoroscopic Access

Both ultrasound (US) and fluoroscopy have been used to aid in the initial renal puncture, and this choice is dependent on surgeon preference and experience. In the fluoroscopic approach, dilute (1:1) iodinated contrast is instilled in a retrograde fashion through the previously placed externalized ureteral stent. The opacified calyces, stone/s, and their relationship to the overlying ribs allow the surgeon to target the appropriate calyx. Steady infusion pressure on the syringe during retrograde opacification can dilate the system, allowing a larger target for puncture. Overly zealous retrograde instillation can result in contrast extravasation and blur subsequent fluoroscopic images. Some instill dilute methylene blue with the contrast agent to help confirm entry into the collecting system.

On choosing a calyx, an 18-gauge or smaller Chiba needle is introduced under real-time fluoroscopy. Very small needles (<18 gauge) may not advance in a straight trajectory and thus are not routinely used by the authors. For lower pole punctures, a skin incision is made two finger breadths caudal to the 12th rib and two fingerbreadths lateral to the paraspinous border. The C-arm is placed such that the beam is directed in a anterior–posterior fashion. The needle is initially placed over the intended trajectory to the targeted calyx. The approximate angle for needle insertion depth can be approximated by aiming for the contralateral mid axillary line. The needle is then advanced in line with the target, and the depth can be fine tuned by rotating the C-arm towards the surgeon in a more horizontal orientation. If the tip of the needle is underneath the targeted stone then the trajectory should be steeper, and if the tip of the needle is above the targeted stone the trajectory should be more superficial. When all three axes are confirmed, the stylet is removed and the needle aspirated, demonstrating successful puncture. More commonly urine is not successfully aspirated and placing a J-tipped guidewire will confirm entry into the collecting system. In some cases, an air-contrast pyelogram is chosen as opposed to a contrast pyelogram, because air should outline the posterior calyces. Although this is theoretically an attractive method, the authors have found that it is not reliable.

Upper pole renal access on the other hand commonly requires a 12th rib supracostal approach. In this case, the C-arm's X-ray beam is oriented directly anterior–posterior, in line with the targeted upper pole calyx. The puncture site is frequently at the lateral edge of the paraspinous muscle. The skin incision is made, and the Chiba needle is advanced while keeping it exactly in line, parallel to the X-ray beam. The needle can be held with a ring forcep to reduce radiation exposure to the surgeon's hands. The biplanar C-arm is then rotated to a more horizontal orientation to confirm depth of the needle. Calyceal entry may be facilitated by small staccato advancements of the needle through the relatively tougher fasciae, renal capsule, and cortex. Entry is confirmed in a similar fashion to lower calyceal access.

If gross arterial blood or frank pus is expressed, the surgeon should consider placement of a nephrostomy, with a planned staged procedure. If the wire cannot be passed across the ureteropelvic junction (UPJ) even with the help of an angled angiographic catheter, the wire should be coiled in the renal pelvis. Confirmation of entry into the collecting system is a prerequisite to tract dilation.

Sonographic Access

Interventional radiologists commonly use US to insert percutaneous nephrostomy tubes and similarly, many urologists rely on US for the initial needle puncture in PNL *(27)*. A potential downside of using US is that the collecting system may be nondistended. In fact, one of the benefits of retrograde opacification for fluoroscopic-guided renal puncture is that the collecting system can be dilated, making the target larger. Acoustic shadowing from calculi may hinder ultrasonic visualization of the collecting system. Acoustic shadowing also may be due to bowel gas and it is important to differentiate where the acoustic shadows are originating from.

Nevertheless, US is the modality of choice in select populations, such as in pediatric urolithiasis, pregnant patients and those with transplanted kidneys *(28,29)*.

In small children, retrograde ureteral access may be impossible, and US may be the only imaging modality that can be used for initial access. Once sonographically assisted renal access is established, routine fluoroscopy is preferable for tract dilation using antegrade pyelography. In the renal transplant patient, urolithiasis can present as acute anuria, graft tenderness, or recurrent infection *(12,28–31)*. The allograft's superficial location may simplify renal access, yet the severe peri-renal inflammation typically seen in such situations can make the dilation challenging. US is strongly recommended for the initial puncture owing to the potential for overlying bowel.

Although US is attractive because ionizing radiation is avoided, there are several important limitations. US is operator-dependent and although larger intrarenal stones and hydroureteronephrosis are visible, smaller stones and those in the ureter may be missed. Furthermore, US cannot differentiate nephrocalcinosis from nephrolithiasis.

In the sonographic approach, the US probe is first used to explore the entire kidney and the collecting system's orientation. Once the calyx of choice is identified, the probe is fixed while the 18-gauge Chiba needle is advanced. Hyperechoic needle tips can be seen entering the anechoic calyx, and entry can be confirmed with urine visualization after stylet removal or with appropriate guidewire advancement. A coaxial wire is then introduced into the collecting system to secure renal access. Antegrade pyelography opacifies the system to aid in tract dilation.

TRACT DILATION

Once initial wire access has been established, the tract must be dilated to allow placement of a safety wire. A 12-Fr fascial dilator is used to dilate the tract to accommodate a safety wire introducer. Thin 6- or 8-Fr fascial dilators may kink while attempting to advance over the initial guidewire. Some centers insist on always passing the safety wire through the UPJ and coiling it inside the bladder. Others routinely coil the wire inside the renal collecting system, and found that crossing the UPJ is neither mandatory nor advantageous, and needlessly increases radiation exposure.

Once both wires are secured, the working wire is used to dilate the tract. There are a variety of methods available, including balloon dilation *(32)*, Alken telescoping dilators *(33)*, and semirigid Amplatz dilators *(34)*. Balloon dilation has been demonstrated to be quick and safe, but more expensive *(35)*. Facility with alternate means of dilation is prudent, because balloon dilation may be impossible in reoperative cases *(36)*. Another useful adjunct is the fascial incising blade that can be advanced coaxially over the working wire to incise the obstructing fascia (Cook Urological, Spencer, IN), in cases with significant perirenal fibrosis.

Several points of technique are worth mentioning here, to ensure safety and success. First, the vector force used to advance the dilator should be in the same direction as the introduced wires. Second, the radio-opaque tip of the dilator should be advanced just millimeters beyond the tip of the fornix, as deeper advancement can crack the infundibulum resulting in significant hemorrhage. Third, if the working wire does not move easily back and forth a few millimeters while advancing the dilator, the wire may be kinked, and the appropriate vector force may thus be inaccurate and the dilator may not follow the wire into the collecting system. Instead, the dilator may take a "false passage" into perirenal tissues.

After tract dilation, the working Amplatz sheath is advanced into the collecting system. In some institutions, a working sheath is not placed at all, and the rigid nephroscope is placed directly into the collecting system through the dilated tract. Although this closed sheathless system keeps the tract smaller and allows better hydrodistension of the collecting system, concerns for systemic absorption of irrigant and loss of renal access have led the authors to routinely use an Amplatz sheath. Furthermore, in the supracostal approach, inadvertent pleural injury and sheathless PNL may lead to massive hydropneumothorax.

Usually, a 30-Fr Amplatz sheath is used to accept a 26-Fr nephroscope, but there have been reports of successful mini-perc PNL using smaller Amplatz sheaths. In one extreme case, a 13-Fr ureteral access sheath was used *(37)* to decrease the morbidity for the patient. Many surgeons routinely use a 30-Fr sheath without problems. The smaller sheaths are useful in small pediatric patients.

Once the sheath is in place, the fluoroscopic arm should be moved out of the field, the nephroscope prepared, and lithotripsy probe readied. The irrigant of choice at this juncture is normal saline, because systemic absorption of dilute solutions may cause hyponatremia.

STONE FRAGMENTATION AND EXTRACTION

On initial insertion of the rigid nephroscope, vision may be obscured by blood clots in the sheath. They can be removed using suction and intermittent activation of the ultrasonic lithotripter. By following the guidewire in the sheath, the leading edge of the stone is usually found. If the collecting system is difficult to find, most commonly looking at the 12 o'clock position will help locate the collecting system. At this point, retrograde instillation of dilute methylene blue may aid in finding the collecting system. If the stone is less than 1 cm in size, a grasper can be used to remove it through the 30-Fr sheath. However, most stones requiring PNL will be larger than 1cm, and a variety of lithotripsy techniques will be required.

Ultrasonic Lithotripsy

Ultrasonic energy is the most commonly used method for intracorporeal lithotripsy owing to its demonstrated safety and efficacy *(38)*. The piezoelectric effect creates vibrational ultrasonic energy which is transmitted down the shaft of the probe *(39)*. These probes are always rigid, therefore rigid nephroscopy is required and its use is limited to calyces which can only be safely reached without undue torquing of the kidney. Although solid probes are available, hollow ultrasonic probes are preferred because of the ability to suction simultaneously. They range from 3 to 12 Fr in size, with the hollow designs being larger in diameter.

Under direct vision, the surgeon gently presses the tip of the probe against the stone. As the surgeon activates the probe, the assistant or activation pedal modulates the suction, thereby balancing visibility by hydrodistending the system with evacuation of broken fragments. Stone graspers are used intermittently to remove fragments less than 1 cm.

Lithoclast

Another major energy source is the pneumatic lithotrite, or Swiss Lithoclast *(40)*. This device has a generator, hand piece, and foot pedal. When activated, compressed air propels a metal projectile inside the hand piece into the base of the probe. Pressures of up to 3 atm are generated, and this ballistic energy is transmitted along the probe onto the stone. No heat is generated, a potential advantage over ultrasonic energy.

Although this technology required rigid probes in the past, flexible probes are available in modern pneumatic lithotrites. Another advance is the merging of ultrasonic and pneumatic capabilities into a single probe, which may significantly decrease PNL operative times *(41)*.

On rare occasions, ultrasonic lithotripsy will be unable to fragment very hard stones, such as cystine, calcium oxalate monohydrate or brushite stones. More frequently, the ultrasonic lithotripter is out of order, requiring the surgeon to turn to other sources of energy. Furthermore, there is consensus that antegrade pyeloscopy should be performed in every PNL to ensure complete stone clearance. For these reasons, electrohydraulic lithotripsy (EHL) or Holmium:YAG laser *(24)* should be available for use.

Electrohydraulic Lithotripsy and Holmium:YAG laser

EHL probes range from 2 to 10 Fr in size, and a spark is generated between the insulated metal cores of the probe *(42)*. Heat generated by this spark causes fluid vaporization, formation of a cavitation bubble and creation of a hydraulic shock-wave.

The Holmium:YAG laser generates a beam with a wavelength of 2100 nm and pulse duration of 250 μs. This wavelength is highly absorbed by water, thus the laser fiber must be placed directly on the stone. Fibers range in size from 200 to 1000 microns, and the power generated by the machine is controlled by modulating the energy (Joules) and frequency (Hertz) of each pulse.

The benefits of using EHL or Holmium laser are that very hard stones can be broken, and that flexible nephroscopy can be used with these energy sources. However, a significant downside compared to ultrasonic lithotrites is that suctioning cannot be performed simultaneously. However, one recent report used an innovative suctioning device together with the Holmium laser *(43)*.

Flexible Nephroscopy

It is widely accepted that flexible nephroscopy should be performed before concluding PNL because only the most rudimentary collecting systems can be completely inspected with rigid scopes. Certainly, flexible nephroscopy is required during a second look, and EHL or laser fibers will allow fragmentation if residual stones are seen. Smaller fragments may be removed using baskets or flexible graspers.

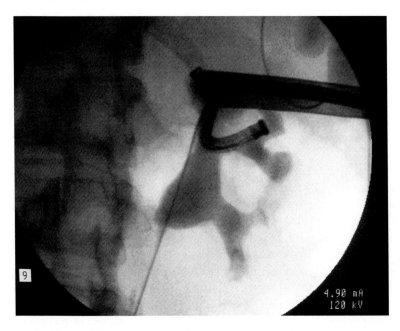

Fig. 3. Intraoperative flexible nephroscopy through a supracostal puncture. Antegrade contrast injection opacifies all the calyces to be examined.

Nephroscopy is performed using a conventional 14-Fr flexible cystoscope. Fluoroscopy will demonstrate suspicious areas of calcification within the renal shadow, and the surgeon should aim to inspect all such areas. Intermittently, contrast is infused through the scope to outline the calyceal anatomy and to convince the surgeon that all calyces have been thoroughly examined (Fig. 3). The proximal ureter should also be examined for residual fragments, and antegrade contrast infused into the ureter should demonstrate free flow into the bladder.

DRAINAGE AFTER PERCUTANEOUS NEPHROLITHOTOMY

Traditionally, a nephrostomy tube is placed at the conclusion of every PNL *(44)*. This allows maximal drainage of the kidney, maintains renal access if second look nephroscopy is required, and tamponades any bleeding points. However, some investigators have tested the feasibility of tubeless PNL in well-selected cases *(45,46)*. Candidates for this approach include patients in whom there is minimal intraoperative bleeding, and patients with a small stone burden and thus requiring minimal manipulation. Nonetheless, the authors routinely use nephrostomy drainage after all PNLs, and therefore drainage options are presented here.

There are myriad choices in nephrostomy drainage, and the final choice is dictated by surgeon experience and discretion. Self-retaining tubes (balloon-Foley, Malecot, Cope loop) are preferred over simple, nonself-retaining tubes such as red rubber Robinson catheters or modified chest tubes because the latter can be easily dislodged. Patient discomfort is greatest with large supracostal nephrostomy drainage tubes. If bleeding is of minimal concern, a 10–12 Fr Cope loop placed through a lower pole puncture will likely be most comfortable.

If second-look nephroscopy is planned for substantial residual stone burden, a nephroureteral catheter is prudent for easy, rapid access *(44,47,48)*. One option is to place a Malecot re-entry catheter, consisting of a Malecot tube with a filiform-like ureteral stent extending from its tip. The Malecot wings are positioned in the renal pelvis whereas the filiform-like ureteral stent traverses the UPJ and rests in the midureter. Another option is to place an antegrade single-J, 7 Fr ureteral stent or a routine 5 Fr angiographic exchange catheter to the bladder. Over these tubes, a 20 Fr Council tip catheter is positioned in the renal pelvis for maximal urinary drainage and secure renal access.

When multiple punctures have been performed, many frequently place a nephroureteral stent across the UPJ and into the bladder for maximal drainage. Alternatively, for the two tracts which have been dilated, an angiographic catheter can be placed from one to the other. Then, two self-retaining nephrostomy tubes can be placed coaxially from either end of this angiographic, creating a U-loop configuration. In cases of significant bleeding postoperatively, the Kaye tamponade nephrostomy *(49)* is an option before pursuing angiographic embolization. Most hemorrhage however can be controlled with clamping the nephrostomy tube/s for a short period postoperatively. Rarely, if bleeding is noted around the clamped tubes angiographic studies should be undertaken.

Twelve to 48 h after the percutaneous procedure, antegrade nephrostograms are typically performed. Complete scout radiographs should be performed to exclude residual stone fragments. Contrast should delineate upper tract anatomy and drain freely into the bladder. Hopefully there are no stones noted and there is free drainage into the bladder. In these situations the nephrostomy may be clamped and removed after a few hours or removed immediately after the study. If there are fragments large enough to be of clinical concern, the surgeon has the option of recommending shock-wave lithotripsy or second-look nephroscopy *(50)*.

Second-look nephroscopy has been performed under sedation, but the authors prefer light general anesthetic owing to airway concerns and the need for patient immobility. Some investigators perform routine postoperative abdominal CT, and this gives them an idea of the size and location of any residual fragments *(50–52)*. Laser lithotripsy and basket extraction is possible using a flexible scope passed through the previously dilated tract.

In this procedure, the patient is positioned in a prone fashion and a safety wire is placed under fluoroscopy. All stents and nephrostomy tubes are then removed, allowing a flexible cystoscope to be passed alongside the wire through a relatively well established tract. In cases of multiple residual fragments or in supracostal punctures, a small Amplatz sheath can be placed into the tract to prevent significant fluid extravasation. If a short second-look is expected in a lower pole puncture, a sheathless approach with a safety wire is sufficient.

COMPLICATIONS OF PERCUTANEOUS NEPHROLITHOTOMY

Bleeding, sepsis, and injury to adjacent structures are the most common and dreaded complications of PNL. Each complication has risk factors associated with it. For example, bleeding may be more likely after multiple punctures or larger stone burdens. Sepsis is more likely if active infection is present; adjacent organs may be injured depending on the percutaneous approach chosen.

Patients should be informed that contemporary published transfusion rates range from 1 to 10% *(8,53)*. Although conservative measures such as bed rest and hydration are the

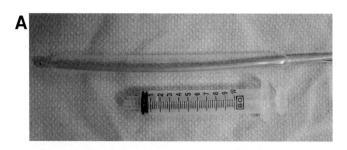

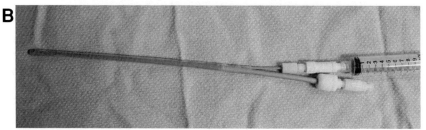

Fig. 4. (A) The Kaye tamponade nephrostomy tube can be inflated for compression of the nephrostomy tract in cases of severe hemorrhage. **(B)** Dual lumen of Kaye tamponade nephrostomy, allowing placement under wire guidance, antegrade nephrostograms, and hemostatic compression of nephrostomy tract.

first line of therapy for hemorrhage, patients should be informed of the possible need for angiographic embolization *(53)* and in extremely rare instances, renal exploration. Open exploration is the therapy of last resort as this typically results in partial or total nephrectomy.

Significant bleeding can manifest intraoperatively or postoperatively. During initial access, common mistakes are poorly targeted punctures or over-advancement of the dilator/s. These maneuvers may injure the infundibulum or cause frank perforation, resulting in excessive bleeding. If significant bleeding persists during lithotripsy, the surgeon should consider aborting the procedure, placing a self-retaining balloon-type nephrostomy, and returning to the operating room another day. If hemorrhage continues, the first step is to clamp the nephrostomy tube and allow the collecting system to tamponade for a few hours. A specially-designed "Kaye" nephrostomy tamponade catheter may be used for more brisk bleeding *(49)* (Fig. 4). More commonly, however, the dilation balloon and working Amplatz sheath tamponade these vessels allowing completion of the procedure. In unusual cases, brisk bleeding can recur at the conclusion of the procedure, once the tamponading effect of the Amplatz sheath is lost. In this situation, bed rest, transfusion and self-retaining clamped nephrostomy drainage typically control the hemorrhage.

Postoperatively, bleeding can occur on removal of nephrostomy tube or several days to months later after patient discharge. Bleeding that occurs at the time of nephrostomy tube removal requires immediate tube re-insertion, and consideration of angiographic embolization. Delayed hemorrhage typically presents as sudden gross hematuria, which requires immediate readmission to the hospital. Initial management consists of conservative measures such as bed rest and transfusion if necessary. Renal angiography is required to rule out a pseudoaneurysm or arteriovenous fistula. If this fails, embolization may be necessary for delayed arterial bleeding or possibly arteriovenous fistula.

Sepsis has been reported in up to 3% of PNL cases *(54,55)*. Sepsis may be minimized by instituting culture-specific antibiotics 1–2 wk before PNL. Perioperative intravenous antibiotics should be continued in those with renal infection, and intra-renal urine should be sent for culture during PNL if the surgeon suspects persistent urinary infection. This is an active area of research, and recent data have shown that intrarenal cultures can differ significantly from routine midstream voided cultures *(56)*. In the postoperative period, blood cultures, broad-spectrum antibiotics, critical care support including vigorous intravenous hydration, and maximal drainage with nephrostomy and/or ureteral stents are paramount if sepsis occurs.

Reported injury to an adjacent organ occurs rarely, between 1 and 4% of cases *(5,7, 26,57–60)*. Intraperitoneal extravasation can occur and may lead to physiologically significant intra-abdominal compression. Paracentesis or exploratory laparotomy may be required. In right sided PNLs, liver injury can occur whereas splenic injury has been reported during left sided PNLs. This can be dramatically reduced by studying preoperative CT scans. Conservative therapy is usually sufficient, although exploration has been reportedly necessary in some cases.

Supracostal puncture is being used more frequently. This has up to a 37% risk of pleural injury, with supra 11th rib approaches being associated with a significantly higher risk. The incidence of hydropneumothorax after PNL was studied by Ogan et al. in 89 consecutive patients *(25)*. In this study, 58% underwent supracostal puncture, and seven patients required intervention for hydropneumothorax. Two cases of hydropneumothorax were discovered during intraoperative chest fluoroscopy, and four by symptoms alone. In their institution, unenhanced abdominal CT was routinely obtained on postoperative day 1, and intervention was instituted in one individual with a significant effusion seen at the lung base. Furthermore, in no case was intervention made on the basis of immediate postoperative chest X-ray if intraoperative fluoroscopic images were negative. The authors concluded that routine postoperative chest radiography was neither necessary nor cost-effective in patients who had routine intraoperative chest fluoroscopy. In general, management is driven by patient evaluation. If the patient is stable, observation alone typically results in spontaneous resolution. Alternatively, one-time aspiration may be adequate whereas in more severe cases, a tube thoracostomy may be required for a few days.

PERCUTANEOUS NEPHROLITHOTOMY IN PATIENTS WITH DYSMORPHIC BODIES

Another common scenario for urologists is the neurologically deficient patient with scoliosis (Fig. 5) or body contractures. In these patients, there may be significant distortions to the bony and skin landmarks usually used for percutaneous access. Therefore, prevention of injury to adjacent solid or hollow viscera becomes an important consideration. Assimos and colleagues published a recent paper demonstrating the utility of CT guided renal access in the radiology suite *(19)*. In their multi-institutional study, six patients underwent successful PNL using this approach for patients with recognized spina bifida and retrorenal colon (Fig. 6).

Once access has been successfully obtained, PNL has been shown to be as effective and as safe *(61,62)* as PNL in patients without spinal cord issues. However, some special precautions are necessary, including the increased risk of infected renal units *(63)* and possibility of autonomic hyperreflexia *(64)*.

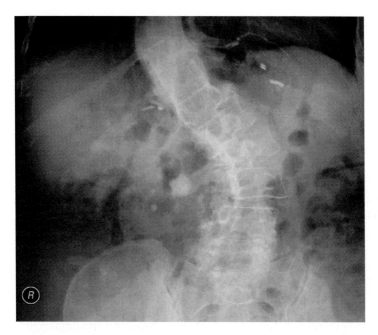

Fig. 5. Right renal nephrolithiasis in a patient with severe lumbar kyphoscoliosis.

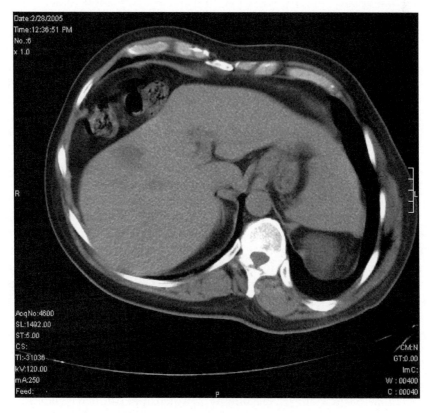

Fig. 6. CT scan of adult patient with myelomeningocele. Note the dysmorphia of the left abdominal cavity and significant pleura overlying the upper pole of the left kidney.

PERCUTANEOUS NEPHROLITHOTOMY
IN THE TRANSPLANTED KIDNEY

Stones in renal allografts or autografts are rare *(30)* but mandate early aggressive treatment because these are solitary renal units *(31)*. Shock-wave lithotripsy has been used for small stones, but the urologist should strongly consider PNL to render the kidney stone-free *(28,29)*. A close working relationship with the transplant nephrologists is wise to monitor immunosuppression and infectious complications in these potentially complex patients.

Percutaneous access to transplanted kidneys is not extremely complex, because of its anterior position *(12)*. The authors favor an US-guided renal access to ensure a tract free of bowel loops *(29)*. Once needle access is obtained, antegrade opacification allows PNL to be completed in the standard fashion *(12)*.

PERCUTANEOUS NEPHROLITHOTOMY
IN THE MORBIDLY OBESE

As morbid obesity becomes more prevalent in the United States, this may have an impact on the incidence of stones. The "metabolic syndrome" of obesity, systolic hypertension and glucose intolerance has recently been linked to urolithiasis *(65)*. In addition, whereas older studies have shown a 3 to 1 male to female predominance, recent updates demonstrate strong trends towards equalization of these rates. Investigators have hypothesized that the increasing obesity rate in women explains this trend.

Thus, urologists are frequently confronted with the difficult scenario of managing a large stone in the significantly obese patient. Shock-wave lithotripsy may be impossible in these cases owing to poor visualization on fluoroscopy, or the stone may be beyond the F_2 focal point *(66)*. Ureteroscopy is an alternative, but complications rise and stone-free rates drop dramatically as stone dimensions increase. PNL may be the most effective means to render the patient stone free, albeit at the cost of higher anxiety for the surgical team. Despite the increased complexity of PNL in the obese, studies have shown no difference in overall success and morbidity compared with nonobese patients *(67–69)*. Indeed, one study stratified PNL outcome by body mass index *(68)*, ranging from <25, 25–30, 30–40, and >40 kg/m^2 and found no differences in outcome. This was not likely to be a result of low statistical power, because success rates were remarkably similar, ranging from 76 to 83%.

Special anesthetic and surgical technical considerations have to be made when planning PNL in the obese. The CT scan should be used to measure the distance from the skin to the stone to determine if longer instruments will be required. Prone positioning can impair ventilation and crush injuries such as rhabdomyolysis have been reported. More than one operating table may be required to support the patient *(68)*, and the surgeon may need to work around poorer fluoroscopic images, inadequately short puncture needles and difficult tract dilation. Others have successfully used the flank position, which may result in less ventilatory compromise *(70)* and movement of the pannus away from the posterior abdominal wall. In the very obese with a very thick pannus, Curtis et al. *(71)* introduced a special method whereby a larger skin incision is made, followed by dissection down to the fascia. Once the fascia is encountered, the puncture needle is introduced at that level to access the kidney. Tract dilation can then be performed in the conventional fashion, but stay sutures should be placed on the outer end of the sheath to prevent it from advancing in the subcutaneous fat.

Manufacturers now offer longer sheaths and nephroscopes for PNL in the obese. Nevertheless, available instrumentation may still be inadequate in super-obese individuals. In such extreme cases, placing a percutaneous nephrostomy may passively dilate the tract allowing flexible nephroscopy at a second stage *(72)*.

CONCLUSIONS

PNL is an important surgical procedure for urologists caring for patients with nephrolithiasis. Successful stone eradication and patient safety are the most important goals, and this begins with proper patient selection, preoperative imaging and a skilled surgeon. It is critical that the surgeon is knowledgeable about various technical options at each step of PNL, and the potential pitfalls of this operation.

When performed on a regular basis, PNL is a versatile operation that can be used for staghorns, calyceal diverticula, transplant urolithiasis, and in special populations such as the obese or elderly.

REFERENCES

1. Fernstrom I, Johansson B. Percutaneous pyelolithotomy. A new extraction technique. Scand J Urol Nephrol 1976; 10: 257.
2. Allen D, O'Brien T, Tiptaft R, et al. Defining the learning curve for percutaneous nephrolithotomy. J Endourol 2005; 19: 279.
3. Hollowell CM, Patel RV, Bales GT, et al. Internet and postal survey of endourologic practice patterns among American urologists. J Urol 2000; 163: 1779.
4. Preminger GM, Assimos DG, Lingeman JE, et al. Chapter 1: AUA guideline on management of staghorn calculi: diagnosis and treatment recommendations. J Urol 2005; 173: 1991.
5. Culkin DJ, Wheeler JS, Jr, Canning JR. Nephro-duodenal fistula: a complication of percutaneous nephrolithotomy. J Urol 1985; 134: 528.
6. Gerspach JM, Bellman GC, Stoller ML, et al. Conservative management of colon injury following percutaneous renal surgery. Urology 1997; 49: 831.
7. Ghai B, Dureja GP, Arvind P. Massive intraabdominal extravasation of fluid: a life threatening complication following percutaneous nephrolithotomy. Int Urol Nephrol 2003; 35: 315.
8. Stoller ML, Wolf JS, Jr, St Lezin MA. Estimated blood loss and transfusion rates associated with percutaneous nephrolithotomy. J Urol 1994; 152: 1977.
9. Cadeddu JA, Chen R, Bishoff J, et al. Clinical significance of fever after percutaneous nephrolithotomy. Urology 1998; 52: 48.
10. Rudnick DM, Stoller ML. Complications of percutaneous nephrostolithotomy. Can J Urol 1999; 6: 872.
11. Ng MT, Sun WH, Cheng CW, et al. Supine position is safe and effective for percutaneous nephrolithotomy. J Endourol 2004; 18: 469.
12. Lu HF, Shekarriz B, Stoller ML. Donor-gifted allograft urolithiasis: early percutaneous management. Urology 2002; 59: 25.
13. Calvert RC, Burgess NA. Urolithiasis and obesity: metabolic and technical considerations. Curr Opin Urol 2005; 15: 113.
14. Smith RC, Rosenfield AT, Choe KA, et al. Acute flank pain: comparison of non-contrast-enhanced CT and intravenous urography. Radiology 1995; 194: 789.
15. Heneghan JP, McGuire KA, Leder RA, et al. Helical CT for nephrolithiasis and ureterolithiasis: comparison of conventional and reduced radiation-dose techniques. Radiology 2003; 229: 575.
16. Amis ES, Jr. Epitaph for the urogram. Radiology 1999; 213: 639.
17. Heneghan JP, Kim DH, Leder RA, et al. Compression CT urography: a comparison with IVU in the opacification of the collecting system and ureters. J Comput Assist Tomogr 2001; 25: 343.
18. Raj GV, Auge BK, Weizer AZ, et al. Percutaneous management of calculi within horseshoe kidneys. J Urol 2003; 170: 48.

19. Matlaga BR, Shah OD, Zagoria RJ, et al. Computerized tomography guided access for percutaneous nephrostolithotomy. J Urol 2003; 170: 45.

20. Bird VG, Fallon B, Winfield HN. Practice patterns in the treatment of large renal stones. J Endourol 2003; 17: 355.

21. Kekre NS, Gopalakrishnan GG, Gupta GG, et al. Supracostal approach in percutaneous nephrolithotomy: experience with 102 cases. J Endourol 2001; 15: 789.

22. Netto NR, Jr, Ikonomidis J, Ikari O, et al. Comparative study of percutaneous access for staghorn calculi. Urology 2005; 65: 659.

23. Ng CS, Herts BR, Streem SB. Percutaneous access to upper pole renal stones: role of prone 3-dimensional computerized tomography in inspiratory and expiratory phases. J Urol 2005; 173: 124.

24. Wong C, Leveillee RJ. Single upper-pole percutaneous access for treatment of greater then or equal to 5-cm complex branched staghorn calculi: is shockwave lithotripsy necessary? J Endourol 2002; 16: 477.

25. Ogan K, Corwin TS, Smith T, et al. Sensitivity of chest fluoroscopy compared with chest CT and chest radiography for diagnosing hydropneumothorax in association with percutaneous nephrostolithotomy. Urology 2003; 62: 988.

26. Munshi CA, Bardeen-Henschel A. Hydropneumothorax after percutaneous nephrolithotomy. Anesth Analg 1985; 64: 840.

27. Osman M, Wendt-Nordahl G, Heger K, et al. Percutaneous nephrolithotomy with ultrasonography-guided renal access: experience from over 300 cases. BJU Int 2005; 96: 875.

28. Challacombe B, Dasgupta P, Tiptaft R et al. Multimodal management of urolithiasis in renal transplantation. BJU Int 2005; 96: 385.

29. Francesca F, Felipetto R, Mosca F, et al. Percutaneous nephrolithotomy of transplanted kidney. J Endourol 2002; 16: 225.

30. Benoit G, Blanchet P, Eschwege P, et al. Occurrence and treatment of kidney graft lithiasis in a series of 1500 patients. Clin Transplant 1996; 10: 176.

31. Fabbian F, Catalano C, Rizzioli E, et al. Acute renal failure due to a calculus obstructing a transplanted kidney. Nephron 2002; 91: 742.

32. Safak M, Gogus C, Soygur T. Nephrostomy tract dilation using a balloon dilator in percutaneous renal surgery: experience with 95 cases and comparison with the fascial dilator system. Urol Int 2003; 71: 382.

33. Alken P. [Percutaneous nephrolithotomy]. Urologe A 1984; 23: 20.

34. Clayman RV, Surya V, Miller RP, et al. Percutaneous nephrolithotomy. An approach to branched and staghorn renal calculi. JAMA 1983; 250: 73.

35. Davidoff R, Bellman GC. Influence of technique of percutaneous tract creation on incidence of renal hemorrhage. J Urol 1997; 157: 1229.

36. Joel AB, Rubenstein JN, Hsieh MH, et al. Failed percutaneous balloon dilation for renal access: incidence and risk factors. Urology 2005; 66: 29.

37. Jackman SV, Docimo SG, Cadeddu JA, et al. The "mini-perc" technique: a less invasive alternative to percutaneous nephrolithotomy. World J Urol 1998; 16: 371.

38. Pietrow PK, Auge BK, Zhong P, et al. Clinical efficacy of a combination pneumatic and ultrasonic lithotrite. J Urol 2003; 169: 1247.

39. Kuo RL, Paterson RF, Siqueira TM, Jr, et al. In vitro assessment of ultrasonic lithotriptors. J Urol 2003; 170: 1101.

40. Kuo RL, Paterson RF, Siqueira TM, Jr, et al. In vitro assessment of lithoclast ultra intracorporeal lithotripter. J Endourol 2004; 18: 153.

41. Olbert P, Weber J, Hegele A, et al. Combining Lithoclast and ultrasound power in one device for percutaneous nephrolithotomy: in vitro results of a novel and highly effective technology. Urology 2003; 61: 55.

42. Miller RA, Payne SR, Wickham JE. Electrohydraulic nephrolithotripsy: a preferable alternative to ultrasound. Br J Urol 1984; 56: 589.

43. Cuellar DC, Averch TD. Holmium laser percutaneous nephrolithotomy using a unique suction device. J Endourol 2004; 18: 780.

44. Kim SC, Tinmouth WW, Kuo RL, et al. Using and choosing a nephrostomy tube after percutaneous nephrolithotomy for large or complex stone disease: a treatment strategy. J Endourol 2005; 19: 348.

45. Gupta NP, Kesarwani P, Goel R, et al. Tubeless percutaneous nephrolithotomy. A comparative study with standard percutaneous nephrolithotomy. Urol Int 2005; 74: 58.

46. Lee DI, Uribe C, Eichel L, et al. Sealing percutaneous nephrolithotomy tracts with gelatin matrix hemostatic sealant: initial clinical use. J Urol 2004; 171: 575.

47. Goel A, Aron M, Gupta NP, et al. Relook percutaneous nephrolithotomy: a simple technique to re-enter the pelvicalyceal system. Urol Int 2003; 71: 143.

48. Marcovich R, Jacobson AI, Singh J, et al. No panacea for drainage after percutaneous nephrolithotomy. J Endourol 2004; 18: 743.

49. Kaye KW, Clayman RV. Tamponade nephrostomy catheter for percutaneous nephrostolithotomy. Urology 1986; 27: 441.

50. Denstedt JD, Clayman RV, Picus DD. Comparison of endoscopic and radiological residual fragment rate following percutaneous nephrolithotripsy. J Urol 1991; 145: 703.

51. Pearle MS, Watamull LM, Mullican MA. Sensitivity of noncontrast helical computerized tomography and plain film radiography compared to flexible nephroscopy for detecting residual fragments after percutaneous nephrostolithotomy. J Urol 1999; 162: 23.

52. Waldmann TB, Lashley DB, Fuchs EF. Unenhanced computerized axial tomography to detect retained calculi after percutaneous ultrasonic lithotripsy. J Urol 1999; 162: 312.

53. Martin X, Murat FJ, Feitosa LC, et al. Severe bleeding after nephrolithotomy: results of hyperselective embolization. Eur Urol 2000; 37: 136.

54. Moskowitz GW, Lee WJ, Pochaczevsky R. Diagnosis and management of complications of percutaneous nephrolithotomy. Crit Rev Diagn Imaging 1989; 29: 1.

55. Gehring H, Nahm W, Zimmermann K, et al. Irrigating fluid absorption during percutaneous nephrolithotripsy. Acta Anaesthesiol Scand 1999; 43: 316.

56. Mariappan P, Smith G, Bariol SV, et al. Stone and pelvic urine culture and sensitivity are better than bladder urine as predictors of urosepsis following percutaneous nephrolithotomy: a prospective clinical study. J Urol 2005; 173: 1610.

57. Green DF, Lytton B, Glickman M. Ureteropelvic junction obstruction after percutaneous nephrolithotripsy. J Urol 1987; 138: 599.

58. Hussain M, Hamid R, Arya M, et al. Management of colonic injury following percutaneous nephrolithotomy. Int J Clin Pract 2003; 57: 549.

59. Miller RA, Kellett MJ, Wickham JE. Air embolism, a new complication of percutaneous nephrolithotomy. What are the implications? J Urol (Paris) 1984; 90: 337.

60. Vallancien G, Capdeville R, Veillon B, et al. Colonic perforation during percutaneous nephrolithotomy. J Urol 1985; 134: 1185.

61. Lawrentschuk N, Pan D, Grills R, et al. Outcome from percutaneous nephrolithotomy in patients with spinal cord injury, using a single-stage dilator for access. BJU Int 96: 379, 2005.

62. Rubenstein JN, Gonzalez CM, Blunt LW, et al. Safety and efficacy of percutaneous nephrolithotomy in patients with neurogenic bladder dysfunction. Urology 2004; 63: 636.

63. Culkin DJ, Wheeler JS, Nemchausky BA, et al. Percutaneous nephrolithotomy: spinal cord injury vs. ambulatory patients. J Am Paraplegia Soc 1990; 13: 4.

64. Chang CP, Chen MT, Chang LS. Autonomic hyperreflexia in spinal cord injury patient during percutaneous nephrolithotomy for renal stone: a case report. J Urol 1991; 146: 1601.

65. Abate N, Chandalia M, Cabo-Chan AV, Jr, et al. The metabolic syndrome and uric acid nephrolithiasis: novel features of renal manifestation of insulin resistance. Kidney Int 2004; 65: 386.

66. Delakas D, Karyotis I, Daskalopoulos G, et al. Independent predictors of failure of shockwave lithotripsy for ureteral stones employing a second-generation lithotripter. J Endourol 2003; 17: 201.

67. Nguyen TA, Belis JA. Endoscopic management of urolithiasis in the morbidly obese patient. J Endourol 1998; 12: 33.

68. Koo BC, Burtt G, Burgess NA. Percutaneous stone surgery in the obese: outcome stratified according to body mass index. BJU Int 2004; 93: 1296.

69. Pearle MS, Nakada SY, Womack JS, et al. Outcomes of contemporary percutaneous nephrostolithotomy in morbidly obese patients. J Urol 1998; 160: 669.

70. Kerbl K, Clayman RV, Chandhoke PS, et al. Percutaneous stone removal with the patient in a flank position. J Urol 1994; 151: 686.

71.   Curtis R, Thorpe AC, Marsh R. Modification of the technique of percutaneous nephrolithotomy
       in the morbidly obese patient. Br J Urol 1997; 79: 138.
72.   Giblin JG, Lossef S, Pahira JJ. A modification of standard percutaneous nephrolithotripsy tech-
       nique for the morbidly obese patient. Urology 1995; 46: 491.

33   Open Stone Surgery

Elizabeth J. Anoia, MD and Martin I. Resnick, MD

CONTENTS

Key Words: Nephrolithiasis; surgery; anatrophic nephrolithotomy; open surgery.

INTRODUCTION

Urinary lithiasis is a disease process that predates the Hippocratic Oath *(1)*. It afflicts males three times more frequently than females with a peak age incidence occurring in the twenties to forties. Most cases of stone disease are not linked to a specific genetic defect and their development is related to multiple external factors, including diet. The main types of stones are composed of calcium, struvite, uric acid, and cystine; the composition of each stone is unique owing to the variety of etiology and patient response to the different therapies available *(2)*. Medical, as well as surgical therapies, are both used as effective forms of treatment. This chapter will focus specifically on the role of open stone surgery in the treatment of patients with urinary lithiasis.

The surgical treatment of urolithiasis has undergone a rapid evolution over the past 25 yr. Before the introduction and refinement of extracorporeal, endourologic, and percutaneous techniques, urinary stones required major open surgical procedures, which had a significant morbidity and potential for renal loss. The advent of these newer less invasive techniques has resulted in a shift in the manner in which all types of stones are managed.

From: Current Clinical Urology, *Urinary Stone Disease:*
A Practical Guide to Medical and Surgical Management
Edited by: M. L. Stoller and M. V. Meng © Humana Press Inc., Totowa, NJ

One open surgical treatment option is termed anatrophic nephrolithotomy. Anatrophic nephrolithotomy is a procedure that has been used by urologists for over 30 yr for the removal of staghorn renal calculi. The original description was by Smith and Boyce in 1968 and was based on the principle of placing the nephrotomy incision through a plane of the kidney that is relatively avascular—between the anterior and posterior segmental arteries. This approach avoids damage to the renal vasculature and subsequent atrophy of the renal parenchyma, hence the term *anatrophic (3)*.

Other types of open stone surgery include radial nephrotomies, pyelolithotomy, extended pyelolithotomy, and ureterolithotomy. Pyelolithotomy refers to the incision of the renal pelvis. Radial nephrotomy describes a procedure in which multiple parenchymal incisions are made over the calculus to effect its removal. A simple pyelolithotomy can be used for partial staghorn stones or multiple 1–2 cm stones that extend into the calyces. An extended pyelolithotomy, also referred to as the Gil-Vernet approach, is indicated for more complex stones that extend into infundibula *(4)*. Ureterolithotomy can be performed throughout the entire length of the ureter when extracorporeal shockwave lithotripsy (SWL) or endoscopic techniques fail. The surgical approach depends on the location of the stone—at the ureteropelvic junction, in the proximal half, or in the distal half.

INDICATIONS FOR OPEN STONE SURGERY

Struvite stones are often associated with urinary tract infections, and the coexistence of these two conditions makes it difficult to eradicate either. Definitive treatment of these stones is generally advocated because of the significant morbidity and mortality associated with untreated infected calculi. Blandy and Singh found that patient survival is reduced with untreated staghorn calculi, with a mortality rate of 28% at 10 yr *(5)*. The American Urologic Association Nephrolithiasis Clinical Guidelines Panel in 1994 recommends a percutaneous procedure with or without SWL as an initial treatment for complex staghorn calculi *(6)*. However, in specific situations anatrophic nephrolithotomy remains the optimal treatment option for renal calculi and thus has maintained an important, albeit smaller, role in the treatment of these large complex stones. Anatrophic nephrolithotomy involves not only removal of the stone but also reconstruction of the intrarenal collecting system to eliminate anatomic obstruction. Thus, this procedure would improve urinary drainage, thereby reducing the likelihood of urinary tract infection, which would prevent recurrent stone formation.

The indications for all open stone surgeries have changed somewhat with advances in minimally invasive methods of treating stones; however, the inability to successfully eradicate a stone with less invasive methods remains an important indication. In 1994, Assimos *(7)* outlined specific anatomic clinical scenarios for open renal or ureteral surgery. Calyceal diverticular stones can be difficult to treat percutaneously when the diverticula are intimately associated with the hilar vessels or have an extrarenal extension. Open surgical pyelolithotomy and pyeloplasty has been recommended in kidneys with stones and a ureteropelvic junction obstruction if there is a large redundant pelvis that necessitates tapering, a high ureteral insertion, a long segment of stricture, if the obstruction is associated with an aberrant lower pole artery, and in patients with solitary kidneys. Patients with other forms of nephroureteral obstruction which require stone treatment in conjunction with anatomic correction are often better served with an open definitive procedure.

Ureteral stones associated with ureterocele, ectopic ureters, obstructing congenital megaureter, or kidney with severe infundibular stenosis are examples that could be treated with a ureterolithotomy (7). Stones in the presence of an ileal conduit present a treatment challenge, especially if there is a Wallace ureterointestinal anastomosis (8). Overall, less than 3% of all upper ureteral stones will require an open procedure. Characteristics more common to this group are moderate to severe hydronephrosis and larger stone size (9).

Emphysematous pyelonephritis associated with stones that have been unsuccessfully treated percutaneously is another indication for an open approach. Ectopic kidneys or pelvic horseshoe kidneys may require an open surgery if the major stone burden is in extremely anterior pelvis that limits adequate shockwave focusing or percutaneous access. A preoperative abdominal angiogram is recommended as the blood supply can vary (7).

Certain stone compositions (calcium oxalate monohydrate and brushite) may not be as effectively treated with SWL therapy, and open procedures may be required if they are refractory after multiple attempts. Impacted stones may also require an open salvage procedure (2,7,9).

Anatrophic nephrolithotomy or other open procedures can also be the first line treatment in patients requiring stone removal but have a body habitus that makes the less invasive procedures difficult to impossible (7,10). The presence of limb contractures, stones in a transplant kidney (11), and obesity often present challenges for positioning and access. These include an inability to reach stones with traditional instruments, the risk of severe tissue necrosis secondary to positioning, and technical issues. SWL can only be performed in patients in whom the stone–skin distance equals the approximate focal length of the specific machine. Percutaneous nephrolithotomy (PCNL) also requires adequate fluoroscopic penetration to visualize the stone.

Despite the need for open surgery, these procedures come with their own set of risks. There can be difficulty in identifying anatomic landmarks and inadvertent incisions have been made above the 10th rib. Other problems are awkward positions for the surgeons, well-vascularized subcutaneous tissue leading to excessive bleeding from skin incisions, intraoperative rhabdomyolysis resulting in temporary renal failure, and wound infection (10).

Other relative indications include select cases of complex stone disease, previous renal surgery, comorbid disease, and patient preference (12,13). Before deciding on a treatment strategy, the above factors, the urologist's preference and access to equipment, and the patient's individual situation must be considered.

If a patient's clinical presentation does not mandate open surgery, other important variables in deciding between open procedures and other less invasive modalities must be considered. Each option has its own advantages, disadvantages, and different stone free rate. Studies have compared the cost and morbidity of percutaneous vs open flank procedures. Percutaneous procedures involved less anesthesia time, less duration of hospitalization, less recuperative time, decreased transfusion requirements, less postoperative need for narcotics, and less total cost without an increased risk for renal parenchymal damage (14,15). However this may not be the case when unsuccessful percutaneous procedures are considered, demonstrating the importance of the learning curve and the stone burden (15). Larger stones require more manipulation, longer procedures, and often multistage approaches.

SURGICAL TECHNIQUE

Incisions

There are several approaches for open stone surgery, depending on the location of the stone and patient and physician preferences previously described: the commonly used flank approach, the posterior approach, and the most invasive transperitoneal approach. The basic surgical principles of stone extraction are similar; the difference lies in how access to the kidney and ureter is obtained. The flank approach may be subcostal or intercostal; this approach provides better access to the renal hilum and the upper pole *(16)*. The posterior approach is an excellent procedure for pyelolithotomy and upper third ureterolithotomy with decreased postoperative pain and shorter hospital stay *(17)*. The transabdominal approach is reserved for patients that are difficult to position or for patients who have undergone multiple previous surgical procedures *(16)*. In any case after the administration of appropriate preoperative intravenous antibiotics and induction of general anesthesia, a Foley catheter is placed in the bladder.

For the flank approach the patient is placed in the standard flank position with elevation of the kidney rest and flexion of the operating table to achieve adequate spacing between the lower costal margin and the iliac crest. Three-inch-wide adhesive tape applied at the shoulders and hips is often used to secure the patient to the table. Adequate padding should be used to protect pressure points. The incision can be placed through the bed of either the 11th or 12th rib, depending on the estimated position of the kidney and the location of the stone, and can be extended as far medially as the lateral border of the rectus sheath. If a previous flank incision has been made for renal surgery, it is preferable to place the incision above the old scar, ensuring that access to the kidney can be achieved through unscarred tissue. After rib identification and resection when access has been gained into the retroperitoneal space, Gerota's fascia is visualized overlying the kidney *(16)*.

The technique for the posterior approach is as follows. The patient is placed in the lateral position with the table flexed to extend the lumbar region. A vertical lumbar incision along the lateral margin of the sacrospinalis muscle is made starting superiorly at the upper margin of the 12th rib extending laterally to the iliac crest inferiorly. The incision is carried down through the lumdodorsal fascia to the sacrospinalis and quadratus lumborum muscles. These are then medially retracted to approach the renal fossa, avoiding the morbidity of a muscle-splitting incision. If greater superior exposure is needed, the 12th rib can be resected or the costovertebral attachment of this rib severed. A selfretaining retractor is then inserted, being careful to avoid injury to the pleura and subcostal vessels. After Gerota's fascia is incised, excellent exposure is gained to the renal pelvis and upper ureter for simple or extended pyelolithotomy or ureterolithotomy *(17)*.

Anatrophic Nephrolithotomy

In the classic description of anatrophic nephrolithotomy *(3)* Gerota's fascia is incised in a cephalad–caudal direction, which facilitates returning the kidney to its fatty pouch at the end of the operation. The kidney is fully mobilized and the perinephric fat is carefully dissected off the renal capsule with care taken not to disrupt the capsule. Should the capsule become inadvertently incised, it can be closed at that time with fine chromic catgut sutures. The kidney is now free to be suspended in the operative field by utilizing

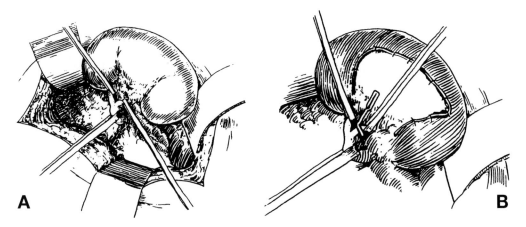

Fig. 1. Anatrophic nephrolithotomy. **(A)** Main renal artery and branches are isolated. **(B)** The posterior segmental artery is occluded, and methylene blue is administered intravenously. The resulting demarcation between pale ischemic and bluish perfused parenchyma defines a relatively avascular nephrotomy plane.

a broad umbilical tape at each pole. At this point a preliminary portable plain radiograph is obtained to identify the position and size of the stone(s).

For the renal hilar dissection, the main renal artery and the posterior segmental branch are approached posteriorly, carefully identified, and dissected (Fig. 1A). The renal pelvis and ureter should be identified, but not dissected. The avascular plane is identified by temporarily clamping the posterior segmental artery and injecting 20 mL of methylene blue intravenously. This results in the blanching of the posterior renal segment while the anterior portion turns blue, allowing identification and marking of the avascular plane (Fig. 1B) *(18)*. Placing the nephrotomy incision through this plane will achieve maximal renal parenchymal preservation and minimize blood loss. The avascular plane can also be identified with the use of a Doppler to localize the area of the kidney with minimal blood flow.

More extensive renal hilar dissection can be avoided by utilizing a modification of the original procedure described by Smith and Boyce. Redman and associates relied on the relatively constant segmental renal vascular supply in the identification of Brodel's line. They advocated placing the incision at the expected location of the avascular plane after clamping the renal pedicle with a Satinsky clamp, in an effort to prevent vasospasm of the renal artery and warm ischemia *(19)*. This modification can be time-saving and spare extensive dissection of the renal hilum.

More recently, McAninch et al. have added another modification to this classic description in an attempt to maximally preserve renal function. In their description the renal capsule is incised over the lateral convex surface of the kidney and a parenchymal incision is made 1–2 cm posterior to the capsulotomy. This location approximates the "avascular plane" and allows access to the collecting system directly over the stone burden. The two potential advantages are avoiding overlying suture lines and ready access to the collecting system *(20)*.

Just before occluding the renal artery, 25 g of intravenous mannitol is administered. This promotes a postischemic diuresis and prevents the formation of intratubular ice

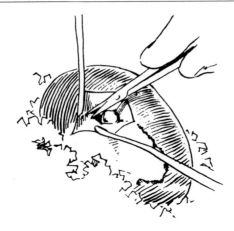

Fig. 2. The collecting system is carefully incised.

crystals by increasing the osmolarity of the glomerular filtrate. The main renal artery is occluded with an atraumatic bulldog vascular clamp. A bowel bag is quickly placed around the kidney, and it is insulated from the body wall and peritoneal contents with dry packs. Hypothermia is then initiated with iced saline slush covering the kidney. The kidney should be cooled for 10–15 min before the nephrotomy incision is made. This should allow achievement of a core renal temperature of 15–20°C, which will allow safe ischemic times from 60 to 75 min and minimizes renal parenchymal damage *(21)*. The ice slush should be continuously reapplied as needed throughout the procedure.

The renal capsule is incised sharply over the previously identified line, being careful to avoid extension into the upper and lower poles. The renal parenchyma is bluntly dissected with the back of the scalpel handle which minimizes injury to the intrarenal arteries that are traversed. Small bleeding vessels can be controlled with 4-0 or 5-0 chromic catgut figure-eight suture ligature. If renal back bleeding continues to be a problem despite these measures, the main renal vein can be occluded.

As the nephrotomy incision proceeds toward the renal hilum, the ideal location to enter the collecting system is at the base of the posterior infundibula. The intraoperative radiograph can be used as a guide to the pelvis and the base of the calyx. Occasionally, with large posterior calyceal calculi, a dilated posterior calyx will be entered initially. The remainder of the collecting system is identified with a probe and opened. If a posterior infundibulum is entered first, the incision is then carried toward the renal pelvis (Fig. 2). The stone is visualized and all ramifications of the stone are exposed by opening adjacent infundibula into the calyces. In order to minimize stone fragmentation and retained calculi, the stone should not be manipulated or removed until all of the calyceal and infundibular extensions are appropriately identified and incised. This allows for complete visualization and mobilization of the collecting system and calculi. Ideally, the stone or stones should be removed without fragmentation; however, often it is inevitable that there will be some piecemeal extraction. If this is necessary, a ureteral stent can be inserted to prevent stone migration down the ureter during manipulation. Each calyx should usually be inspected for stone fragments. After removal of all stone fragments, the renal pelvis and calyces are copiously irrigated with cold saline and the irrigant is aspirated. A nephroscope can be used to look for residual fragments. A

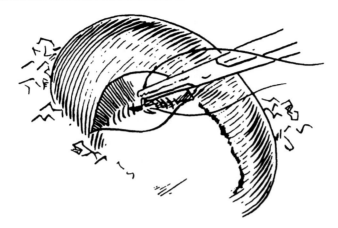

Fig. 3. The renal pelvis is closed with a running 6-0 chromic suture.

plain radiograph or ultrasonography are also options. At this time, a "double-J" ureteral stent is passed from the renal pelvis into the bladder if this was not done at the time of stone manipulation. The routine use of internal ureteral catheters is encouraged. They provide good urinary drainage, protect the freshly reconstructed collecting system, and minimize postoperative urinary extravasation.

The next step in the procedure is the reconstruction of the intrarenal collecting system with correction of coexistent anatomic abnormalities that may be present. Infundibular stenosis or stricture, which results in obstruction promoting urinary stasis and recurrent stone formation, should be corrected with caliorrhaphy or calicoplasty. All intrarenal reconstructive suturing is accomplished with 5-0 or 6-0 chromic catgut sutures. When suturing the mucosal edges, it is important to avoid incorporation of underlying interlobular arteries, thus preventing ischemia. The renal pelvis is then closed, first with reinforcing corner sutures and then with a running 6-0 chromic catgut suture (Fig. 3). Before closing the renal capsule bleeding points are identified and ligated with 4-0 or 5-0 chromic figure-eight sutures. The renal capsule is closed with a running lock stitch of 4-0 chromic catgut suture or mattress sutures over bolsters can be used.

McAninch et al. have also created a modification involving renal reconstruction after nephrolithotomy. Traditionally, the infundibula are reconstructed and the collecting system is formally closed. The modification simplifies this closure by not reconstructing the infundibula; instead, the capsular and parenchymal staggered incisions are closed with nonoverlapping suture lines forming a watertight renal closure. When postoperative renal function results are compared there is a slight decrease in renal function in McAninch's series; however, overall findings are comparable to Smith and Boyce *(20)*.

After the capsule is closed and adequate hemostasis has been achieved, the renal artery is unclamped and the kidney is observed for good hemostasis and return of pink color and turgor. It is then returned into Gerota's fascia, and the kidney and proximal ureter are covered with some perirenal fat to minimize postoperative scar formation. If Gerota's fascia is unavailable because of previous surgery, omentum can be mobilized through a peritoneal opening and wrapped around these structures. The peritoneal opening should be sutured to the omentum to prevent herniation of the abdominal viscera.

A Penrose or suction-type drain is placed within Gerota's fascia and brought out through a separate stab incision. This drain is left in place until minimal drainage occurs, usually by the third or fourth postoperative day. Nephrostomy tubes are generally avoided because of their potential for causing infection or further renal damage. The flank musculature and skin are closed in the standard fashion.

Pyelolithotomy

A pyelolithotomy also begins with mobilization of the kidney after Gerota's fascia is incised. The degree of mobilization is dependent on the size of the stone. If a smaller, more centrally located renal pelvis stone is anticipated, it is not necessary to dissect the renal artery. The renal pelvis and upper ureter are identified and the pelvis is approached posteriorly to avoid injury to the renal vein. Two stay sutures are placed in the renal pelvis using 4-0 chromic suture and a longitudinal incision made. Care must be taken to avoid extension into the ureteropelvic junction so as to reduce the risk of subsequent scarring and the development of ureteropelvic junction obstruction. After the successful removal of all stones, the renal pelvis is closed with a 4-0 chromic continuous suture. Drainage of the system is performed as described previously *(16)*.

Extended Pyelolithotomy

In an extended pyelolithotomy described by Gil-Vernet *(4)*, the dissection is more extensive. The thin layer of connective tissue that extends from the renal capsule onto the renal pelvis must be carefully incised in order to gain access to the renal hilum and infundibula. The dissection is carried subparenchymally to expose the renal pelvis and the infundibula. A curvilinear pyelotomy incision is made over the stone and then extended to the superior and inferior calyces. The stone is freed from the mucosa and removed. Once one is confident that all fragments have been removed with the aid of radiographs and nephroscopy, the collecting system is closed with a continuous 4-0 chromic catgut suture as described above. The infundibular incisions will be covered by the renal parenchyma; therefore it is not necessary to completely close them *(22)*. Drainage of the flank is again performed.

Ureterolithotomy

Ureterolithotomy can be performed via multiple approaches. The flank or posterior lumbotomy incision can be used for the upper ureter, an anterior extraperitoneal muscle-splitting incision can adequately expose the mid-ureter, and the lower ureter can be accessed via a Gibson, Pfannenstiel, or midline suprapubic incision *(8)*. Once the approach is decided, radiographs are obtained to confirm stone position. For an upper ureterolithotomy Gerota's fascia is opened and the upper ureter is identified. A Babcock forceps or vessel loop is placed on the ureter above the stone for traction and to prevent stone migration. Dissection is carried downward to provide adequate exposure, being careful not to devascularize the ureter or injure the muscularis layer. A vertical ureterotomy is made over the stone without injuring the posterior ureteral wall. After careful stone extraction the entire ureter is irrigated and a double J stent may be placed. The incision is closed longitudinally with simple interrupted 5-0 sutures placed 1–2 mm apart. A Penrose or suction drain is used to drain the area of the ureterotomy. The principles of stone extraction remain the same in a distal ureterolithotomy; however, exposure of the ureter requires certain other maneuvers. Identifying the iliac vessels and dividing the obliterated umbilical vessels can help. The bladder is reflected medially and kept decompressed with a Foley catheter *(8,23)*.

Postoperative Management

Postoperative management after anatrophic nephrolithotomy, pyelolithotomy, or ureterolithotomy should follow the same principles that guide management after other major operations. Intravenous fluids are maintained to achieve brisk urine output and until the patient is able to tolerate a clear liquid diet. Broad-spectrum intravenous antibiotics are administered perioperatively and continued postoperatively for 5–7 d. Antibiotic coverage is guided by preoperative urine culture and sensitivity findings. The ureteral stent is removed cystoscopically at approx 7 d postoperatively in uncomplicated cases. A urine culture is checked for persistence of infection. At 1–2 mo a follow-up intravenous pyelogram is obtained.

RESULTS

Stone free rates with staghorn calculi show that 21% of percutaneous procedures required additional procedures to clear the stone burden. In contrast only 4% of patients required further intervention after anatrophic nephrolithotomy. Residual stone disease leading to multiple procedures is one of the significant drawbacks of PCNL *(14)*. Less than 10 yr after its development SWL monotherapy was found to have a 61% stone-free rate at 8 mo of follow-up *(24)*. PCNL or PCNL–SWL sandwich therapy stone free rates were reported as 54–95% depending on stone volume and collecting system dilatation *(7)*. Endoscopic therapy of renal and ureteral stones with the Holmium:YAG laser is reported to have an overall stone free rate of 95% when combined with other types of lithotripsy *(25)*. Overall, anatrophic nephrolithotomy stone free rates range from 80–100% depending on collecting system dilatation and stone burden *(12,26)*.

Open pyelolithotomy has a stone-free rate that approaches 100% if there is a single stone. However if a staghorn stone is present or if there are multiple calyceal stones, the stone-free rate decreases to approx 90% *(16)*. A retrospective study by Paik et al. in 1998 reported an initial stone free rate of 93% in patients with large renal pelvic stones undergoing simple or extended pyelolithotomy *(13)*.

In 1997, the American Urologic Association published a meta-analysis on the currently available methods for treating ureteral calculi. Stone free rates for ureterolithotomy vary from 84–100% depending on stone size and location *(9,27)*. SWL had a 57% stone-free rate with one-third of patients requiring second procedures. Endoscopic procedures were more successful with an initial stone-free rate of 74% and a final clearance rate of 95% after additional procedures *(9)*. Overall, the goals of open stone surgery should be to remove all calculi and fragments, to improve urinary drainage of any obstructed intrarenal collecting system, to eradicate infection, to preserve and improve renal function, and to prevent stone recurrence *(28)*.

As open stone surgery accounts for <5% of treatment modalities for staghorn and other complex stones, there are now other less invasive techniques either alone or in combination that have replaced these procedures. Despite impressive advances with the less invasive techniques, anatrophic nephrolithotomy, pyelolithotomy, or ureterolithotomy remain viable treatment options for large or staghorn calculi not expected to be eliminated with a reasonable number of less invasive procedures. Staghorn stones associated with anatomic abnormalities also require open surgical correction.

COMPLICATIONS

Complications resulting from open stone surgery are similar to other forms of open surgery, for example wound infections and postoperative fevers. Pulmonary complications are common including atelectasis, pneumothorax, and pulmonary embolism. Patients with a history of pulmonary disease should likely undergo preoperative evaluation with pulmonary function testing and initiation of vigorous pulmonary toilet before surgery. Postoperatively, patients should be encouraged to breathe deeply, and use of an incentive spirometer should be routine to prevent atelectasis. Early ambulation will also be beneficial.

Pneumothorax should occur in fewer than 5% of patients *(28)*. A patient with a history of pyelonephritis or previous renal surgery is at increased risk. Inadvertent opening of the pleura, usually during incision and resection of a rib, should be identified and repaired intraoperatively with a running chromic catgut suture. The lung is hyperinflated just before the final suture is placed to ensure re-expansion of the lung. Chest tubes are not routinely used but may be necessary if any question remains regarding the reliability of the pleural closure. A chest radiograph should be obtained in the recovery room for any patient who undergoes repair of a pleural defect. Pulmonary embolism remains a potential complication of any major surgery. Routine use of support hose and sequential-compression stockings can lower the risk of deep venous thrombosis. Encouragement of early ambulation is also an important preventive measure.

Significant postoperative renal hemorrhage after anatrophic nephrolithotomy should occur in fewer than 10% of patients. Assimos and associates reported an incidence of 6.4%. Bleeding usually occurs immediately or approx 1 wk postoperatively. Extensive intrarenal reconstruction, older age, impaired renal function, and presence of blood dyscrasias were found to be significant risk factors. Slow bleeding will usually resolve on its own; management includes correction of any bleeding abnormalities and replacement with blood products as necessary. Oral aminocaproic acid can be successful in certain cases. Bleeding that is brisk or cannot be adequately treated conservatively will require a more aggressive approach. A renal arteriogram can help identify the lesion, and an attempt at arteriographic embolization should be considered. Re-exploration may be required in the remainder of the cases, with reinstitution of hypothermia and suture ligation of the bleeding vessel(s). Persistent hematuria 1–4 wk postoperatively should alert the clinician to the possibility of renal arteriovenous fistula formation or a false aneurysm *(29)*. Other possible complications that can result from arterial clamping include renal injury and hypertension.

Urinary extravasation with any procedure should occur infrequently with the routine use of perinephric drains and ureteral catheter drainage. Should drainage recur or persist following removal of the drain and/or ureteral stent, replacement of the ureteral stent should be considered to decompress the system and relieve any obstruction. Flank abscess as a result of extravasation is an unusual complication that can usually be managed conservatively with percutaneous drainage or may require open drainage *(15)*.

Open ureterolithotomy has a complication rate ranging from 17–34% via the posterior lumbotomy and flank approaches, respectively *(9)*. A few complications that are unique to this procedure include loss of the stone intraoperatively, fistulas, and strictures *(8)*. Preoperative localization and immobilization of the stone can decrease the risk of stone loss. Fistulas, although uncommon, can occur with ureteral damage or infection. In 1993 a ureterofallopian fistula, manifesting as complete urinary incontinence, occurred after open surgery for a distal calculus *(30)*. Ureteral stricture formation can occur with calculus disease after any form of manipulation. This complication has decreased from 5% to less than 1% with refinement of technology. Risk factors that have been associated with strictures are ureteral perforation, incomplete stone removal, and impaction greater than 2 mo *(31)*.

CONCLUSIONS

When performed for appropriate indications and with meticulous technique, open stone surgery can achieve successful removal of all calculi, preservation of renal function, improved urinary drainage, and eradication of infection. Stone-free rates greater than 90% should be achieved. Stone recurrence rates following anatrophic nephrolithotomy have been reported from 5% to 30% *(28)*. Recurrent calculi usually form in those with persistent urinary tract infections, persistent urinary drainage impairment, and those with previously unidentified or refractory metabolic disturbances *(32)*.

We believe that for large or complex staghorn calculi, especially those associated with some anatomic abnormality leading to impaired urinary drainage, open stone surgery remains an important treatment option. This modality achieves comparable or better stone-free rates and the achievement of a stone-free state with a single operative procedure. In the long term, treatment of these complex calculi with anatrophic nephrolithotomy, pyelolithotomy, or ureterolithotomy should preserve renal function in the involved kidney and, in a majority of patients, eradicate stone disease and chronic urinary tract infection.

REFERENCES

1. Clendening, L. Source Book of Medical History. Dove Publications, New York, NY, 1942.
2. Van Arsdalen KN, Banner MP, Pollack HM. Radiographic imaging and urologic decision making in the management of renal and ureteral calculi. Urol Clin North Am 1990; 17(1): 171.
3. Smith MJV, Boyce, W.H.: Anatrophic nephrotomy and plastic calyrhaphy. J Urol 1968; 99: 521.
4. Gil-Vernet JM. New surgical concepts in removing renal calculi. Urol Int 1965; 20: 255.
5. Blandy JP, Singh M. The case for a more aggressive approach to staghorn stones. J Urol 1976; 115: 505.
6. Segura JW, Preminger GM, Assimos DG, et al. Nephrolithiasis Clinical Guidelines Panel summary report on the management of staghorn calculi. J Urol 1994; 151: 1648.
7. Assimos DG. Should one perform open surgery in 1994? Semin Urol 1994; 12: 26.
8. Cohen JD, Persky L. Ureteral stones. Urol Clin North Am 1983; 10(4): 699.
9. Liong ML, Clayman RV, Gittes RF, Lingeman JE, Huffman JL, Lyon ES. Treatment options for proximal ureteral urolithiasis: Review and recommendations. J Urol 1989; 141: 504.
10. Hofmann R, Stoller ML. Endoscopic and open stone surgery in morbidly obese patients. J Urol 1992; 148: 1108.
11. Caldwell TC, Burns JR. Current operative management of urinary calculi after renal transplantation. J Urol 1988; 140: 1360.
12. Paik ML, Resnick MI. Is there a role for open stone surgery? Urol Clin North Am 2000; 27(2): 323.
13. Paik ML, Wainstein MA, Spirnak JP, Hampel N, Resnick MI. Current indications for open stone surgery in the treatment of renal and ureteral calculi. J Urol 1998; 159: 374.
14. Snyder JA, Smith AD. Staghorn calculi: percutaneous extraction vs anatrophic nephrolithotomy. J Urol 1986; 136: 351.
15. Brown MW, Carson III CC, Dunnick NR, Weinerth JL. Comparison of the costs and morbidity of percutaneous and open flank procedures. J Urol 1986; 135: 1150.
16. Fitzpatrick JM. Pyelolithotomy. In: Glenn's Urologic Surgery, (Graham SD, Jr, Glenn JF, eds.). Lippincott-Raven, Philadelphia, PA, 1998, pp. 155–161.

17. Novick AC. Posterior surgical approach to the kidney and ureter. J Urol 1980; 124: 192.
18. Myers RP. Brodel's line. Surg Gynecol Obstet 1971; 132: 424.
19. Redman JF, Bissada NK, Harper DL. Anatrophic nephrolithotomy: experience with a simplification of the Smith and Boyce technique. J Urol 1979; 122: 595.
20. Morey AF, Nitahara KS, McAninch JW. Modified anatrophic nephrolithotomy for management of staghorn calculi: Is renal function preserved? J Urol 1999; 162: 670.
21. McDougal WS. Renal perfusion/reperfusion injuries. J Urol 1988; 140:1325.
22. Spirnak JP, Resnick MI. Pyelolithotomy. In: Stewart's Operative Urology, (Novick AC, Streem SB, Pontes JE, eds.). Williams & Wilkins, Baltimore, MD, 1989, pp. 184–190.
23. Hodge EE. Operations on the Ureter. In: Stewart's Operative Urology, (Novick AC, Streem SB, Pontes JE, eds.). Williams & Wilkins, Baltimore, MD, 1989, pp. 368–380.
24. Winfield HN, Clayman RV, Chaussy CG, Weyman PJ, Fuchs GJ, Lupu AN. Monotherapy of staghorn renal calculi: a comparative study between percutaneous nephrolithotomy and extracorporeal shock wave lithotripsy. J Urol 1988; 139: 895.
25. Razvi HA, Dendstedt JD, Chun SS, Sales JL. Intracorporeal lithotripsy with the holmium:YAG laser. J Urol 1996; 156: 912.
26. Assimos DG, Wrenn JJ, Harrison LH, et al. A comparison of anatrophic nephrolithotomy and percutaneous nephrolithotomy with and without extracorporeal shock wave lithotripsy for management of patients with staghorn calculi. J Urol 1991; 145: 710.
27. Segura JW, Preminger GM, Assimos DG, et al. Ureteral Stones Clinical Guidelines Panel summary report on the management of ureteral calculi. J Urol 1997; 158: 1915.
28. Spirnak JP, Resnick MI. Anatrophic nephrolithotomy. Urol Clin North Am 1983; 10(4): 665.
29. Assimos DG, Boyce WH, Harrison LH, Hall JA, McCullough DL. Postoperative anatrophic nephrolithotomy bleeding. J Urol 1986; 135: 1153.
30. Braslis KG, Stephens DA. Uretero-fallopian fistula: An unusual complication of open ureterolithotomy. J Urol 1993; 150: 1900.
31. Roberts WM, Cadeddu JA, Micali S, Kavoussi LR, Moore RG. Ureteral stricture formation after removal of impacted calculi. J Urol 1998; 159: 723.
32. Russell JM, Harrison LH, Boyce WH. Recurrent urolithiasis following anatrophic nephrolithotomy. J Urol 1981; 125: 471.

34 Laparoscopic Approach to Urinary Stone Disease

Anup P. Ramani MD *and Inderbir S. Gill* MD, MCH

Contents

Key Words: Laparoscopy; calculus; kidney; ureter

INTRODUCTION

Minimally invasive antegrade and retrograde techniques combined with extracorporeal shockwave lithotripsy (SWL) have virtually eliminated open surgery for stone disease. Success rates for treating renal calculi with the above combination approach 100%. The availability of finer instruments with better optical resolution has made the endourological approach the standard of care today. Nevertheless, there exists a category of stones that fail endourologic therapy and thus are candidates for open surgical intervention.

The advantages of laparoscopy over open surgery have been described before and include reduced operative time, blood loss, hospital stay, morbidity, and faster return to activities of daily living. Laparoscopy has been successfully applied to the management of almost every aspect of urinary tract disease and can be equally efficacious in patients failing endourologic therapy or in whom endourologic therapy is contraindicated because of size or location characteristics of the stone. The spectrum of options with the laparoscopic approach varies with the stone size, location, and status of the contralateral kidney and includes laparoscopic pyelolithotomy with or without pyeloplasty, laparoscopic ure-

From: Current Clinical Urology, *Urinary Stone Disease:*
A Practical Guide to Medical and Surgical Management
Edited by: M. L. Stoller and M. V. Meng © Humana Press Inc., Totowa, NJ

terolithotomy, laparoscopic anatrophic nephrolithotomy, laparoscopic calyceal diverticular repair, and laparoscopic ureterocalycostomy. All steps of open surgery are duplicated with strict adherence to principles of stone surgery.

PATIENT EVALUATION

Laboratory Studies

Recurrence rates for renal stones vary from 50% to 100%. Given this high probability of subsequent stone formation, it is plausible to argue that all patients with renal stone should undergo a complete evaluation. Metabolic work-up forms an important part of the evaluation. Certainly, men between the ages of 20 and 50, patients with a strong family history, nephrocalcinosis, and gout deserve a through metabolic work-up before treatment can be initiated. Typical strategies to evaluate stone formers are well documented in literature and are beyond the scope of this chapter *(1)*.

Imaging Studies

Radiographic evaluation of the patient has to be tailored to provide accurate information on size and location of calculi and the degree of renal functional and morphologic impairment. Other causes of urinary obstruction, such as tumor, intraluminal blood clot, sloughed papillae, or infected aggregates must always be considered in the differential diagnosis.

The standard radiographic evaluation revolves around the plain radiograph, the intravenous urogram, computerized tomographic scan, and the ultrasound evaluation. The plain film of the abdomen or kidneys, ureter, bladder (KUB) is usually the first investigation in many scenarios. Most but not all calcifications are visible in the plain film. These however also show non renal calcifications, which may cloud the issue. Typical examples include gallstones, calcified mesenteric lymph nodes, phleboliths, and other artifacts. About 90% of calculi greater than 2 or 3 mm can be picked up on the plain film. Intravenous urography is a standard and well accepted investigation to document urinary obstruction and renal function in patients with renal lithiasis. Sonography is quick, cost effective, and can demonstrate renal parenchymal and collecting system pathology without injecting contrast. Indeed in patients with acute abdominal pain, sonography is invaluable as an initial investigation to rule out a majority of other abdominal causes. Noncontrast helical or spiral CT today is the most innovative and cost effective investigation for a renal colic. With a sensitivity and specificity of over 97% it easily outperforms other modalities of investigation *(1)*.

As such a combination of these tests as well as other tests are routinely employed in evaluating a patient. Investigations are tailored to each individual depending on stone characteristics.

LAPAROSCOPIC PYELOLITHOTOMY

Introduction

Pyelolithotomy is occasionally necessary in patients with pelvic and renal calculi who fail ESWL and percutaneous nephrolithotomy (PCNL) or have a complex stone. About 4–6% patients with renal stones fall into this category. Laparoscopic pyelolithotomy combines the advantages of open surgery with the minimally invasive nature of laparoscopy. Laparoscopic pyelolithotomy can be performed by either the transperitoneal or the retroperitoneal route. In addition, concurrent pyeloplasty can be performed at the same time if needed.

Gaur et al. reported the first laparoscopic pyelolithotomy in 1994, a series of eight patients with a 62.5% stone clearance *(2)*. Literature is scant about long term results of laparoscopic pyelolithotomy given the fact that only a small percentage of patients require a formal pyelolithotomy in the era of SWL and PCNL. However the success of laparoscopy with other pathologies of the urinary tract points to favorable outcomes in this category of patients.

Transperitoneal Laparoscopic Pyelolithotomy

PATIENT POSITION

After general anesthesia, the patient is placed in the 45–60 ° flank position. Extreme care is taken with padding and positioning. The table is flexed somewhat, an axillary roll placed and the patient is secured to the table with 6-in cloth tape and safety belt.

PORT PLACEMENT

Peritoneal access is gained using a Veress needle. The abdomen is insufflated with carbon dioxide to a pressure of 25 mmHg. The first port (10 mm) is placed mid way between the umbilicus and the anterior superior iliac spine, at the level of the umbilicus. The second port (5 mm) is placed at the angle between the costal margin and the lateral border of the ipsilateral rectus muscle. The third port (10 or 12 mm) is placed between these two ports, closer to the upper port than the lower one, so as to allow a direct vision of the renal hilum. This port, which houses the 30 ° laparoscope, may alternatively be placed in the umbilicus.

IDENTIFICATION OF THE PELVIS

Mobilization of the colon is performed by incising along the line of Toldt, up to the liver on the right and the splenic ligaments on the left. This allows the colon, spleen, and pancreas to be reflected away from the left kidney. On either the left or the right side, the anterior surface of Gerota's fascia is visualized by reflecting the mesocolon in an avascular plane. The psoas muscle is an important landmark, which guides the laparoscopic surgeon's orientation and must always be visualized horizontally at the base of the field. As such the psoas muscle must be identified between the ureter and gonadal vein (lateral) and the ipsilateral great vessel (medial). The ureter is now identified above the psoas muscle and dissected up to it's insertion in the renal pelvis. The renal pelvis is dissected free from adjacent tissues so that the anterior and the posterior aspects of the pelvis are exposed. A U-shaped pyelotomy is created on the pelvic wall and the pelvis opened. The stone is identified and gently grasped with a laparoscopic grasper and delivered out. The stone is placed in an endo-catch bag and positioned aside for later removal. After confirming complete removal of the stone, the pelvic defect is sutured with interrupted Vicryl 3-0 sutures. All sutures are free hand. Placement of a double-J stent is only necessary in patients with an unsatisfactory closure of the pelvis or severe pelvic wall edema. A Jackson-Pratt drain is inserted with its tip away from the anastomotic site. The endo-catch bag is delivered out from one of the port sites. The port site incision may be enlarged if necessary to facilitate delivery of the stone. Once the procedure is complete, laparoscopic exit is performed. The port sites are closed with the help of a Carter Thomasson needle and skin approximated with subcuticular sutures.

Perioperative antibiotics are administered for 24 h after surgery. Analgesics are administered as required. The patient is usually discharged within 24 h. The Jackson-Pratt drain is removed after drainage reduces to less than 60 mL/d.

Patients with a coexisting ureteropelvic junction obstruction (primary or secondary), may also undergo concomitant laparoscopic pyeloplasty. One of the advantages of laparoscopic pyeloplasty over antegrade and retrograde endourologic techniques is that it can address anatomical nuances like high inserting ureter, crossing vessel, and redundant pelvis at the same time. Laparoscopic pyeloplasty entails mobilization of the pelvis and the upper ureter, excision of the pathologic segment of the pelvis and the ureter, spatulation of the ureter laterally, free hand suture of the ureter to the pelvis with two continuous 3-0 monocryl sutures on a CT-1 needle, over a double-J stent.

Retroperitoneal Technique

Port Placement

Our standard three-port retroperitoneal laparoscopic access is achieved. A 1-cm incision is made at the tip of the 12th rib in the midaxillary line. The incision is deepened up to the dorsolumbar fascia. An incision is made in the dorsolumbar fascia and a finger inserted into the retroperitoneal space. This is confirmed by palpating the psoas muscle and the lower pole of the kidney. A balloon dilator is introduced into the retroperitoneal space and the balloon inflated 50 mL. The balloon is now hitched up against the abdominal wall and inflated an additional 700 mL. This maneuver pushes the peritoneum forward and out of the operative field. The balloon is removed and replaced by a 10- or 12-mm port. The retroperitoneum is now inspected and correct access confirmed. Insufflation is initiated at 25 mmHg. The second port (5 mm) is placed at the angle of the 12th rib and the paraspinal muscles. The third port (5 mm) is placed in the anterior axillary line, three fingerbreadths above the anterior superior iliac spine.

Mobilization of the Kidney

The initial step is to identify the ureter below the lower pole of the kidney as it lies above the psoas. The ureter is then dissected cephalad, leaving a good amount of periureteral tissue, till the ureteropelvic junction is reached. The peripelvic fat and the Gerota's fascia are opened and the pelvis exposed. The pelvis is completely freed and pyelolithotomy is carried out in the above fashion.

Results of Laparoscopic Pyelolithotomy

Jordan et al. in 1997, reported an operative time of 2.5 h (3). Blood loss was 5 mL. Patients were discharged within 24 h. Ramakumar et al. reported a combination of laparoscopic pyelolithotomy and pyeloplasty with a mean operating time of 4.6 h, blood loss of 145 mL (4). Mean hospital stay was 3.4 d and patients returned to activity by 3 wk. They had no intraoperative complications.

LAPAROSCOPIC URETEROLITHOTOMY

Introduction

As for pelvic calculi, the advent of endourological techniques and SWL has almost eliminated the need for open surgery in patients with ureteral calculi. Success rates of ureteroscopy for lower and middle third ureteral calculi approach 100%. Success rates of percutaneous surgery and SWL for upper third calculi are similar. Open or laparoscopic ureterolithotomy is still however indicated in patients with large, long-standing and hard ureteral calculi, particularly those that cross into the pelvis. As mentioned before, the laparoscopic option has significant advantages over open surgery.

The first laparoscopic retroperitoneal ureterolithotomy was described by Wickham in 1979 and popularized by Gaur in the 1990s (5–7). The first transperitoneal laparoscopic ureterolithotomy was performed by Raboy et al. in 1992 (8). Success rates of 88–100% have been quoted in literature. With the retroperitoneal route, the risk of visceral injury is lower, abdominal adhesions from previous surgeries do not interfere with the surgery and there is no need to mobilize the colon. At the author's institution, the retroperitoneal route is preferred.

Technique

Patient position, access via the transperitoneal or the retroperitoneal route and initial mobilization are performed in the standard fashion as described before. In the transperitoneal approach, once the colon has been mobilized, the ureter is identified above the psoas muscle. The segment of the ureter with the stone is approached and freed of the overlying fat. Careful dissection is necessary at this juncture to avoid stripping the ureter of its investing layers for a long segment. This jeopardizes ureteral vascular supply.

The stone, if not immediately apparent, can be localized by sounding the ureter with the tip of a grasper. Once the stone is localized, the ureter over the stone is incised in a linear fashion for adequate length. The stone is carefully freed from its attachments to the ureteral mucosa and delivered out. A double-J stent is then inserted over a guide wire, which has been passed down the ureter from one of the ports. After the stent is in position, the ureteral defect is closed with interrupted 3-0 vicryl or monocryl sutures. The sutures are just tight enough to approximate the edges of the defect without undue tension. Hemostasis is confirmed. A Jackson-Pratt drain is usually not necessary if the suture line is satisfactory, however it can be left in place if there is any doubt about the integrity of the anastomosis. The stent can be removed between 4 and 6 wk after surgery. Laparoscopic exit is performed in the standard fashion.

Result

Harewood et al. in their experience of nine patients reported a mean patient age of 55.5 yr, mean stone size of 13.2 mm (5). The mean operative time was 158 min. One patient developed a postoperative urine leak. The mean hospital stay was 5.2 d. Feyaerts et al. reported a series of 24 patients who underwent laparoscopic ureterolithotomy (6). The mean operating time was 140 min. There was no intraoperative complication and no blood transfusions were required. Mean hospital stay was 3.8 d. All patients were followed up with intravenous pyelogram and demonstrated success at 6-mo intervals.

LAPAROSCOPIC MANAGEMENT OF CALYCEAL DIVERTICULAR CALCULI

Introduction

A calyceal diverticulum is a cystic intrarenal cavity lined by nonsecretory urothelium that communicates with the collecting system via a narrow neck and is typically located at a calyceal fornix or infundibulum. Although usually asymptomatic, they are prone to urinary stasis and stone formation. Although over the last decade, shockwave lithotripsy, ureterorenoscopy, and percutaneous endoscopic techniques have been highly successful in treating this entity, laparoscopy has emerged as an attractive treatment option for caliceal diverticular stones. Apart from stone extraction, laparoscopy allows plastic repair of the caliceal diverticulum to prevent a caliceal fistula.

Technique

Laparoscopic Access

With the patient in the dorsal lithotomy position a 6 Fr open-ended ureteral catheter is inserted into the renal pelvis via cystoscopy and secured to a 16 Fr urethral catheter. The patient is then placed in the standard flank position with the kidney rest elevated and the table flexed. Our standard three-port retroperitoneoscopic approach is used as previously described.

Stone Localization and Extraction

Gerota's fascia is incised to identify and mobilize the kidney. Complete examination of the kidney surface is then done via laparoscopy. If the diverticulum is not immediately apparent, indigo carmine dye may be injected through the ureteral catheter. This discolors the thin parenchyma over the diverticulum. Alternatively, either intraoperative fluoroscopy or intraoperative ultrasonography with a laparoscopic, flexible, color Doppler probe may be used to localize the stone. Using electrosurgical scissors or J-hook electrocautery a longitudinal nephrotomy incision is made perpendicular through the thinnest area of the parenchyma over the stone or along the avascular plane of Brodel's line at the posterior lateral aspect of the convex surface of the kidney. The calculus or calculi are gently extracted using endoscopic graspers. They are then immediately entrapped in an endoscopy bag and the area is then copiously irrigated with 2–3 L of antibiotic solution. The diverticulum is inspected to rule out residual stone or a tumor.

Definitive Management of Calyceal Diverticulum

Indigo carmine is now injected through the ureteral catheter to identify the site of communication with the pelvicalyceal system or the diverticular neck. This site is then either fulgurated if small or sutured using interrupted figure-eight sutures with 3-0 polyglactin on a CT-1 needle. Repeat injection of indigo carmine dye is performed to ensure closure of the fistula. The rest of the diverticular epithelium is then fulgurated using the argon beam or the J-hook. Adjacent perirenal fat is mobilized to fill the defect in the parenchyma. Gerota's fascia is re-approximated with interrupted sutures. A Jackson-Pratt drain is positioned outside the Gerota's fascia, exiting the anterior port. The stone is extracted in the endoscopy bag through the 12-mm port site. The patient is then repositioned in the dorsal lithotomy position and the ureteral catheter exchanged for a double-J stent. A urethral Foley catheter is then placed.

Results

Miller et al. reported a series of five patients who underwent laparoscopic extraction of calyceal diverticular calculi *(9)*. The mean age was 47.4 yr, mean operative time was 133.8 min and the mean blood loss was less than 50 mL. Average hospital stay was 36.4 h. There were no intraoperative complications.

LAPAROSCOPIC URETEROCALICOSTOMY

Introduction

Ureterocalicostomy is a reconstructive option in the rare patient with a failed, difficult ureteropelvic junction obstruction secondary to stones and an intrarenal pelvis. Laparoscopy is a viable option for the surgical management of this entity. Gill et al. reported the first laparoscopic ureterocalycostomy in 2004 *(10)*.

Technique

Under general anesthesia, a 4.7-Fr, 26-cm J-stent is cystoscopically inserted into the ipsilateral renal pelvis. With the patient positioned in a 45–60° flank position, a three- or four-port transperitoneal approach is employed as described previously. Colon is reflected medially and the renal hilar vessels are mobilized en bloc for possible Satinsky clamping subsequently. The kidney is mobilized within Gerota's fascia, and the thinned lower pole parenchyma is exposed. The ureter with adequate periureteral tissue is dissected cephalad towards the renal pelvis. A circular rim of the tip of the lower pole renal parenchyma is excised using J-hook electrocautery exposing the dilated lower calyx. The calculi are immediately collected in an endoscopic bag and the area flushed with an antibiotic (gentamycin) solution.

Laparoscopic ultrasonography is performed to rule out any residual calculi. The ureteropelvic junction is now transected and the pelvis is suture ligated. The ureter is spatulated laterally taking care to preserve the J-stent. End-to-end ureterocalyceal anastomosis is performed in a mucosa-to-mucosa fashion using two hemi-circular running sutures (3-0 vicryl on RB-1 needle). Free-hand intracorporeal suturing and knot-tying techniques are employed. At this point, intravenous indigo carmine dye is injected to confirm a watertight repair. A Jackson-Pratt drain is inserted and laparoscopic exit performed.

LAPAROSCOPIC ANATROPHIC NEPHROLITHOTOMY

Introduction

Anatrophic nephrolithotomy was first described by Boyce and Smith, who used renal anatomic and physiologic principles and reconstructive surgical techniques to perform this surgery. The procedure involves incising the renal parenchyma along an avascular plane to remove a large, complex renal stone. Open surgical anatrophic nephrolithotomy provides 91–94% stone free rates. Because the advent of minimally invasive techniques, anatrophic nephrolithotomy is today reserved for a small group of patients with complex staghorn renal calculi.

The American Urological Association's guideline panel has laid down the current indications for this surgery *(11)*. These include struvite staghorn calculi not expected to be removed by a reasonable number of percutaneous lithotripsy and/or ESWL. These patients usually have a large stone load as well as complex collecting systems. Another group of patients considered candidates for anatrophic nephrolithotomy are obese individuals (600 lb or greater) with staghorn calculi, as in these patients access may be difficult or impossible.

With increasing experience, laparoscopy is today being applied to almost every urological pathology at many centers in the world. Certainly, the advantages of laparoscopy over open surgery are well documented in literature. Laparoscopic anatrophic nephrolithotomy provides all the advantages of minimally invasive surgery coupled with the success rates of open surgery.

Anatrophic nephrolithotomy is contraindicated in patients with uncorrected coagulopathy and sepsis. Severe chronic renal insufficiency is a relative contraindication.

Technique

LAPAROSCOPIC ACCESS

After general anesthesia, patient is placed in the flank position and secured to the operating table. A four-port transperitoneal approach is employed.

RENAL HILUM CONTROL

The kidney is mobilized circumferentially, and the renal hilum is dissected so as to allow optimal application of a Satinsky clamp. After adequate hydration, 12.5 g of manitol and 10 mg of Lasix are administered intravenously. En-bloc clamping of the renal artery and vein is achieved using a laparoscopic Satinsky clamp.

LATERAL INCISION OF RENAL PARENCHYMA AND COLLECTING SYSTEM

Intraoperative laparoscopic ultrasonography may be used to identify the site of thinnest parenchyma along the lateral border of the kidney. Doppler signal can be used to locate further an avascular plane through the thinned parenchyma. The incision is carried deep into the renal calyces.

STONE EXTRACTION

The staghorn calculus is fragmented using either a mechanical or an ultrasonic lithotriptor. The stone fragments are extracted and retrieved within a 10-mm endo-catch bag. Laparoscopic ultrasonography is repeated or flexible endoscopy of the calyceal system and upper ureter is performed to identify and retrieve any residual stones to achieve complete stone clearance.

INTRACORPOREAL WATERTIGHT SUTURE-REPAIR OF THE INCISED COLLECTING SYSTEM AND RENAL PARENCHYMA

The collecting system is continuously sutured (No. 2.0 polygalactic acid-absorbable suture on a GS-21 needle) in a watertight manner. In a second layer, the renal parenchyma is reconstructed using interrupted sutures (No. 1 polygalactic acid absorbable suture on a GS-25 needle) placed in a hemostatic fashion.

A nephrostomy tube is positioned to drain the kidney only if there is any doubt about the integrity of the anastomosis. Usually, a double-J stent is considered enough to secure adequate renal drainage for 4–6 wk post surgery. An abdominal drain is kept for 24–48 h depending on the drainage.

Results

Kaouk et al. described the first laparoscopic anatrophic nephrolithotomy in 2003 *(12)*. This was performed based on studies in a porcine model *(13)*. After injection of polyurethane into the renal pelvis to simulate a complete staghorn calculus, laparoscopic anatrophic nephrolithotomy was performed. The mean warm ischemia time was 30 min with complete "stone" removal in 70% of animals. Nuclear renal scans documented an improvement in glomerular filtration rate after relief of obstruction and stone removal. To date, the clinical experience in humans remains limited *(14)*.

CONCLUSION

The laparoscopic approach to renal and ureteral calculi represents an effective and minimally invasive modality to manage these calculi. It allows for correction of any underlying anatomical abnormality thus reducing risk for recurrent stone formation. Appropriate patient selection is however of paramount importance. With experience, laparoscopy can be applied to the management of most renal and ureteral calculi, which fail or are unsuitable for endourologic and shockwave management. As more centers overcome the learning curve, laparoscopy will be widely available for managing appropriate renal calculi in the near future.

REFERENCES

1. Begun FP, Foley WD, Peterson A, White B. Patient evaluation: Laboratory and imaging studies. Urol Clin North Am 1997; 1: 97–115.
2. Gaur DD, Agarwal DK, Purohit KC, Darshane AS. Retroperitoneal laparoscopic pyelolithotomy. J Urol 1994; 151: 927.
3. Jordan GH, McCammon KA, Robey EL. Laparoscopic pyelolithotomy. Urology 1994; 49: 131–134.
4. Ramakumar S, Lancini V, Chan DY, Parsons JK, Kavoussi LR, Jarrett TW. Laparoscopic pyeloplasty with concomitant pyelolithotomy. J Urol 2002; 167: 1378–1380.
5. Harewood LM, Pope AJ. Laparoscopic ureterolithotomy: the results of an initial series, and evaluation of it's role in the management of ureteric calculi. Br J Urol 1994; 74: 170–176.
6. Feyaerts A, Rietbergen J, Navarra S, Vallancien G, Guillonneau B. Laparoscopic ureterolithotomy for ureteral calculi. J Urol 2001; 40: 609–613.
7. Wickham JEA. The surgery of renal lithiasis. In: Urinary Calculus Disease. Churchill Livingstone, Edinburgh, 1979: 145–198.
8. Raboy A, Ferzli GS, Ioffreda R, Albert PS. Laparoscopic ureterolithotomy. Urology 1992; 39: 223–225.
9. Miller SD, Ng CS, Streem SB, Gill IS. Laparoscopic management of caliceal diverticular calculi. J Urol 2002; 167: 1248–1252.
10. Gill IS, Cherullo EE, Steinberg AP, Desai MM, Abreu SC, Ng C, Kaouk JH. Laparoscopic ureterocalicostomy: initial experience. J Urol 2004; 171: 1227–1230.
11. Assimos DG. Anatrophic nephrolithotomy. Urology 2001; 57: 161–165.
12. Kaouk JH, Gill IS, Desai MM, et al. Laparoscopic anatrophic nephrolithotomy. J Urol 2003; 169: 691–696.
13. Kaouk JH, Banks KL, Desai MM, et al. Laparoscopic anatrophic nephrolithotomy. J Urol 2001; 165(2): 376, abstract 1542.
14. Deger S, Tuellmann M, Schoenberger B, et al. Laparoscopic anatrophic nephrolithotomy. Scand J Urol Nephrol 2004; 38: 263.

35

Stones of the Urethra, Prostate, Seminal Vesicle, Bladder, and Encrusted Foreign Bodies

Bradley F. Schwartz, DO, FACS

Contents

Key Words: Calculus; bladder stone; encrustation; foreign body.

INTRODUCTION

Renal and ureteral calculi comprise the majority of genitourinary calcifications encountered clinically. Significant morbidity, however, may occur from less common urologic calculi. Although treatment of most stones remains uncomplicated, etiology and prevention prove elusive. Mandel hypothesized that most if not all extraosseous calcifications in the body arise from a nidus of carbonate apatite *(1)*. If this is true, inhibition of the initial crystallization may help prevent formation of most genitourinary stones. Hopefully, future research and investigation will help us understand and eventually direct nonsurgical treatment of these calculi. This chapter discusses the etiology, symptoms, diagnosis, treatment, and prevention of stones found in the urethra, prostate, seminal vesicle, and bladder. The management and prevention of encrusted foreign bodies is also presented.

From: Current Clinical Urology, *Urinary Stone Disease:*
A Practical Guide to Medical and Surgical Management
Edited by: M. L. Stoller and M. V. Meng © Humana Press Inc., Totowa, NJ

URETHRAL CALCULI

Etiology

Most urethral calculi originate in the kidney or urinary bladder *(2–4)*. A review of 271 urethral calculi demonstrates a clear male predominance (253 to 18) with the majority occurring in the posterior urethra *(2–15)*. Koga *(2)* treated 56 patients with urethral calculi and found a 32% incidence of simultaneous renal and ureteral calculi. A similar study from the Sudan reported 33% of their 36 patients suffered from upper tract calculi *(15)*, both studies emphasizing the importance of upper urinary tract evaluation in patients with urethral calculi. The normal diameter of the adult human urethra of 30 Fr should allow stones ≤10 mm to pass spontaneously, but stone configuration, previous surgery, or radiation therapy, and anatomical abnormalities such as diverticulae and strictures may prevent such passage.

Stones that do not originate in the urethra are usually composed of calcium. Paulk *(3)* reported on 47 patients referred to the Mayo Clinic with urethral stones, 21 of whom had stone analysis performed. Twenty of 21 (95%) were calcium based and one was struvite. In contrast, a study from Turkey published the authors' results on 60 children with urethral stones *(5)*. Stone analysis was available on only 12 patients, and all of them were struvite. Those studies reporting urine culture results found that 68% of isolates were urease-splitting organisms *(3,7)*. Calcium oxalate, calcium phosphate, and uric acid urethral stones have been associated with the use of the hypercholesterolemia agent cholestyramine *(6)*. In general, stones found in Western societies that originate in the upper urinary tract are noninfectious, calcium-based calculi, and those encountered in non-Western cultures developing in abnormal urinary tracts are usually ammonium acid urate or struvite.

The pediatric patient often presents a different set of etiological circumstances. Hypospadias, cloacal and bladder exstrophy, bladder neck reconstruction procedures, and posterior urethral valves predispose this population to urethral calculi formation *(5,7–9)*. A detailed history should be sought in these patients.

Symptoms

Patients with urethral calculi may present with a wide range of symptoms (Table 1). Virtually all patients with urethral calculi have pain with or without lower urinary tract symptoms (LUTS). Urinary retention, especially in children, is a common presentation, and urethral calculi should be suspected when a history of lower urinary tract surgery is elicited. A palpable mass along the course of the urethra warrants a high index of suspicion, as does a perineal cutaneous fistula, and should prompt either radiographic or cystoscopic evaluation.

Diagnosis

A thorough history should be obtained and a genitourinary physical examination should be performed. Because most primary urethral stones form in an abnormal urethra, either from obstruction or stasis, information regarding previous surgery or the presence of lower urinary tract symptoms such as urinary urgency, intermittency, dysuria, decreased force of stream, or incontinence should be sought. Although some urethral calculi are diagnosed serendipitously by radiographic studies, the single best diagnostic modality remains urethroscopy. Endoscopic evaluation of the lower urinary

Table 1
Symptoms of 271 Patients
Presenting With Urethral Calculi [a]

Symptoms	Number of patients
Pain	167
Lower urinary tract symptoms	104
Urinary retention	92
Palpable mass	60
Hematuria	26
Incontinence	22
Fistula	10
Bilharziasis	7
Urinary tract infection	5
Urethralgia	2

[a] Some patients had more than one symptom, comorbidity and treatment. Also, some articles did not provide complete information. As a result, not all categories add up to 271.
Data from References 2–15.

Table 2
Comorbid Conditions of 271 Patients
Presenting With Urethral Calculi [a]

Comorbid conditions	Number of patients
Urethral stricture	55
Prostatectomy	26
Recurrent urinary tract infection	20
Prostatism	20
Other surgery	11
Diverticulum	10
Neurogenic bladder	10
Phimosis	6
Posterior urethral valves	4
Trauma	4
Renal colic	4
Exstrophy/hypospadias	2

[a] Some patients had more than one symptom, comorbidity and treatment. Also, some articles did not provide complete information. As a result, not all categories add up to 271.
Adapted from References 2–15.

tract will also enable the urologist to identify other comorbid conditions that may impact the treatment (Table 2). A retrograde urethrogram may be helpful before endoscopy to provide anatomic detail of the urethra and help plan potential surgical procedures. Urethral stricture disease, previous surgery, urinary tract infection, prostatism, and diverticulae are the most commonly associated conditions found on radiographs and endoscopy.

Table 3
Treatment of 271 Patients Presenting With Urethral Calculi [a]

Treatment	Number of patients
Push into bladder and treat	105
Internal urethrotomy and stone extraction	51
Endoscopic *in situ*	41
Meatotomy	27
Open removal with repair of underlying disease	17
Open removal	17
Spontaneous passage	7
Lost to follow-up	4
Extracorporeal shockwave lithotomy	1

[a] Some patients had more than one symptom, comorbidity and treatment. Also, some articles did not provide complete information. As a result, not all categories add up to 271.

Adapted from References *2–15*.

Treatment

Treatment of urethral stones depends on the location and cause of the stone and may range from spontaneous passage to lithotomy with repair of the underlying pathology (Table 3). In the male, proximal stones are usually pushed into the bladder and treated by conventional modalities such as laser or ultrasonic lithotripsy *(2,3)*. Middle and distal urethral stones are typically endoscopically extracted, sometimes with the aid of a meatotomy *(3)*. Stones trapped at the fossa navicularis can be extracted using a safe and rapid technique that requires only local anesthesia and basic surgical instruments *(16)*.

Stones found within a urethral diverticulum, whether male or female, require surgical excision with diverticulectomy and stone extraction. Similarly, urethral stricture disease may be managed with urethrotomy or open repair when encountered. Pathologic investigation for occult malignancy should be obtained.

The tools available for endoscopic treatment are similar to those used in other parts of the urinary tract. Laser, electrohydraulic, pneumatic, ultrasonic, extracorporeal shockwave, and manual lithotripsy can be used to treat urethral stones. Which modality is used depends on the technology available, preference and experience of the surgeon, cost considerations, and anesthetic availability. There have been no studies directly comparing various modalities to declare a clear benefit of one over another in the management of urethral calculi.

Prevention

Prevention of urethral calculi is aimed at treatment of the underlying disease. If the stone is believed to arise from the upper urinary tract, a metabolic evaluation including serum calcium and uric acid levels and a 24-hr urine collection should be performed. Appropriate dietary counseling and medical therapy are provided based on these results. Because urinary infection is a common finding, culture selective antibiotics should be used when infection is diagnosed. Aggressive treatment of prostatism and urethral stricture disease is recommended. The aim of treatment for these diseases is to reduce postvoid residual urine volumes, enhance bladder emptying, and reduce the risk of infection.

Finally, routine surveillance and appropriate intervention of known upper tract stones may prevent future episodes of "urethral colic."

PROSTATIC CALCULI

Etiology

Although the clinical manifestations of primary prostatic calculi are different from bladder calculi, their pathogenesis may provide insight to lithogenesis in the urinary tract. Historically, their pathogenesis is attributed to obstruction of the prostatic ducts, formation of corpora amylacea, and accumulation of debris. This debris binds to the calcium present in high concentrations in prostatic secretions forming stones that may grow *(17)*. Many investigators have found that prostatic secretions have a high calcium concentration but concurrently high citrate levels bind the calcium making it unavailable to precipitate mimicking the situation in the kidney and bladder *(18,19)*. Multiple studies have shown that prostatic calculi are composed almost exclusively of hydroxyapatite *(18–20)*. Fox determined the incidence of prostatic calculi to be 14% based on 3510 abdominal radiographs *(17)* although histopathological studies indicate a 70% prevalence *(21)*.

The relationship of bacteria to prostatic calculi has been postulated by Meares *(24)*. He reported on three men with prostatism, who were found to have prostatic calculi and persistent positive urine cultures. Open prostatectomy in two and transurethral resection in one were curative of their symptoms and sterilized their urine. Finally, Sonergaard and colleagues evaluated 300 prostates obtained from autopsy *(25)*. They found 99% of the glands contained stones. Also, the stones increased in size and number with age suggesting their formation is a normal part of the aging process.

Symptoms

Prostatic calculi are rarely symptomatic and are usually diagnosed during prostatic ultrasonography performed during prostate biopsy or pelvic computed tomography performed for unrelated complaints. If the stones are related to bacterial growth, symptoms such as urgency, frequency, intermittency, and dysuria are likely to be present. Chronic pelvic pain and perineal discomfort may be related to prostate stones but a definite relationship has not been established.

Diagnosis

The vast majority of prostatic calculi are discovered incidentally during transrectal ultrasonography or computed abdominal tomography performed for unrelated complaints. Transrectal ultrasonography can also be used intraoperatively to guide transurethral resection of the offending calculi. Digital rectal examination can occasionally suggest the presence of large peripheral stones. The relationship between serum prostate specific antigen and prostatic calculi has not been established. It should be stressed that the diagnosis of prostatic calculi does not warrant treatment. If it is determined that lower urinary tract symptoms are originating from infected prostatic calculi attempts at removal should be undertaken.

Treatment

Most prostatic calculi require no treatment. Occasionally men with lower urinary tract symptoms or chronic infection may require definitive treatment. Mears performed open perineal and retropubic prostatectomy and transurethral resection in three patients with infectious stones. We have employed ultrasound-assisted transurethral prostatectomy in two patients with pelvic pain syndrome and large prostatic calculi (unpublished data). Directed resection resulted in an improvement in symptoms in both men. Because there are inadequate reports in the literature to make unequivocal treatment recommendations regarding prostatic calculi, patient treatment should be individualized and routine culture, cancer, and outlet obstruction investigation should be performed.

Prevention

Because of the infrequent occurrence of symptomatic prostatic calculi, significant efforts at prevention have not been undertaken. Further investigation of prostatic calculi may help elucidate the origin of other nonosseous stones. At this time there are no recognized preventative measures.

SEMINAL VESICLE CALCULI

Calculi of the seminal vesicle, ejaculatory duct, and vas deferens are uncommon and rarely of clinical significance. Since 1965, the English literature has produced eight case reports of clinically significant seminal vesicle stones *(26–33)*. The etiology, symptoms, diagnosis, and treatment can be seen in Table 4. Figures 1 and 2 demonstrate an ejaculatory duct stone managed endoscopically. These stones occur so infrequently it is difficult to make recommendations on their clinical management. Sound urologic principles of relieving obstruction, eradicating infection, and providing unimpeded urinary drainage will usually prove successful in their treatment.

Recent advances in and increased use of lower genitourinary tract imaging have identified calculi in the prostate, seminal vesicles, and ejaculatory ducts with increasing frequency. Kuligowska performed transrectal ultrasound on 276 men with low ejaculate-volume and azoospermia *(34)*. Twelve (4.4%) men had stones: five (42%) in the ejaculatory ducts, four (33%) in the vas deferens, and three (25%) in the seminal vesicles. Cho performed magnetic resonance imaging in 17 men presenting with hemospermia *(35)*. Nineteen calculi were observed: five in the prostate, eight in the seminal vesicle, four in the ejaculatory ducts, and two in müllerian duct cysts. Engin used magnetic resonance imaging and transrectal ultrasound to evaluate 218 infertile men with low ejaculate-volumes *(36)*. Ejaculatory duct calcifications were found in 27% of the azoospermic men and 6% of the nonazoospermic men. These studies suggest the use of imaging to look for clinically significant calculi in men with infertility, especially low-volume azoospermia. The significance of these calcifications and their affect on spermatozoa are currently unknown.

BLADDER CALCULI

Etiology

Bladder calculi have afflicted man for thousands of years. Archeologists discovered a stone resting in the pelvis of an ancient Egyptian skeleton dating back more than 7000 yr *(37)*. Fortunately, over the last 50 yr, the incidence of vesical calculi in developed countries has declined significantly and currently represents roughly 5% of all urinary calculi in the Western world *(38,39)*. Underdeveloped societies still suffer from endemic bladder calculi, especially children, usually owing to diets rich in cereals and grains and deficient in animal proteins. A high acid-ash and low-phosphate diet in conjunction with dehydration from chronic diarrhea and malnutrition results in low urinary pH with

Table 4
Eight Patients With Seminal Vesicle or Ejaculatory Duct Calculi

Age	Presenting complaint	Previous surgery	Imaging	Stone analysis	Treatment
7	• Recurrent epididymo-orchitis	• None	• Abdominal radiograph + • Abdominal ultrasound + • Computed tomography + • Digital rectal examination palpable	• Not available	• Open seminal vesiculolithotomy
10	• Recurrent epididymo-orchitis	• Anorectal malformation • Urethral fistula • Bladder diverticulectomy • Ureteral reimplant	• Abdominal radiograph + • Digital rectal examination palpable • Computed tomography + • Intravenous pyelogram normal	• Not available	• Open seminal vesiculolithotomy
12	• Inability to self catheterize	• Myelomeningocele • Spina bifida	• Retrograde urethrogram ejaculatory duct reflux	• Calcium phosphate	• Laser lithotripsy • Ejaculatory duct fulguration
25	• Painful ejaculation	• None	• Transrectal ultrasonograph + • Digital rectal examination normal	• Not available	• Spontaneous passage
26	• Asymptomatic pyuria	• Ureteral reimplant • Bladder neck repair • Incision ureterocele	• Abdominal radiograph + • Retrograde urethrogram ejaculatory duct reflux	• Not available	• Observation
32	• Azoospermia	• None	• Digital rectal examination palpable • Transrectal ultrasonograph + • magnetic resonance imaging +	• Calcium phosphate	• Transurethral resection of the ejaculatory ducts
41	• Renal colic • Irritative voiding symptoms	• None	• Intravenous pyelogram ectopic ureter entering into the seminal vesicle	• Carbonate • Urate • Phosphate • Struvite	• Open nephro-ureterectomy • Seminal vesiculectomy
53	• Orchalgia • Perineal pain	• Two previous open seminal vesiculolithotomy	• Digital rectal examination palpable • Abdominal radiograph + • Intravenous pyelogram normal	• Not available	• Transrectal excision

Adapted from References 26–33.

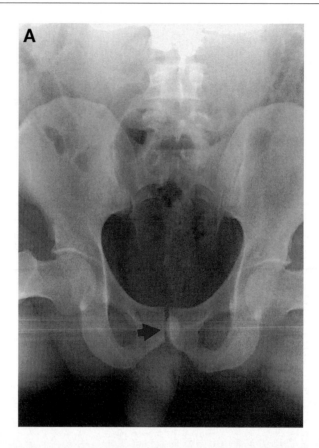

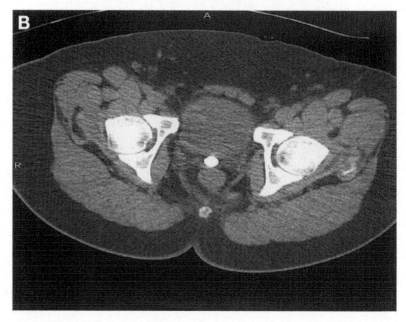

Fig. 1. (A) Plain abdominal radiograph demonstrating a large calcification (arrow) overlying the symphysis pubis; and **(B)** computed tomography of the pelvis confirming the location of the stone within the ejaculatory duct.

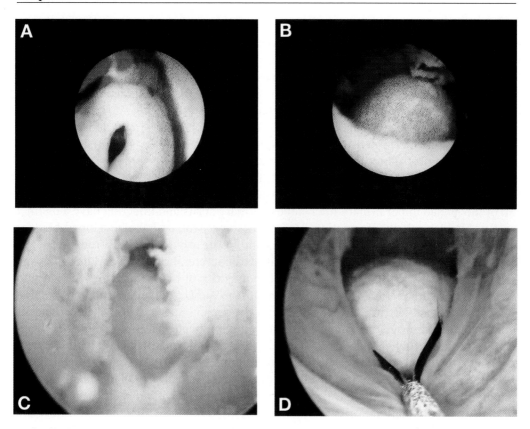

Fig. 2. (A) Cystoscopic view of the verumontanum with a stone visible in the left ejaculatory duct. **(B)** A pediatric cystoscope was used to enter the ejaculatory duct to better visualize the stone. **(C)** At a second setting the ejaculatory duct was incised with Collins knife exposing the stone. **(D)** A 3 Fr tipless four-wire basket engaging the stone. The stone was extracted from the duct and fragmented with the holmium laser.

subsequent uric acid or ammonium acid urate stone formation. Magnesium ammonium phosphate stones are also common in underdeveloped nations owing to high infection rates and limited antibiotic therapy available in these areas. Western series report a high incidence of calcium-based stones, reflecting compositions similar to those of upper urinary tract calculi. A recent comprehensive review of 1440 children with urinary calculi support the historical data presented above. Interestingly, they documented that bladder stones were present in 60% of cases in the mid-1980s but decreased to 15% in the mid-1990s *(40)*.

Attempts to identify the inciting event in bladder stone formation have yielded interesting results. African investigators analyzed nuclei and multiple layers of 42 pediatric bladder stones using infrared spectrometry *(41)*. The major constituents were ammonium acid urate and calcium oxalate monohydrate. Eighty per cent of the nuclei contained ammonium acid urate whereas 50% had calcium oxalate. Struvite and calcium phosphate nuclei were not found in any of their stones. Analysis of the concentric layers, however, revealed large amounts of struvite and calcium phosphate indicating that infection may not be required for stone initiation, but once crystallization has started, it may be a significant promoter of stone growth.

It is uncommon for bladder stones to form in the absence of obstruction, infection, or stasis. In one of the largest reviews to date, Takasaki reviewed 273 bladder calculi from 220 males and 53 females aged 2–89 yr *(42)*. Overall, 142 (52%) of the stones contained magnesium ammonium phosphate (MAP) with or without calcium. Calculi in women were composed of MAP 71.6% (38/53) of the time compared to 47.2% of the males. No uric acid calculi were found in women compared to 17 (7.7%) males. Calcium was the major constituent in 101 (45.9%) calculi: 92 (41.8%) men and 10 (18.9%) women. Associated lower urinary tract disorders consisted of 98 (44.6%) patients with bladder outlet obstruction secondary to an enlarged prostate or previous prostate surgery and 26 (11.8%) with a neurogenic bladder. Interestingly, 59 of 120 patients with calcium stones (39.6% of the whole series) had no lower urinary tract abnormalities and 30 of the 59 had upper urinary tract stones. Urinary stasis and infection have a distinct role in bladder calculus formation. However, some patients have developed bladder calculi in the absence of upper tract stones and lower urinary tract disorders.

Bladder stones have been associated with vesicoureteral reflux in children *(43)* and in spinal cord injury (SCI) patients *(44)*. The majority of bladder calculi secondary to female pelvic surgery *(45–48)* or genital prolapse *(49–54)* result either from obstruction or foreign bodies left in the bladder during the repair. Stasis of urine, poor bladder emptying, and neurogenic bladder physiology are implicated as etiologic factors. Douenias et al. identified predisposing factors in 100 patients with bladder calculi; 83 were attributed to various prostatic diseases or operations *(55)*. Fifty per cent of the patients had uric acid stones. They attributed this high percentage to the diet of the mostly Jewish population they served. Gutman observed a high predilection of uric acid urinary calculi in the Jewish population attributable to genetics and diet *(56)*. In contrast, Smith and O'Flynn found uric acid stones in 5.4% of 648 cases *(57)*. Stones resulting from obstruction may be composed of several different constituents. Pickworth reported recovering "thousands" of small bladder calculi while performing a transurethral resection of the prostate *(58)*. They were composed of calcium, ammonium, magnesium, carbonate, oxalate, and phosphate without a central nidus.

Spinal cord injury increases the risk of bladder calculi formation. Hall et al. found 261 of 898 (29%) SCI patients to have bladder stones at their institution *(59)*. Of those with bladder calculi, 62.5% were managed with indwelling Foley catheters. The remainder wore external appliances for urinary collection. Of 40 female tetraplegics with permanent catheter drainage, Singh and Thomas found 22 (55%) who required treatment for recurrent bladder calculi *(60)*. DeVivo and colleagues looked at 500 SCI patients being followed at their institution *(61)*. Thirty-six per cent developed bladder calculi over an 8-yr period with the greatest risk occurring in the first 3 mo after injury. Three factors were significant in the predisposition of bladder calculi: a complete neurologic lesion, urinary tract infection caused by *Klebsiella* species, and Caucasian race. There was not a significant difference in bladder stone formation based on the methods of bladder management. Statistical significance was not reached because patients regularly changed bladder management from clean intermittent catheterization (CIC), external condom catheter collection, and indwelling Foley catheter drainage. Bladder management in this group of patients remains a challenge and should be a focus in their counseling.

Leunissen et al. reported 4 of 80 (5%) renal transplant patients suffered from bladder calculi *(62)*. All of them formed on the ends of vicryl suture used in the ureterovesical anastomosis. In a series of 312 renal transplant recipients, seven (2.2%) developed bladder calculi *(63)*. The first 196 patients underwent ureteroneocystostomy with polypropylene suture. The following 116 anastomoses were performed with absorbable polydioxanone (PDS) suture. All of the calculi formed on the nonabsorbable polypropylene suture material and all seven were stone free after electrohydraulic lithotripsy (EHL) and endoscopic removal of the suture nidus. Of 300 simultaneous kidney pancreas transplants, nine (3%) developed bladder calculi *(64)*. All of the stones developed on nonabsorbable suture material exposed to urinary constituents and were successfully treated with EHL and endoscopic suture removal. The only case of nonsuture related calculus formation was felt to arise from dystrophic calcification of an ischemic portion of the cuff of the allograft ureter *(65)*.

Various drugs have been implicated in bladder calculi formation. Nakano et al. report a bladder stone made of tosufloxacin, an oral fluoroquinolone, in a woman on CIC for a neurogenic bladder *(66)*. The sole report of a triamterene bladder calculus in the absence of upper tract stones or abnormalities was in a patient with significant infravesical obstruction and high post void residuals from benign prostatic hyperplasia *(67)*. The protease inhibitor indinavir sulfate (Crixivan) has been shown to cause renal lithiasis *(68,69)*. It is possible that with the increased use of this drug, and the increasing frequency of urinary manifestations of the acquired immunodeficiency syndrome, indinavir bladder calculi may be encountered in the future.

Symptoms

Patients with bladder calculi present similarly to those with urethral calculi. Stranguria, decreased force of stream, recurrent urinary tract infection, dysuria, urgency, frequency, and intermittency are common presenting complaints in patients who have bladder calculi. Often, microscopic or gross hematuria are the presenting signs of bladder calculi. Three patients with postoperative dysuria, urgency, and pain following a Stamey anti-incontinence procedure were found to have calculi on the ends of intravesical sutures *(48)*.

Diagnosis

Most patients with bladder calculi have either gross or microscopic hematuria. As a result, both radiographic and cystoscopic evaluations are usually performed. Despite the accuracy of modern imaging, the diagnosis of bladder calculi is best confirmed with cystoscopy. The anatomy of the urethra, prostate, and bladder as well as the presence of coinciding pathology can be identified.

Treatment

Although the ancient Greeks described the perineal vesicolithotomy 3000 yr ago, it was not until the fifth century BCE that Hippocrates thoroughly documented vesicolithiasis. The first true "lithotomists," Ammonius of Alexandria, emerged about 200 BCE. He used the perineal approach and invented the hand held lithotrite *(70)*. The latter half of the 20th century saw a technological explosion in lithotripsy technology. The emergence of laser, pneumatic, ultrasonic, and extracorporeal shockwave lithotripsy devices has lessened the need for open surgery and made the handheld lithotrite almost obsolete. Historically, manual lithalopaxy with or without cystoscopic assistance was the only treatment method available short of open cystolithotomy. As early as 1963, routine open cystolithotomy was challenged as the optimal treatment for vesical calculi *(71)*. As late as 1990, tactile lithalopaxy was employed in a series of 45 patients with a 91.1% success rate but a complication rate of 31% including one bladder perforation *(72)*.

Bladder neck contracture after open prostatectomy was the cause of a large dumbbell shaped calculus reported in a 67-yr-old man 12 mo postoperatively *(73)*. The authors combined extracorporeal shockwave lithotripsy (SWL) and percutaneous suprapubic ultrasonic lithotripsy. They were able to fragment the prostatic calculus with SWL, push the remainder of the stone into the bladder, and then perform the suprapubic procedure. Some time later, the patient underwent transurethral incision of the bladder neck contracture. The stone consisted of struvite and hydroxyapatite.

The use of SWL has revolutionized the management of urinary calculi. Its use in the upper tracts is undeniable. However, its success and practicality in treating bladder calculi has been questioned. Thirty-six males underwent SWL monotherapy with the HM-4 lithotriptor (Dornier Medical Systems, Inc., Marietta, GA) achieving a 72% stone-free rate *(74)*. Ten (28%) patients required eventual cystoscopic removal of non- or poorly fragmented calculi. Husain et al. performed primary bladder stone reduction therapy with the HM-3 (Dornier Medical Systems) in 24 patients *(75)*. This procedure was followed immediately by cystolitholapaxy with a manual lithotrite in all patients. They reported an 83% success rate with minimal complications. However, the mean hospital stay was 3.5 d.

Treating large calculi over 4 cm in diameter have traditionally been surgical. Two reports using the Holmium:yttrium-aluminum-garnet (Ho:YAG) laser have been reported recently. Grasso treated 12 patients with calculi averaging 55.8 mm in one sitting with no complications *(76)*. Teichman et al. successfully cleared 14 patients of their stones averaging 6 cm and none less than 4 cm without complications *(77)*. The laser is a very effective tool to manage bladder calculi. The fiber is flexible and comes in different sizes. They can fit through virtually any endoscope. The laser machines are small and mobile. Although there is limited data in the literature, the laser is the author's preferred choice for treatment of bladder stones because of its unparalleled power and ability to "dust" large stones efficiently.

Pneumatic lithotripsy is a relatively new technology that has proven quite effective in fragmenting large, hard calculi with minimal tissue injury. The Swiss Lithoclast (EMS Lithoclast, Nyon, Switzerland) was used in 17 patients with neurogenic bladder and bladder calculi *(78)*. Stones cleared within 1 wk in all patients. One patient suffered bleeding requiring continuous irrigation for 3 d. The biggest limitation to pneumatic lithotripsy is the inability to clear the large remnants that remain. The introduction of the Lithoclast Ultra lithotriptor (Boston Scientific, Natick, MA), which combines pneumatic and ultrasonic lithotripsy with suction capabilities, should prove exceptional in treating bladder calculi. One drawback to this technology is the need for an offset scope to perform cystoscopy.

There are two reports in the literature that compare various methods of cystolithotripsy. Bhatia and Biyani reviewed 128 bladder calculi treated with open cystolithotomy (5), manual lithalopaxy (80), and SWL (43) *(79)*. Open surgery resulted in 100% stone removal at one setting but required the longest hospital stay (5.2 d). The only complication was a fever of greater than 100°F in one patient. Manual lithotripsy had a complication rate of 25% and included urethral stricture, bladder perforation and failure. Hospitalization averaged 2.4 d and intraoperative bleeding resulting in poor visualization required retreatment in two patients. SWL had the shortest hospital stay (20 h) but suffered two cases of urethral fragment impaction (4.8%). Four patients required two

SWL sessions for complete fragmentation. Razvi et al. compared manual lithotripsy (53), ultrasonic lithotripsy (17), electrohydraulic lithotripsy (16), and pneumatic lithotripsy (20) *(80)*. The success rates were 90%, 88%, 63%, and 85% respectively whereas the complication rates were 10%, 2.5%, 8%, and 10% respectively. Finally, a host of novel percutaneous and "laparoscopic" methods of stone extraction have been reported recently *(81–84)*.

When determining the optimal treatment modality for bladder calculi, there are several considerations: size and composition of stone, underlying etiology, comorbid conditions, previously operated lower urinary tract, patient morphology, cost, patient compliance and follow-up risk, available instrumentation, experience of the surgeon, and risk to the patient for each option being considered. All of these items need to be fully evaluated and the risks weighed against each other to eradicate the stone and the underlying condition with the least complication and cost.

Prevention

Removing a bladder calculus is not usually difficult. On diagnosis of a bladder calculus, the initial thought is to remove it. The most important principle of treating bladder calculi, however, is prevention and eradication of the underlying cause. Relieving obstruction, eliminating infection, meticulous surgical technique, and accurate diagnosis are paramount in treating bladder calculi.

The necessity to perform intraoperative cystoscopy during anti-incontinence surgery cannot be over emphasized. Likewise, it is imperative that women who present after urogynecological procedures with significant lower urinary tract symptoms with or without recurrent urinary tract infections undergo a thorough cystoscopic examination to rule out inadvertent intravesical suture placement. If the suture is observed before stone formation, it may be cut without significant morbidity. Calculogenesis in these patients is secondary to the foreign body in contact with urine.

The key to prevention of prostate disease-related bladder calculi is relief of obstruction. Any procedure performed on the bladder neck, prostate or prostatic urethra may result in obstructive changes, incomplete bladder evacuation, secondary infection, and calculus formation. Aggressive medical and/or surgical therapy aimed at decreasing high postvoid residuals, enhanced bladder emptying, and decreased voiding pressures will help prevent bladder stone formation.

Bladder calculi reported in transplant patients have been associated with a foreign body or tissue ischemia. Transplant recipients do not have an increased risk of bladder stone formation if care is taken to limit intravesical sutures and minimize perivesical clips. Diagnosis of bladder calculi in these patients can be difficult and should be suspected in patients with irritative voiding symptoms, unexplained urinary tract infection, or stranguria. Dietary modifications and antibiotic therapy will help prevent bladder calculi formation in those areas where they are endemic.

Pediatric bladder stones deserve special mention. The most interesting aspect of pediatric cystolithiasis is the pathophysiology of stone formation. In the absence of obstruction, infection or neurologic disease, pediatric stones can be considered endemic in certain geographic areas and most likely result from multiple factors. Johnson looked at Ethiopian children and found a significant increase in bladder stones in males of low socioeconomic classes *(85)*. Nutritional deficiencies in vitamin A, magnesium, phosphate, and vitamin B6 combined with a low protein and high carbohydrate diet is implicated in lithogenesis. The majority of his patients consumed minimal meat and a staple of carbohydrates: injera, kotcho, and sorghum.

It is known that the saturation of uric acid in solution is bimodal with 50% ionization at a pH of 5.5 and 90% solubility at a pH greater than 7.0. Dehydration, diarrhea, fever, and infection decrease urine production, thereby increasing the concentration of uric acid and enhancing crystallization. These conditions, in addition to decreased phosphorous intake and a carbohydrate staple, acidify the urine, further compounding the problem. Increased conversion of glutamine to ammonia in combination with the already saturated uric acid environment will precipitate ammonium acid urate calculi. These factors increase calcium oxalate excretion leading to calcium oxalate precipitation. The resulting calculi are composed of a mixture of varying amounts of calcium oxalate and ammonium acid urate (86).

Hydration remains important in bladder stone formation. The effect of water constituents and additives on vesicolithiasis has been addressed. Twenty children with endemic stones and 20 age-matched controls were evaluated for the effect of fluoride on stone formation (87). No differences were found in the composition of the drinking water, daily dietary intake constituents, plasma biochemistry parameters, or urinary excretion parameters between the two groups. Also, the fluoride content in the center of the stones was no different than the periphery, indicating fluoride does not act as a nidus in stone formation.

Finally, there is a fascinating concept pioneered by researchers in Thailand. Bladder stones are endemic in the north and northeast regions of the country. Suphiphat et al. evaluated the effect of pumpkin seeds, a dietary staple in this region, on the incidence of bladder calculi (88). Consumption of dietary phosphorous is only 35% of the recommended level in Thai adolescents. Pumpkin seeds are very rich in phosphorous and are cheaper than other sources. The levels of the crystal inhibitors, urinary pyrophosphates and glycosaminoglycans, were significantly higher in the pumpkin seed group. Unfortunately, urinary pH decreased, and urinary oxalate levels increased significantly in the same study group creating an acid-urine rich in oxalates. A long prospective trial is needed to determine if pumpkin seed supplementation lessens the occurrence of bladder calculi in this population.

In the absence of anatomic abnormalities, obstruction, and infection, one must consider dysfunctional voiding as a cause of bladder calculi. In a series of 100 children with bladder calculi from the United States, three (3%) exhibited dysfunctional voiding patterns (89). Hassan identified 5 of 22 (23%) Nigerian children with bladder calculi have no predisposing factors (90). He does not specifically address dysfunctional voiding, however, it is quite possible these children suffered from some type of abnormal voiding habits predisposing them to bladder calculi formation. The use of diapers in western countries may promote frequent and complete emptying of the urinary bladder in children. Developing countries may ostracize those children who remain wet discouraging them to void more frequently leading to larger post void residuals and chronic urinary retention. When a child presents with a bladder calculus it is imperative to rule out voiding dysfunction as a cause.

If infectious, obstructive and neurogenic conditions can be addressed early, bladder calculi can be avoided in most situations. The addition of phosphorous, protein, vitamins, and magnesium to the diets of children where stones are endemic can significantly decrease the incidence and attendant morbidity of pediatric vesical calculi. Treatment of dehydration states is crucial in the prevention of such stones.

ENCRUSTED FOREIGN BODIES

The initial event in stone formation is probably crystallization. There are two types of nucleation in crystal development: homogeneous and heterogeneous. In the presence of a foreign body, heterogeneous nucleation occurs. Additionally, aggregation is required for crystal growth and proliferation and eventual stone formation. It is imperative to remove the foreign body and the calculus if further stone formation is to be prevented.

The most common foreign bodies to calcify in the urinary tract are Foley catheters, ureteral stents, nephrostomy tubes, and suprapubic catheters. There are a host of other objects that have been reported to be a nidus for stone formation. Removal of these "stones" can be challenging.

It is well known that indwelling Foley catheters place patients at risk for urinary infection, bladder and urethral erosion, and calculus formation. A recent study looked at the prevalence and morbidity of long-term catheterization (indwelling urethral Foley catheter greater than 3 mo) in a population approaching one million people *(91)*. A total of 773 patients were identified as utilizing long-term catheterization, a prevalence of 0.07% (0.5% for patients greater than 75 yr of age). The reasons for catheterization varied but the majority were spinal cord injured patients. Seventeen patients (2.2%) with chronic indwelling catheters were found to have bladder calculi.

Derry reported formation of a vesical calculus forming over a hair nidus in a spinal cord injured patient undergoing frequent catheter changes *(92)*. The follicle was presumably introduced during one of the catheter exchanges emphasizing attention to detail when performing this procedure.

There are numerous reports in the literature concerning migration of intrauterine devices and intravaginal gynecological accessories including pessaries, diaphragms, and cerclages into the bladder *(93–100)*. Insight into crystal growth on foreign bodies was provided by Khan and Wilkinson *(97)*. They performed open cystolithotomy on a 24-yr-old woman who had an IUD placed 4 yr earlier. Scanning electron micrography revealed deposits of calcium phosphate crystals along various parts of the IUD. Stones grew individually around each nidus in different areas until they coalesced into one large stone. The stone also contained struvite, indicating that the nidus became secondarily infected with urease-splitting organisms. This may help explain the "spread" of crystal "growth."

Autoerotic behavior has been practiced by all ages and sexes for centuries. Dalton reported a large assortment of items found in bladders of patients practicing autoeroticism including chewing gum, hairpins, and thermometers *(101)*. Basu reported a case of bladder rupture secondary to calculus formation around an unidentified foreign body introduced in the urethra 14 yr earlier *(102)*. Fishing line has been implicated in two cases *(103,104)*. Finally, there is the case of a 23-yr-old male who practiced autoerotic manipulation with a 25-cm piece of polyethylene tubing. The bladder stone surrounding the tubing measured 7.5 cm × 7.5 cm × 5 cm. Unfortunately, the embarrassment of seeking medical attention led to his ultimate demise caused by pyelonephritis, pneumonia, and sepsis *(105)*.

Bladder calculi have been reported as complications of several nonurologic surgical procedures, all caused by foreign body migration from the original surgery. Cholevesical lithiasis resulted from a dropped gallstone during a laparoscopic cholecystectomy. During the case, several stones were dropped and presumably landed in the retrovesical location causing an intense inflammatory reaction and eventual fistula formation. Cystoscopic extraction of several cholesterol stones and long-term antibiotics were curative *(106)*.

Maier reported the intravesical migration of a surgical clip used in a laparoscopic hernia repair causing stone formation *(107)*. Removal was performed endoscopically with pneumatic lithotripsy and the analysis revealed 100% calcium phosphate.

Encrustation is a well-known complication of indwelling ureteral stents. The relatively new urethral stents can also stimulate intravesical lithogenesis. Squires reported a 6-cm bladder calculus that formed on the proximal portion of a titanium stent that protruded into the bladder *(108)*. Analysis revealed 100% struvite implying an infectious etiology.

Edwards removed a 156-g hour-glass-shaped bladder calculus protruding through a 2-cm midline abdominal hernia presumably from a midline cesarean section performed 40 yr earlier *(109)*. She presented with recurrent urinary tract infections and the stone was composed entirely of magnesium ammonium phosphate.

Eroding foreign bodies may find their way into the bladder and promote stone formation. An inflatable penile prosthesis reservoir from a patient who had symptomatic relief by inflating the prosthesis was reported by Dupont *(110)*. The stones were removed at the same time as the device explant. Pomerantz reported a large calculus formation on an eroded ilioiliac arterial graft placed 4 yr previous *(111)*. On electrohydraulic lithotripsy of the bladder calculus, a large rush of blood was encountered and emergent laparotomy performed. The calculus was removed and immediate axillofemoral bypass was required.

Methylmethacrylate cement, used in orthopedic surgery, was found to be the cause of "bladder stones" in a 71-yr-old male with recurrent urinary tract infections. The chronically infected hip fistulized to the bladder, facilitating cement migration. Interestingly, the *Staphylococcus aureus* repeatedly growing out of his hip wound was never cultured from the urine. Only Gram-negative organisms were recovered from his urinary tract *(112)*. Finally, Pajor reported a 38-yr-old imprisoned women who attempted suicide by swallowing a knife blade *(113)*. After 4 yr of being asymptomatic, she was evaluated for lower urinary tract symptoms. Abdominal radiograph and cystoscopy confirmed that the calcified knife blade had perforated the bowel and came to rest in the bladder. The patient refused surgery and 2 d later, the "knifestone" passed through a vesicovaginal fistula without incident!

Encrusted ureteral stents are of particular interest to those managing urologic patients (Figs. 3 and 4). There are a number of excellent articles in the literature describing complex problems managed with a multifaceted approach *(114–116)*. The most recent review emphasizes the multimodal approach necessary to treat encrusted ureteral stents *(117)*. Four patients with a mean stone burden of 807 mm^2 and an indwelling stent underwent two to four procedures each to render them stone-free. Extracorporeal shockwave lithotripsy, cystolitholapaxy, antegrade, and retrograde ureteroscopy, and percutaneous nephrolithotomy were used in combination to treat these stones. Open surgery is reserved for those calculi and stents not removable endoscopically.

In summary, any foreign body placed within the urinary tract has lithogenic potential. Most stones are mixed composition and if infection is present, struvite is a major constituent. The processes of heterogeneous nucleation and aggregation are central to the formation of calculi that form on foreign bodies. As a result, the best treatment of these stones is prevention.

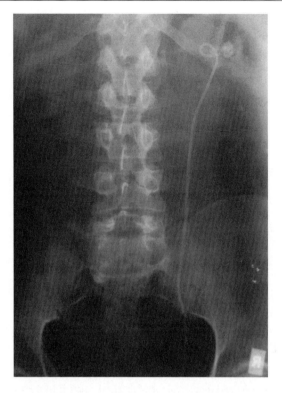

Fig. 3. Original stone for which a stent was placed before extracorporeal shockwave lithotripsy

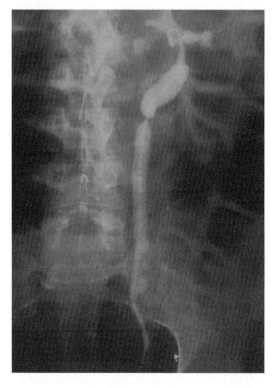

Fig. 4. Forgotten stent 5 yr after insertion. He presented in renal insufficiency and left flank pain.

REFERENCES

1. Mandel N. Mechanism of stone formation. Sem Nephrol 1996; 16: 364.
2. Koga S, Arakaki Y, Matsuoka M, Ohyama C. Urethral calculi. Br J Urol 1990; 65: 288, 289.
3. Paulk SC, Khan AU, Malek RS, Greene LF. Urethral calculi. J Urol 1976; 116: 436–439.
4. Noble JG, Chapple CR. Formation of a urethral calculus around an unusual foreign body. Br J Urol 1993; 72: 248, 249.
5. Salman B. Urethral calculi in children. J Ped Surg 1996; 31(10): 1379–1382.
6. Courtney SP, Wightman JAK. Urethral calculi caused by cholestyramine. Br J Urol 1991; 68: 654.
7. Hassan I, Mahammed I. Urethral calculi: A review. East Afr Med J 1993; 70: 523–525.
8. Walker BR, Hamilton BD. Urethral calculi managed with transurethral holmium laser ablation. J Ped Surg 2001; 36: 16, 17.
9. Giordano DR, Carnevale M, Ascione A, Franzese C, Giordano DS, Petrarola F. Ambulatory treatment by extracorporeal shock-wave lithotripsy for an urethral stone in a hypospadiac boy. Child Neph Urol 1988–1989; 9: 239, 240.
10. Suzuki Y, Ishigooka M, Hayami S, Nakada T, Mitobe K. A case of primary giant calculus in female urethra. Int Urol Neph 1997; 29: 237–239.
11. Melekos MD, Veronikis DK, Siamplis D, Kalfarentzos F. Diverticulum of the male urethra with a giant stone and multiple calculi. Urol Int 1989; 44: 184–186.
12. Durazi MH, Samiei MR. Ultrasonic fragmentation in the treatment of male urethral calculi. Br J Urol 1988; 62: 443, 444.
13. Selli C, Barbagli G, Carini M, Lenzi R, Masini G. Treatment of male urethral calculi. J Urol 1984; 132: 37–39.
14. Hemal AK, Sharma DK. Male urethral calculi. Urol Int 1991; 46: 334–337.
15. Sharfi AR. Presentation and management of urethral calculi: Br J Urol 1991; 68: 271, 272.
16. Jezior JR, Schwartz BF. Urethral calculus extraction using a penile ring block anesthetic. Tech Urol 1998; 4: 165, 166.
17. Fox M. The natural history and significance of stone formation in the prostate gland. J Urol 1963; 89: 716–721.
18. Huggins C, Bear RS. The course of the prostatic ducts and the anatomy, chemical and x-ray diffraction analysis of prostatic calculi. J Urol 1944; 51: 37.
19. Huggins C, Johnson AA. The analysis and pathogenesis of prostatic calculi. Am J Physiol 1933; 103: 573.
19a. Magura CE, Spector M. Scanning electron microscopy of human prostatic corpora amylacea and corpora calculi, and prostatic calculi. Scanning Electron Microscopy 1979; III: 713–720.
20. Magura CE, Spector M, Allen R, Turner WR. Brushite encrustation and lithiasis of the prostatic bed after transurethral resection of the prostate. J Urol 1980; 123: 294–297.
21. Smith MJV, Chir B. Prostatic corpora amylacea. Monogr Surg Sci 1966; 3: 209–265.
22. Kovi J, Heshmet MY, Jackson MA, Rao MS, Akberzie ME, Ogunmuyiwa TA. Incidence of prostatic calcification in blacks in Washington D.C. and selected African cities. Urology 1979; 14: 363–369.
23. Hassler O. Calcifications in the prostate gland and adjacent tissues: a combined biophysical and histological study. Pathol Microbiol 1968; 31: 97–107.
24. Meares Jr EM. Infection stones of prostate gland: Laboratory diagnosis and clinical management. Urology 1974; 4: 560–566.
25. Sonergaard G, Vetner M, Christensen PO. Prostatic calculi. Acta Path Microbiol Scand Section A 1987; 95: 141–145.
26. Gordon Z, Monga M. Endoscopic extraction of an ejaculatory duct calculus to treat obstructive azoospermia. J Endo 2001; 15: 949:950.
27. Tackett LD, Minevich E, Wacksman J, Sheldon CA. Holmium laser lithotripsy for ejaculatory duct calculi. J Urol 2000; 164: 2067.
28. Corriere JN. Painful ejaculation due to seminal vesicle calculi. J Urol 1997; 157: 626.
29. Li YK. Diagnosis and management of large seminal vesicle stones. Br J Urol 1991; 68: 322–323.
30. Wesson L, Steinhardt G. Case profile: seminal vesicle stones. Urology 1983; 22: 204, 205.

31. Carachi R, Gobara O. Recurrent epidiymo-orchitis in a child seconday to a stone in the seminal vesicle. Br J Urol 1997; 79: 997.
32. Wilkinson AG. Case report: calculus in the seminal vesicle. Ped Rad 1993; 23: 327.
33. Orquiza LS, Bhayani BN, Derry JL, Bahlen CP. Ectopic opening of the ureter into the seminal vesicle. J Urol 1970; 104: 532.
34. Kuligowska E, Fenlon HM. Transrectal US in male infertility: Spectrum of findings and role in patient care. Radiology 1998; 207: 173–181.
35. Cho IN, Lee MS, Rha RH, Hong SJ, Park SS, Kim MJ. Magnetic resonance imaging in hemospermia. J Urol 1997; 157: 258–262.
36. Engin G, Kadioglu A, Orhan I, Akdol S, Rozanes I. Transrectal ultrasound and endorectal MR imaging in partial and complete obstruction of the seminal duct system. Acta Radiol 2000; 41: 288–295.
37. Shattock SG. A prehistoric or predynastic Egiptian calculus. Trans Path Soc Lon 1905; 56: 275.
38. Takasaki E, Murahashi I, Nagata M. A four-year retrospective study of urolithiasis. Dokkyo J Med Sci 1979; 6: 120.
39. Yoshida O. A chronological and geographical study on urolithiasis in Japan. Jpn J Endourol ESWL 1990; 3: 5.
40. Rizvi SAH, Naqvi SAA, Hussain Z, et al. Pediatric urolithiasis: Developing nation perspectives. J Urol 2002; 168: 1522–1525.
41. Vanwaeyenbergh J, Vergauwe D, Verbeeck RMH. Infrared spectrometric analysis of endemic bladder stones in Niger. Eur Urol 1995; 27: 154.
42. Takasaki E, Suzuki T, Honda M, et al. Chemical compositions of 300 lower urinary tract calculi and associated disorders of the urinary tract. Urol Int 1995; 54: 89.
43. Roberts JP, Atwell JD. Vesicoureteric reflux and urinary calculi in children. Br J Urol 1989; 64: 10.
44. Hall MK, Hackler RH, Zampieri TA, et al. Renal calculi in spinal cord-injured patient: association with reflux, bladder stones, and foley catheter drainage. Urology 1989; 34: 126.
45. Zderic SA, Burros HM, Hanno PM, et al. Bladder calculi in women after urethrovesical suspension. J Urol 1988; 139: 1047.
46. Borgaonkar SS, Hackman BW. Neodymium:YAG laser removal of stone formed on nonabsorbable suture used previously in colposuspension. J Urol 1996; 156: 472.
47. Chamary VL. An unusual cause of iatrogenic bladder stone. Br Jurol 1995; 76: 138.
48. Evans JWH, Chapple CR, Ralph DJ, et al. Bladder calculus formation as a complication of the Stamey procedure. Br J Urol 1990; 65: 580.
49. Bera SK, De KC, Chakrabarty B. A rare case of cystolithiasis in procidentia. J Indian Med Assoc 1996; 94: 84.
50. Chambers CB. Uterine prolapse with incarceration. Am J Obstet Gynecol 1975; 122: 459.
51. Johnson CG. Giant calculus in the urinary bladder associated with complete uterine prolapse. Report of a case. Obstet Gynecol 1958; 11: 579.
52. Mahran M. Vesical calculi complicating uterovaginal prolapse. J Obstet Gynecol Brit Commw 1972; 79: 145.
53. Nieder AM, Chun TY, Nitti VW. Total vaginal prolapse with multiple vesical calculi after hysterectomy. J Urol 1998; 159: 983.
54. Pranikoff K, Cockett TK, Walker LA. Procidentia incarcerated by vesical calculi. J Urol 1982; 127: 320.
55. Douenias R, Rich M, Badlani G, et al. Predisposing factors in bladder calculi. Review of 100 cases. Urology 1991; 37: 240.
56. Gutman AB, Yu TF. Uric acid nephrolithiasis. Am J Med 1968; 45: 756.
57. Smith JM, O'Flynn JD. Transurethral removal of bladder stones: the place of litholapaxy. Br J Urol 1977; 49: 401.
58. Pickworth FE, Dubbins PA, Choa RG. Case report: Limey urine. Clin Rad 1992; 45: 345.
59. Hall MK, Hackler RH, Zampieri TA, et al. Renal calculi in spinal cord-injured patient: association with reflux, bladder stones, and foley catheter drainage. Urology 1989; 34: 126.
60. Singh G, Thomas DG. The female tetraplegic: an admission of urological failure. Br J Urol 1997; 79: 708.

61. DeVivo MJ, Fine PR, Cutter GR, et al. The risk of bladder calculi in patients with spinal cord injuries. Arch Int Med 1985; 145: 428.
62. Leunissen KM, Weil EH, Mooy JM, et al. Bladder stones as an unusual cause of post-transplant macroscopic hematuria. Transplantation 1987; 44: 582.
63. Klein FA, Goldma MH. Vesical calculus: an unusual complication of renal transplantation. Clin Transplantation 1997; 11: 110.
64. Hahnfeld LE, Nakada SY, Sollinger HW, et al. Endourologic therapy of bladder calculi in simultaneous kidney-pancreas transplant recipients. Urology 1998; 51: 404.
65. O'Dey MJ, Zincke H, Riveras TA, et al. Occurrence of vesical calculus following renal transplantation. Br J Urol 1975; 47: 424.
66. Nakano M, Satoshi I, Takashi D, et al. Fluoroquinolone associated bladder stone. J Urol 1997; 157: 946.
67. Hollander JB. Triamterene bladder calculus. Urology 1987; 30: 154.
68. Gentle DL, Stoller ML, Jarrett TW. Protease inhibitor-induced urolithiasis. Urology 1997; 50: 508.
69. Kopp JB, Miller KD, Mican JA. Crystalluria and urinary tract abnormalities associated with Indinavir. Ann Int Med 1997; 127; 119.
70. Shelley HS. Cutting for the stone. J Hist Med 1958; 13: 50.
71. Barnes RW, Bergman RT, Worton E. Lithalopaxy vs cystolithotomy. J Urol 1963; 89: 680.
72. Kaur P, Garg KM, Bhandari NS. Lithalopaxy: a fading art. J Indian Med Assoc 1990; 88: 163.
73. Melone F, Lardani T, Azzaroli G. Dumbell stone of prostatic fossa after prostatectomy. A combined ESWL and suprapubic percutaneous treatment. Acta Urol Belg 1996; 64: 27.
74. Kostakopoulos A, Stavropoulos NJ, Makrichortis C. Extracorporeal shock wave lithotripsy monotherapy for bladder stones. Int Urol Neph 1996; 28: 157.
75. Husain I, El-Faqih SR, Shamsuddin AB. Primary extracorporeal shock wave lithotripsy in management of large bladder calculi. J Endourology 1994; 8: 183.
76. Grasso M. Experience with the Holmium laser as an endoscopic lithotrite. Urology 1996; 48: 199.
77. Teichman JMH, Rogenes VJ, McIver BJ. Holmium:yttrium-aluminum-garnet laser cystolithotripsy of large bladder calculi. Urology 1997; 50: 44.
78. Vespasiani G, Pesce F, Agro EF. Endoscopic ballistic lithotripsy in the treatment of bladder calculi in patients with neurogenic voiding dysfunction. J Endourol 1996; 10: 551.
79. Bhatia V, Biyani CS. Vesical lithiasis: open surgery versus cystolithotripsy versus extracorporeal shock wave lithotripsy. J Urol 1994; 151: 660.
80. Razvi HA, Song TY, Denstedt JD. Management of vesical calculi:comparison of lithotripsy devices. Kid Int 1995; 48: 876.
81. Adsan O, Yildiz O, Ozturk B, et al. A giant bladder stone: managed with osteotome. Int Urol Neph 1996; 28: 163.
82. Batislam E, Germiyanoglu C, Karabulut A. A new application of laparoscopic instruments in percutaneous bladder stone removal. J Lap Adv Surg Tech 1997; 7: 241.
83. Elder JS. Percutaneous cystolithotomy with endotracheal tube tract dilation aftetr urinary tract reconstruction. J Urol 1997; 157: 2298.
84. Van Savage JG, Khoury AE, McLorie GA. Percutaneous vacuum vesicolithotomy under direct vision: a new technique. J Urol 1996; 156 (Suppl): 706.
85. Johnson O. Vesical calculus in Ethiopian children. Ethiop Med J 1995; 33: 31.
86. Teotia M, Teotia SPS. Endemic vesical stone: nutritional factors. Indian Ped 1987; 24: 117.
87. Teotia M, Rodgers A, Teotia SPS, et al. Fluoride metabolism and fluoride content of stones from children with endemic vesical stones. Br J Urol 1991; 68: 425.
88. Suphiphat V, Morjaroen N, Pukboonme I, et al. The effect of pumpkin seed snack on inhibitors and promoters of urolithiasis in Thai adolescents. J Med Assoc Thai 1993; 76: 488.
89. Choi H, Snyder HM, Duckett JW. Urolithiasis in childood: current management. J Ped Surg 1987; 22: 158.
90. Hassan I, Mabogunje OA. Urinary stones in children in Zaria. Ann Trop Ped 1993; 13: 269.
91. Kohler J, Ockmore J, Feneley RCL. Long-term catheterization of the bladder: prevelence and morbidity. Br J Urol 1996; 77: 347.
92. Derry E, Nuseibeh I. Vesical calculi formed over a hair nidus. Br J Urol 1997; 80: 965.

93. Chow S, LaSalle MD, Rosenberg GS. Urinary incontinence secondary to a vaginal pessary. Urology 1997; 49: 458.

94. Cumming GP, Bramwell SP, Lees DAR. An unusual case of cystolithiasis: a urological lesson for gynecologists. Br J Obstet Gynecol 1997; 104: 117.

95. Ehrenpreis MD, Alarcon JA, Firfer R. Case profile: Large bladder calculus postcervical circlage. Urology 1986; 27: 366.

96. El Diasty TA, Shokeir AA, El-Gharib MS, et al. Bladder stone: a complication of intravesical migration of Lippes Loop. Scand J Urol Nephrol 1993; 27: 279.

97. Khan SR, Wilkinson EJ. Bladder stone in a human female: The case of an abnormally located intrauterine contraceptive device. Scanning Microscopy 1990; 4: 395.

98. Mahazan P. Secondary vesical calculus following translocated IUCD in urinary bladder. J Ind Med Assoc 1995; 93: 326.

99. Maskey CP, Rahman M, Sigdar TK, et al. Vesical calculus around an intra-uterine contraceptive device. Br J Urol 1997; 79: 654.

100. Staskin D, Malloy T, Carpiniello V, et al. Urological complications secondary to a contraceptive diaphragm. J Urol 1985; 134: 142.

101. Dalton DC, Hughes J, Glenn JF. Foreign bodies and urinary stones. Urology 1975; 6: 1.

102. Basu A, Mojahid I, Williamson EPM. Spontaneous bladder rupture resulting from giant vesical calculus. Br J Urol 1994; 74: 385.

103. Elder JS, Young LW. Radiological case of the month. Am J Dis Child 1986; 140: 55.

104. Williams RJL, Freeman A, Brendler CB. Acute renal failure secondary to fishing line. Br J Urol 1985; 57: 590.

105. Sivaloganathan S. Catheteroticum: fatal late complication following autoerotic practice. Am J Forensic Med Path 1985; 64: 340.

106. Chia JKS. Gallstones exiting the urinary bladder: a complication of laparoscopic cholecystectomy. Arch Surg 1995; 130: 677.

107. Maier U, Treu TM. Bladder stone as a rare complication one year after laparoscopic herniorrhaphy. Surgery 1996; 119: 110.

108. Squires B, Gillat DA. Massive bladder calculus as a complication of a titanium prostatic stent. Br J Urol 1995; 75: 252.

109. Edwards DP, Vedi V, Barber PA, et al. Giant stone in a partially herniated hour-glass bladder presenting as incarcerated incisional hernia. Br J Urol 1997; 80: 157.

110. Dupont MC, Hochman HI. Erosion of an inflatable penile prosthesis reservoir into the bladder, presenting as bladder calculi. J Urol 1988; 139: 367.

111. Pomerantz PA. Giant vesical calculus formed around arterial graft incorporated into bladder. Urology 1989; 33: 57.

112. Radford, PJ, Thomson DJ. A case of methylmethacrylate bladder stone. Acta Orthop Scand 1989; 60: 218.

113. Pajor L, Szabo V. Bladder stone formation on a swallowed knife blade and spontaneous passage through a vesicovaginal fistula. Br J Urol 1995; 76: 659.

114. Mohan-Pillai K, Keeley FX Jr, Moussa SA. Endourological management of severely encrusted ureteral stents. J Endourology 1999; 13: 377–379.

115. Schulze KA, Wettlaufer JN, Oldani G. Encrustation and stone formation: complication of indwelling ureteral stents. Urology 1985; 25: 616–618.

116. Somers WJ. Management of forgotten or retained indwelling ureteral stents. Urology 1996; 47: 431–433.

117. Borboroglu PG, Kane CJ. Current management of severely encrusted ureteral stents with a large associated stone burden. J Urol 2000; 164: 648–650.

Index